Cerebral Revascularization

Microsurgical and Endovascular Techniques

Thieme

Cerebral Revascularization

Microsurgical and Endovascular Techniques

Eric S. Nussbaum, MD
Chair
National Brain Aneurysm Center
St. Joseph's Hospital
St. Paul, Minnesota

J Mocco, MD, MS
Assistant Professor
Department of Neurosurgery
University of Florida
Gainesville, Florida

Thieme
New York • Stuttgart

Thieme Medical Publishers, Inc.
333 Seventh Ave.
New York, NY 10001

Executive Editor: Kay Conerly
Managing Editor: Dominik Pucek
Editorial Assistant: Judith Tomat
Editorial Director, Clinical Reference: Michael Wachinger
Production Editor: Grace R. Caputo, Dovetail Content Solutions
International Production Director: Andreas Schabert
Vice President, International Marketing and Sales: Cornelia Schulze
Chief Financial Officer: James W. Mitos
President: Brian D. Scanlan
Compositor: Maryland Composition
Printer: Leo Paper Group

Library of Congress Cataloging-in-Publication Data

Cerebral revascularization : microsurgical and endovascular techniques / edited by Eric S. Nussbaum and J Mocco.
p. ; cm.
Includes bibliographical references.
ISBN 978-1-60406-263-2
1. Cerebral revascularization. 2. Cerebrovascular disease—Surgery. I. Nussbaum, Eric S. II. Mocco, J
[DNLM: 1. Cerebral Revascularization—methods. WL 355]
RD594.2.C465 2011
617.4'81—dc22

2010034334

Printed in China

978-1-60406-263-2

Contents

Foreword

The stimulating monography, divided into five distinct sections, encompasses twenty-three competently written chapters by internationally renowned experts. The comprehensive contributions describe the open neuromicrovascular surgery and neuroendovascular treatments, complementary to each other in the detailed appraisal of individual aspects of brain revascularization. Each chapter is rich in documents with informative visualization, pictures of operations, and more than a hundred excellent educative artistic drawings. The two current treatment options for recanalization and revascularization of brain arteries and venous sinuses are accorded full and impartial representation.

I am convinced that this stimulating monography will not only capture the interest of neurovascular experts, but data expressed here will also attract, in particular, the young generation of neuroscientists, who will be challenged by the effective treatment avenues being pursued in this broad and immense field of neurovascular diseases.

It is well known that in the second half of the nineteenth century, advances in scientific technology subsequently provoked those involved in medicine and general surgery to aspire to innovations in their respective specialties and subspecialties. In the field of neurosciences, the sophisticated visualization and recording technologies that reveal the various and multidimensional structures and functions of the central nervous system definitely supported the creative development of neuromicrosurgical and neuroendovascular approaches and treatments. In the 1960s, the availability of a universal operating microscope, micro-instruments, temporary vessel-clips, and particularly the punctual coagulation facility with perfected bipolar coagulation technology of Len Malis have been essential tools in the development of microvascular procedures on brain arteries in animal laboratories and, in 1967, in human operating theaters. The sophisticated modalities of CT-scan and MRI, transcranial Doppler flowmetry evolved in the following decades, and more recently Indocyanine Green (ICG) technology represent important armamentarium for diagnostic and treatment procedures for neurovascular diseases.

Besides these gratifying technologic innovations, the enhanced knowledge concerning the specific anatomy and physiology of the brain vasculature is of great value for each microneurosurgical procedure. The arteries and veins of the central nervous system are arranged in numerous segments each with different, distinct histologic, biochemical, and immunologic properties. They have no vasa vasorum and no lymph vessels. The outer third of the arterial wall is in close metabolic-nutritional connection with CSF. The vessels of the central nervous system can therefore be compared to submarines, for they are surrounded by circulating waves of cerebrospinal fluid with rhythmical changes in pressure, in a circa-diem fashion. The arteries are encased within the compartments of cisterns by numerous arachnoidal-pial fibers and membranes containing also autonomous nerves. The arteries, suspended in fibers, are not completely immobile; they have some degree of undulating movements by their pulsations with certain effects to the cerebrospinal fluid circulation. Therefore, exploration of either short or longer segments of arteries and veins requires proficiency, paying attention to meticulous microdissection techniques and tactics. Further, the mastery of cisternal exploration of lesions along the veins and arteries is a skill that can only be acquired during intense training in the laboratory. The ability to explore and repair brain vessels will give confidence to young colleagues and establish the aptitude to perform each type of neuromicrosurgical procedure for the treatment of aneurysms, AVMs, cavernomas, extrinsic and intrinsic tumors, as well as extra-intracranial and intra-intracranial bypass surgery.

This monograph, under the editorship and authorship of Drs. Eric S. Nussbaum and J Mocco documents successful accomplishments designed and executed routinely by well-trained experts.

M. Gazi Yasargil, MD
Professor of Neurosurgery
University of Arkansas for Medical Sciences
Little Rock, Arkansas

Preface

Open microsurgical bypass techniques have always held a particular fascination for neurosurgeons, probably owing to their anatomic elegance and technically demanding nature. After the disappointing findings of the Cooperative Trial were published in the mid 1980s, the number of bypass procedures being performed declined so significantly that it appeared the operation might become a historical footnote in the medical literature. But this was not the end of the story. Over time it became clear that, using sophisticated physiologic imaging, we could identify selected patients with ischemic cerebrovascular disease who would benefit from bypass. In addition, a new and expanded role for bypass emerged in the management of intracranial aneurysms, including giant, unclippable lesions, as well as increasingly prevalent previously coiled recurrent aneurysms. For these reasons, and because of an ever more aggressive attitude toward the management of acute ischemic stroke, there has been a resurgence of interest in extracranial–intracranial (EC-IC) bypass surgery during the past decade.

Initially, a short monograph focusing on open surgical bypass had been envisioned in response to a perceived growing interest by younger neurosurgeons who wished to learn the all-but-forgotten art of brain bypass surgery. But as the idea for a "how-to" text on EC-IC bypass began to crystallize, it became clear that a book focused only on open surgery would be missing at least half the story. Today, a large percentage of cerebral revascularization procedures are being performed not in the operating room but in the catheterization laboratory. Neurosurgical trainees are exposed to endovascular procedures on a routine basis, and many are as comfortable performing carotid angioplasty as they are traditional endarterectomy. This has resulted in a completely "new" area of medicine, and a tremendous interest in this burgeoning field has developed. It seems surprising that, until now, no book has been dedicated to cerebral revascularization, pairing a thorough description of the current state-of-the-art for open surgery with that for endovascular therapy.

Thus emerged *Cerebral Revascularization*, a work that covers the entire spectrum of the field, detailing technical options, indications, complications, and outcomes of the various forms of open and endovascular surgery. The editors are an open vascular microsurgeon with extensive expertise in surgical revascularization techniques and a neurosurgeon with dedicated subspecialty expertise in endovascular therapy. An entire section has been devoted to perioperative critical care, prepared by an expert neurointensivist, in the hopes of emphasizing the important role that ICU management occupies in these cases and to help readers optimize their patients' outcomes. To maximize the impact and usefulness of the work, we have collected a group of contributors who are internationally acclaimed experts, thereby amassing in one book a truly unique collective experience in cerebral revascularization.

By combining our complementary experiences, we have attempted to create a dynamic work that will provide the reader with a thorough grasp of revascularization options, ranging from carotid endarterectomy to carotid angioplasty and stenting, from STA-MCA anastomosis to saphenous vein grafting, and from intracranial angioplasty to innovative options, such as excimer laser–assisted nonocclusive anastomosis (ELANA) techniques.

As such, *Cerebral Revascularization* should be of interest to a wide variety of readers. Neurosurgery and neurology residents learning about and taking part in these procedures will find clear descriptions and case examples in each chapter. Critical care physicians being called on to prepare these patients for surgery and to monitor them afterward can focus on the critical care section. Operating room and catheterization laboratory nurses and technologists may be interested to learn more about the procedures in which they participate on a routine basis. Neurosurgeons and neurologists who are not themselves focused on cerebral revascularization will be able to learn thoroughly about the state-of-the-art therapies that open surgery and endovascular therapy can offer. This may be particularly helpful when faced with patients in an emergency setting or when preparing for board recertification examinations. Even experts subspecializing in this area may enjoy the unique collection of cases provided by the respected authors of this book.

Cerebral Revascularization is not an encyclopedic, heavily referenced text, doomed to be left on the shelf collecting dust, only to be opened when researching the bibliography for a new manuscript. It is highly visual, with operative photos, color illustrations, and rich imaging examples. Take this book into the operating room! Read it the night before a giant aneurysm procedure is planned. Study the angiographic images when contemplating the treatment options for a complex case of intracranial atherosclerosis. Should an open bypass procedure be chosen, or would an endovascular approach be more reasonable?

Ultimately, we believe that cerebral revascularization plays a critical role in the neurosurgical management of patients with ischemic and complex cerebrovascular disease, and that readers will find this to be a practical text that can be used both to plan procedures and to avoid problems. It is our hope that this work will contribute in a meaningful way to the cerebrovascular field and will encourage younger neurosurgeons to further explore the potential options available to revascularize the brain.

Acknowledgments

A number of neurosurgeons have shaped my professional career either directly or indirectly. For as long as I can remember, my uncle, Dr. Ira Kasoff, has been the consummate neurosurgeon. My earliest steps as a medical student were guided by Dr. Daniele Rigamonti, who has remained a friend and a moral compass. I cannot imagine training under a more supportive and encouraging chairman than Dr. Roberto Heros. His skill and honesty both in and out of the operating room have remained an ongoing reference point throughout my career. Dr. Donald Erickson sat by patiently while I performed my first STA-MCA anastomosis. Probably the only poorly executed maneuver I can think of to attribute to Don was his authoring of an ill-fated book on revascularization for stroke that came to publication immediately after the release of the Cooperative Study. Upon his retirement, he gave me a rare "collector's edition" with an inscription that read, "You will need to decide whether this book goes on the history shelf or the practice shelf." I hope the current work helps to answer his challenge.

Dr. Charles Drake may well have been the most humble and understated neurosurgeon I have ever met. His temerity in the operating room, his neverending quest for excellence, and the monumental work he accomplished are a source of ongoing inspiration to all neurosurgeons. Early in my career, I would often call him to ask his thoughts on a particularly challenging aneurysm, and the enthusiasm he demonstrated for every single case left an indelible impression on me. The wonderful experience I had in London, Ontario, working with outstanding surgeons like John Girvin, Gary Ferguson, and Steve Lownie forever shaped my surgical abilities. Finally, over the past 10 years I have had the privilege of developing a professional relationship with Dr. Robert Spetzler, whose body of work stands as a testament to what a singularly talented individual can accomplish in the field of neurosurgery. When I have felt outmatched by a complex case, he has always been available.

I could not have achieved anything without the support of my family. To my wife, Leslie, a talented neurosurgeon in her own right, and to our five children, Josef Tobias, Penelope Elizabeth, Frank Morris, Heather Adina, and Bailey Rivka, I extend my love and thanks for their indulgence as I worked on this book and for all the late nights and weekends my profession has required.

I must thank Jody Lowary, an extraordinary nurse practitioner, colleague, and friend who always provides patients with attention that goes well beyond what anyone could possibly expect. And, finally, to all the patients who have allowed me the honor of participating in their care as a neurosurgeon, I express my deepest gratitude and admiration. There is no such thing as a "theoretical" neurosurgeon. Only through repeated operative endeavor can the neurosurgeon hope to perfect his craft. Nowhere is this more evident than in the area of cerebral revascularization, a uniquely demanding surgical niche that remains as much (and possibly more) art than science. It is hoped that this book will enhance the reader's understanding of this fascinating field and will stand as a reference for those wishing to acquire the skills necessary to revascularize the brain.

—ESN

My sincere thanks and appreciation go to the team at Thieme, in particular, Dominik and Kay. Without your support, effort, and timely reminders, this book would never have come to fruition. I would also like to thank Dr. Eric Nussbaum for involving me in this worthwhile endeavor. Lastly, my love and eternal gratitude to my family, Wendy, Finn, and Michael, who are my source of strength and who provide the support that allows me to pursue this career with such passion . . . thank you.

—JM

Contributors

Section Editors

Neuro-Critical Care
Tariq Janjua, MD, FCCP, FAASM
Medical Director
Neurocritical Care Medicine
National Brain Aneurysm Center
St. Joseph's Hospital
St. Paul, Minnesota

Endovascular Revascularization Techniques
J Mocco, MD, MS
Assistant Professor
Department of Neurosurgery
University of Florida
Gainesville, Florida

Surgical Revascularization Techniques
Eric S. Nussbaum, MD
Chair
National Brain Aneurysm Center
St. Joseph's Hospital
St. Paul, Minnesota

Contributing Authors

H. Huntington Batjer, MD, FACS
Chair, Department of Neurological Surgery
Feinberg School of Medicine
Northwestern University
Chicago, Illinois

Bernard R. Bendok, MD
Associate Professor of Neurological Surgery and Radiology
Feinberg School of Medicine
Northwestern University
Chicago, Illinois

Jeffrey A. Bennett, MD
Assistant Professor
Department of Radiology
College of Medicine
University of Florida
Gainesville, Florida

Sharatchandra S. Bidari, MD
Department of Radiology
College of Medicine
University of Florida
Gainesville, Florida

Paul T. L. Chiam, MBBS, MRCP, FACC
Consultant Cardiologist
National Heart Centre Singapore
Republic of Singapore

Ziad Darkhabani, MD
Medical Resident
School of Medicine and Biomedical Sciences
University at Buffalo, State University of New York
Millard Fillmore Gates Hospital, Kaleida Health
Buffalo, New York

Gregory A. Dumanian, MD, FACS
Professor of Surgery and Neurosurgery
Division of Plastic Surgery
Feinberg School of Medicine
Northwestern University
Northwestern Memorial Hospital
Chicago, Illinois

Christopher S. Eddleman, MD, PhD
Department of Neurological Surgery
Feinberg School of Medicine
Northwestern University
Chicago, Illinois

Giuseppe Esposito, MD
Institute of Neurosurgery
Catholic University School of Medicine
Rome, Italy

Manuel Ferreira, Jr., MD, PhD
Senior Fellow/Acting Instructor
Department of Neurological Surgery
University of Washington
Harborview Medical Center
Seattle, Washington

David Fiorella, MD, PhD
Interventional Neuroradiologist
Department of Neurological Surgery
Stony Brook University Medical Center
Stony Brook, New York

James Kyle Goddard III, MD
Interventional Neuroradiologist
St. Paul Radiology
St. Paul, Minnesota

Erik F. Hauck, MD, PhD
Department of Neurosurgery
University Texas Southwestern
Galveston, Texas

Brian Hoh, MD, FACS, FAHA
William Merz Assistant Professor of Neurological Surgery
Department of Neurosurgery
College of Medicine
University of Florida
Gainesville, Florida

L. Nelson Hopkins, MD
Chairman and Professor
Department of Neurosurgery
University at Buffalo, State University of New York
UB Neurosurgery, Inc.
Millard Fillmore Gates Hospital
Buffalo, New York

Jeffrey P. Lassig, MD
Interventional Neuroradiologist
St. Paul Radiology and National Brain
Aneurysm Center
St. Joseph's Hospital
Medical Director
Interventional Neuroradiology
Nasseff Neuroscience Center
United Hospital
St. Paul, Minnesota

Michael T. Lawton, MD
Professor of Neurological Surgery
Chief, Cerebrovascular and Skull Base
Surgery Programs
Vice Chairman, Department of Neurological Surgery
Tong Po Kan Endowed Chair
Principal Investigator, Center for Cerebrovascular
Research
University of California, San Francisco
San Francisco, California

Elad I. Levy, MD, FACS, FAHAa
Professor of Neurosurgery and Radiology
School of Medicine and Biomedical Sciences
University at Buffalo, State University of New York
Department of Neurosurgery
Millard Fillmore Gates Hospital, Kaleida Health
Buffalo, New York

William J. Mack, MD
Assistant Professor
Department of Neurosurgery
Keck School of Medicine
University of Southern California
Los Angeles, California

Michael T. Madison, MD
Medical Director
Interventional Neuroradiology
National Brain Aneurysm Center
St. Joseph's Hospital
St. Paul, Minnesota

Edward M. Manno, MD
Head, Neurocritical Care
Cleveland Clinic
Cleveland, Ohio

Thomas J. Masaryk, MD
Department of Neurological Surgery
Cleveland Clinic
Cleveland, Ohio

Fredric B. Meyer, MD
Professor and Chair
Department of Neurologic Surgery
Mayo Clinic
Rochester, Minnesota

Sabareesh K. Natarajan, MD, MS
Department of Neurological Surgery
University of Washington
Harborview Medical Center
Seattle, Washington

Leslie A. Nussbaum, MD, PhD
Director, Cyberknife Center
St. Joseph's Hospital
St. Paul, Minnesota

Joshua Olson, BA
National Brain Aneurysm Center
St. Joseph's Hospital
St. Paul, Minnesota

Dinesh Ramanathan, MD, MS
Fellow
Department of Neurological Surgery
University of Washington
Harborview Medical Center
Seattle, Washington

Luca Regli, MD, PhD
Professor and Chairman
Rudolf Magnus Institute of Neuroscience
Department of Neurology and Neurosurgery
University Medical Center Utrecht
Utrecht, the Netherlands

Gary S. Roubin, MD, PhD
Chairman, Cardiovascular Medicine
Lenox Hill Heart and Vascular Institute
New York, New York

Nader Sanai, MD
Director, Neurosurgical Oncology
Director, Barrow Brain Tumor Research Center
Barrow Neurological Institute
Phoenix, Arizona

R. Michael Scott, MD
Professor of Surgery (Neurosurgery)
Harvard Medical School
Neurosurgeon-in-Chief
Department of Neurosurgery
Children's Hospital Boston
Boston, Massachusetts

Laligam N. Sekhar, MD, FACS
Vice-Chairman and William Joseph Leedom and Bennett Bigelow Professor
Director, Cerebrovascular Surgery
Co-Director, Skull Base Surgery
Department of Neurological Surgery
University of Washington
Harborview Medical Center
President, World Federation of Skull Base Societies
Seattle, Washington

Adnan H. Siddiqui, MD, PhD
Assistant Professor of Neurosurgery and Radiology
School of Medicine and Biomedical Sciences
University at Buffalo, State University of New York
Buffalo, New York

Edward R. Smith, MD
Director, Pediatric Cerebrovascular Surgery
Department of Neurosurgery
Children's Hospital Boston
Harvard Medical School
Boston, Massachusetts

Robert F. Spetzler, MD
Director and J. N. Harber Chairman of Neurological Surgery
Barrow Neurological Institute
Phoenix, Arizona
Professor, Department of Surgery
Section of Neurosurgery
University of Arizona College of Medicine
Tuscon, Arizona

Maria M. Toledo, MD
Assistant Professor
Department of Neurosurgery
University of Puerto Rico School of Medicine
University District Hospital
San Juan, Puerto Rico

Aquilla S. Turk, DO
Associate Professor
Department of Radiology and Radiological Science
Director, Neurointerventional Radiology
Medical University of South Carolina
Charleston, South Carolina

Albert van der Zwan, MD, PhD
Rudolf Magnus Institute of Neuroscience
Department of Neurosurgery
University Medical Center Utrecht
Utrecht, The Netherlands

Tristan P. C. van Doormaal
Rudolf Magnus Institute of Neuroscience
Department of Neurosurgery
University Medical Center Utrecht
Utrecht, The Netherlands

Gregory J. Velat, MD
Department of Neurosurgery
College of Medicine
University of Florida
Gainesville, Florida

Fernando Viñuela, MD
Professor of Radiology
Director, Interventional Neuroradiology Division
Department of Radiological Sciences
Ronald Reagan UCLA Medical Center
Los Angeles, California

I

Background

Chapter 1

Microsurgical Cerebral Revascularization: A Historical Perspective

Leslie A. Nussbaum and Eric S. Nussbaum

Although the usefulness of iatrogenic surgical vascular occlusion had been described by the renowned Scottish surgeon John Hunter in the 1700s, it was not until the early 20th century that direct vascular reconstruction using arterial anastomotic techniques became recognized. In 1902, the French surgeon Alexis Carrel who has been considered the father of modern vascular surgery described the first arterial end-to-end anastomosis with suture.[1,2] Following this, early attempts at cerebral revascularization in the first half of the 20th century met with little success.

It is not surprising that some of the first procedures suggested for revascularizing the ischemic brain were indirect operations that relied on the delayed ingrowth of blood vessels from the temporalis muscle to the exposed brain. In the earliest reported examples of encephaloduromyosynangiosis (EDMS), German and Taffel used vascularized muscle flaps that were applied directly onto the cerebral cortex in dogs and primates.[3] Soon thereafter, Kredel attempted this procedure in humans, but was discouraged by the high incidence of perioperative seizures.[4] In 1949, Beck described a technique for revascularizing the brain by creating a cervical carotid-jugular fistula in pediatric patients, but the efficacy of the procedure was difficult to establish.[5]

Around this time, C. Miller Fisher popularized the idea that many strokes actually resulted from cervical carotid atherosclerotic disease. He also suggested the possibility of distal vascular reconstruction to prevent ischemic injury.[6] Perhaps, in part, in response to his prophetic comments, several groups reported the first cervical carotid reconstruction procedures in the early 1950s.[7] These first examples of extracranial carotid artery reconstruction paved the way for carotid endarterectomy, which has become one of the most commonly performed operations today. Since then, vast numbers of patients have been spared the devastating disability of ischemic stroke by this simple and elegant procedure.

In the 1960s, great interest began to develop around the use of the operating microscope in neurosurgery. At this time, Jacobson and Suarez described their seminal experience with the anastomosis of small vessels using the microscope.[8] While Yasargil was working in Donaghy's laboratory at the University of Vermont perfecting surgical anastomoses in animal models, early reports of creative cerebral revascularization in patients began to emerge.[9] In 1963, Worriger and Kunlin reported the first common carotid artery to intracranial internal carotid artery (ICA) long saphenous vein graft, although the patient did not survive.[10] That same year, Chou described a successful embolectomy of the middle cerebral artery.[11] In 1965, Pool and Potts reported an ingenious attempt to revascularize the distal anterior cerebral artery (ACA) by connecting a plastic tube from the superficial temporal artery (STA) to the ACA in the management of a large ACA aneurysm. Although the graft clotted, the patient did well.[12] Then in 1967, Yasargil took a giant step forward, successfully performing the first STA-MCA (superficial temporal artery to middle cerebral artery) anastomosis procedures for ICA occlusion.[13,14] Shortly thereafter, he reported success using similar bypasses for moyamoya disease in children.[13,14]

In the 1970s, technical expertise in the creation of extracranial-intracranial (EC-IC) bypasses developed exponentially. Several surgeons amassed considerable experience with EC-IC bypasses, demonstrating high patency and low morbidity rates associated with the procedure.[15–18] Spetzler added the occipital artery to an MCA graft as an option; Ausman reported the use of the radial artery as an alternative donor graft. Tew and Story described their growing experiences with long saphenous vein grafting to replace the ICA.[2,19–22] At the same time, revascularization options for the posterior circulation began to emerge with Sundt refining a variety of techniques including long saphenous vein grafts to the posterior cerebral artery, and Ausman describing the use of the occipital artery to revascularize the posterior inferior cerebellar artery and anterior inferior cerebellar artery as well as the STA to reconstruct the superior cerebellar artery.[19,23,24]

Sadly, the tremendous promise and great technical surgical mastery embodied by these creative operations failed to show anticipated results. In 1985, the Cooperative Study on EC-IC Bypass was unable to demonstrate benefit from bypass in the prevention of subsequent stroke.[25] The study, widely criticized as poorly designed and not properly empowered to generate meaningful subgroup analyses, found that some patient subgroups actually fared worse with bypass when compared with their medically treated counterparts.

Following these disappointing results, EC-IC bypass was largely abandoned in the treatment of ischemic disease except at select centers that continued to use the operation in severe cases that failed nonsurgical management options.[2,26,27] Although limited anecdotal success continued to be described in this setting, it has only been over the past decade that interest in this operation has once again grown, in large part because of the development and refinement of ancillary radiologic testing to better assess cerebral blood flow and cerebrovascular reserve.[28] Such testing which may help select those patients at the highest risk for stroke and thus those who might potentially benefit from surgery, has sparked a renewed interest in the use of bypass for ischemic disease.

At the same time, larger centers treating complex intracranial aneurysms and skull base tumors continued to use revascularization techniques in the management of complex and giant, unclippable aneurysms and those tumors that surrounded the carotid and vertebral arteries.[29–31] In addition, revascularization surgery gained an accepted and important role in the management of moyamoya disease, particularly in the pediatric population. Indirect procedures such as encephalomyosynangiosis, encephaloduroarteriosynangiosis, and pial synangiosis, as well as direct EC-IC bypass have been demonstrated reproducibly to decrease the morbidity and mortality of patients in this setting.[32–34]

Today, neurovascular surgeons agree on the important role of bypass in the treatment of complex aneurysms, skull base tumors, and moyamoya disease. A growing recognition of subsets of patients with ischemic disease that may benefit from bypass has emerged as well. As expertise with EC-IC bypass continues to grow and with the development of newer techniques to refine these operations, it is likely that open microsurgical revascularization surgery will continue to hold an important and unique place in the field of neurovascular surgery.

References

1. Carrel A. Nobel Prize in Physiology or Medicine 1912. Amsterdam: Elsevier; 1967
2. Hayden MG, Lee M, Guzman R, Steinberg GK. The evolution of cerebral revascularization surgery. Neurosurg Focus 2009;26(5):E17
3. German WJ, Taffel W. Surgical production of collateral intracranial circulation: an experimental study. Yale J Biol Med 1941;13(4):451–460
4. Kredel FE. Collateral cerebral circulation by muscle graft: technique of operation with report of 3 cases. Southern Surgeon 1942;10:235–244
5. Beck CS, McKhann CF, Belnap WD. Revascularization of the brain through establishment of a cervical arteriovenous fistula; effects in children with mental retardation and convulsive disorders. J Pediatr 1949;35(3):317–329
6. Fisher CM. Occlusion of the internal carotid artery. Arch Neurol Psychiatry 1951;65:346–377
7. Eastcott HHG, Pickering GW, Rob CG. Reconstruction of internal carotid artery in a patient with intermittent attacks of hemiplegia. Lancet 1954;267(6846):994–996
8. Jacobson JH II, Suarez EL. Microsurgery in anastomosis of small vessels. Surg Forum 1960;11:243–245
9. Donaghy RM. The history of microsurgery in neurosurgery. Clin Neurosurg 1979;26:619–625
10. Woringer E, Kunlin J, Worringer E, Kunlin J. Anastomose entre le carotide primitive et la carotid intra-cranienne ou las sylvienne par griffon selon la technique de la suture suspendue. [Anastomosis between the common carotid and the intracranial carotid or the Sylvian artery by a graft, using the suspended suture technique.] Neurochirurgie 1963;200:181–188
11. Chou SN. Embolectomy of the middle cerebral artery. J Neurosurg 1963;20:161–163
12. Pool DP, Potts DG. Aneurysms and Arteriovenous Anomalies of the Brain: Diagnosis and Treatment. New York: Harper & Row; 1965
13. Yasargil MG. Diagnosis and indications for operations in cerebrovascular occlusive disease. In: Yasargil MG. ed, Microsurgery Applied to Neurosurgery. Stuttgart: Georg Theime Verlag; 1969:95–118
14. Yasargil MG, Yonekawa Y. Results of microsurgical extra-intracranial arterial bypass in the treatment of cerebral ischemia. Neurosurgery 1977;1(1):22–24
15. Chater N. Neurosurgical extracranial-intracranial bypass for stroke: with 400 cases. Neurol Res 1983;5(2):1–9
16. Gratzl O, Schmiedek P, Spetzler R, Steinhoff H, Marguth F. Clinical experience with extra-intracranial arterial anastomosis in 65 cases. J Neurosurg 1976;44(3):313–324
17. Schmiedek P, Gratzl O, Spetzler R, et al. Selection of patients for extra-intracranial arterial bypass surgery based on rCBF measurements. J Neurosurg 1976;44(3):303–312
18. Sundt TM Jr, Whisnant JP, Fode NC, Piepgras DG, Houser OW. Results, complications, and follow-up of 415 bypass operations for occlusive disease of the carotid system. Mayo Clin Proc 1985;60(4):230–240
19. Ausman JI, Chou SN, Lee M, Klassen A. Occipital to cerebellar artery anastomosis for brainstem infarction from vertebral basilar occlusive disease. Stroke 1976;7:13
20. Spetzler R, Chater N. Occipital artery–middle cerebral artery anastomosis for cerebral artery occlusive disease. Surg Neurol 1974;2(4): 235–238
21. Story JL, Brown WE, Eidelberg E, Arom KV, Stewart JR. Cerebral revascularization: proximal external carotid to distal middle cerebral artery bypass with a synthetic tube graft. Neurosurgery 1978;3(1):61–65
22. Tew JM Jr. Reconstructive intracranial vascular surgery for prevention of stroke. Clin Neurosurg 1975;22:264–280
23. Ausman JI, Diaz FG, Vacca DF, Sadasivan B. Superficial temporal and occipital artery bypass pedicles to superior, anterior inferior, and posterior inferior cerebellar arteries for vertebrobasilar insufficiency. J Neurosurg 1990;72(4):554–558
24. Sundt TM Jr, Whisnant JP, Piepgras DG, Campbell JK, Holman CB. Intracranial bypass grafts for vertebral-basilar ischemia. Mayo Clin Proc 1978;53(1):12–18
25. The EC/IC Bypass Study Group. Failure of extracranial-intracranial arterial bypass to reduce the risk of ischemic stroke: results of an international randomized trial. N Engl J Med 1985;313(19):1191–1200
26. Amin-Hanjani S, Butler WE, Ogilvy CS, Carter BS, Barker FG II. Extracranial-intracranial bypass in the treatment of occlusive cerebrovascular disease and intracranial aneurysms in the United States between 1992 and 2001: a population-based study. J Neurosurg 2005;103(5): 794–804
27. Nussbaum ES, Erickson DL. Extracranial-intracranial bypass for ischemic cerebrovascular disease refractory to maximal medical therapy. Neurosurgery 2000;46(1):37–42, discussion 42–43
28. Grubb RL Jr, Derdeyn CP, Fritsch SM, et al. Importance of hemodynamic factors in the prognosis of symptomatic carotid occlusion. JAMA 1998;280(12):1055–1060

29. Peerless SJ, Ferguson GG, Drake CG. Extracranial-intracranial (EC/IC) bypass in the treatment of giant intracranial aneurysms. Neurosurg Rev 1982;5(3):77–81

30. Sekhar LN, Kalavakonda C. Cerebral revascularization for aneurysms and tumors. Neurosurgery 2002;50(2):321–331

31. Spetzler RF, Fukushima T, Martin N, Zabramski JM. Petrous carotid-to-intradural carotid saphenous vein graft for intracavernous giant aneurysm, tumor, and occlusive cerebrovascular disease. J Neurosurg 1990;73(4):496–501

32. Marsushima T, Fujiwara S, Nagata S, et al. Surgical treatment for pediatric patients with moya moya disease by indirect revascularization procedures (EDAS, EMS, EMAS). Acta Neurochir 1988;98:135–140

33. Matsushima Y, Aoyagi M, Suzuki R, Nariai T, Shishido T, Hirakawa K. Dual anastomosis for pediatric moya moya patients using the anterior and posterior branches of the superficial temporal artery. Childs Nerv Syst 1993;18:27–32

34. Scott RM. Surgical treatment of moyamoya syndrome in children, 1985. Pediatr Neurosurg 1995;22(1):39–46

Chapter 2

Indications for Microsurgical Cerebral Revascularization

Eric S. Nussbaum

◆ Background

Extracranial-intracranial (EC-IC) bypass represents one of the most refined microsurgical procedures performed today. Over time, the specific indications for various forms of bypass surgery have evolved, and endovascular techniques for revascularizing the brain have emerged. Following its introduction in the late 1960s, EC-IC bypass assumed an important role in the surgical management of ischemic cerebrovascular disease.[1–3] At that time, it was assumed that "more" was necessarily "better." Thus, it was widely held that the augmentation of blood flow via bypass could only serve to decrease the risk of future stroke in patients who were felt to be at increased risk for ischemic injury. It was also conjectured that increasing blood flow to the brain might reverse neurodegenerative conditions including various forms of dementia.

In the mid 1980s, the Cooperative Study on EC-IC bypass raised questions about the true efficacy of the operation to decrease the risk of ischemic stroke.[4] Subsequently, the volume of bypass procedures decreased sharply.[1,5] Over time, more sophisticated techniques for imaging the physiologic status of the brain began to shed greater light on impaired cerebral blood flow and cerebrovascular reserve.[6,7] As such, it has become increasingly possible to predict which patients might benefit the most from revascularization. Nevertheless, the exact indications for bypass in the setting of cerebral ischemia remain uncertain and highly controversial.

Today, there is general agreement that cerebral revascularization is indicated in the management of selected complex, unclippable intracranial aneurysms as well as certain skull base tumors.[8,9] Although most neurovascular surgeons believe that there are patients with occlusive cerebrovascular disease that will benefit from bypass, there is little solid scientific data to establish firm criteria for patient selection. This chapter covers both accepted and controversial indications for microsurgical cerebral revascularization.

◆ Occlusive Cerebrovascular Disease

In the setting of ischemic disease, EC-IC bypass is generally considered as an option in the subacute or chronic phase in patients presenting with transient ischemic events and/or watershed ischemic injury. These patients may suffer from borderline cerebral hypoperfusion, becoming symptomatic at times of particular hemodynamic stress. In our practice, we have considered patients to be candidates for bypass only when they demonstrate clear evidence of cerebral ischemia in a distribution referable to an anatomic lesion not amenable to carotid endarterectomy. We have generally deferred surgery in patients who are asymptomatic or who have only vague, nonspecific symptoms such as dizziness or lightheadedness unless they are very young with overwhelming evidence of hypoperfusion on magnetic resonance imaging (possibly demonstrating areas of silent ischemic injury) and physiologic imaging studies. Young patients with moyamoya may also be an exception and will be addressed below and in a separate chapter.

In all cases, diagnostic angiography should be performed to exclude the presence of good collateral supply to the affected territory. The patient with a symptomatic high-grade stenosis of the internal carotid artery (ICA) at the carotid bifurcation should undergo endarterectomy rather than bypass. Also, the patient with a cervical ICA occlusion who presents with a transient ischemic attack but who has robust collateral across the anterior communicating artery or from the posterior communicating artery is much more likely to have suffered symptoms from a small embolic insult rather than a hypoperfusion injury and would probably be best served by antiplatelet or anticoagulant therapy rather than surgery.

With rare exception, we have recommended that patients undergo a trial of antiplatelet and/or anticoagulation therapy prior to consideration for surgical bypass. In addition, we have evaluated numerous patients who presented with intermittent ischemic symptoms that fully resolved when their aggressive antihypertensive regimens were changed. These simple medical maneuvers will obviate the need for surgery in a surprising number of patients (**Fig. 2.1**).

At this point, one is left with a subgroup of patients who suffer from ischemic symptoms referable to a particular vascular territory that is clearly underperfused with limited collateral supply based on cerebral angiography. Functional, physiologic testing now becomes important to stratify these patients into appropriate risk categories for future ischemic injury. As a general rule, those patients with ongoing ischemic symptoms compatible with hypoperfusion of the involved vascular territory and/or a watershed-type insult may benefit from revascularization. Ancillary testing with computed tomography (CT) or MR perfusion or positron emission tomography (PET) confirming hypoperfusion with impaired reserve provides important supporting evidence that bypass may be appropriate. In addition, younger patient age and good general health may be helpful factors in recommending revascularization.

Finally, it is worthwhile to note that surgical revascularization can play a rare role in the management of acute ischemic stroke. In selected cases, emergency embolectomy of the middle cerebral artery (video) or emergency EC-IC bypass can be contemplated when endovascular therapy is contraindicated or unsuccessful and when no intervention is likely to result in a devastating injury.[10] A good example might include a young patient with an acute M1 occlusion not amenable to endovascular treatment who has poor leptomeningeal collateral flow and presents with severe deficit but only limited watershed ischemic injury on an early MRI scan (**Fig. 2.2**). In addition, patients who undergo attempted but failed endovascular therapy may be considered for open surgery as a rescue, "salvage" maneuver in select instances.[10]

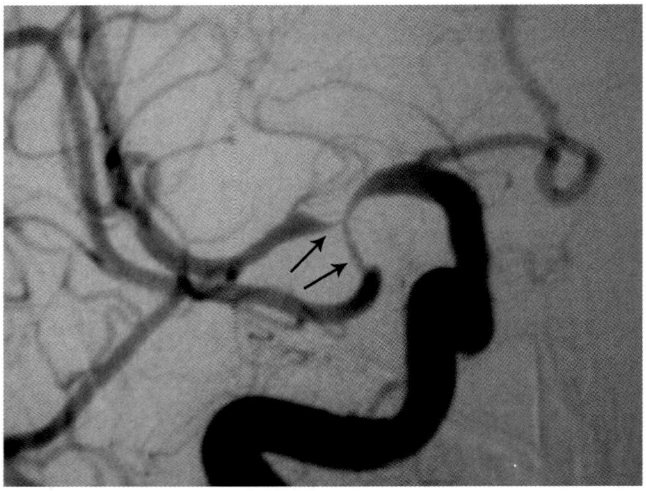

Fig. 2.1 A critical stenosis of the distal M1 segment and both M2 branches (*arrows*) of the middle cerebral artery is identified on this arteriogram obtained in an 81-year-old woman who presented with a flurry of transient ischemic attacks resulting in contralateral arm and leg weakness. The patient was anticoagulated and then converted to antiplatelet therapy with complete cessation of her symptoms. Given her age, nothing further was done, and the patient remained symptom-free at 2-year follow-up.

Anatomic Localization

Patients with ischemic disease that may benefit from surgical revascularization can be divided based on the anatomic location of their stenosis or occlusion. Most individuals with cervical ICA occlusion tolerate the occlusion without symptoms. In fact, over 80% of patients tolerate unilateral ICA occlusion without suffering a significant ischemic event. Some patients with no collateral supply present with a devastating infarct, obviating consideration for bypass. Nevertheless, a small percentage of patients have adequate collateral supply to prevent severe, irreversible ischemic injury during most ordinary circumstances but will become symptomatic during periods of hypotension or high hemodynamic stress. Patients with cervical ICA occlusion tend to be older and often have good collateral supply, but when they are symptomatic due to watershed hypoperfusion, bypass may be a useful adjunct to decrease future risk of stroke (**Fig. 2.3**). It is specifically this population that is being investigated by the Carotid Occlusion Surgery Study (COSS), which uses oxygen extraction fraction based on PET evaluation to attempt to select those patients at highest risk for stroke and to randomize these individuals to bypass versus medical management.[6]

Patients with petrous or cavernous ICA stenosis or occlusion will present with similar clinical pictures. When the carotid is stenotic, endovascular options may be useful (as described in separate chapters), particularly for older patients who may be poor surgical candidates. Because the ICA in these segments does not give rise to critical perforators and is relatively large in caliber, these lesions can be treated with bypass but may also be addressed with endovascular angioplasty and stenting.

In our experience, patients with supraclinoid ICA stenosis or occlusion tend to be younger and the pathologic process is often an arterial dissection rather than atherosclerotic. If the stenosis is above or across the origin of the posterior communicating artery, one important source of collateral supply may be compromised. These patients may present with a highly unstable picture, and we have found bypass to be extremely effective in arresting progressive ischemic symptoms in this population.

Middle cerebral artery (MCA) stenosis or occlusion (MCAO) represents a dangerous condition because the only collateral supply distal to the anatomic lesion is typically from leptomeningeal vessels derived from the anterior (ACA) and posterior cerebral artery (PCA) territories. Despite this, it is surprising how frequently patients will tolerate unilateral MCAO without significant ischemic injury. We have found these patients

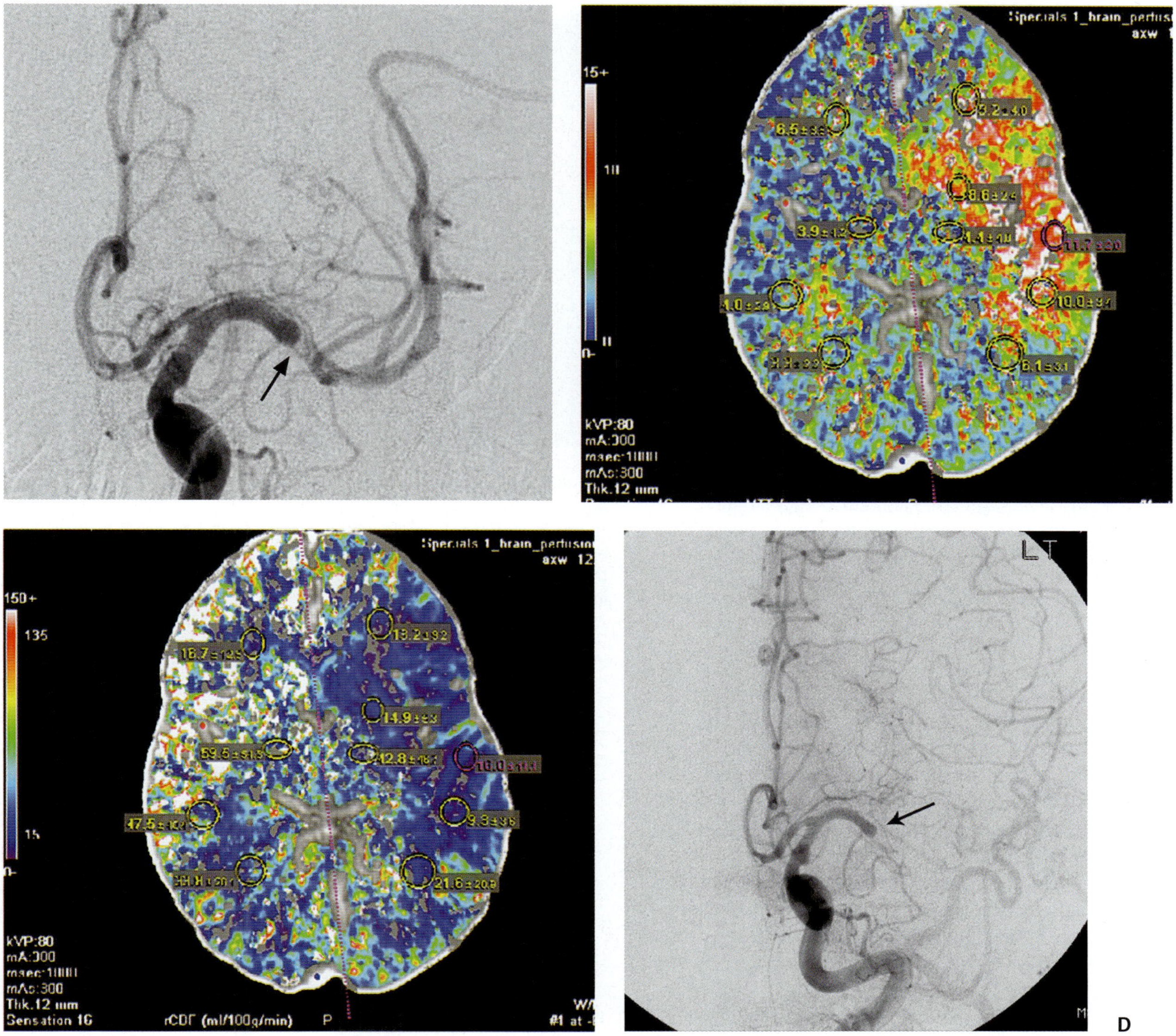

A B C D

Fig. 2.2 A 41-year-old right-handed man presented with fluctuating speech difficulty and right-sided weakness. He was transferred to our center after cerebral angiography performed at an outside facility revealed significant stenosis of the left M1 segment (*arrow*) compatible with an acute arterial dissection **(A)**. Dynamic perfusion CT images revealed significant elevation in mean transit time **(B)** and decreased regional cerebral blood flow **(C)** in the involved left hemisphere. Over the next 6 hours, the patient developed severe dysphasia and profound right-sided hemiparesis, and repeat angiography revealed M1 occlusion (*arrow*) **(D)**. MRI demonstrated only a small area of watershed injury, and the patient underwent emergency superficial temporal artery–middle cerebral artery anastomosis with rapid correction of his preoperative deficit and a good ultimate recovery.

to fall into two distinct categories. Older patients with atherosclerotic narrowing or occlusion of the MCA often present with a significant ischemic insult. Most patients either have adequate collateral supply to obviate the need for a bypass or suffer a severe injury making bypass unnecessary. A second group of younger patients seem to present with high-grade stenosis of the MCA, probably related to an acute or subacute arterial dissection. These patients present with watershed ischemic injury on MRI and may have fluctuating ischemic symptoms. We have found many of these patients to benefit from bypass, including some who have been treated successfully on an emergency basis.[10]

One distinct group of patients that deserves mention includes those individuals suffering from moyamoya disease. Although moyamoya classically affects children and young adults, we have encountered this disease or a variant thereof in patients of all ages and of all ethnic backgrounds. There is significant controversy regarding the optimal form of revascularization in these patients, and indirect methods for revascularization are detailed in a separate chapter. We have favored direct superficial temporal artery to middle cerebral artery (STA-MCA) anastomosis when feasible in this population to immediately restore blood flow to the affected hemisphere. Nevertheless, there is excellent evidence,

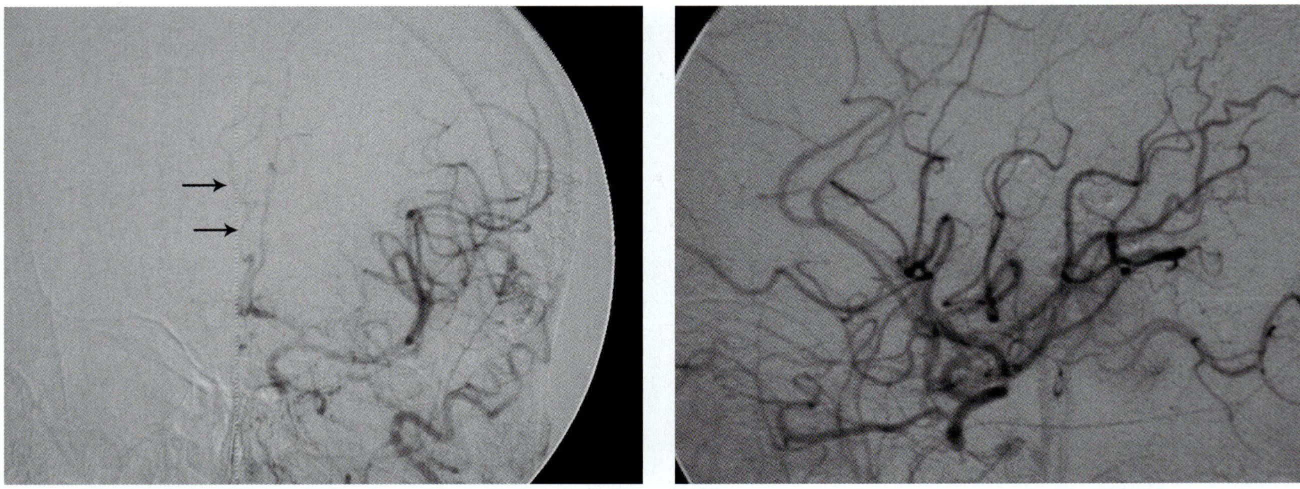

A B

Fig. 2.3 A 61-year-old man with bilateral internal carotid artery occlusions presented with repeated left hemispheric TIAs despite cessation of antihypertensive agents and institution of anticoagulation and antiplatelet therapy. He underwent left-sided superficial temporal artery–middle cerebral artery bypass. Interestingly, in addition to complete cessation of his TIAs, the patient reported rapid improvement in ipsilateral leg weakness, which had been present for more than 2 years. Postoperative AP **(A)** and lateral **(B)** external carotid arteriographic images reveal dramatic filling of the left hemispheric circulation through the bypass. Of note, the contralateral anterior carotid artery (*arrows*) fills from the graft as well, which may explain the improved, long-standing ipsilateral lower extremity paresis.

particularly in children, that indirect forms of revascularization can be extremely effective.[11,12] As a rule, when the STA is of reasonable caliber, we have dissected out the STA and then explored the cortical surface for an adequate recipient vessel. If the cortical MCA branches are small, flattened, and pale, we have performed an encephaloduroarteriosynangiosis (EDAS) procedure. If a healthy-appearing MCA branch is encountered, a direct bypass is performed. Still, delayed postoperative angiography has often revealed the development of indirect collateral supply through the craniotomy that is equal to or more robust than that provided by the anastomosis.

On occasion, patients present with multiple arterial occlusions challenging surgeons to develop innovative techniques to revascularize the brain. Patients with common carotid artery occlusion requiring bypass may be treated with a long saphenous vein graft from the subclavian artery to the MCA or with a "bonnet" bypass.[13] As an alternative, we have occasionally utilized the STA which may itself be open through collateral supply from the contralateral side in reverse fashion to revascularize the brain in just this setting. In addition, we have encountered several patients with Takayasu arteritis including one who was managed with an aorto-carotid bypass performed in conjunction with our cardiothoracic colleagues (**Fig. 2.4**).

◆ Vertebrobasilar Disease

Patients with posterior circulation ischemic disease should be mentioned as an entirely separate category. Although we have continued to rely heavily on open surgical revascularization in patients with anterior circulation disease, we have increasingly used endovascular therapy for patients with posterior circulation involvement. Stenosis of the cervical vertebral artery or the basilar artery is often well treated with angioplasty and stenting. This often affects an older population with severe advanced atherosclerotic disease, and these patients may be at high risk for complications during open microsurgery.

In select cases, when endovascular therapy is not an option or is considered to carry an excessive risk, open surgery can be considered. Proximal vertebral artery stenosis is well treated with vertebral transposition or carotid to vertebral bypass, and patients with bilateral vertebral occlusion may benefit from a cervical carotid to vertebral bypass or from an occipital posterior inferior cerebellar artery (PICA) bypass (**Fig. 2.5**). Patients with mid to upper basilar stenosis not amenable to angioplasty can be offered STA-SCA or STA-PCA bypass, although this is generally a hard operation on this fragile patient population.[14,15] Alternatively, an occipital to PCA bypass may be a reasonable option in some patients (**Fig. 2.6**). Finally, patients with subclavian steal syndrome may require open surgery, which can be curative in properly selected cases (**Fig. 2.7**).

Endovascular Options

With the progressive refinement of endovascular techniques including angioplasty and intravascular stent placement, many of the lesions that were previously treated with microsurgical bypass can now be addressed by endovascular therapy. At our center, every case is reviewed by the neurovascular team, and all such lesions are considered for conservative, open surgical, and endovascular therapy. It should be remembered that cases

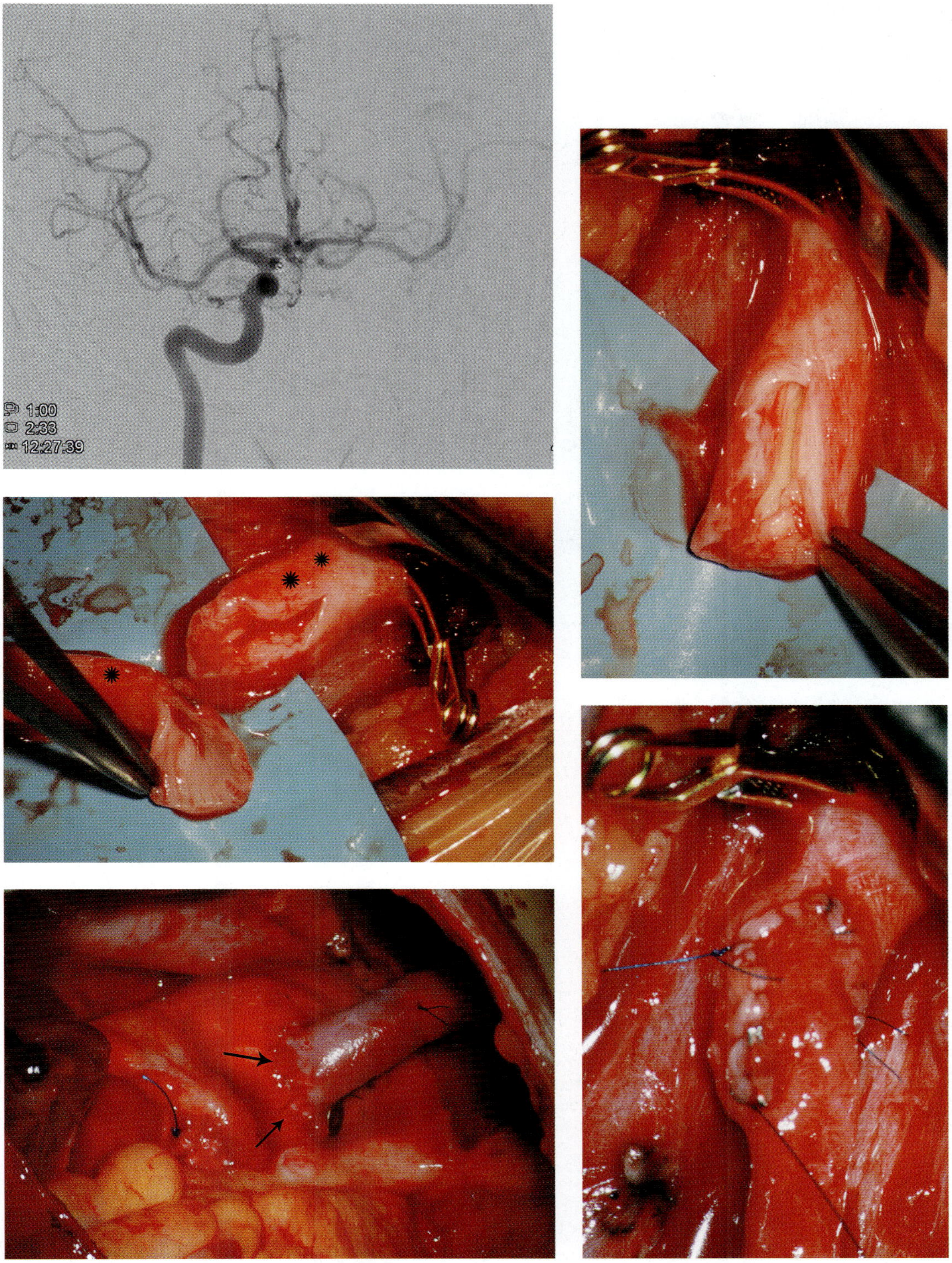

Fig. 2.4 This 32-year-old woman with Takayasu arteritis presented with a subarachnoid hemorrhage from a ruptured superior hypophyseal aneurysm. The aneurysm arose on her right internal carotid artery (ICA), which was the only patent vessel supplying intracranial flow. An AP right internal carotid angiographic image **(A)** shows filling of the entire anterior circulation as well as both posterior cerebral arteries and the upper basilar artery from the right ICA. The aneurysm was coiled, and once the patient had recovered, an aorto-carotid bypass was performed with a saphenous vein graft. At the time of surgery, the common carotid artery was exposed and sectioned repeatedly moving upward toward the bifurcation until a reasonable lumen was encountered. The end of the distal cervical CCA is exposed **(B)**, revealing the thickened and irregular wall. The distal end of the saphenous vein graft (single star) has now been introduced alongside the CCA (*double star*) **(C)**. A running anastomosis was performed **(D)**. The saphenous vein anastomosed (*arrows*) to the aorta is shown **(E)**. *(continued)*

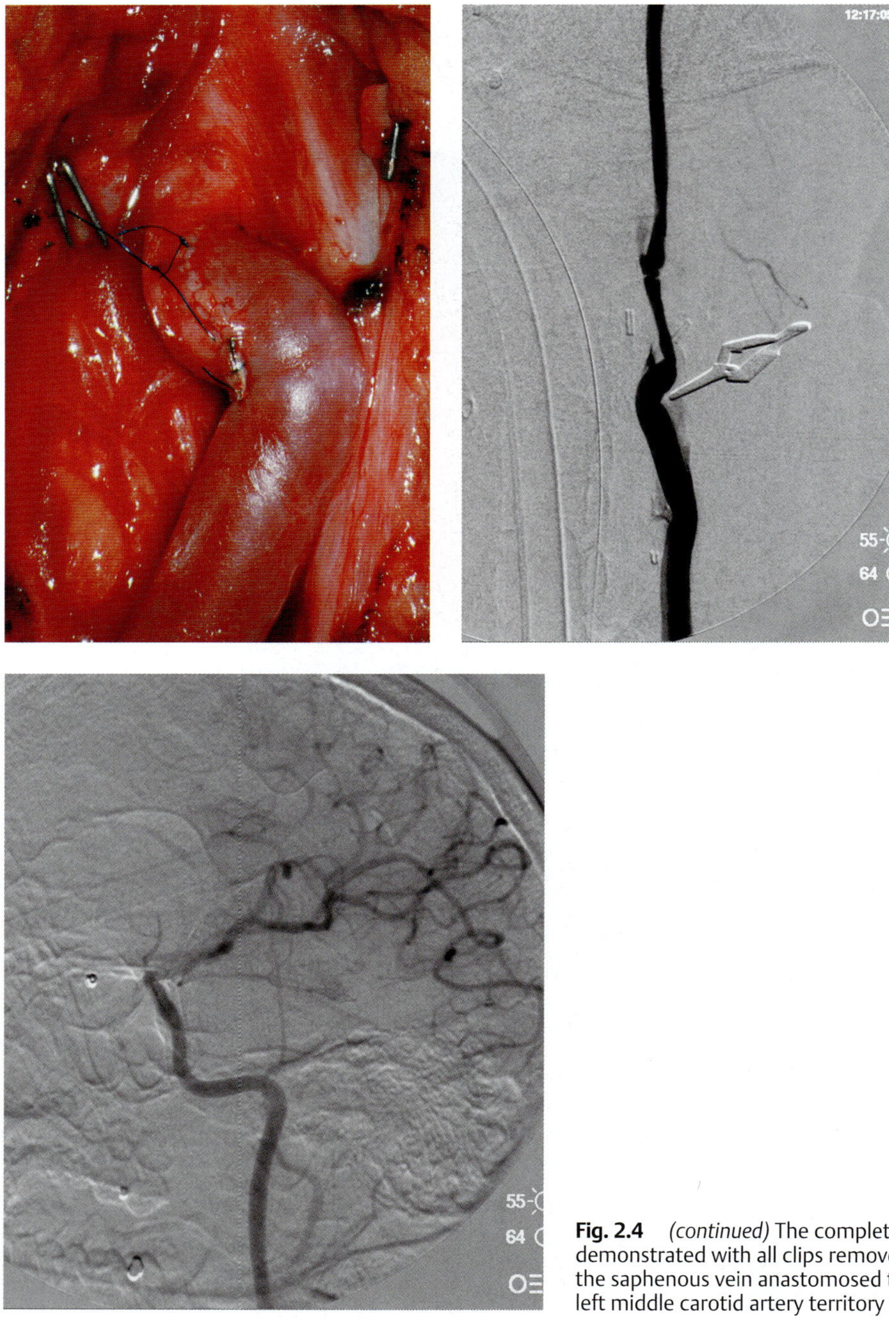

F G H

Fig. 2.4 *(continued)* The completed anastomosis to the cervical CCA is demonstrated with all clips removed **(F)**. Intraoperative angiography demonstrates the saphenous vein anastomosed to the distal CCA **(G)** and the graft now filling the left middle carotid artery territory **(H)**.

must be considered on an individual basis. For certain entities such as an M1 segment dissection, the actual procedural morbidity and mortality rates may well be lower with EC-IC bypass when the operation is performed by an experienced neurovascular surgeon. The risks of acute arterial dissection or rupture during angioplasty are not a factor with open bypass. In addition, the extremely high restenosis rates that have been associated in particular with anterior circulation angioplasty and stenting represent a real limitation of endovascular technology at the present time.[16,17] Although there is a general appeal associated with the less-invasive endovascular options, it is critical that each team individually assess every patient based on their own complication rates when choosing the optimal treatment in a given case.

As discussed above, at our center, we continue to rely on microsurgical bypass in a significant percentage of symptomatic patients with anterior circulation disease. On the other hand, we consider posterior circulation microsurgical revascularization only when our endovascular colleagues feel that they cannot offer treatment with reasonable safety and efficacy.

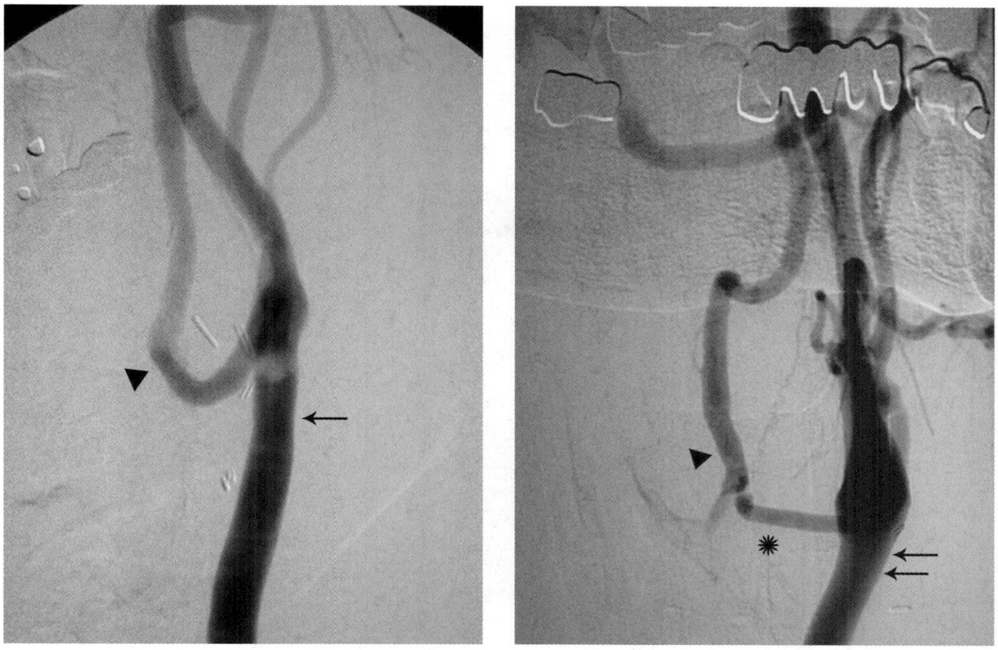

Fig. 2.5 Two angiograms illustrating revascularization options for proximal vertebral artery occlusion are shown. In this setting, the vertebral artery (*arrowhead*) may be transposed and anastomosed to the CCA (*arrow*) **(A)**, or a short segment saphenous vein graft (*star*) may be used to perform a jump graft from the CCA (*arrows*) or proximal ECA to the midcervical vertebral artery (*arrowhead*), which is exposed in the vertebral artery canal **(B)**.

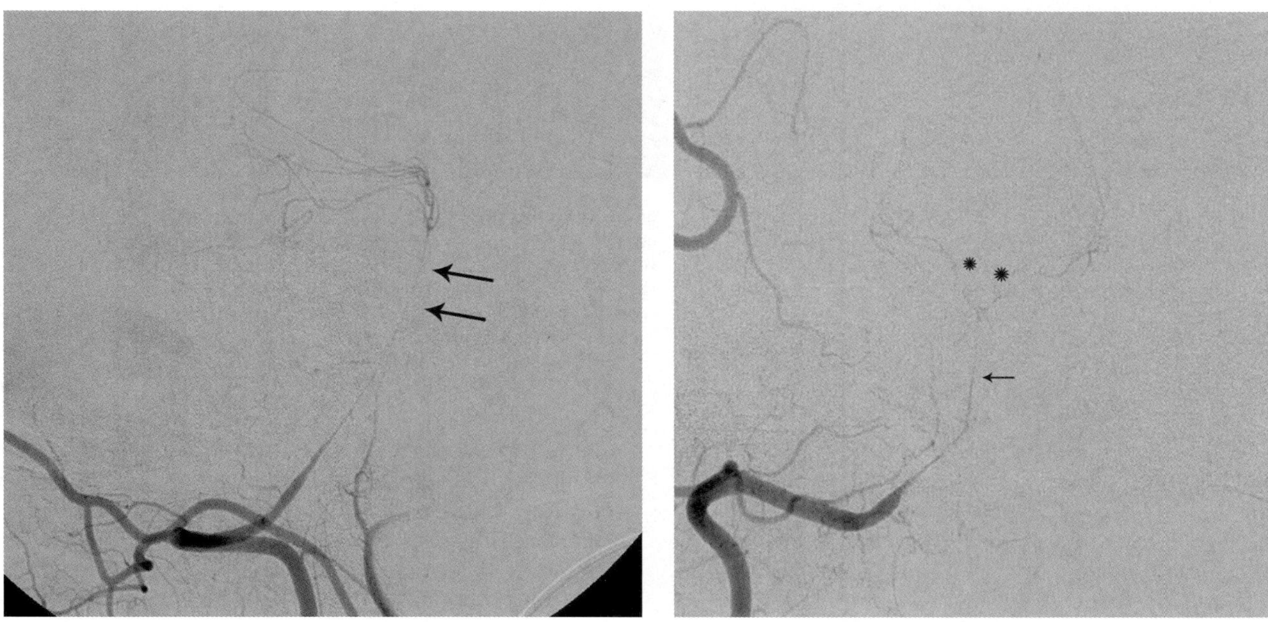

Fig. 2.6 In this fascinating case, a 45-year-old man presented with progressive obtundation 1 month after suffering acute bacterial meningitis. He was found to have severe vasospasm or vasculitis involving the intracranial vasculature and particularly the posterior circulation. Lateral **(A)** and AP **(B)** vertebral angiograms reveal severe narrowing of the basilar artery (*arrows*) and both posterior cerebral arteries (PCAs) (*stars*). *(continued)*

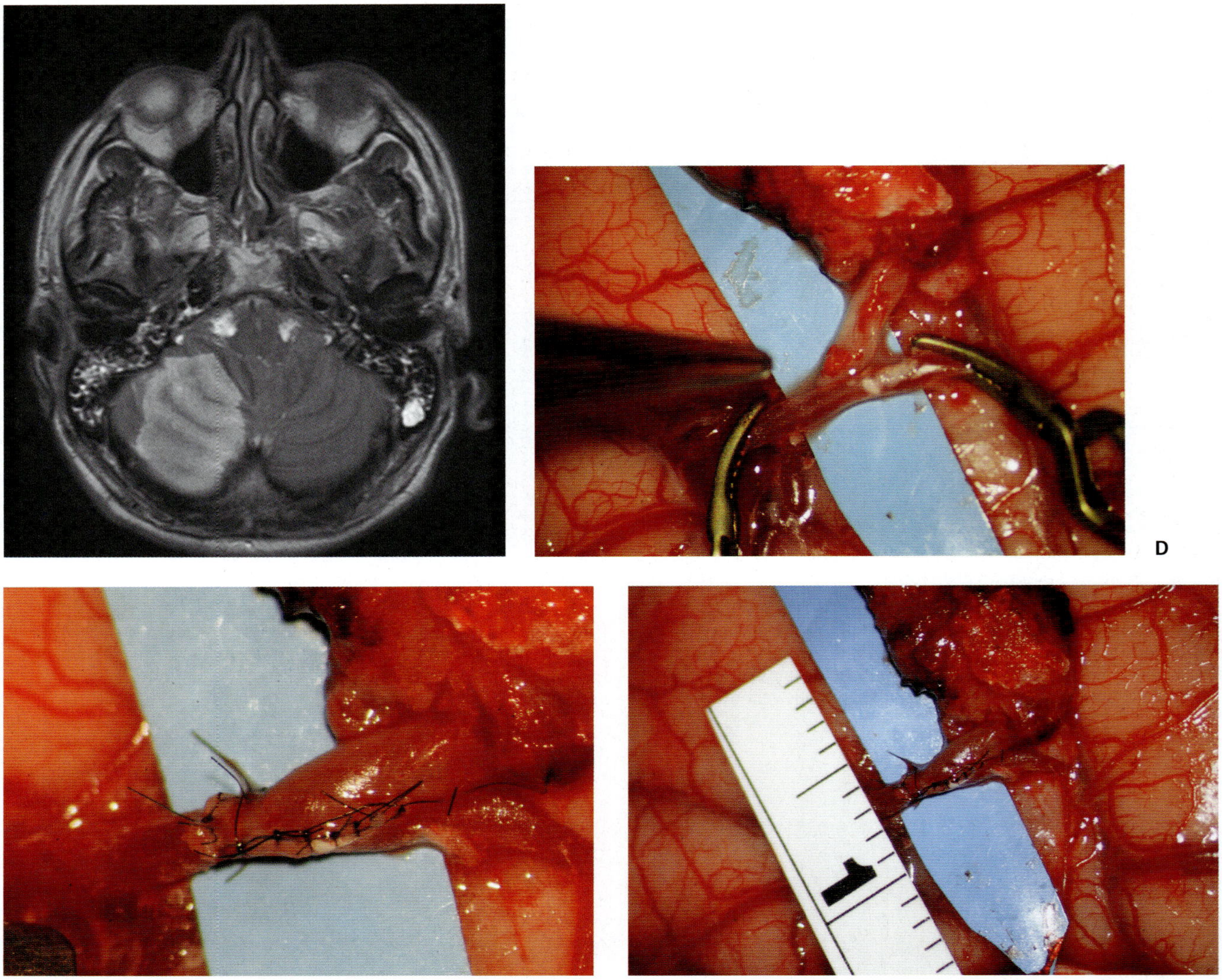

Fig. 2.6 *(continued)* T2-weighted axial MRI **(C)** reveals a large cerebellar infarct. The development of multiple areas of ischemia within the cerebellum and occipital lobes necessitated a posterior fossa decompression for cerebellar edema. At the same time, an occipital artery to PCA bypass was performed to augment flow to the posterior circulation. The cortical PCA branch and dissected occipital artery are shown prepared for anastomosis **(D)**. The anastomosis has been completed and clips removed **(E)**. Note the use of interrupted 11-0 sutures throughout, which we have found particularly useful when dealing with very small vessels. The small size of the vessels is highlighted by the superimposed ruler for scale **(F)**. Following surgery, the patient suffered no further ischemic events and ultimately made an excellent recovery.

◆ Revascularization and Intracranial Aneurysms

Cerebral revascularization may represent a reasonable treatment option in the management of complex intracranial aneurysms that cannot be repaired using direct microsurgical clipping or endosaccular coil therapy.[8,9,18] In these instances, trapping of the aneurysm segment (if that segment is free of critical perforators) or proximal occlusion (if the segment has critical perforators that cannot be sacrificed) may be combined with distal revascularization to treat the aneurysm. In our experience, various forms of revascularization, often creatively combined with microsurgery or endovascular techniques have allowed us to manage with excellent results some aneurysms that would have otherwise been essentially untreatable (**Figs. 2.8**, **2.9**, and **2.10**).[19]

The need for revascularization in this setting depends heavily on the experience and expertise of the surgeon. Although some giant MCA aneurysms can be treated with temporary arterial occlusion and aneurysmorrhaphy, these same lesions can be treated with distal revascularization and proximal occlusion, often with less risk of ischemic injury, again depending on the skills of the surgeon. Giant dissecting or dolichoectatic basilar aneurysms and giant basilar apex aneurysms, particularly those filled

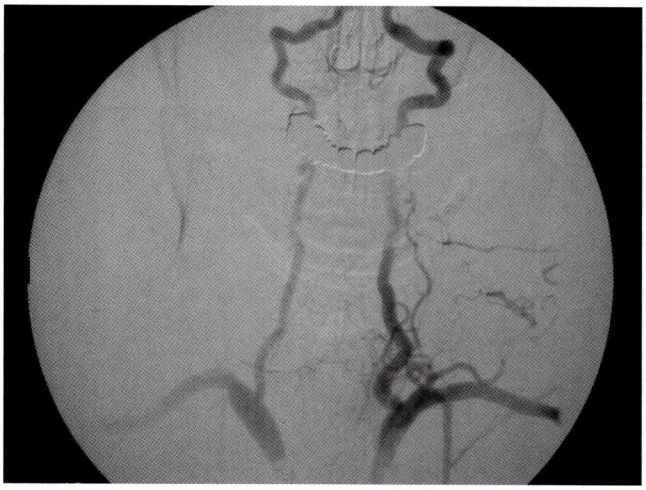

A

Fig. 2.7 This 58-year-old woman presented with classic symptoms of subclavian steal syndrome. A left vertebral artery injection arteriogram **(A)** demonstrates retrograde filling down the right vertebral artery to fill the right subclavian artery. At surgery, the atheromatous subclavian artery has been exposed and opened **(B)**. A synthetic graft has been anastomosed from the proximal CCA to the subclavian artery **(C)**. Also, a right carotid endarterectomy was performed with a patch (*arrowheads*), as can be seen in **C**, at the same time for a 75% asymptomatic carotid stenosis.

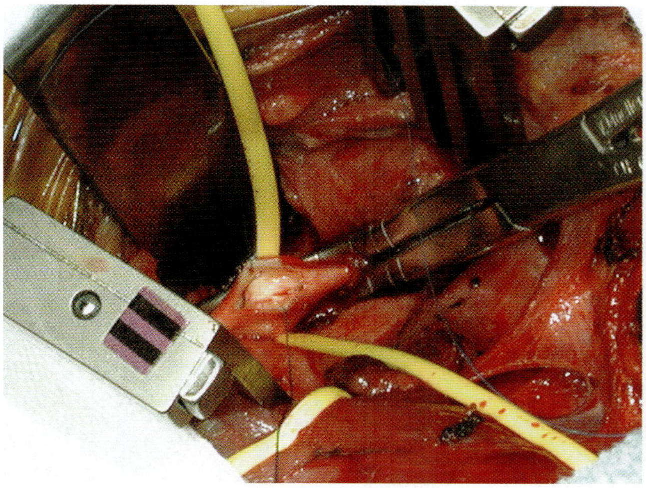

B

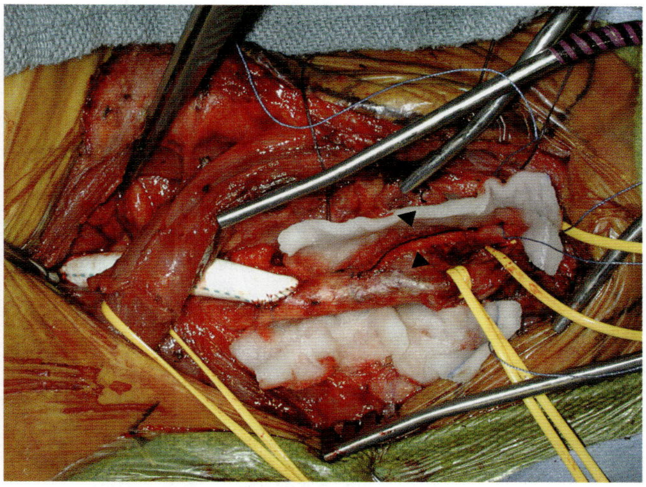

C

with coils, are daunting lesions that can only rarely be clipped successfully and only by the most experienced neurovascular surgeons. In our experience, proximal or distal basilar occlusion with a PCA or SCA bypass (if the native collateral supply via the posterior communicating arteries is inadequate) represents a reasonably low-risk alternative that has often resulted in an excellent outcome (**Fig. 2.11**).

In our experience, we have utilized some form of revascularization in a large percentage of giant and truly fusiform aneurysms (**Figs. 2.12** and **2.13**).[19] In addition, we have performed preliminary EC-IC bypass in several giant or complex aneurysms when we suspected that we would be able to successfully clip the aneurysm but when we also thought that the temporary arterial occlusion time necessary to clip the aneurysm would likely exceed ischemic tolerance limits. In these select cases, the bypass (whose patency was confirmed with intraoperative angiography prior to proceeding with temporary occlusion to address the aneurysm) provided both a safety net and great comfort to the surgeon during the procedure. In fact, having the bypass in place completely transforms the temporary arterial occlusion period from a highly stressful time when one is "working against the clock" to a much more relaxed opportunity to carefully open the aneurysm, evacuate thrombus and atheroma, and then properly apply clips as necessary to reconstruct the segment. In 2 of 18 such cases, we could not achieve a satisfactory clip construct, and the aneurysm was simply trapped, relying on the bypass that prevented any associated ischemic injury.

Whenever vascular sacrifice is contemplated to treat an aneurysm, a trial balloon test occlusion may be useful to assess the patient's native collateral circulation and to better understand the necessity of revascularization. In our experience, we have adopted a relatively aggressive policy favoring some form of revascularization in most patients undergoing iatrogenic occlusion of the ICA. Our algorithm is outlined in **Fig. 2.14**, which illustrates some of the factors influencing the decision for bypass and the choice between a high flow and low flow graft.

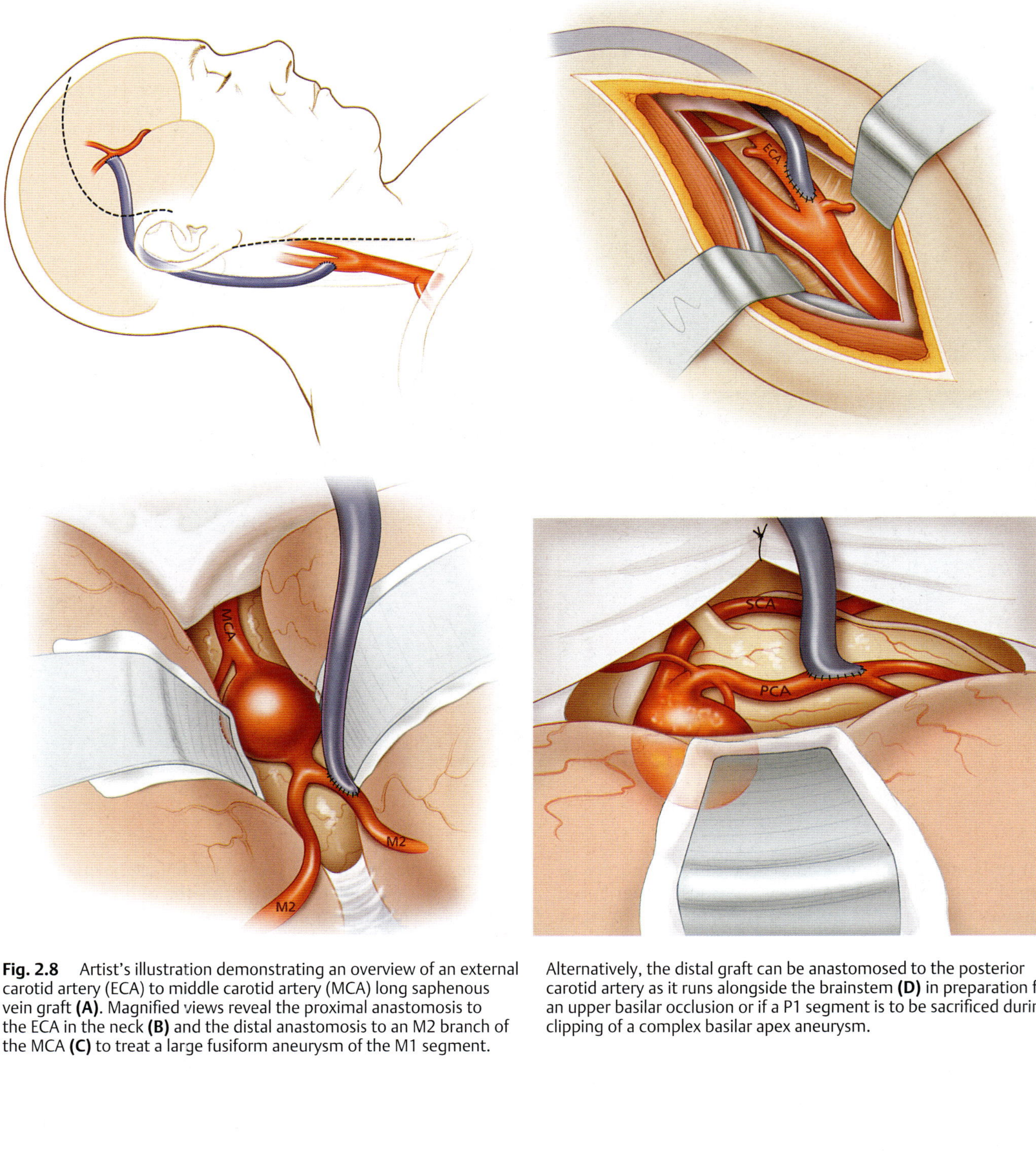

Fig. 2.8 Artist's illustration demonstrating an overview of an external carotid artery (ECA) to middle carotid artery (MCA) long saphenous vein graft **(A)**. Magnified views reveal the proximal anastomosis to the ECA in the neck **(B)** and the distal anastomosis to an M2 branch of the MCA **(C)** to treat a large fusiform aneurysm of the M1 segment. Alternatively, the distal graft can be anastomosed to the posterior carotid artery as it runs alongside the brainstem **(D)** in preparation for an upper basilar occlusion or if a P1 segment is to be sacrificed during clipping of a complex basilar apex aneurysm.

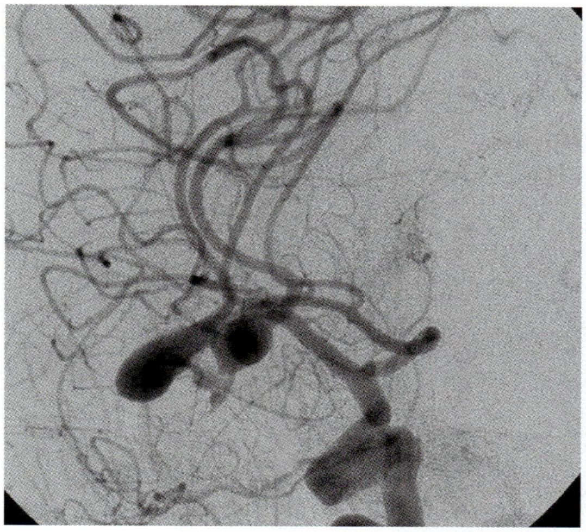
A

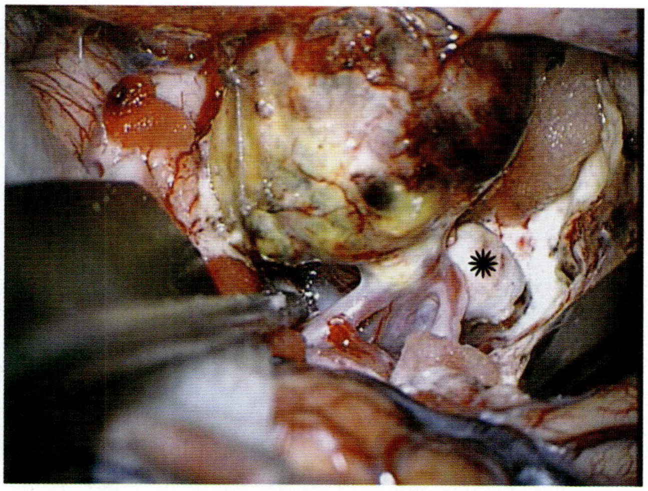
B

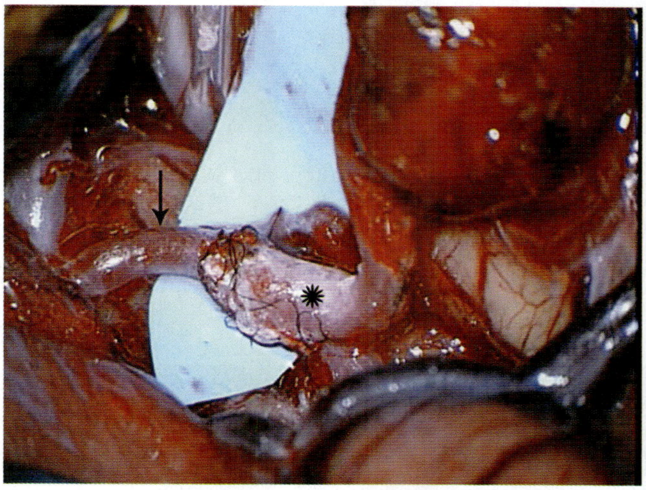
C

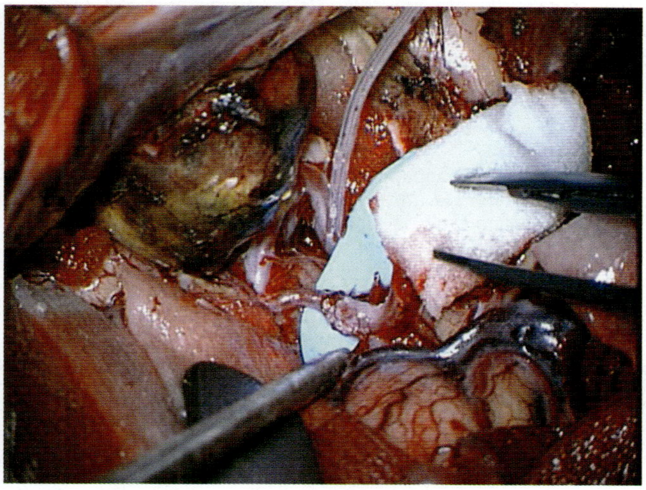
D

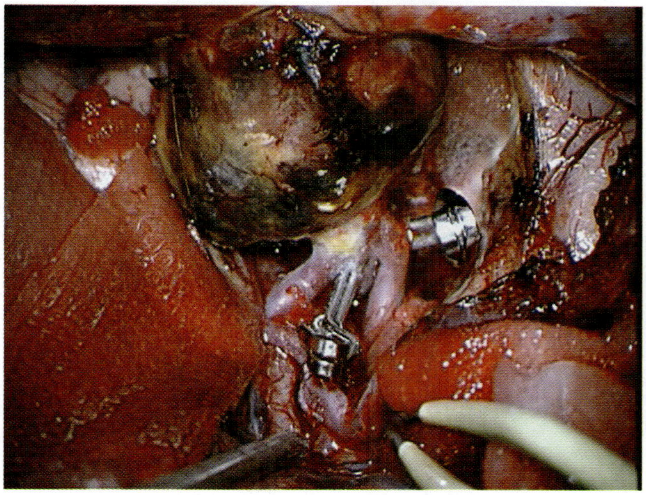
E

Fig. 2.9 This 62-year-old man presented with hemispheric edema and seizures from this giant, partially thrombosed aneurysm of the middle cerebral artery (MCA). Preoperative AP right carotid arteriogram **(A)** demonstrates the giant, partially filling MCA aneurysm. The giant aneurysm as well as a smaller neighboring aneurysm (*star*) arising from the opposite side of the MCA bifurcation have been exposed **(B)**. The superficial temporal artery (STA) (*star*) has been anastomosed to a large MCA branch (*arrow*) within the Sylvian fissure **(C,D)**. The distal M1 has been sacrificed, and the second, smaller aneurysm has been occluded with a separate clip **(E)**. *(continued)*

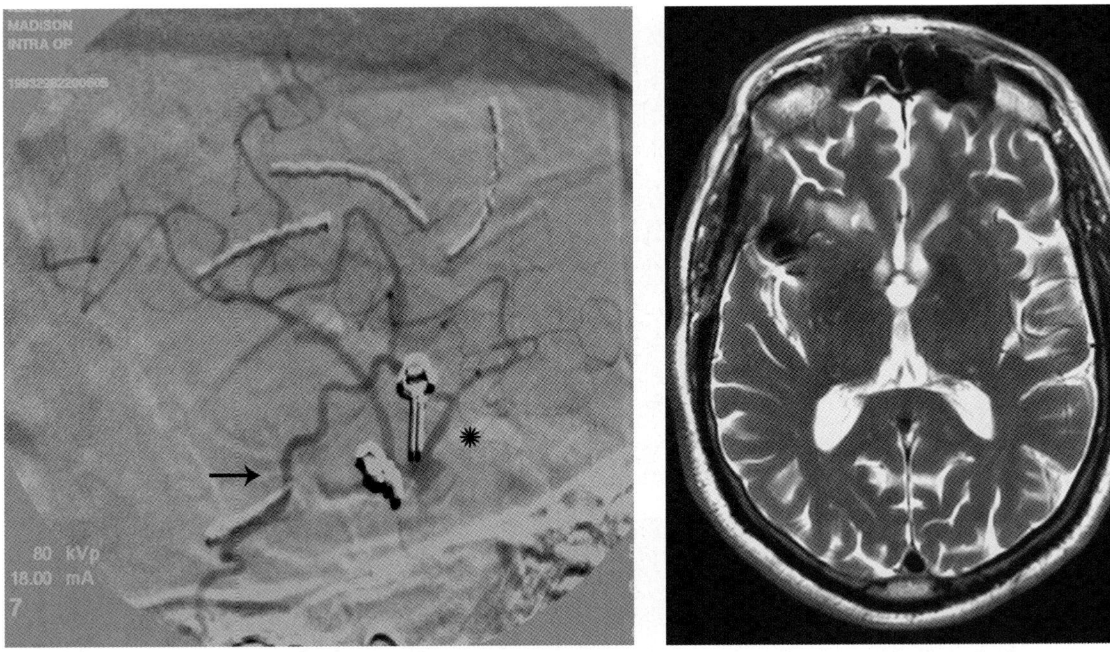

F G

Fig. 2.9 *(continued)* Intraoperative external carotid artery (ECA) angiogram reveals the STA (*arrow*) filling the distal MCA vasculature with retrograde filling of a small portion of the giant aneurysm neck (just below the *star*) **(F)**. Delayed postoperative axial T2-weighted MRI demonstrates resolution of the preoperative edema without ischemic injury **(G)**.

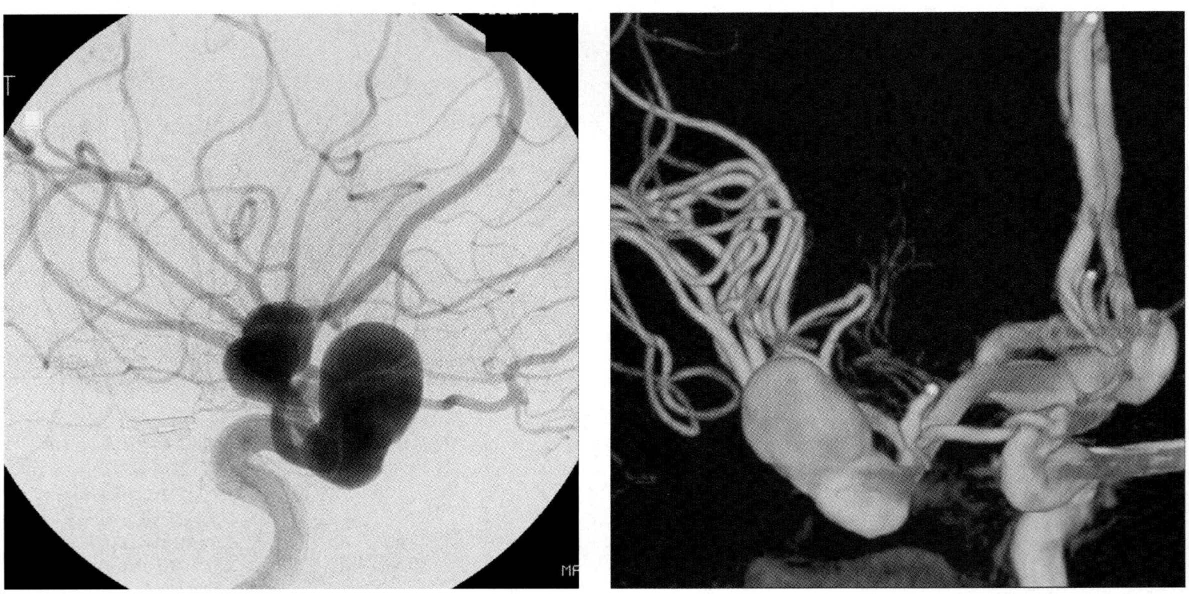

A B

Fig. 2.10 A 54-year-old man had previously undergone microsurgical clipping of a large, ruptured basilar apex aneurysm, and returned 10 years later with the de novo development of giant partially thrombosed aneurysms involving the right supraclinoid internal carotid artery (ICA) and middle carotid artery (MCA) bifurcation **(A,B)**. *(continued)*

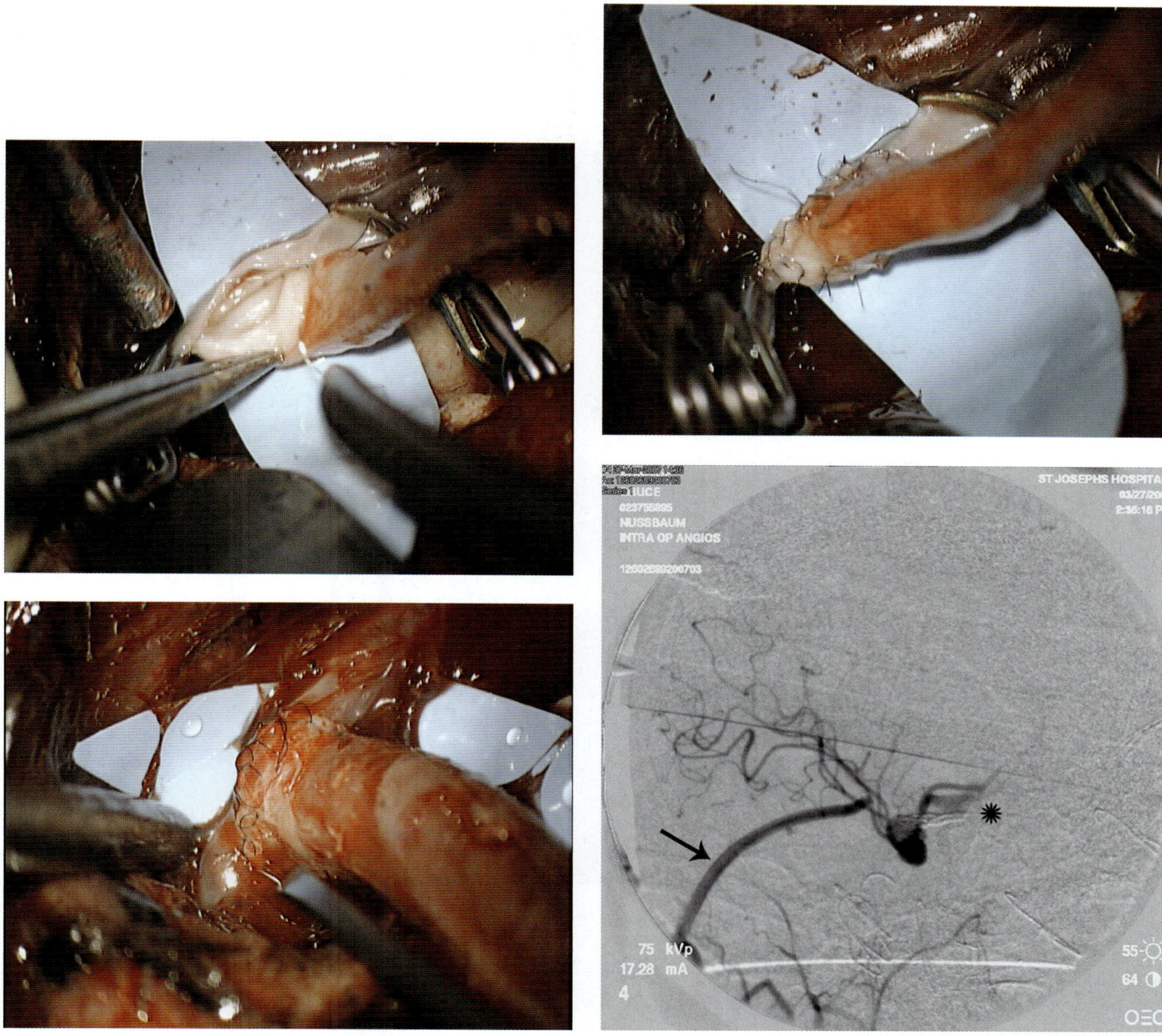

C D E F

Fig. 2.10 *(continued)* A decision was made to perform a distal saphenous vein graft to the middle cerebral artery followed by clip occlusion of the ICA just proximal to the carotid aneurysm. Intraoperative photomicrographs demonstrate the distal end of the saphenous vein graft being anastomosed to the M2 branch with the front wall **(C)**, back wall **(D)**, and completed anastomosis **(E)** shown. Intraoperative angiogram demonstrates the saphenous vein graft (*arrow*) perfusing the MCA territory and filling the ICA retrograde to the clip (*star*) with immediate significant decreased filling of both aneurysms **(F)**.

◆ Skull Base and Head and Neck Tumors

The field of skull base surgery has evolved dramatically over the past 25 years. As the benefits and efficacy of stereotactic radiosurgery have become increasingly clear, fewer tumors are being treated with radically aggressive resection that would necessitate intentional vascular occlusion. Nevertheless, we still encounter, on occasion, the young patient with a skull base or head and neck tumor that can only be completely resected with carotid sacrifice and that is relatively resistant to radiotherapy and/or chemotherapy. In this setting, revascularization must be considered to allow for optimal tumor resection (**Fig. 2.15**).

In our experience, we have considered vascular sacrifice with revascularization when maximally aggressive tumor resection would require carotid sacrifice, and when such an aggressive approach clearly offered a potential benefit to the patient. In these cases, we have generally relied on therapeutic balloon occlusion testing to assess the patients' tolerance to vascular sacrifice preoperatively. It is important

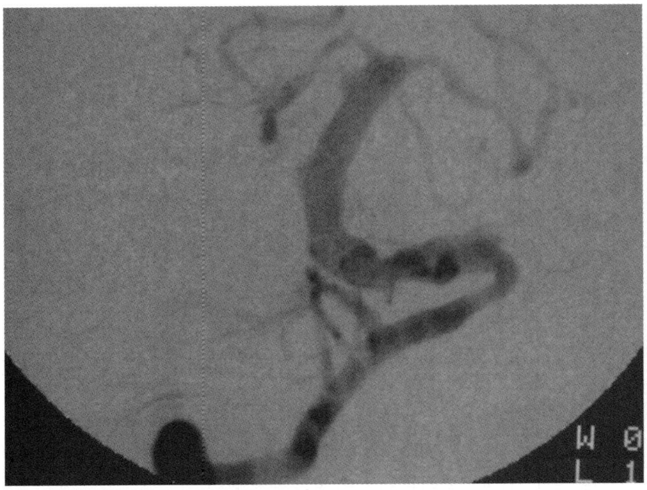

A

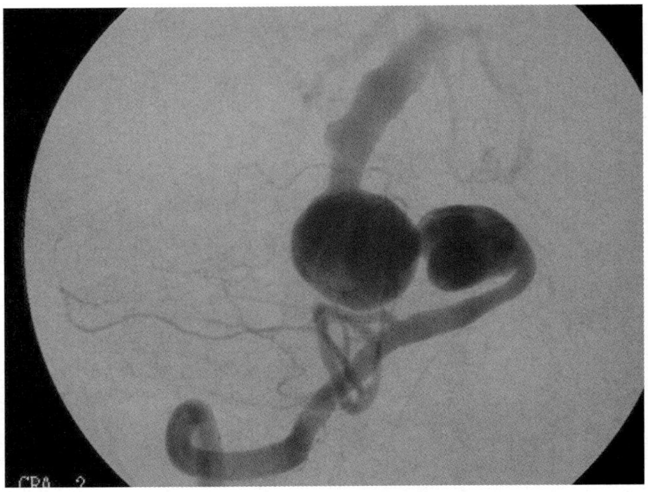

B

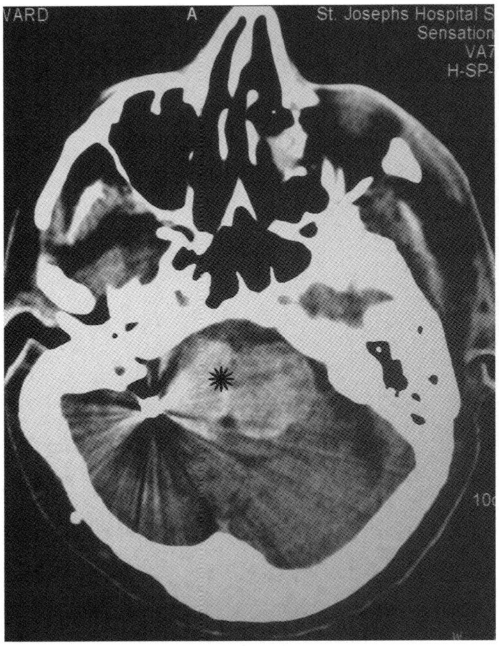

C

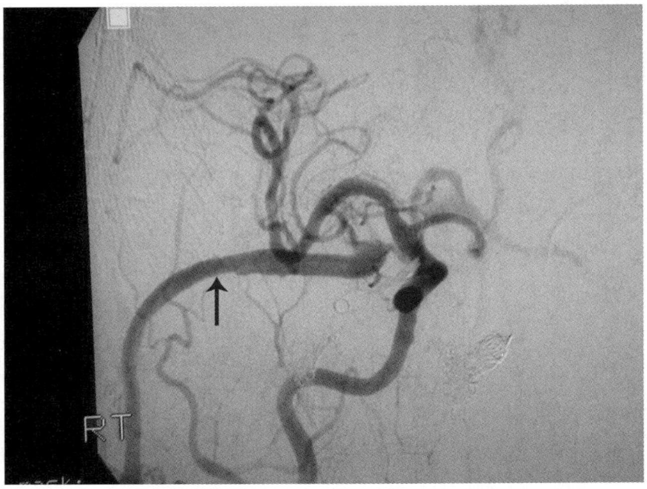

D

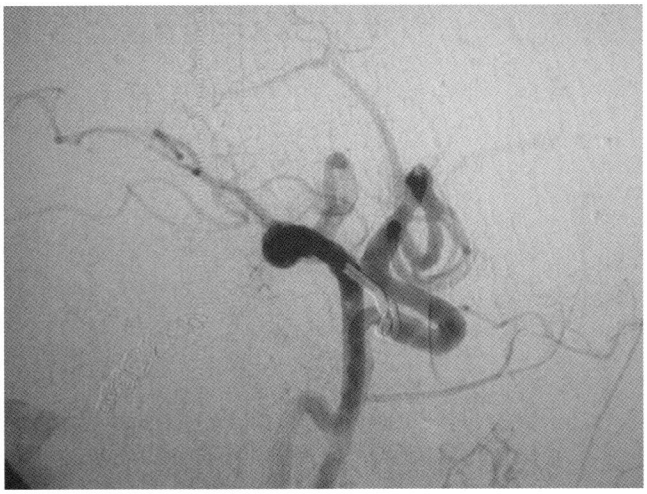

E

Fig. 2.11 This 68-year-old man initially presented with a brainstem transient ischemic attack and was found to have a dolichoectatic basilar artery **(A)**. He was started on antiplatelet therapy and did well. Five years later, the patient returned with progressive gait and swallowing difficulty as well as incoordination and lethargy. He was found to have significant enlargement of a multilobulated fusiform dolichoectatic aneurysm of the basilar artery as shown on an AP vertebral angiogram **(B)** as well as a mass lesion (*star*) resulting in significant brainstem compression on an axial CT image **(C)**. The patient underwent staged vertebral artery occlusions (one endovascular, the second surgical) after a saphenous vein graft (*arrow*) was anastomosed from the cervical carotid to the right posterior carotid artery as seen on the AP **(D)** and lateral common carotid **(E)** arteriograms.

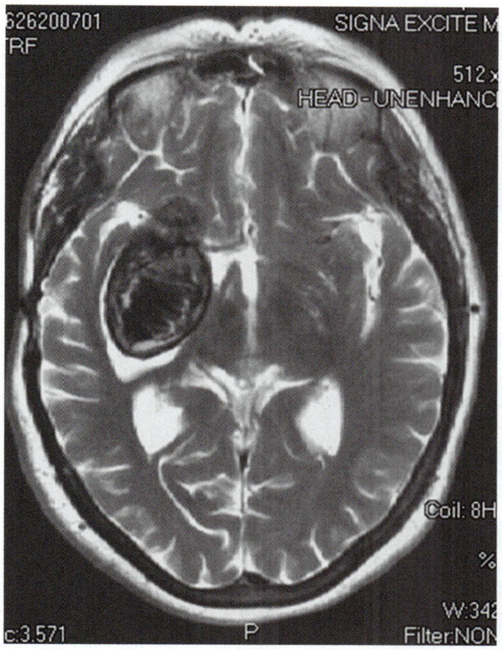

A

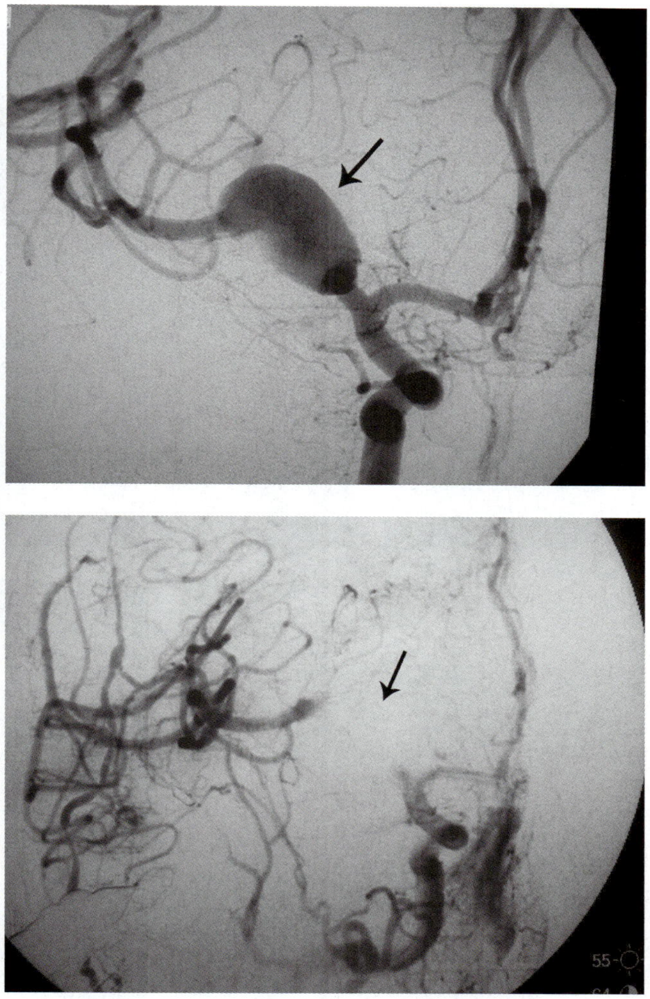

B

C

Fig. 2.12 A 62-year-old woman was found to have a giant MCA aneurysm measuring over 6 cm in maximal diameter on a routine screening MRI **(A)**. Amazingly, the lesion was asymptomatic. Angiography revealed a partially thrombosed, fusiform lesion (*arrow*) **(B)**. Extracranial-intracranial bypass was performed in preparation for a proximal M1 occlusion. Intraoperative angiography **(C)** to assess patency of the graft revealed immediate thrombosis of the aneurysm without obvious filling of the M1 segment (*arrow*) of the middle carotid artery, which was confirmed with delayed angiography as well. The patient has remained neurologically intact during more than 5 years of follow-up.

to remember that blood loss may be a real concern during surgical resection of some of these tumors. As a result, even patients who pass balloon occlusion testing may be at risk for stroke if they suffer significant intraoperative hypotension or hemodilution related to blood loss.

As an interesting alternative for head and neck tumors encasing the cervical internal carotid artery, we have previously described a novel technique of "carotid extarterectomy," which combines endovascular and open surgical therapy.[20] In these cases, a stent is placed in the internal carotid artery several weeks before surgery. Endothelialization of the stent then allows for the subsequent removal of the tumor en bloc along with the external wall of the ICA, which has almost always been invaded by the malignancy. The endothelialized stent has been sufficient to limit bleeding following careful removal of the ICA wall and the stent is then wrapped with an artificial material or a vein graft to add reinforcement. This technique represents a good illustration of how a combined, team approach can offer innovative solutions to manage complex problems.

◆ Intraoperative Misadventures

Although surgeons prefer to avoid discussing this scenario, even excellent neurovascular surgeons occasionally have an unexpected problem that may result in an ischemic injury if left untreated. Examples include inadvertent arterial injury during microdissection of an aneurysm or skull base tumor. In such a setting, facility with cerebral revascularization techniques may provide an opportunity to sidestep a potential disaster by revascularizing the distal "at risk" territory.

In our experience, we have encountered three cases during which sharp microdissection at the neck of an aneurysm resulted in a tear. Clipping techniques alone could have stopped the bleeding only by severely narrowing or occluding the parent artery. Instead, we were able to temporarily trap the segment and strategically place several 10-0 sutures. This, in turn, allowed us to subsequently clip the aneurysm in proper fashion without any associated ischemic injury.

In two cases, we encountered inadvertent arterial injury (an AICA during removal of an acoustic neuroma and an A2

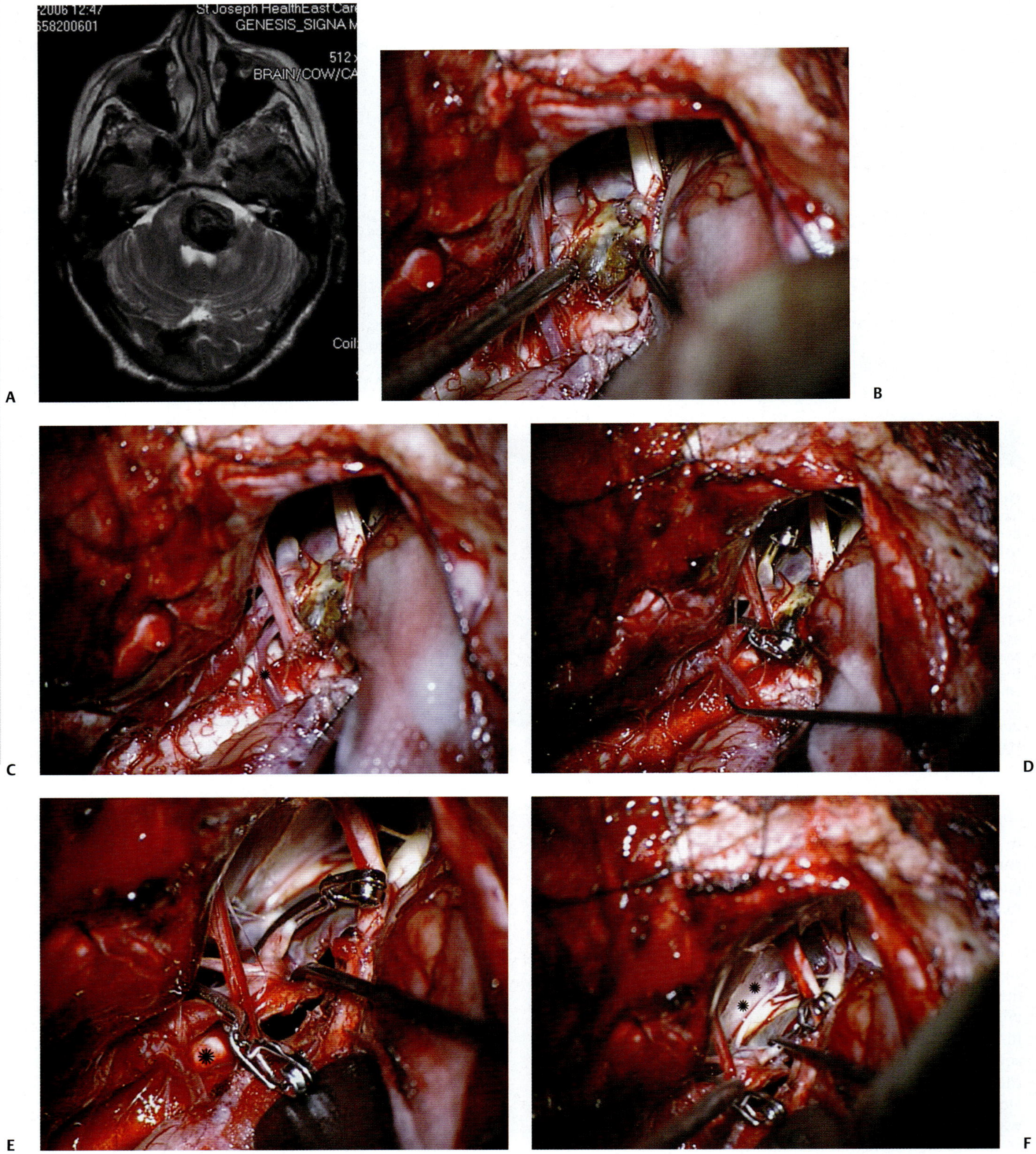

Fig. 2.13 This 76-year-old woman presented with progressive gait difficulty and swallowing trouble and was found to have a giant, largely thrombosed aneurysm of the PICA. MRI demonstrated significant brainstem compression **(A)**. A far-lateral suboccipital exposure **(B)** allowed for proper dissection of the aneurysm, and the posterior inferior cerebellar artery (PICA) (*star*) was found to be intimately involved in the neck of the aneurysm **(C)**. A decision was made to divide the proximal PICA, which was then reanastomosed to the vertebral artery proximal to the aneurysm. The reimplanted PICA is indicated by the microdissector **(D)**, and the proximal and distal vertebral artery segments are visible along with the lower cranial nerves and the VII–VIII nerve complex. The aneurysm was then trapped, opened, and evacuated of thrombus to decompress the brainstem **(E)** with the reimplanted PICA (*star*) filling from the proximal vertebral artery. At this point, even the sixth nerve (*stars*) following its course into Dorello's canal could be seen with limited retraction **(F)**.

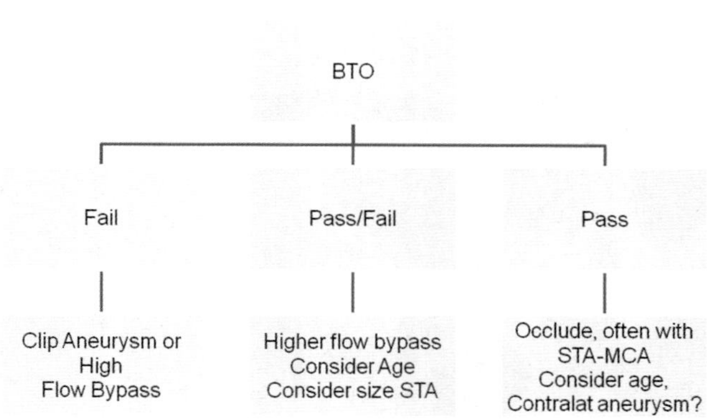

Fig. 2.14 Flow diagram illustrating management algorithm for patients with complex aneurysms who may require carotid sacrifice. "Pass/ Fail" denotes those patients who pass the balloon test occlusion (BTO) clinically but have minimal abnormality on SPECT imaging mandating a bypass that should be higher flow in younger patients. Patients who pass the BTO are considered for low-flow bypass in most cases, particularly when young or when contralateral aneurysms are present. STA-MCA, superficial temporal artery–middle cerebral artery.

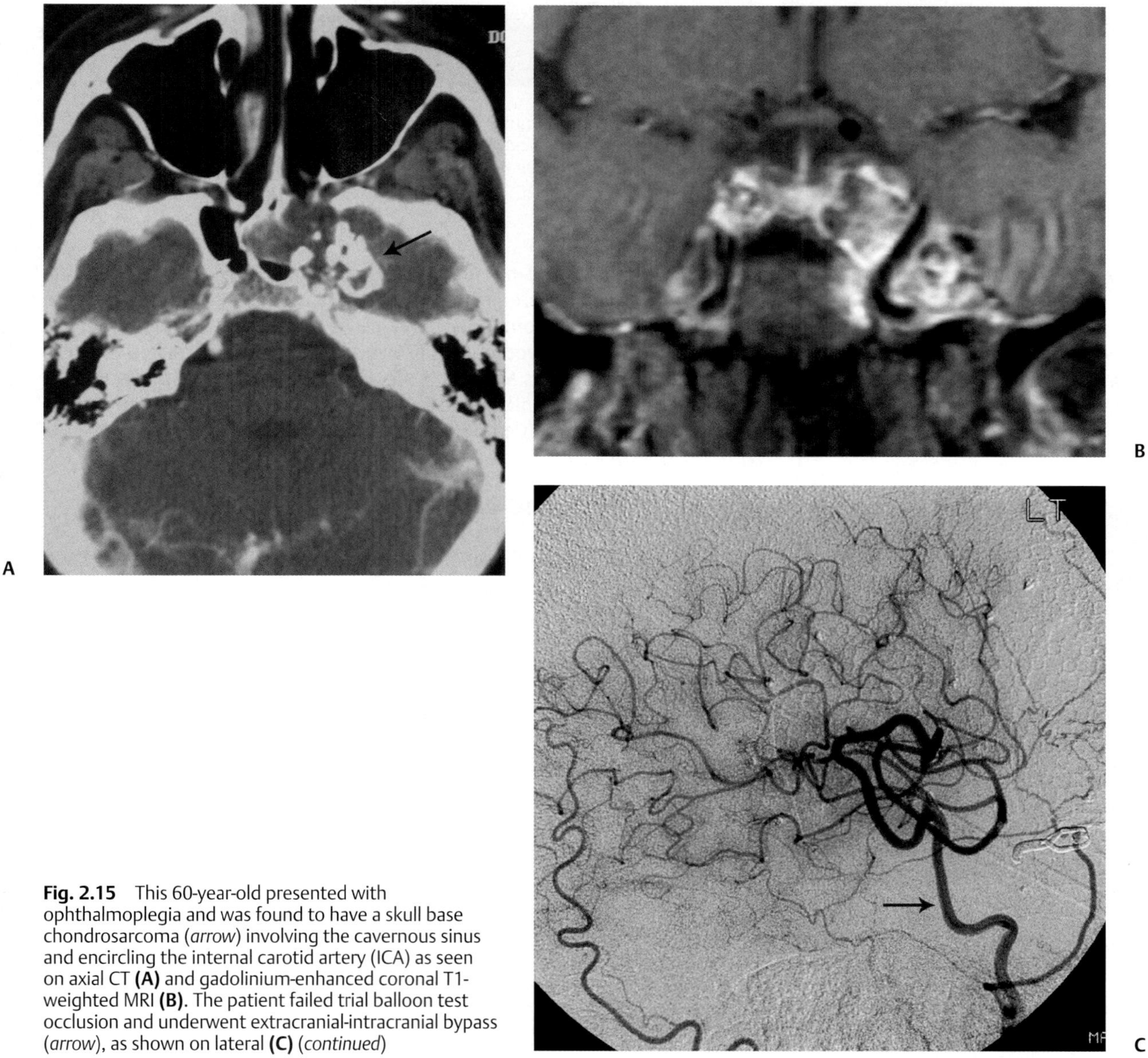

Fig. 2.15 This 60-year-old presented with ophthalmoplegia and was found to have a skull base chondrosarcoma (*arrow*) involving the cavernous sinus and encircling the internal carotid artery (ICA) as seen on axial CT **(A)** and gadolinium-enhanced coronal T1-weighted MRI **(B)**. The patient failed trial balloon test occlusion and underwent extracranial-intracranial bypass (*arrow*), as shown on lateral **(C)** (*continued*)

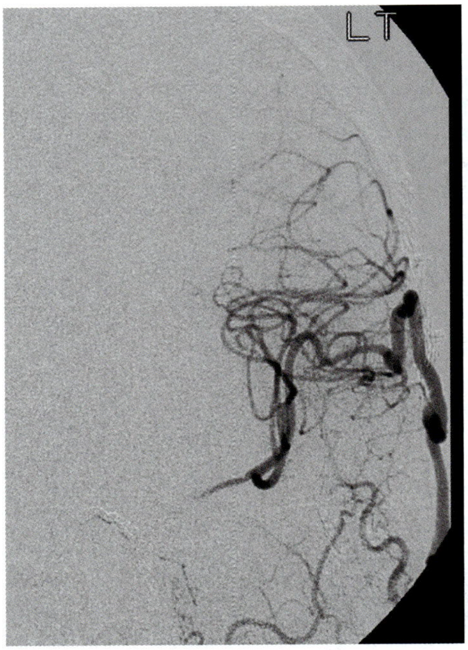

D

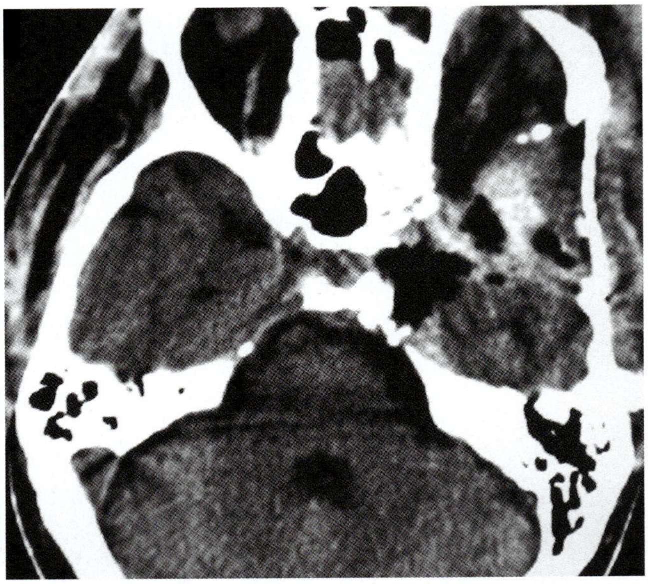

E

Fig. 2.15 (*continued*) and AP **(D)** angiographic images. Two days later, an aggressive resection of the tumor was performed via an expanded orbitozygomatic approach including resection of the involved segment of the ICA. Postoperative CT demonstrates aggressive tumor resection **(E)**. The patient did well for 5 years then suffered a local recurrence requiring reoperation and radiosurgery. It has now been 8 years since his original operation.

segment of the ACA during removal of a recurrent interhemispheric meningioma) during removal of a tumor (**Fig. 2.16**). To prevent a possible ischemic injury, we applied temporary clips to the cut ends of the vessel and reanastomosed the vessels in end-to-end fashion. Postoperative angiography confirmed patency of the vessels, and the patients did well without any ischemic injury on MRI. We have also described a case of microvascular repair of a large cortical draining vein injured during removal of a large atypical parasagittal meningioma.[21] Although it is uncertain whether collateral supply would have prevented an infarction related to these problems, we have generally preferred "not to find out," and simple microsurgical revascularization techniques can be extremely important in these settings.

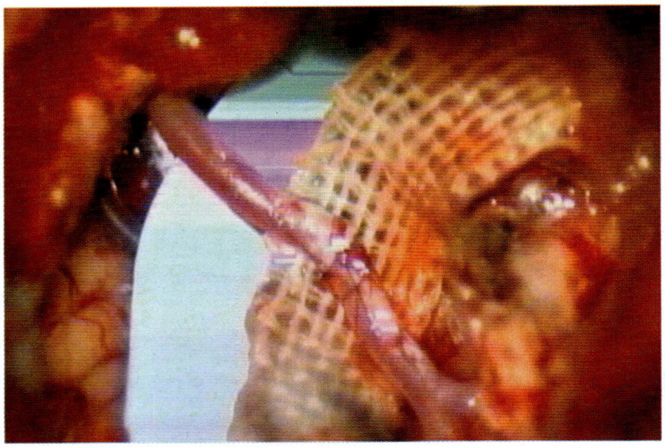

Fig. 2.16 During a translabyrinthine exposure of a previously operated, previously irradiated acoustic neuroma, our neurotology colleagues inadvertently injured a large branch of the anteroinferior cerebellar artery. After expeditious removal of the tumor, the vessel was divided cleanly, reanastomosed end-to-end, and then wrapped with gauze. Postoperative angiography confirmed patency of the vessel, and the patient suffered no adverse effects.

◆ Conclusions

Indications for microsurgical cerebral revascularization continue to evolve. At present, it is clear that selected aneurysms and skull base tumors may be treated best using a variety of creative revascularization options as described in this and other chapters in this book. In addition, most neurovascular surgeons feel strongly that there are selected patients with occlusive cerebrovascular disease that may benefit from revascularization. As endovascular techniques continue to improve, the role of open microsurgery has changed. Nevertheless, there remains an important role for open revascularization in the management of these complex and challenging cases.

References

1. Ausman JI, Diaz FG. Critique of the extracranial-intracranial bypass study. Surg Neurol 1986;26(3):218–221
2. Chater N. Neurosurgical extracranial-intracranial bypass for stroke: with 400 cases. Neurol Res 1983;5(2):1–9

3. Nussbaum ES, Erickson DL. Extracranial-intracranial bypass for ischemic cerebrovascular disease refractory to maximal medical therapy. Neurosurgery 2000;46(1):37–42
4. The EC/IC Bypass Study Group. Failure of extracranial-intracranial arterial bypass to reduce the risk of ischemic stroke: results of an international randomized trial. N Engl J Med 1985;313(19): 1191–1200
5. Amin-Hanjani S, Butler WE, Ogilvy CS, Carter BS, Barker FG II. Extracranial-intracranial bypass in the treatment of occlusive cerebrovascular disease and intracranial aneurysms in the United States between 1992 and 2001: a population-based study. J Neurosurg 2005;103(5): 794–804
6. Grubb RL Jr, Derdeyn CP, Fritsch SM, et al. Importance of hemodynamic factors in the prognosis of symptomatic carotid occlusion. JAMA 1998;280(12):1055–1060
7. Schmiedek P, Gratzl O, Spetzler R, et al. Selection of patients for extra-intracranial arterial bypass surgery based on rCBF measurements. J Neurosurg 1976;44(3):303–312
8. Sekhar LN, Kalavakonda C. Cerebral revascularization for aneurysms and tumors. Neurosurgery 2002;50(2):321–331
9. Spetzler RF, Fukushima T, Martin N, Zabramski JM. Petrous carotid-to-intradural carotid saphenous vein graft for intracavernous giant aneurysm, tumor, and occlusive cerebrovascular disease. J Neurosurg 1990;73(4):496–501
10. Nussbaum ES, Janjua TM, Defillo A, Lowary JL, Nussbaum LA. Emergency extracranial-intracranial bypass surgery for acute ischemic stroke. J Neurosurg 2010;112(3):666–673
11. Matsushima T, Fujiwara S, Nagata S, et al. Surgical treatment for paediatric patients with moyamoya disease by indirect revascularization procedures (EDAS, EMS, EMAS). Acta Neurochir (Wien) 1989;98 (3–4):135–140
12. Matsushima Y, Aoyagi M, Suzuki R, Nariai T, Shishido T, Hirakawa K. Dual anastomosis for pediatric moya moya patients using the anterior and posterior branches of the superficial temporal artery. Childs Nerv Syst 1993;18:27–32
13. Spetzler RF, Roski RA, Rhodes RS, Modic MT. The "bonnet bypass": case report. J Neurosurg 1980;53(5):707–709
14. Ausman JI, Diaz FG, Vacca DF, Sadasivan B. Superficial temporal and occipital artery bypass pedicles to superior, anterior inferior, and posterior inferior cerebellar arteries for vertebrobasilar insufficiency. J Neurosurg 1990;72(4):554–558
15. Sundt TM Jr, Whisnant JP, Piepgras DG, Campbell JK, Holman CB. Intracranial bypass grafts for vertebral-basilar ischemia. Mayo Clin Proc 1978;53(1):12–18
16. Levy EI, Turk AS, Albuquerque FC, et al. Wingspan in-stent restenosis and thrombosis: incidence, clinical presentation, and management. Neurosurgery 2007;61(3):644–650
17. Turk AS, Levy EI, Albuquerque FC, et al. Influence of patient age and stenosis location on wingspan in-stent restenosis. AJNR Am J Neuroradiol 2008;29(1):23–27
18. Peerless SJ, Ferguson GG, Drake CG. Extracranial-intracranial (EC/IC) bypass in the treatment of giant intracranial aneurysms. Neurosurg Rev 1982;5(3):77–81
19. Nussbaum ES, Madison MT, Goddard JK, Lassig JP, Nussbaum LA. Peripheral intracranial aneurysms: management challenges in 60 consecutive cases. J Neurosurg 2009;110(1):7–13
20. Nussbaum ES, Levine SC, Hamlar D, Madison MT. Carotid stenting and "extarterectomy" in the management of head and neck cancer involving the internal carotid artery: technical case report. Neurosurgery 2000;47(4):981–984
21. Nussbaum ES, Defillo A, Janjua TM, Nussbaum LA. Microvascular repair of an injured cortical draining vein. Surg Neurol 2009;72(5):530–531

Chapter 3

Indications for Endovascular Revascularization

Michael T. Madison, James K. Goddard, Jeffrey P. Lassig, Joshua Olson, and Eric S. Nussbaum

During the past 20 years, endovascular options for revascularizing the ischemic brain have revolutionized the management of patients either suffering from or at risk for ischemic stroke. The progressive improvements in catheter-based technologies as well as the development of newer, more flexible stents and distal protection devices have created greater opportunities for intervention while improving safety as well as overall patient outcomes. Our dedicated endovascular practice represents a multidisciplinary team approach incorporating the expertise of interventional neuroradiology, stroke neurology, neurovascular surgery, and neurocritical care. All patients are assessed using a team approach to decide on the optimal management paradigm. Over time, it has become clear that despite the varied technologies at our disposal, careful judgment and thoughtful planning often remain our most valuable tools when treating patients with occlusive cerebrovascular disease.

◆ Cervical Carotid and Extracranial Vertebral Angioplasty and Stenting

Percutaneous transluminal angioplasty was first introduced in the 1960s by Dotter and Judkins.[1] The earliest reports of carotid and vertebral angioplasty appeared some 20 years later.[2,3] Although it was initially felt that carotid angioplasty and stenting (CAS) would likely carry stroke rates much higher than carotid endarterectomy (CEA), improved technology, specifically easily deployed distal protection devices have significantly decreased complication rates to a level below 5%. In our practice, we have generally considered CEA the gold standard treatment for traditional atherosclerotic disease involving the carotid bifurcation. Nevertheless, we have used CAS successfully in selected patient populations, including those with recurrent stenosis following prior CEA, with radiation-induced carotid disease, in the very elderly, and in patients with significant comorbidities that increase the surgical risk of CEA. We have also treated patients felt to be reasonable candidates for CEA who have carefully reviewed their options and decided to pursue CAS. Most of our patients have presented with symptomatic narrowing of the carotid artery while asymptomatic patients are currently being treated as part of the SAPPHIRE (Stenting and Angioplasty with Protection in Patients at High Risk for Endarterectomy) trial.

At our center, we perform CAS in the neurointerventional suite using conscious sedation as necessary following pretreatment with antiplatelet therapy. We generally attempt to deploy the stent first, and then postdilate the vessel if there is a greater than 50% residual stenosis after stenting. If the stenosis is too tight to place the stent as a first-line maneuver, balloon predilation is performed, followed by stenting, and then postdilation as necessary. A distal protection device is used in all cases. Although cardiac irregularities have been rare in our experience, all patients have an external pacer placed at the beginning of the procedure. Particularly during the postdilation portion of the procedure, patients may be prone to transient bradycardia and hypotension. To limit this, we generally pretreat patients with 0.2 mg Robinul (Pfizer Pharmaceuticals, New York, NY) and keep atropine available. Roughly 20% of our patients have demonstrated limited but persistent hypotension, which may require pharmacologic treatment and may last for 1 to 3 days in some cases. Following the procedure, all patients are maintained on antiplatelet therapy, generally a combination of aspirin and Plavix (Bristol-Myers Squibb, New York, NY) for at least 3 months. A baseline carotid ultrasound study is obtained the day after the procedure prior to patient discharge. This is compared with a follow-up ultrasound that is obtained 6 months later (**Fig. 3.1**).

In contrast to the cervical carotid arteries, the extracranial vertebral arteries are prone to atherosclerotic narrowing particularly at their origins from the great vessels. The majority of endovascular treatment of the extracranial vertebral arteries has

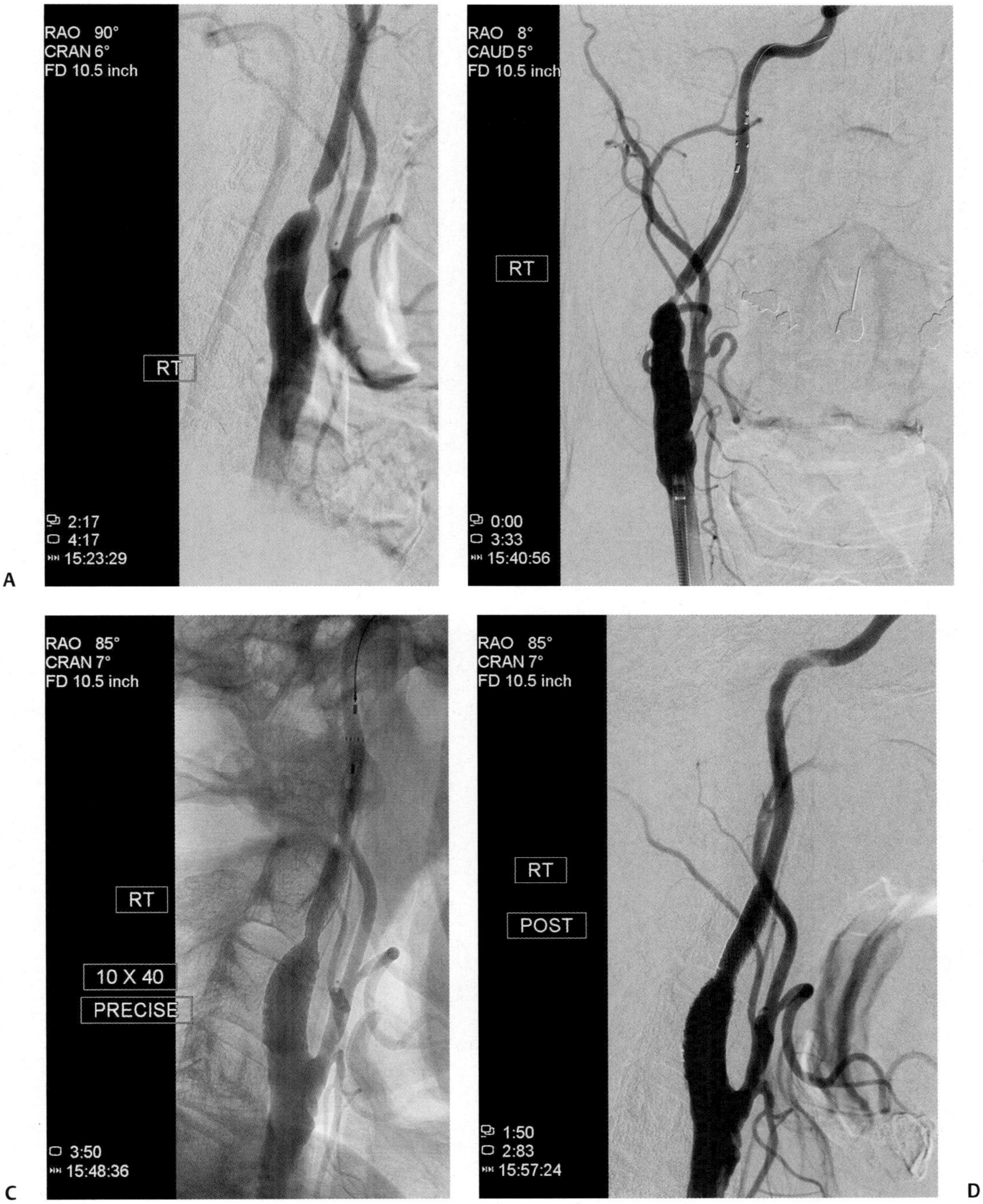

Fig. 3.1 Carotid angioplasty and stenting. **(A)** Oblique AP right common carotid angiogram of a 63-year-old man with a history of a right carotid endarterectomy 1 year prior and a marked increase in peak systolic velocities on a recent follow-up carotid Doppler examination. Imaging demonstrates a high-grade, 85 to 90% stenosis just distal to the bulb, as measured by North American Symptomatic Carotid Endarterectomy Trial (NASCET) criteria. **(B)** Right CCA angiogram after placement and deployment of a 5-mm Angioguard distal protection device and microguidewire (Cordis, Bridgewater, NJ) in the distal cervical ICA, beyond the stenosis, which was thought to be secondary to clamp injury. **(C)** Right common carotid artery (CCA) angiogram after deployment of a 10 × 40–mm Precise stent (Cordis, Bridgewater, NJ) across the stenosis, demonstrating an ~50% residual stenosis. **(D)** Final right CCA angiogram after angioplasty of the waist point within the stent with a 5 × 20–mm coronary balloon showing a widely patent stent with no significant residual stenosis.

thus been focused on angioplasty and stenting of the vertebral artery origin. In general, we have avoided treating most patients with asymptomatic disease, and most treated patients have some degree of bilateral vertebral artery compromise. Symptoms may occur in the context of atherosclerotic involvement of one vertebral artery when the other vessel is congenitally atretic or terminates in the posterior inferior cerebellar artery (PICA). In these cases and in contrast to patients with carotid disease, most patients have presented with flow-related symptoms rather than embolic stroke (**Fig. 3.2**).

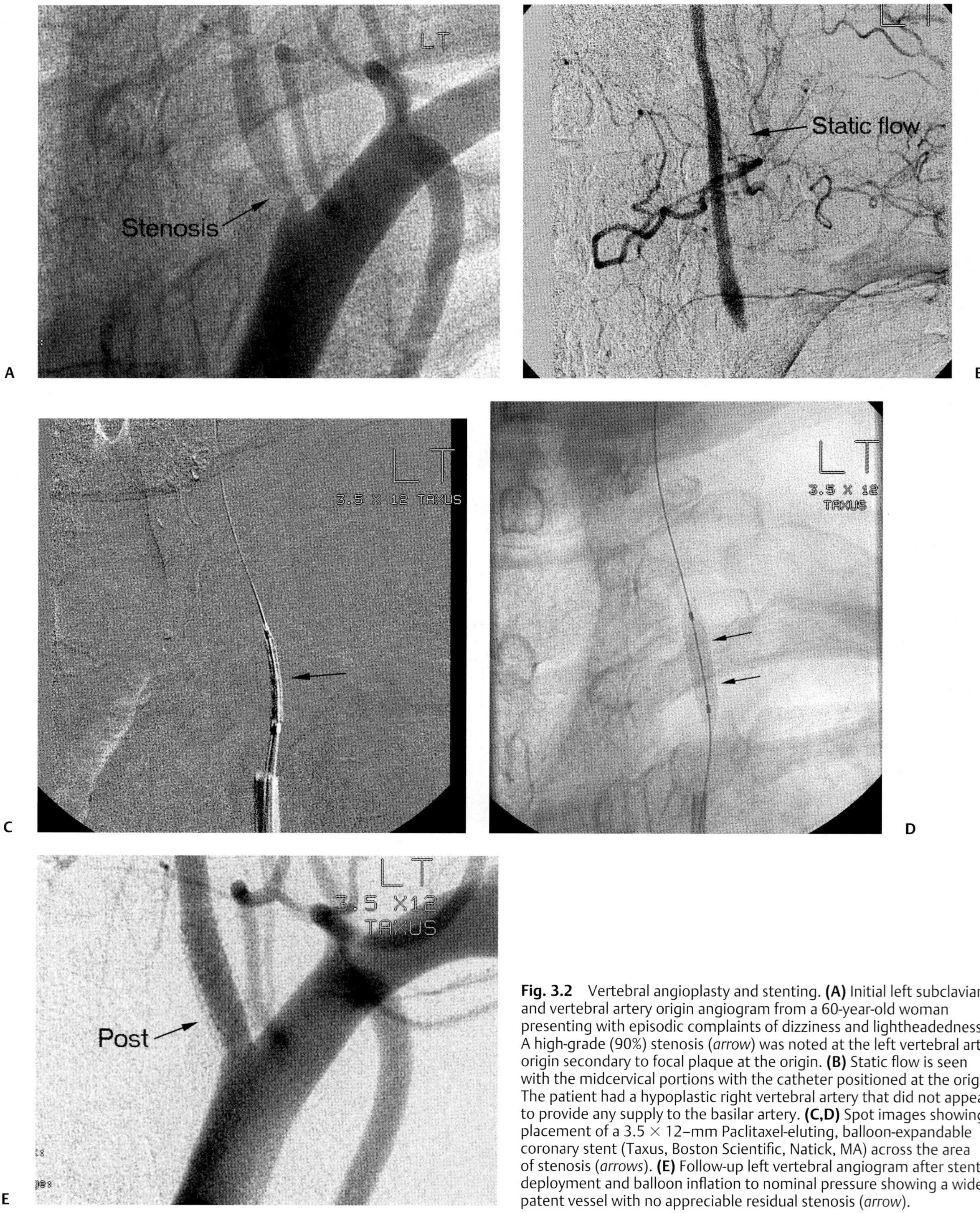

Fig. 3.2 Vertebral angioplasty and stenting. **(A)** Initial left subclavian and vertebral artery origin angiogram from a 60-year-old woman presenting with episodic complaints of dizziness and lightheadedness. A high-grade (90%) stenosis (*arrow*) was noted at the left vertebral artery origin secondary to focal plaque at the origin. **(B)** Static flow is seen with the midcervical portions with the catheter positioned at the origin. The patient had a hypoplastic right vertebral artery that did not appear to provide any supply to the basilar artery. **(C,D)** Spot images showing placement of a 3.5 × 12–mm Paclitaxel-eluting, balloon-expandable coronary stent (Taxus, Boston Scientific, Natick, MA) across the area of stenosis (*arrows*). **(E)** Follow-up left vertebral angiogram after stent deployment and balloon inflation to nominal pressure showing a widely patent vessel with no appreciable residual stenosis (*arrow*).

In general, vertebral angioplasty and stenting is performed without distal protection. We have favored the use of a coated coronary stent technology to limit restenosis rates. Despite this, the greatest risk associated with the procedure in our experience has been restenosis, which has been found in 15 to 20% of our cases. All patients are reimaged using either magnetic resonance angiography (MRA) or formal angiography 6 months after the procedure, and significant and/or symptomatic restenosis may be retreated using repeat angioplasty as warranted. In our experience, such retreatment has often been effective and has not carried a meaningful risk for ischemic complications. Like patients undergoing CAS, those treated with vertebral angioplasty and stenting (VAS) have also been treated after the procedure with a minimum of 3 months of antiplatelet therapy, generally consisting of a combination of aspirin and Plavix.

◆ Intracranial Angioplasty and Stenting

The development of intracranial angioplasty and stenting for atherosclerotic disease has provided a novel option for treatment of a difficult condition that often occurs in patients with multiple comorbidities, which may limit other treatment options. Early options for intracranial stenting required the use of balloon-mounted, stiff coronary stents that often carried significant risk of local arterial injury. Newer, improved technology has made intracranial angioplasty and stenting a more feasible and safer option. In addition, early cases of intracranial angioplasty were performed via a surgical approach with the patients under general anesthesia, whereas most procedures performed today can be performed with the patient awake.[3,4] Although many patients with intracranial stenoses can be managed adequately with various combinations of antiplatelet agents and anticoagulation, some patients will exhibit genuine hypoperfusion related to a significant stenosis in a vascular territory with inadequate collateral circulation. When patients fail aggressive medical therapy, treatment options include open surgical revascularization or endovascular angioplasty and stenting. Again, at our center, these cases are generally reviewed by our multidisciplinary team to assess the various treatment options including the relative risks associated with each approach.

In the anterior circulation, a superficial temporal artery to middle cerebral artery (STA-MCA) bypass may represent a reasonable option in some cases. At the same time, selected patients with narrowing of the intracranial ICA or the M1 trunk have been well-treated by angioplasty and stenting in our experience. We have generally not treated patients with anterior cerebral artery (ACA) stenoses or those with distal MCA stenoses using angioplasty techniques. As a rule, patients have been pretreated with aspirin and Plavix for 5 days when possible. We have generally used the Wingspan stent system (Boston Scientific, Natick, MA). Predilation is accomplished with the Gateway Balloon (Boston Scientific), and then the stent is deployed. On occasion, in the setting of what clearly appears to be a fresh arterial dissection, we have deployed the stent without balloon predilation. We have not generally needed to perform postdilation in this setting (**Fig. 3.3**).

In the posterior circulation, open microsurgical revascularization procedures are more difficult, and we have generally favored endovascular options when possible. We have

A

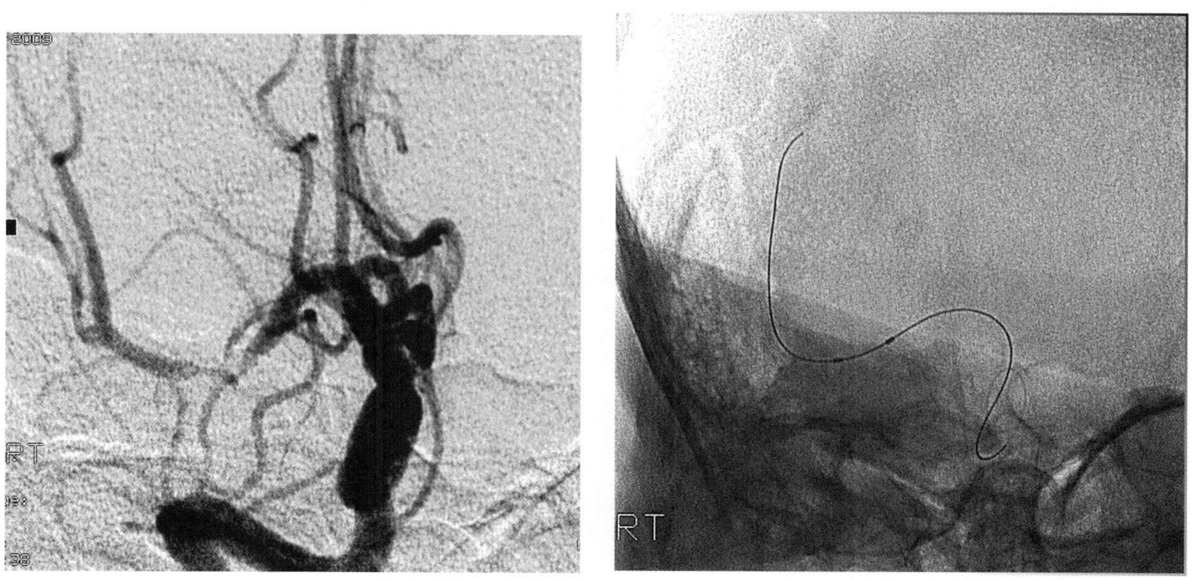

B

Fig. 3.3 M1 angioplasty. **(A)** AP right internal carotid angiogram from a 29-year-old right-handed man with a history of right hemispheric watershed infarcts, including a second ischemic event while on antiplatelet therapy (combination aspirin and clopidogrel). The image shows a focus of plaque within the mid M1 segment of the right middle cerebral artery, extending for upward of 6 to 7 mm, and causing a high-grade, hemodynamically significant stenosis. **(B)** Spot image with a 300-cm Transcend floppy tip wire and an uninflated 2 × 9–mm Gateway intracranial angioplasty balloon (Boston Scientific, Natick, MA) across the stenosis. *(continued)*

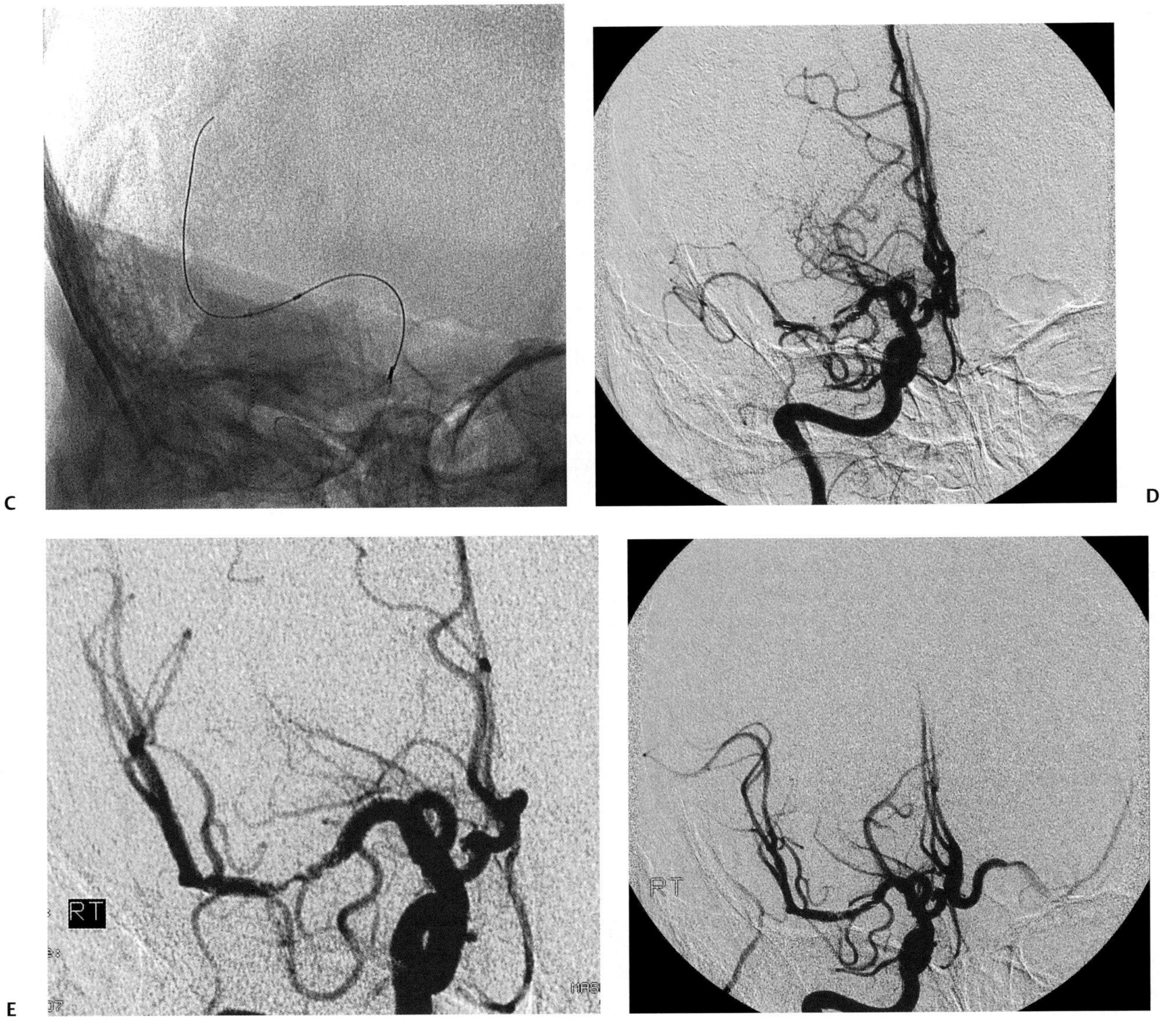

Fig. 3.3 *(continued)* **(C)** Spot image with balloon inflated to nominal pressure (5 atmospheres). **(D)** AP right inferior cerebellar artery (ICA) angiogram several minutes after deployment of a 3 × 15–mm Wingspan stent (Boston Scientific) across the stenosis showing extensive platelet aggregation within the mid-portion of the stent and poor filling of distal branches. **(E)** Follow-up AP right ICA angiogram 7 minutes after administration of a single weight-based bolus of intravenous Integrilin (eptifibatide; Schering-Plough Corp., Memphis, TN) and administration of additional intravenous heparin showing partial but incomplete resolution of platelet aggregation and thrombus. **(F)** Second follow-up angiogram after administration of an additional 8 mg of intraarterial eptifibatide demonstrating nearly complete resolution of platelet aggregation with widely patent M1 segment and markedly improved filling of distal middle cerebral artery (MCA) branches.

had good success treating disease involving the intracranial vertebral arteries or basilar artery, although we have not treated posterior cerebral artery (PCA) stenoses.

Overall, significant complication rates have been low with intracranial angioplasty and stenting (IAS), in our experience, in the range of 6 to 8%. At our center, the greatest risk of therapy has been restenosis, which has been a particular problem in younger patients (below the age of 55 years) undergoing treatment of anterior circulation disease. In the anterior circulation, restenosis rates have ranged from 20 to 25%. In this setting, we have performed a repeat angioplasty of an in-stent stenosis in some cases with success, although some patients have been referred for open surgery when repeated restenosis occurs. Rare but serious complications can occur with IAS, including local arterial dissection, at times resulting in ischemic injury or hemorrhage. When treating basilar artery disease, we have rarely encountered a new small brainstem ischemic insult presumably related to a perforator injury either as a result of the angioplasty forcing plaque across the orifice of a perforator or possibly due to the interstices of a stent crossing a perforator origin. Embolic insult from the angioplasty or the development of acute in-stent thrombus can also occur (**Fig. 3.4**).

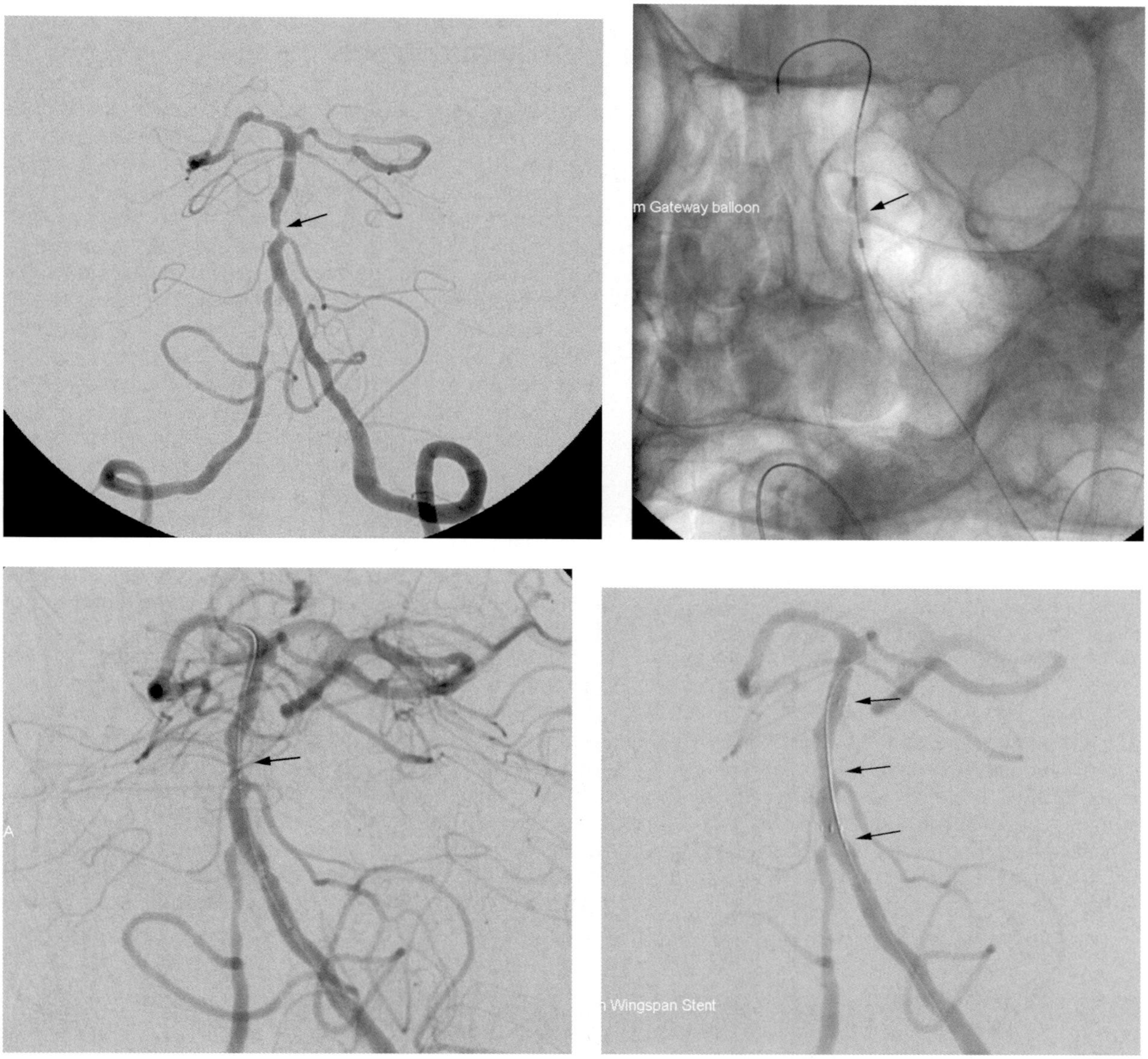

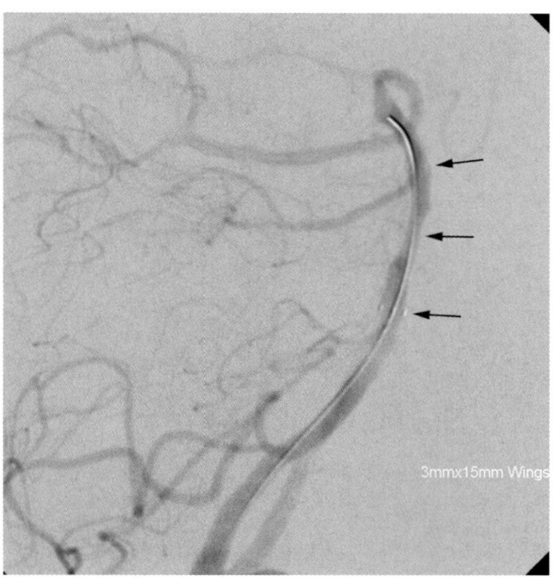

Fig. 3.4 Basilar angioplasty and stenting. **(A)** Initial AP left vertebral artery angiogram from a 72-year-old woman with recurrent symptoms of basilar artery insufficiency, including episodes of dizziness, double vision, and dysarthria while on antiplatelet therapy. Note the high-grade, focal, 80 to 85% stenosis in the midbasilar artery (*arrow*), thought to be atherosclerotic in nature. There is also a high-grade stenosis at the right vertebro-basilar junction. **(B)** Spot image showing placement of a Gateway 2.5 × 15–mm intracranial angioplasty balloon (Boston Scientific, Natick, MA) across the stenosis (*arrow*). **(C)** Postangioplasty angiogram demonstrating excellent postdilatation result, with only minimal residual stenosis (*arrow*). **(D,E)** AP and lateral left vertebral angiograms after deployment of a 3 × 15–mm Wingspan self-expanding stent (Boston Scientific, Natick, MA) across the residual stenosis (*arrows*). *(continued)*

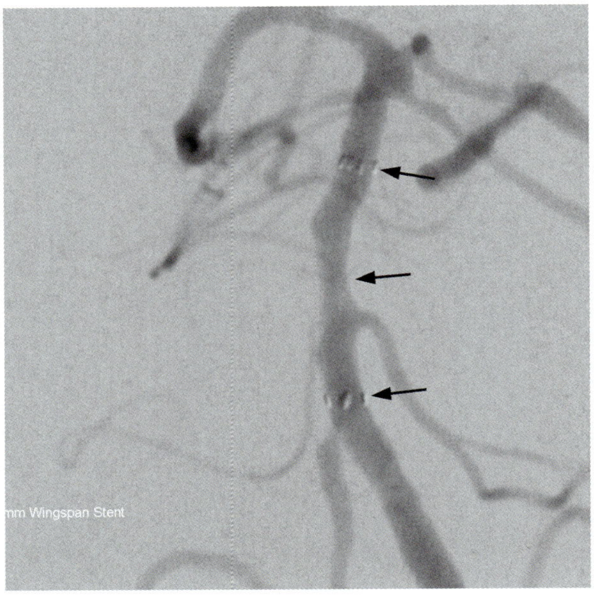

F

Fig. 3.4 *(continued)* **(F)** Final left vertebral AP angiogram showing widely patent stent with no appreciable residual narrowing. *Arrows* point to proximal and distal stent tine markers and the area of previously demonstrated stenosis in the midportion of the stent.

In our practice, we have maintained patients on a combination of aspirin and Plavix for a minimum of 6 months after treatment. Younger patients are often treated with a more prolonged course often exceeding one year in duration. All patients undergo repeat diagnostic angiography 6 months after their initial procedure to assess for in-stent stenosis.

◆ Revascularization Strategies for Acute Ischemic Stroke

The earliest reported series using fibrinolytic and thrombolytic agents in the setting of acute stroke appeared in the late 1950s and early 1960s.[5,6] Since that time, evolving endovascular technology has dramatically changed the management of acute ischemic stroke over the past decade. In general, stroke patients are now managed by multidisciplinary teams trained specifically to assess the acute neurologic event. Treatment options include intravenous thrombolytic infusion, intraarterial pharmacologic or mechanical thrombolysis, and rarely, surgical intervention. In those patients selected for endovascular therapy, our goal has been to reestablish large vessel flow as quickly and safely as possible. Current microcatheter technology allows the interventionalist to address not just acute occlusion of the cervical ICA but also occlusion of the intracranial ICA, the MCA and its branches, as well as the vertebrobasilar system. In our experience, 70% of our treated patients have had M1 occlusion, 20% have occlusion of the distal ICA, and ~10% have vertebral and/or basilar artery occlusion.

Following appropriate cross-sectional imaging, patients are brought immediately to the neurointerventional suite. Diagnostic angiography can generally be accomplished in just minutes to confirm the presence of a vascular occlusion that correlates with the patients' symptoms. We generally begin by injecting 15 to 25 mg of intraarterial tissue plasminogen activator (tPA) as well as a weight-based bolus of a 2B3A-inhibitor such as Integrilin (Schering-Plough Corp., Memphis, TN), delivering the drug beyond, into, and proximal to the clot. By lacing the clot in this fashion, some emboli

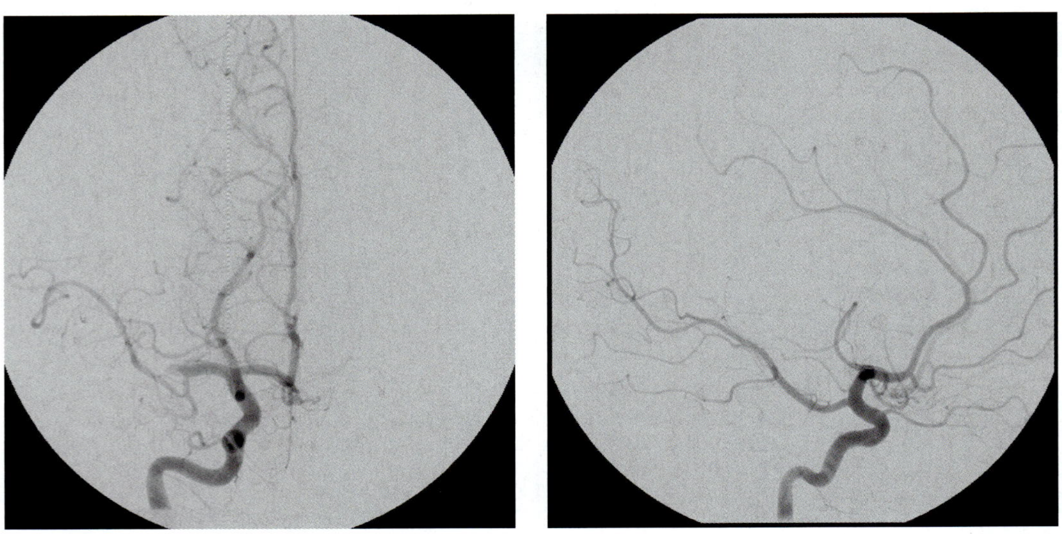

A B

Fig. 3.5 Acute stroke. **(A,B)** Initial AP and lateral right internal carotid angiograms from a 61-year-old male truck driver with a history of atrial fibrillation who drove his semi-trailer truck into a ditch. He was evaluated at a local emergency room and was found to have significant left upper and lower extremity weakness, slurred speech, and left facial palsy, and was subsequently transferred to our institution for further evaluation and management. Images show a patent anterior temporal branch of the right middle cerebral artery, but complete occlusion of antegrade flow at the distal M1 segment, presumably secondary to thromboembolism. *(continued)*

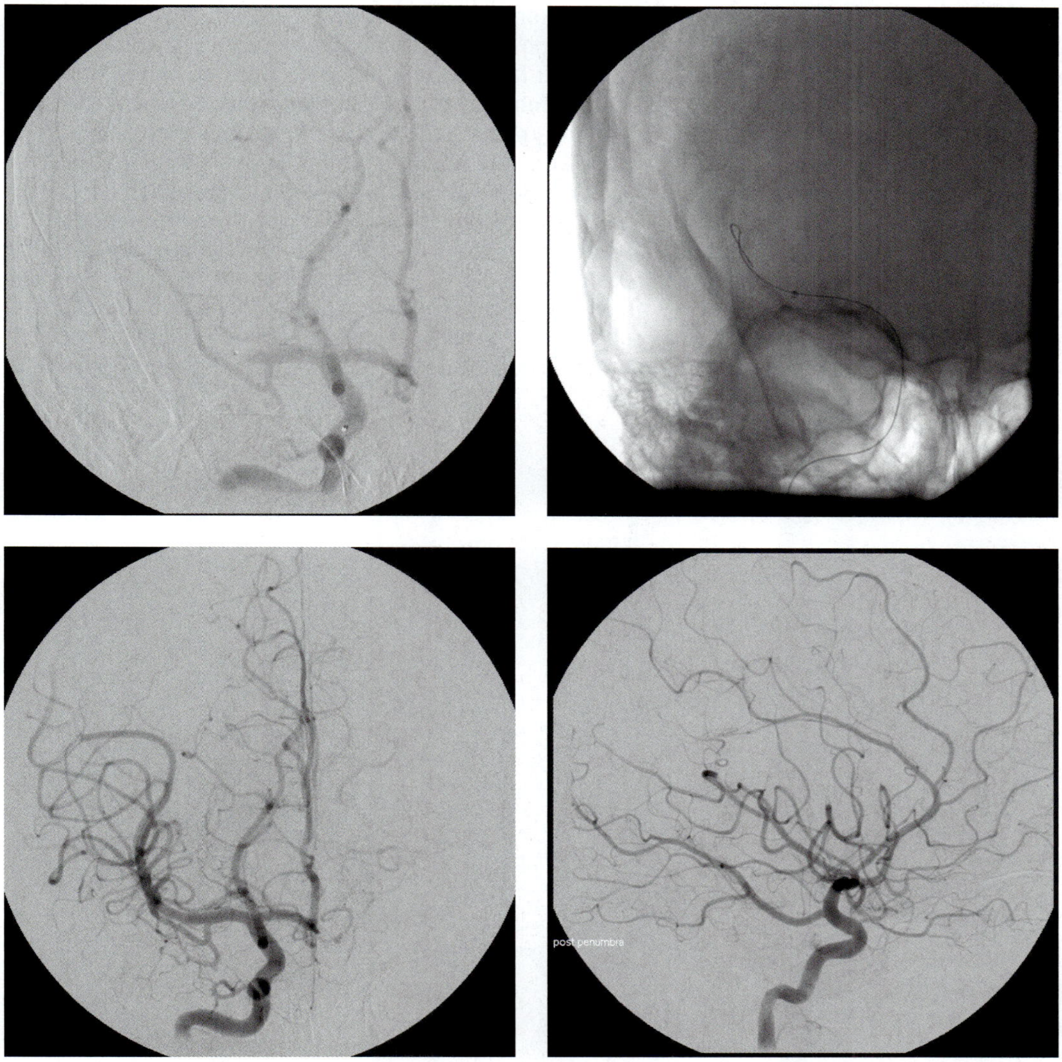

Fig. 3.5 *(continued)* **(C)** Upright ICA angiogram after infusion of 20 mg intraarterial tissue plasminogen activator and 8 mg intraarterial eptifibatide, demonstrating persistent occlusion of the distal right M1 segment. **(D)** Spot image showing Penumbra 0.041 aspiration microcatheter (Penumbra Inc., San Leandro, CA) being advanced over a microguidewire, with the tip positioned at the proximal end of the residual clot. **(E,F)** Final AP and lateral angiograms following 4 minutes of aspiration with the Penumbra system demonstrating near complete recanalization of the right middle cerebral artery. Normal, TIMI 3 flow is now present throughout the M1 and M2 segments of the both and anterior and posterior divisions. A small area of residual embolus is present in a distal M3 branch of the anterior division.

will promptly lyse without further intervention, although this represents the minority of cases. If the clot persists at this point, we generally move immediately to a mechanical thrombectomy device. We have found the Penumbra aspiration catheter system (Penumbra, Inc., San Leandro, CA) to be more effective than the Merci system (Concentric Medical, Mountain View, CA) in our hands (**Fig. 3.5**).

Using this regimen in a series of 177 patients, we have achieved a "Thrombolysis in Myocardial Infarction" (TIMI) score of 2 or 3 flow in over 75% of patients. Of these, 60% have demonstrated significant neurologic improvement over a 24- to 48-hour period, improving from a mean presentation NIH Stroke Scale Score (NIHSS) of 14 to a mean 48-hour NIHSS score of 5.

◆ Treatment Strategies for Cerebral Vasospasm

Endovascular treatment for cerebral vasospasm has expanded the armamentarium of options available for this difficult problem. Zubkov reported the earliest experience with balloon dilatation of vessels narrowed by vasospasm in 1984.[7] Following a subarachnoid hemorrhage (SAH), a significant percentage of patients experience some degree of spasm, with up to 40% of patients who have suffered a severe SAH developing symptomatic spasm. Classic HHH (hypertensive, hypervolemic, hemodilution) therapy remains the gold standard of treatment for both prevention and management of cerebral vasospasm following SAH. Nevertheless, we like others have become progressively more aggressive regarding the use of endovascular techniques when treating patients with spasm, particularly when the narrowing is severe and/or persistent.

In general, we have used intraarterial drug delivery as a first-line measure in this setting. Currently, our preferred option is to use intraarterial verapamil, which can be injected either through a microcatheter or through a diagnostic catheter in the ICA or vertebral artery, delivering 10 to 20 mg per vessel as needed. Treatment often results in improvement of the spasm, but may require daily retreatment for a prolonged period often ranging from 5 to 7 days depending on the severity of vascular narrowing. In refractory cases that fail to respond to drug infusion and in those patients demonstrating progressive areas of ischemia despite maximal medical therapy, balloon angioplasty should be considered as a possible option. In our practice, we generally use a HyperGlide balloon (ev3 Endovascular, Inc., Plymouth, MN) to angioplasty the larger involved vessels; such treatment will often provide a durable improvement in the spasm. Angioplasty does carry some small risk of serious injury in the range of 5% including the possibility of vessel rupture in this setting: this technique remains somewhat controversial as a result. Some centers use angioplasty as an

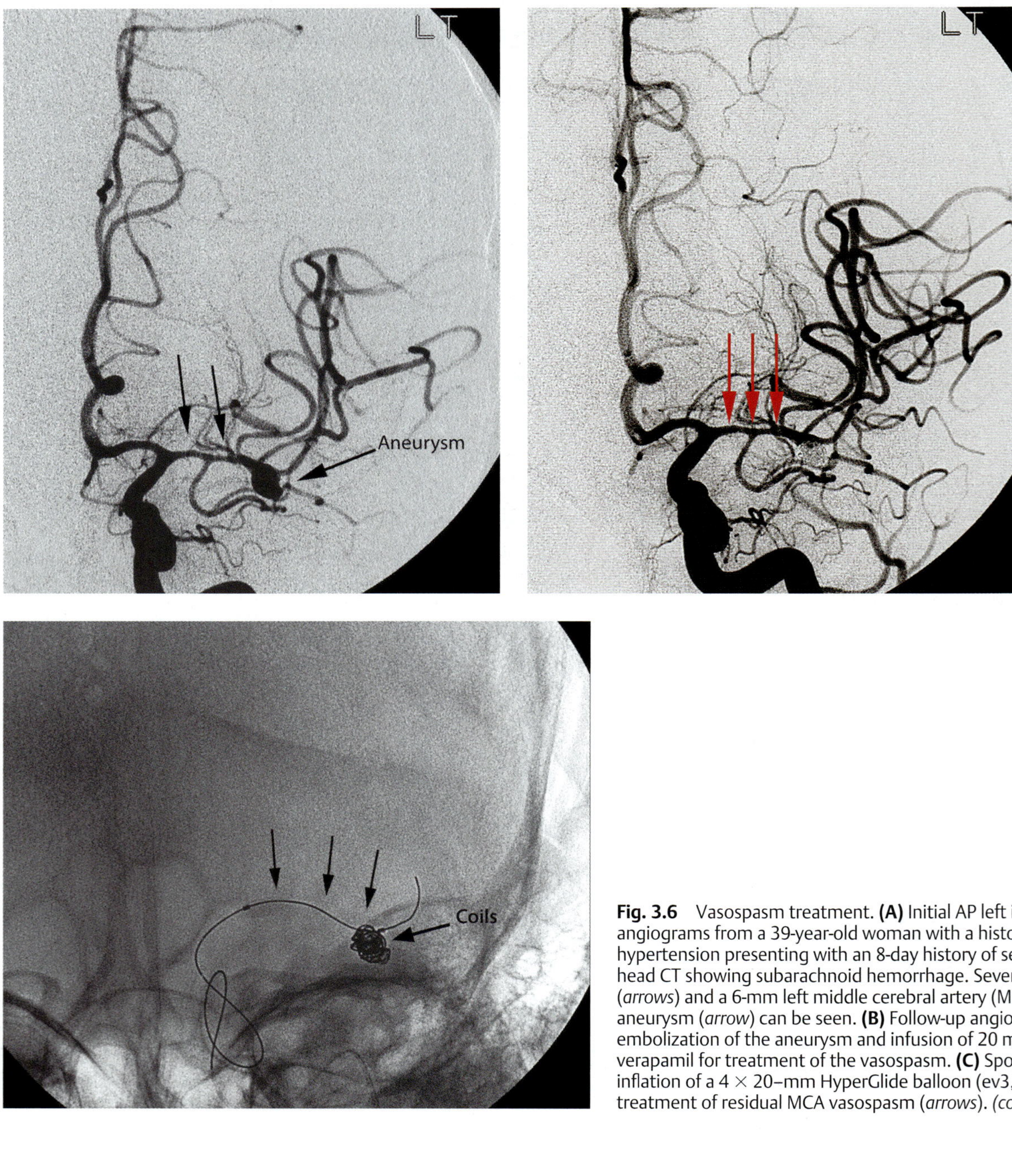

A B C

Fig. 3.6 Vasospasm treatment. **(A)** Initial AP left internal carotid angiograms from a 39-year-old woman with a history of smoking and hypertension presenting with an 8-day history of severe headache and head CT showing subarachnoid hemorrhage. Severe left M1 vasospasm (*arrows*) and a 6-mm left middle cerebral artery (MCA) bifurcation aneurysm (*arrow*) can be seen. **(B)** Follow-up angiogram after coil embolization of the aneurysm and infusion of 20 mg of intraarterial verapamil for treatment of the vasospasm. **(C)** Spot image during inflation of a 4 × 20–mm HyperGlide balloon (ev3, Plymouth, MN) for treatment of residual MCA vasospasm (*arrows*). *(continued)*

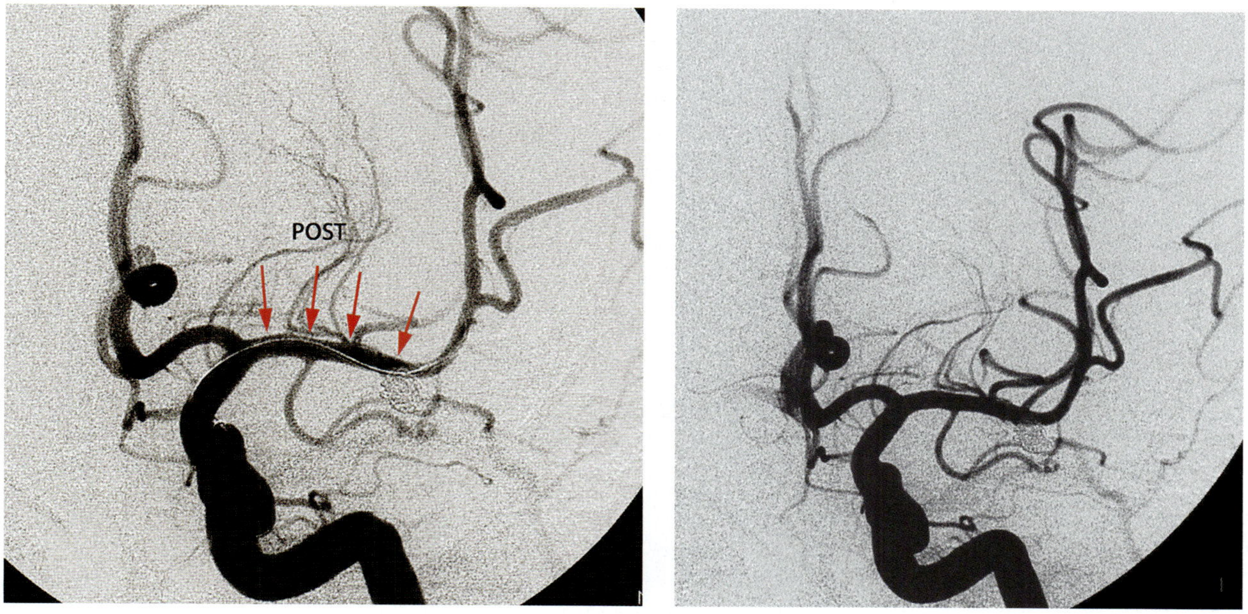

D
E

Fig. 3.6 *(continued)* **(D,E)** Follow-up angiograms after angioplasty show complete resolution of stenosis secondary to vasospasm and dramatically improved filling of left middle cerebral artery branches (*arrows*).

early treatment option, although we have usually reserved angioplasty for patients failing more traditional options (**Fig. 3.6**).

◆ Conclusions

In summary, over a short period of several decades, endovascular techniques have truly revolutionized the management of acute ischemic stroke and occlusive cerebrovascular disease. Options—once dangerous and of limited effectiveness—have become first-line measures in the management of many situations. As the available technology continues to improve, it can be anticipated that endovascular options will expand, and a greater number of patients will benefit from these important techniques.

References

1. Dotter CT, Judkins MP. Transluminal treatment of arteriosclerotic obstruction: description of a new technic and a preliminary report of its application. Circulation 1964;30:654–670
2. Higashida RT, Hieshima GB, Tsai FY, Bentson JR, Halbach VV. Percutaneous transluminal angioplasty of the subclavian and vertebral arteries. Acta Radiol Suppl 1986;369:124–126
3. Kerber CW, Cromwell LD, Loehden OL. Catheter dilatation of proximal carotid stenosis during distal bifurcation endarterectomy. AJNR Am J Neuroradiol 1980;1(4):348–349
4. Sundt TM Jr, Smith HC, Campbell JK, Vlietstra RE, Cucchiara RF, Stanson AW. Transluminal angioplasty for basilar artery stenosis. Mayo Clin Proc 1980;55(11):673–680
5. Meyer JS, Gilroy J, Barnhart MI, Johnson JF. Therapeutic thrombolysis in cerebral thromboembolism. Neurology 1963;13:927–937
6. Sussman BJ, Fitch TS. Thrombolysis with fibrinolysin in cerebral arterial occlusion. J Am Med Assoc 1958;167(14):1705–1709
7. Zubkov YN, Nikiforov BM, Shustin VA. Balloon catheter technique for dilatation of constricted cerebral arteries after aneurysmal SAH. Acta Neurochir (Wien) 1984;70(1–2):65–79

II

Surgical Revascularization Techniques

Chapter 4

Carotid Endarterectomy and Extracranial Carotid Reconstruction

Fredric B. Meyer

The cervical carotid artery pathologies that a neurovascular surgeon will encounter most frequently include carotid stenosis, carotid body tumor, and arterial dissection with delayed pseudoaneurysm formation. Each of these pathologies has its own natural history and hence indications for surgical or endovascular reconstruction. In regard to carotid stenosis, overwhelming data indicate that a carotid endarterectomy is the gold standard for treatment of symptomatic hemodynamically significant carotid artery stenosis.[1] There is also excellent evidence to indicate that in a hemodynamically significant asymptomatic carotid stenosis, a carotid endarterectomy is the treatment of choice as opposed to the natural history of the disease depending on the patient's age and other medical comorbidities.[2] Although it has been suggested through several studies that certain high-risk patients should be preferentially referred for carotid angioplasty, the definition of "high risk" is subjective. In my opinion, the only current indication for carotid angioplasty is for a symptomatic recurrent carotid artery stenosis.[3] Patients who are sometimes termed high risk, such as those with radiation-induced atherosclerosis, a high bifurcation, or contralateral occlusion, or those who are elderly, are in fact surgical candidates.[4–7]

The rare carotid body tumor and cervical carotid artery aneurysm are usually operated on as a growing enlarging mass in the neck.[8,9] As the neck mass increases, the patient may start to have difficulty with swallowing due to either irritation or compromise of the branches of the 10th nerve, specifically the superior laryngeal nerve, or as a result of compression of the trachea.[10–12] These indications are enough to require surgical exploration and resection. Currently, cervical carotid artery dissection is best treated with a combination of anticoagulation and antiplatelet therapy or, more rarely, with stenting with overall good results.[13,14] It is uncommon that a cervical carotid artery dissection requires a reconstruction graft.

◆ Technique

There are some basic principles of carotid surgery that merit emphasis.

First, the surgeon must always be aware of the status of collateral circulation to the ipsilateral cerebral hemisphere. Specifically, during a carotid endarterectomy or reconstruction of a cervical carotid artery aneurysm, it will obviously be necessary to occlude the carotid artery for a given period of time. Accordingly it is essential to ensure that there is sufficient collateral blood flow. During resection of very large carotid body tumors, the external carotid artery (ECA) is often partially encased by the tumor and occasionally it may be advantageous to temporarily occlude the CCA during dissection. During a vertebral artery reconstruction, it is necessary to temporarily occlude at least the side portion of the CCA during the anastomosis. Although it is always useful to monitor patients during a standard carotid artery endarterectomy, some surgeons have reported excellent results in which no shunting is used, a shunt is always placed, or the carotid endarterectomy is done in a very rapid fashion. Placing a shunt routinely does have some issues including the small risk of an embolic event through the shunt from dislodgement of a plaque in the CCA or dissection of a distal intimal flap from insertion of the distal shunt. It can also be difficult to control a shunt in a patient with a very high carotid artery bifurcation. In addition, reconstructing a carotid artery over a shunt for a cervical carotid artery aneurysm adds a degree of complexity that would be beneficial to avoid if at all possible. A useful technique to enhance collateral blood flow in all such circumstances is to increase the mean arterial blood pressure to ~150–170 mm Hg prior to cross clamping the CCA. In my experience, induced hypertension has reduced the need for a shunt based on electroencephalogram (EEG) criteria from ~30% to 5%.

There are many different ways to monitor brain collateral blood flow and activity during carotid artery surgery. Time-proven standards include intraoperative EEG monitoring, somatosensory evoked potential (SSEP) monitoring, and transcranial Doppler. Other less well-documented techniques include stump pressure measurements from the distal ICA and performing carotid surgery while the patient is awake. Each of these monitoring techniques has its advantages and disadvantages. EEG monitoring is effective but requires a trained technician and adds increased costs to an operation. SSEP monitoring is an objective assessment; however, it does not necessarily measure in a broad way cortical activity and hence collateral blood flow to the cortex. Stump pressure measurements correlate poorly with intraoperative EEG and should be avoided. Transcranial Doppler is better at assessing embolic events as opposed to collateral blood flow, and awake monitoring can be used only during a quick carotid endarterectomy and not for complex carotid reconstructions. The important point here is that the surgeon should have a reliable technique for monitoring collateral blood flow during carotid surgery.

A second principle for cervical carotid artery surgery is exposure (**Fig. 4.1**). There are times when it proves necessary to be able to expose the distal carotid artery well up to the skull base. For example, a high carotid bifurcation, a high plaque extending up the distal ICA, a preoperative prediction based on an isolated circulation that a shunt will be necessary, a carotid body tumor and/or cervical carotid artery aneurysm will require consideration and planning for a high neck dissection. Ischemic complications can no doubt be reduced if there is adequate exposure of the distal ICA above the pathology.

There are various ways to obtain good distal exposure, but they all start off with a long linear exposure that extends up to the area underneath the angle of the jaw. This extended incision can be extended posterior toward the mastoid or anterior in front of the ear. The incision in front of the ear offers the advantage of mobilizing the lower component of the facial nerve in the parotid gland. When performing a high dissection, it is necessary to remember the planes that are going to be exposed. It is safest to first identify the CCA then advance the dissection rostral, staying on top of the ICA. This will help prevent inadvertent exposure of the spinal accessory nerve or the vagus nerve, which are at risk with high exposures that are too lateral. Typically, it will be necessary to mobilize and likely sever the descending hypoglossal branch of the 12th nerve to allow upward displacement of the hypoglossal nerve. Commonly, it will also be necessary to ligate a branch or two of the occipital artery, which can act as a tethering band over the hypoglossal nerve. If it is necessary to ligate this ECA branch, it should be done so with suture and not bipolar cautery. After dissecting or sectioning of the descending hypoglossal nerve and perhaps ligating the tethering branches of the ECA, the hypoglossal nerve can be reflected up under the angle of the jaw out of harm's way. There are typically small veins and branches off the facial vein at the skull base that can be easily controlled with bipolar cautery. The main branches of the facial vein should be ligated with a silk suture because it cauterizes poorly. Ligating larger veins in the neck with suture will help prevent postoperative hematoma complications. Fish hook retractors are useful. They can be placed in the fascia of the carotid sheath medial and lateral and then manipulated to pull the carotid artery up into the surgeon's view. A vascular loop can be placed around the ECA and brought downward toward the chest helping pull the bifurcation caudal. For a carotid endarterectomy, it is best not to dissect underneath the carotid bifurcation for two reasons. First, this puts the superior laryngeal nerve at risk, which can lead to swallowing difficulties, and second, dissecting under the bifurcation can lead to an increased risk of embolic complications from dislodgment of plaque. Accordingly, during a high dissection, the distal ICA is dissected free and then if necessary, as a last step the underside of the bifurcation is mobilized. For high exposures, including young patients, a nasal intubation will give a slight increased distal exposure as compared with a typical oral intubation. It may be necessary to use a retractor under the jaw. This should be judiciously placed underneath the digastric muscle. Excessive retraction under the mandible can lead to a palsy of the mandibular branch of the facial nerve, which often does not recover well.

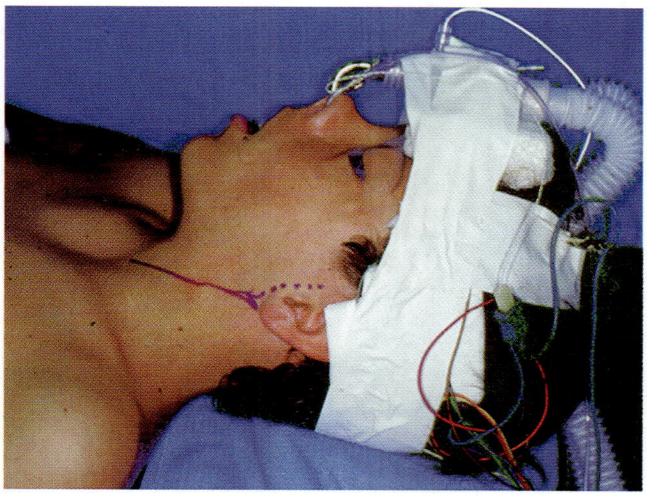

Fig. 4.1 In patients with high bifurcations, aneurysms, or paragangliomas, a high dissection is often required. Illustrated here are some useful techniques, including nasal intubation and an extended cervical incision either in front of or behind the ear depending on surgeon's desired exposure. With high exposures, branches of the facial, spinal accessory, and vagus nerves are at risk, as is the hypoglossal nerve.

The third issue that should be considered is the need for antiplatelet or anticoagulation. There is good evidence that having patients on antiplatelet therapy such as 81 mg of aspirin prior to a carotid endarterectomy decreases perioperative embolic and cardiac complications. In patients who are on a combination of aspirin and Plavix (Bristol-Myers Squibb, New York, NY), platelet dysfunction can be difficult to control intraoperatively with excessive oozing from the skin edges and deeper tissues. In that circumstance, the surgeon might consider keeping the patient intubated overnight, which will help prevent any airway compromise from an expanding hematoma. If there is prophylactic overnight incubation, the patient can still be discharged the next day.

It is standard to give 3000 to 5000 units of heparin prior to cross-clamping, which is not reversed. Older experimentation suggested that heparin at 5000 units was advantageous in preventing thromboembolic complications. However, in the last several thousand carotid endarterectomies, this dose of heparin has been reduced to 3000 without any increased risk of embolic complications and clearly less bleeding postoperatively. This is now especially important when considering discharge of the patient the day after the operation.

◆ Carotid Endarterectomy

The patient's head is slightly extended and rotated to the side opposite the surgeon. Through a gentle S-shaped incision, an incision is carried deep through the platysma muscle to identify the anterior border of the sternocleidomastoid muscle. At the lower end of the incision the surgeon encounters the omohyoid. The omohyoid and sternocleidomastoid muscle form a V, and at the apex of which the CCA can be identified. Identification of the CCA proximal in the neck will help prevent adherent wandering through tissue plains with risk of neurovascular injury. Once the CCA is identified, the surgeon dissects on top of the CCA up to the bifurcation, gently dividing the carotid sheath. This general plain of dissection is avascular except for some small branches, which might include an arterial branch of the sternocleidomastoid muscle that runs across the lower portion of the incision and can be cauterized and divided. At the bifurcation, one encounters the superior thyroid artery running medial and a hemostatic clip can be used to occlude this. A gentle dissection of the bifurcation is then performed to identify the external and internal carotid arteries.

It is best for the surgeon to *gently* palpate the CCA and then the ICA to identify the distal extent of the plaque. This will help guide the length of the dissection. It is prudent to have a dissection at least 1.5 cm above the top of the distal end of the plaque. It is not uncommon to have subendothelial extensions of the plaque, and it might be necessary to place a shunt. Hence, a distal exposure is advantageous. As noted above, dissection under the carotid bifurcation is avoided for several reasons including risk of cranial nerve injury to the superior laryngeal nerve and dislodgement of emboli from a fragile, active plaque (**Fig. 4.2**).

Once the carotid is identified, a vascular loop is placed around the ECA as well as two vascular loops around the CCA. Some surgeons prefer to also place a vascular loop around the distal ICA. Once the vascular loops are placed, the surgeon should check with an anesthesiologist to confirm that the patient's blood pressure has been elevated. Heparin—3000 to 5000 units—is then administered, and the CCA is occluded with a soft-shoed Fogarty clamp. When occluding the CCA with this type of clamp, only one click is required. The surgeon should remember that plaque and thickened intima always extend down to the aortic arch and that too much occlusion pressure across the CCA can lead to a fracture or disruption of the intima with postoperative stenosis or occlusion of the CCA. The ECA is occluded by tensing up on the vascular loop or placing a temporary clip. Likewise, the distal ICA is occluded with a temporary vascular clip.

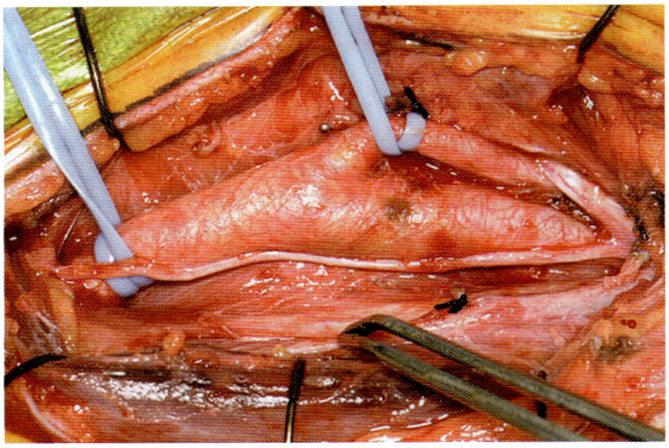

Fig. 4.2 A standard endarterectomy exposure of the right carotid artery illustrating the essential anatomy. The descendens hypoglossi can be followed during the distal dissection to identify and protect the hypoglossal nerve. The atraumatic angles vascular pickup is pointing to the vagus nerve, which sits between the carotid artery and jugular vein. Vascular loops have been placed on the common and external carotid arteries.

An incision is made with a no. 11 blade knife and extended with Potts scissors. During this time, the surgeon's assistant is irrigating with a heparin saline solution and suction tip to allow good visualization of the distal plaque. It is preferable to dissect the plaque out of the distal ICA first. By doing so, one can ensure that the plaque taper is adequate without a distal intimal flap. If one removes the plaque out of the CCA or ECA first, this can lead to a "tail wagging the dog" phenomenon of the plaque taper up the distal ICA creating intimal flaps that can be difficult to remove (**Fig. 4.3**).

When removing the plaque out of the distal ICA, a small spatula can be used to actually push the ICA away from the

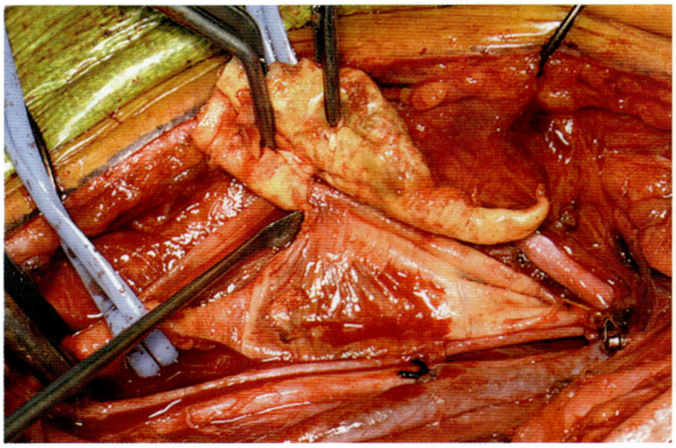

Fig. 4.3 The plaque is meticulously dissected out of the internal carotid artery first. Usually it feathers out of the internal carotid artery. Any small intimal flaps can be teased or pulled off with a jeweler's forceps. Removal of the plaque out of the external carotid artery is usually through an eversion technique. After plaque removal, the endarterectomy bed is irrigated with heparin saline and any debris or small atheroma flaps are removed.

plaque. The surgeon's assistant holds the plaque with some tension caudal. By pushing the artery away from the plaque typically the plaque will gently fracture and taper off without any intimal flaps. With this technique, it is unnecessary to place any tacking sutures. Tacking sutures can lead to arterial stenosis. The dissection is then carried down the CCA, and Potts scissors are used to sharply cleave the plaque from the stump of the CCA. The dissection then extends up into the ECA, where an inverted type of approach is used to pull the plaque out of the ECA orifice.

After removing the plaque, it is absolutely essential to make sure that there are no intimal flaps, which could be the source of thromboembolic complications. The wound is irrigated with heparin, and during that time a small jeweler's forceps is used to peel any little flaps off the bed of the endarterectomy. In particular, the distal ICA is inspected to make sure that there are no intimal flaps and that the distal intima is adherent to the artery. It is important to spend sufficient time to make sure that the transition from the endarterectomy bed to the ICA is smooth without any flaps or intimal tags. It is not uncommon to have some rough edges or flaps at the orifice of the ECA. The jeweler's forceps can be a useful tool to peel little flaps or adherent bits of atheroma. At some point it is important not to be overly aggressive because there is a small potential of punching a hole into the adventitia along the backside of the carotid artery bifurcation.

After plaque removal, the temporary clip on the ICA is released to backflow and flush any debris out of the ICA. It is valuable to visually observe the degree of backflow from the ICA to make sure that it at least appears to be sufficient. If the amount of backflow is poor, even if monitoring suggests good collateral blood flow, a shunt should be considered. If a shunt is necessary, it is easiest to first place the shunt in the CCA and secure it with two vascular loops. The Fogarty clamp is released and air is flushed out of the shunt, which has been previously heparinized. The shunt is then inserted into the ICA gently to prevent any dissection of flaps. The distal ICA clip is then removed, and the shunt is inserted further and secured with a clip. Finally, as the last step the Fogarty clamp is released (**Fig. 4.4**). On restoring flow, it is

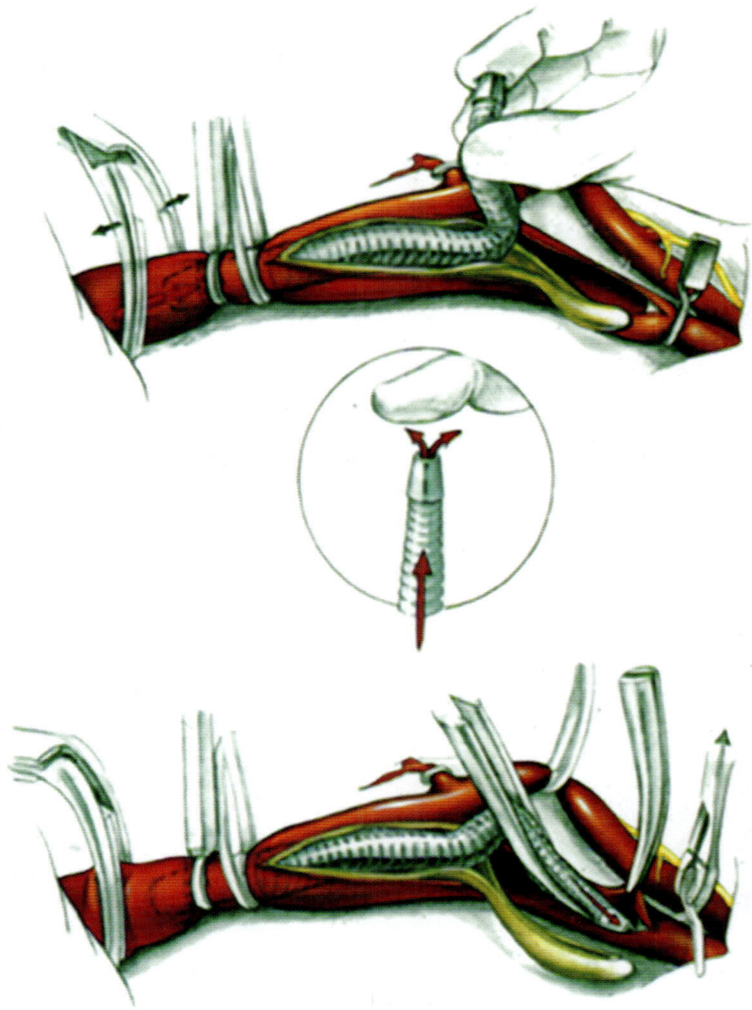

Fig. 4.4 The shunt is first inserted into the proximal carotid artery and secured with several vascular loops. The Fogarty clamp is then released and the shunt is bled to expel any air or debris. Then the common carotid is reoccluded and the distal shunt is inserted into the internal carotid artery and secured. Finally, the Fogarty clamp is released and flow is restored. (From Meyer FB, ed. Atlas of Neurosurgery: Basic Approaches to Cranial and Vascular Procedures. Edinburgh: Churchill Livingstone; 1999. Reprinted with permission.)

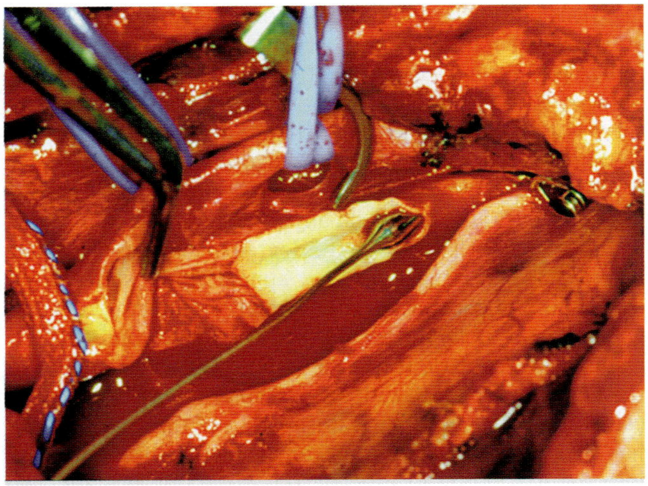

Fig. 4.5 Occasionally, the surgeon will encounter a thin caliber internal carotid artery. In addition to repairing the arteriotomy with a patch graft, the Garrett dilators are useful in enlarging the distal internal carotid artery. Successive enlarging dilators are passed up the internal carotid artery gently to the skull base. The Garrett dilators worked better than Fogarty balloons. Fogarty balloons have a higher tendency to lead to a carotid cavernous fistula or distal internal carotid artery dissection from overinflation of the balloon.

important to confirm with the monitoring technician that there has been improvement in the previously detected attenuation. If not, the surgeon must consider that an intraoperative embolus has occurred. In that circumstance, an intraoperative angiogram via injection through the shunt should be considered. With a small ICA, it can occasionally be beneficial to dilate the artery prior to closure (**Fig. 4.5**).

Once the endarterectomy has been completed, the arteriotomy can be closed in two ways. The traditional way is to close it with a running Prolene 5.0 or 6.0 suture. The less common way is to close the arteriotomy with a patch graft. In the past, saphenous vein was used, but the risk of pseudoaneurysm or rupture caused surgeons who do like to patch to change to a synthetic graft. Currently, the preferred patch is a synthetic collagen-impregnated Dacron-type graft. It has been suggested by some that closing with a patch decreases the risk of recurrent stenosis.[15] However, closure with a patch of some type is a distinctly uncommon practice (**Fig. 4.6**).

It is important to review the technique for restoring flow. Just prior to closure of the arteriotomy, the ICA is briefly backbled and then reoccluded. The Fogarty clamp is then gently released to flush out any proximal debris. It is then reoccluded. After securing the arteriotomy suture knot, the

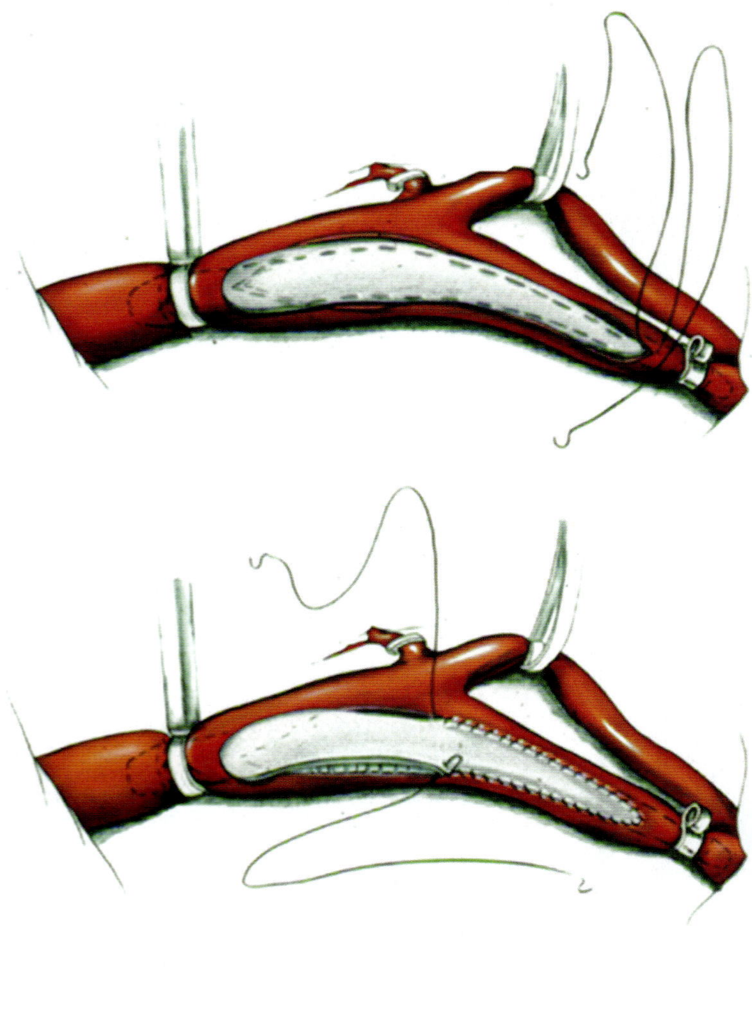

Fig. 4.6 After removal of the plaque, the arteriotomy can be repaired primarily with a running 5.0 suture or a synthetic patch graft, as illustrated here. (From Meyer FB, ed. Atlas of Neurosurgery: Basic Approaches to Cranial and Vascular Procedures. Edinburgh: Churchill Livingstone; 1999. Reprinted with permission.)

surgeon should ensure from the anesthesiologist that the blood pressure has been normalized to help prevent excessive bleeding from the arterial repair and a hyperperfusion syndrome. Thereafter, flow is first restored by releasing the Fogarty clamp followed by release of the ECA loop or clip. The ICA remains occluded. In that way, any possible debris and air is flushed up the ECA system and not to the brain. It should be emphasized that during this sequence of events, at no time has backflow down the ECA been performed. After reestablishing flow, it is useful to palpate the superficial temporal artery. If per chance the patient develops a neurologic deficit in the recovery room or after surgery, the obvious differential diagnosis is either an embolic event versus thrombosis of the endarterectomy site. If there is a good temporal artery pulse that was present at the time of flow restoration, it is quite unlikely that the CCA is occluded; hence, it would be best to consider a diagnostic angiogram and possible endovascular treatment of an intracranial embolus. Alternatively, if there was a superficial temporal artery pulse that has disappeared, the CCA has probably thrombosed and it is reasonable to quickly reopen the endarterectomy in a controlled operating room circumstance to try to reestablish flow. If perchance an endarterectomy was patent, again it would be best to perform intraoperative angiography looking for a distal embolus. Fortunately, the above scenario is exceedingly rare.

Postoperatively, carotid endarterectomy patients should be observed in a monitored setting to make sure that the blood pressure remains under 150 mm Hg. This will help prevent a hyperperfusion syndrome such as hemorrhage or seizures. Typically, the patient is maintained on one aspirin per day and discharged the day after the operation. Long-term follow-up with carotid ultrasound is usually recommended.

◆ Cervical Carotid Artery Aneurysms

With a cervical carotid artery aneurysm (**Figs. 4.7** and **4.8**), it is valuable to perform a preoperative trial balloon occlusion to assess the degree of collateral blood flow because the occlusion time will be significantly longer than a standard carotid endarterectomy. This will help guide the surgeon as to whether a shunt is necessary. It is almost always necessary for cervical carotid artery aneurysms as well as carotid body tumors to have a high cervical exposure. As described above, typically the S-shaped incision for a carotid endarterectomy can be used, but it is often necessary to extend it behind the ear toward the mastoid versus curving anteriorly in front of the ear to mobilize the parotid gland. It is important to recognize that the parotid gland, if dissected free, should be retracted anterosuperiorly and in that way help prevent injury to the lower branches of the facial nerve.

It will often prove necessary to carefully dissect out the belly of the digastric muscle. It is uncommon to have to remove the thyrohyoid process. However, the stylomandibular

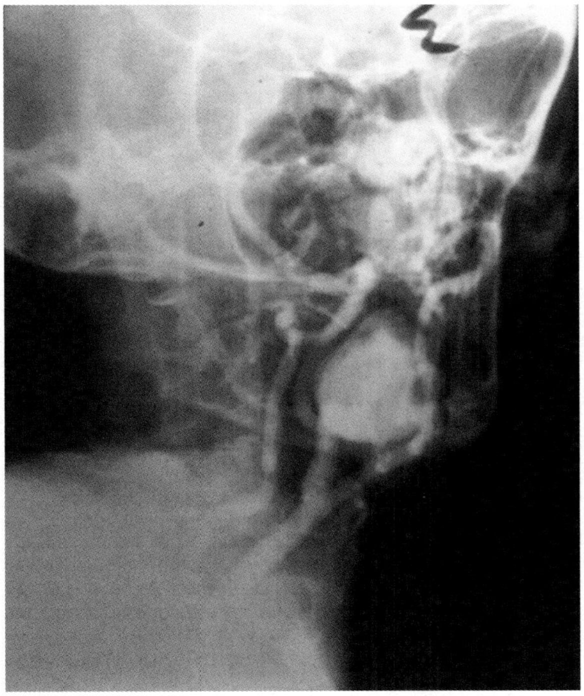

Fig. 4.7 A distal internal carotid artery aneurysm. The surgical plan here was excision of the aneurysm and a direct anastomosis of the redundant distal internal carotid artery to the proximal internal carotid artery.

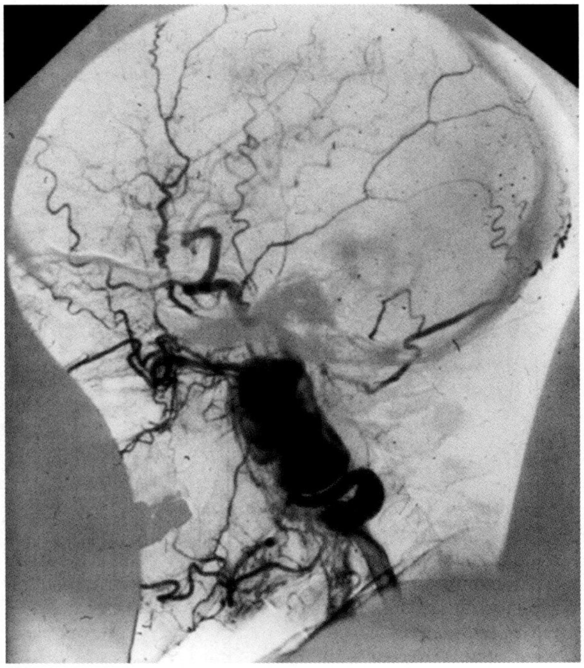

Fig. 4.8 A more complex and large internal carotid artery aneurysm that extends up to the skull base. A far distal carotid exposure was necessary. This artery was reconstructed via excision of the aneurysm and placement of a Gore-Tex graft (W.L. Gore & Associates, Inc., Elkton, MD) between the common carotid and distal internal carotid arteries.

ligament and the digastric muscles might necessarily have to be divided to obtain distal exposure toward the skull base. To mobilize the hypoglossal nerve, the descending hypoglossi branch will often need to be sectioned. Likewise, any tethering branches of the occipital artery off the ECA should be ligated and divided.

For cervical carotid artery aneurysms, the site of vascular occlusion depends greatly on the location of the aneurysm. If the aneurysm is above the bifurcation, a side-biting vascular clamp versus a Fogarty clamp can be used to occlude the ICA just above the bifurcation, thereby allowing continuous flow from the CCA up into the ECA helping to prevent any thrombus within the CCA. The distal ICA is typically occluded with at least one perhaps two temporary aneurysm clips.

For most ICA dissecting type aneurysms, it is typically necessary to excise the diseased segment (**Fig. 4.9**). In doing so, one needs to be cautious about branches of the vagus nerve running along the underside of the ICA. If there is some adhesiveness of the diseased segment of artery, a graft can be placed within the bed of the diseased segment, thereby obviating the need to dissect this segment of artery off the vagus nerve branches.

Two types of grafts can be considered, either a saphenous vein harvested from the proximal thigh or a standard vascular graft. Both work well. It is best to choose a graft that is going to have reasonable size match up with the distal ICA because this is the more difficult anastomosis. There are many different types of anastomosis that can be created along the proximal graft into the bifurcation that allow a good transition into the CCA (**Fig. 4.1**). If one is jumping a graft from the distal ICA to the CCA, then by necessity the ECA should be ligated.

The distal anastomosis should be performed with the operative microscope for superior visualization. Three different types of anastomosis can be considered as illustrative

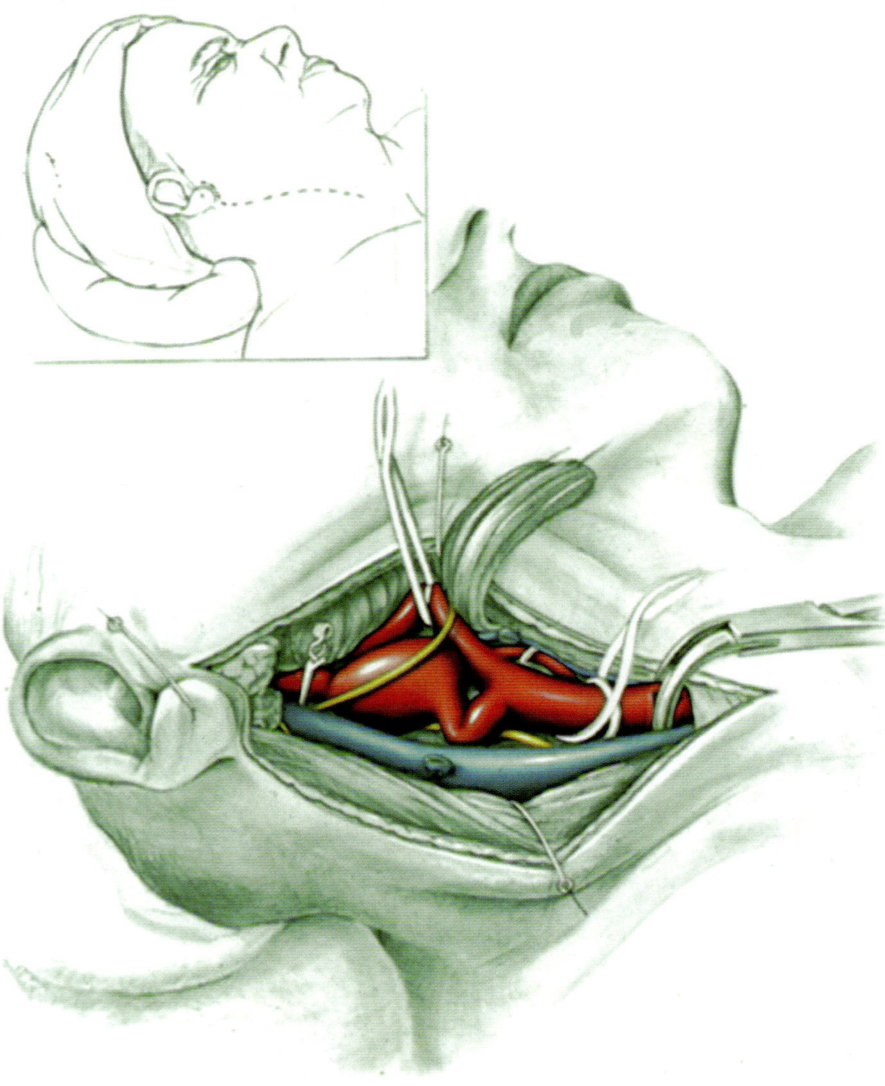

A

Fig. 4.9 **(A)** Illustrated here is exposure of a distal internal carotid artery aneurysm. *(continued)*

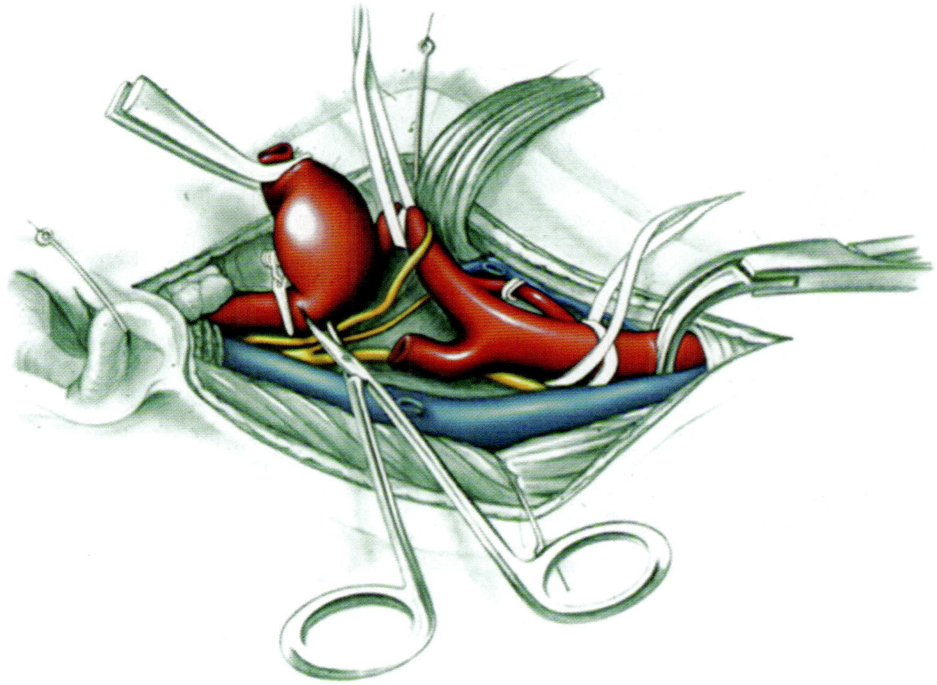

B

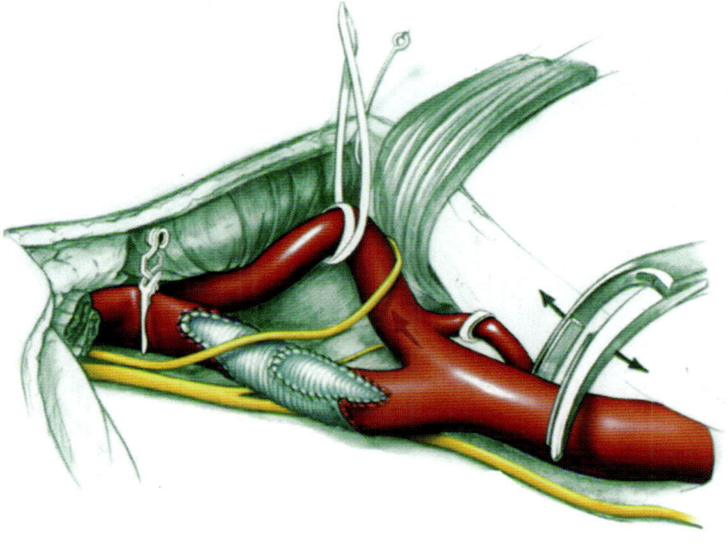

C

Fig. 4.9 *(continued)* **(B)** The distal internal carotid artery has been exposed and the aneurysm is now being excised. **(C)** The artery has been reconstructed with an interposition Gore-Tex graft (W.L. Gore & Associates, Inc., Elkton, MD). A tapered angled anastomosis was used distally and a spatulated patch anastomosis was used proximally to provide better taper of the graft to the larger proximal artery. (From Meyer FB, ed. Atlas of Neurosurgery: Basic Approaches to Cranial and Vascular Procedures. Edinburgh: Churchill Livingstone; 1999. Reprinted with permission.)

(**Fig. 4.10**). Typically, for the distal ICA anastomosis, the angulated approach works best. This is performed with two 5.0 sutures, each being placed 180 degrees with a tacking suture at the apex of the anastomosis then run halfway and secured in the midportion. Usually, the back wall anastomosis is performed first. The angulated anastomosis prevents stenosis of this important distal anastomosis site.

When performing a jump graft, it is important to "stretch" the graft to make sure that it will not kink before anastomosing it to the CCA. The graft chosen will be smaller in caliber than the CCA, and an anastomosis (**Fig. 4.11**) should be considered. This proximal anastomosis is again performed with 5.0 Prolene sutures. It is reasonable to perform a back wall anastomosis first with an everting technique and then repair the roof with

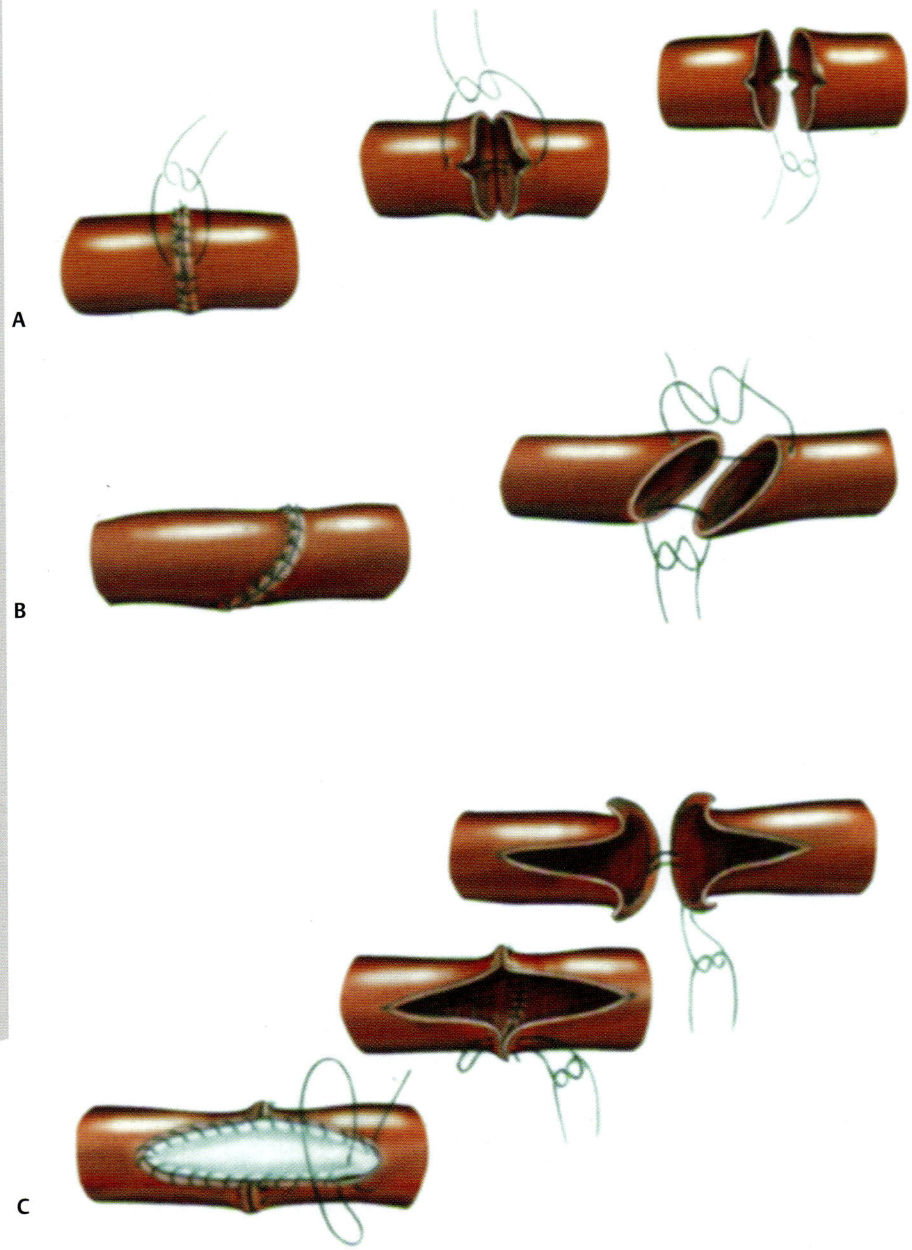

Fig. 4.10 There are three basic anastomoses for vascular reconstructions. **(A)** The first is an everted direct end-to-end anastomosis with either running or interrupted sutures. **(B)** The second is an angulated anastomosis in which two tacking sutures are placed at 180 degrees and then run circumferentially. This angulated anastomosis helps prevent a stenosis. **(C)** This complex anastomosis is useful for providing transition of a smaller graft to a larger proximal vessel. All of the grafts can be either a dilated saphenous vein or standard synthetic grafts. (From Meyer FB, ed. Atlas of Neurosurgery: Basic Approaches to Cranial and Vascular Procedures. Edinburgh: Churchill Livingstone; 1999. Reprinted with permission.)

a separate piece of graft or vein to allow a smooth transition from the CCA to the distal ICA. Just before the last suture knot is tied, backbleeding should be allowed from the ICA and the CCA to flush out any air or debris. Once again heparin administered at the time of the crossclamping is not reversed.

◆ Carotid Body Tumors

Carotid body tumors are benign tumors that arise from the CO_2-sensitive carotid body, which is located along the back wall of the carotid bifurcation in the media. The surgical risk is potential bleeding or injury to the carotid bifurcation. This can be avoided if the dissection is done carefully under magnification. Embolization is typically not necessary, although it is sometimes advocated for very large carotid body tumors. The carotid body tumors will parasitize large blood vessels off the ECA, which can usually be dissected free and controlled early in the dissection (**Fig. 4.12**). In some very large posterior-protecting carotid body tumors, there can be muscular branches from the vertebral artery and in fact embolization of these vessels can be beneficial. As noted above, a temporary trial balloon occlusion is useful to determine whether it is permissible to occlude the CCA if significant bleeding occurred.

The dissection is comparable to that described for the cervical carotid artery aneurysms in that a high dissection

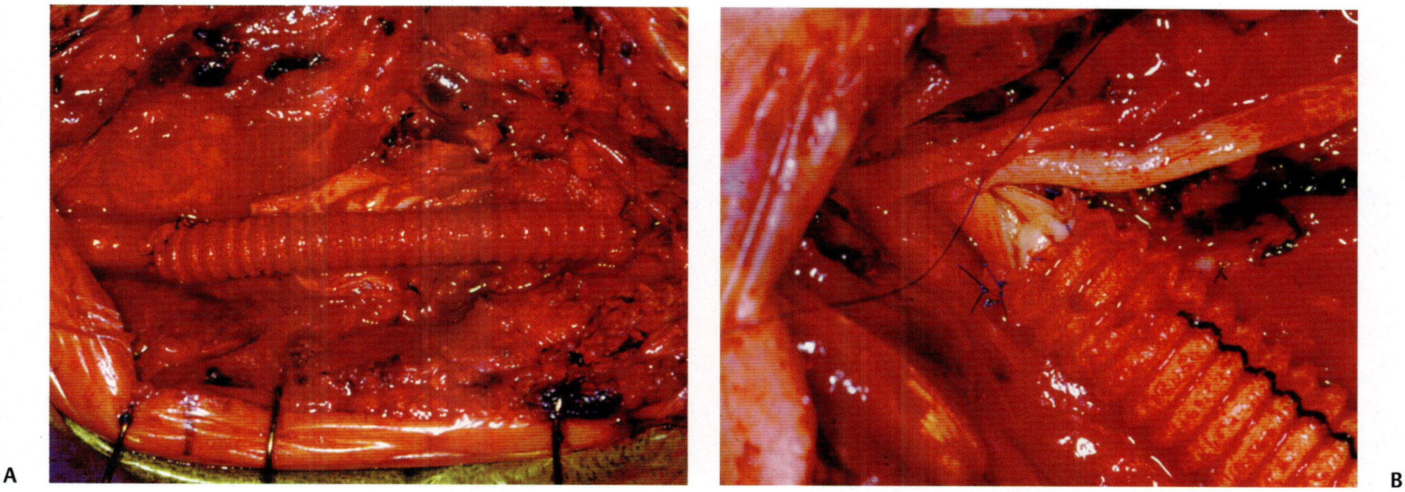

Fig. 4.11 **(A)** Carotid reconstruction with a Gore-Tex (W.L. Gore & Associates, Inc., Elkton, MD) graft following excision of an aneurysm. The graft is actually sitting within the bed of the aneurysm. By leaving the back wall of the aneurysm intact, there is less risk of injury to branches of the vagus nerve. Illustrated here is the proximal anastomosis between the common carotid artery and the Gore-Tex (W.L. Gore & Associates, Inc., Elkton, MD) rip graft. The type of anastomosis used here was an angulated anastomosis. **(B)** Distal anastomosis between the Gore-Tex graft and the distal internal carotid artery. The back wall has been anastomosed together with interrupted 6.0 Prolene sutures in an inverted fashion. A saphenous vein has been harvested from the ankle to provide a patch repair with transition from a larger proximal vessel to a smaller distal internal carotid artery. The 12th nerve sits just above the suture.

is necessary to expose the top side of the tumor. Often the 12th nerve is encased in the capsule of the tumor and must be sharply dissected free. The same is true for branches of the 10th nerve along the underside of the bifurcation.

After exposing the CCA, the dissection then proceeds between the ECA and ICA planes (**Fig. 4.13**). The large branches off the ECA can be cauterized with the bipolar or individually ligated if necessary. Historically, the area of potential vascular risk was at the origin of the carotid body tumor

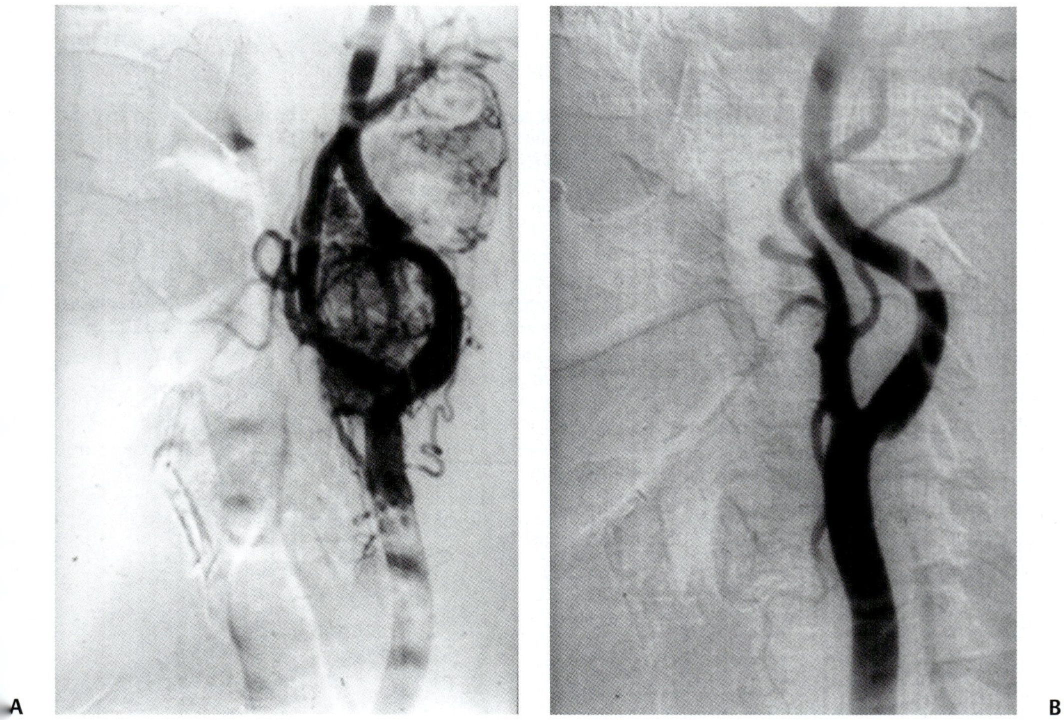

Fig. 4.12 Preoperative **(A)** and postoperative **(B)** images of a standard carotid body tumor. Carotid body tumors tend to widen the bifurcation in a very typical manner. There is dense vascular supply typically off branches of the external carotid artery.

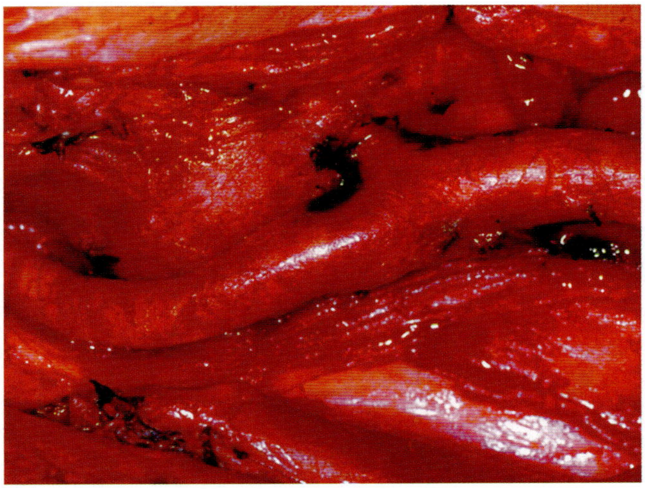

Fig. 4.13 Intraoperative photograph of a carotid body tumor that is encasing the external carotid artery.

along the backside of the bifurcation. This attachment of the carotid body to the underside of the ICA can usually be dissected free without much difficulty. Temporary occlusion of the CCA may prove useful and necessary. The plane off the back wall can be established by simply following the plain established off the distal ECA and distal ICA, both pointing back toward the carotid bifurcation.

Although historically the risk of bleeding or stroke was reported to be significant for carotid body tumors, contemporary experience in fact shows that the only risk is really one of 12th or 10th nerve injury. It is uncommon to have any significant bleeding or ischemic events with resection of these tumors.

◆ Complications

Carotid endarterectomy can usually be performed at very low risk. In my prospective database (1995–2008), ≥1500 patients with an average age of 70 underwent surgery. Sixty percent were symptomatic, and all had hemodynamically significant stenosis of ≥70% on preoperative imaging. In this group, there were two deaths (0.13%), two perioperative transient ischemic attacks (0.13%), one cerebral hemorrhage from hyperperfusion, one minor stroke with full recovery in 2 weeks, five postoperative patients with transient dysphagia (0.4%), and four major strokes (0.2%). Hence, the major morbidity and mortality rate was 0.4%. The long-term follow-up (mean 7 years) in 1000 patients demonstrated a recurrent stenosis rate of just under 0.1%.

The Sundt classification system divides patients into risk for surgery in which a grade 1 patient has no outstanding risks, grade 2 patients have an anatomic risk such as a contralateral carotid stenosis, grade 3 patients have serious cardiac comorbidities, and grade 4 patients are neurologically unstable. In the above cohort of patients, the major morbidity and mortality occurred in the grade 3 and 4 patients.[16]

In the cervical carotid aneurysms and carotid body tumors, the incidence of major stroke has proved to be quite small. Depending on the size of the lesion and extent of dissection, the primary risk continues to be postoperative swallowing difficulties at a 5 to 7% risk.

References

1. Brott TG, Brown RD Jr, Meyer FB, Miller DA, Cloft HJ, Sullivan TM. Carotid revascularization for prevention of stroke: carotid endarterectomy and carotid artery stenting. Mayo Clin Proc 2004;79(9):1197–1208
2. Dodick DW, Meissner I, Meyer FB, Cloft HJ. Evaluation and management of asymptomatic carotid artery stenosis. Mayo Clin Proc 2004;79(7):937–944
3. Meyer FB, Piepgras DG, Fode NC. Surgical treatment of recurrent carotid artery stenosis. J Neurosurg 1994;80(5):781–787
4. Kashyap VS, Moore WS, Quinones-Baldrich WJ. Carotid artery repair for radiation-associated atherosclerosis is a safe and durable procedure. J Vasc Surg 1999;29(1):90–96, discussion 97–99
5. Meyer FB, Fode NC, Marsh WR, Piepgras DG. Carotid endarterectomy in patients with contralateral carotid occlusion. Mayo Clin Proc 1993;68(4):337–342
6. Meyer FB, Meissner I, Fode NC, Losasso TJ. Carotid endarterectomy in elderly patients. Mayo Clin Proc 1991;66(5):464–469
7. Yadav JS, Wholey MH, Kuntz RE, et al, for the Stenting and Angioplasty with Protection in Patients at High Risk for Endarterectomy Investigators. Protected carotid-artery stenting versus endarterectomy in high-risk patients. N Engl J Med 2004;351(15):1493–1501
8. Maher CO, Meyer FB. Surgical treatment of nonatherosclerotic lesions of the extracranial carotid artery. Neurosurg Clin N Am 2000;11(2): 309–322
9. Shamblin WR, ReMine WH, Sheps SG, Harrison EG Jr. Carotid body tumor (chemodectoma): clinicopathologic analysis of ninety cases. Am J Surg 1971;122(6):732–739
10. McCaffrey TV, Meyer FB, Michels VV, Piepgras DG, Marion MS. Familial paragangliomas of the head and neck. Arch Otolaryngol Head Neck Surg 1994;120(11):1211–1216
11. Meyer FB, Sundt TM Jr, Pearson BW. Carotid body tumors: a subject review and suggested surgical approach. J Neurosurg 1986;64(3):377–385
12. Mokri B, Piepgras DG, Sundt TM Jr, Pearson BW. Extracranial internal carotid artery aneurysms. Mayo Clin Proc 1982;57(5):310–321
13. Meissner I, Mokri B. Vascular diseases of the cervical carotid artery. Cardiovasc Clin 1992;22(3):161–188
14. Mokri B, Sundt TM Jr, Houser OW, Piepgras DG. Spontaneous dissection of the cervical internal carotid artery. Ann Neurol 1986;19(2):126–138
15. Ecker RD, Pichelmann MA, Meissner I, Meyer FB. Durability of carotid endarterectomy. Stroke 2003;34(12):2941–2944
16. Sundt TM Jr, Sandok BA, Whisnant JP. Carotid endarterectomy: complications and preoperative assessment of risk. Mayo Clin Proc 1975;50(6):301–306

Chapter 5

Extracranial–Intracranial Bypass: Superficial Temporal Artery to Middle Cerebral Artery Anastomosis

Eric S. Nussbaum

◆ Background

The superficial temporal artery to middle cerebral artery (STA-MCA) bypass represents one of the most refined microsurgical procedures performed today. After its original introduction in the late 1960s by Yasargil and Donaghy, neurosurgeons became facile with this procedure, and some investigators reported large series of patients with low complication and high patency rates.[1–4] Unfortunately, the Cooperative Study published in the *New England Journal of Medicine* in 1985 raised serious concerns as to the ability of the operation to diminish the risk of stroke in patients with occlusive cerebrovascular disease.[5,6] Despite the many flaws associated with the design and execution of this trial, extracranial-intracranial (EC-IC) bypass was all but abandoned at most neurosurgical centers following the Cooperative Study's publication.[7–10]

In the cerebrovascular session of the 2000 meeting of the Congress of Neurological Surgeons, the attendees were polled regarding the frequency with which EC-IC bypass was being performed at individual hospitals or centers. Among the audience members, there was only one person who said they had performed more than five bypass procedures during the previous 12 months. There was one who had performed two, and only a handful had performed even one bypass over the previous year.

A decade later, a renewed interest in bypass surgery has emerged. Practical courses have been developed either as part of major annual meetings or as stand-alone clinical offerings to expose neurosurgeons to the various available techniques. The literature is being repopulated with new studies on bypass surgery, and residents are being exposed to this operation again.

The STA-MCA anastomosis represents the cornerstone of EC-IC bypass. As a training exercise for more complex bypass procedures, STA-MCA anastomosis allows for the development of proper microsurgical dexterity and teaches the delicate handling of tissues necessary to learn the art of cerebral revascularization. The basic microvascular techniques required by this operation should be practiced and then mastered in an appropriately equipped microsurgical laboratory prior to entering the operating room. Once this has been achieved, the procedure can be performed quickly using a reliable and reproducible technique; an experienced surgeon can complete the procedure in under 3 hours. In addition, the operation is performed on the cortical surface, limiting trauma to an already potentially compromised brain.

◆ Surgical Technique

Patient Positioning

STA-MCA anastomosis can be performed with the patient on a donut or secured in a rigid frame. We have favored the use of a frame simply because of the improved ability to reposition the head as needed. The patient is typically supine with the head turned more than 60 degrees. Depending on the particular patient, head rotation up to 90 degrees may be beneficial during the exposure and performance of the anastomosis. We have used a radiolucent head frame and often expose and prepare the groin as well should we elect to perform intraoperative angiography.

Doppler Identification of the Superficial Temporal Artery

At this point, we use a handheld Doppler probe to map out the course of the STA. We typically mark both the frontal and parietal branches. If the parietal branch is to be utilized, as is more often the case, a narrow strip of hair is shaved following the course of this vessel. The mapping is carried above the superior temporal line to be sure an adequate length of the STA is exposed. If the frontal branch is to be used, we typically make a gently curving incision that rises vertically above the ear toward the superior temporal line and then curves anteriorly to reach the hairline, between the midpupillary line and the midline. It is important to differentiate the typical venous signal of the superficial temporal veins from the more classic arterial pulsation of the STA.

Dissection of the Superficial Temporal Artery

The incision is generally started at the level of the zygoma and carried up over a length of several centimeters (**Fig. 5.1**). We do not use lidocaine for the incision as this may injure or cause spasm in the underlying artery. When the scalp is thick, a deeper incision can be made, but in thinner individuals, particularly older women, a shallow incision is made with a knife so as not to injure the vessel inadvertently. We have favored the use of the operating microscope for dissection of the STA. This technique has several advantages. It facilitates proper exposure and dissection of the vessel with minimal trauma to the vessel itself. In addition, the surgeon starts to work under high-power magnification early in the operation, setting the stage for the delicate microsurgery that will become necessary during the anastomosis portion of the operation.

At this point, the root of the STA must be identified. Dissection can be performed with fine scissors such as a tenotomy or iris, or with the use of a fine-tipped monopolar electrocautery. In either case, the vessel must be carefully protected at this point. Often, the superficial temporal vein is overlying or opposed to the artery, and at times, simply stopping the dissection to look for the pulse of the STA will help identify the vessel. If this does not work, the Doppler can be used again to confirm the location and direct the dissection.

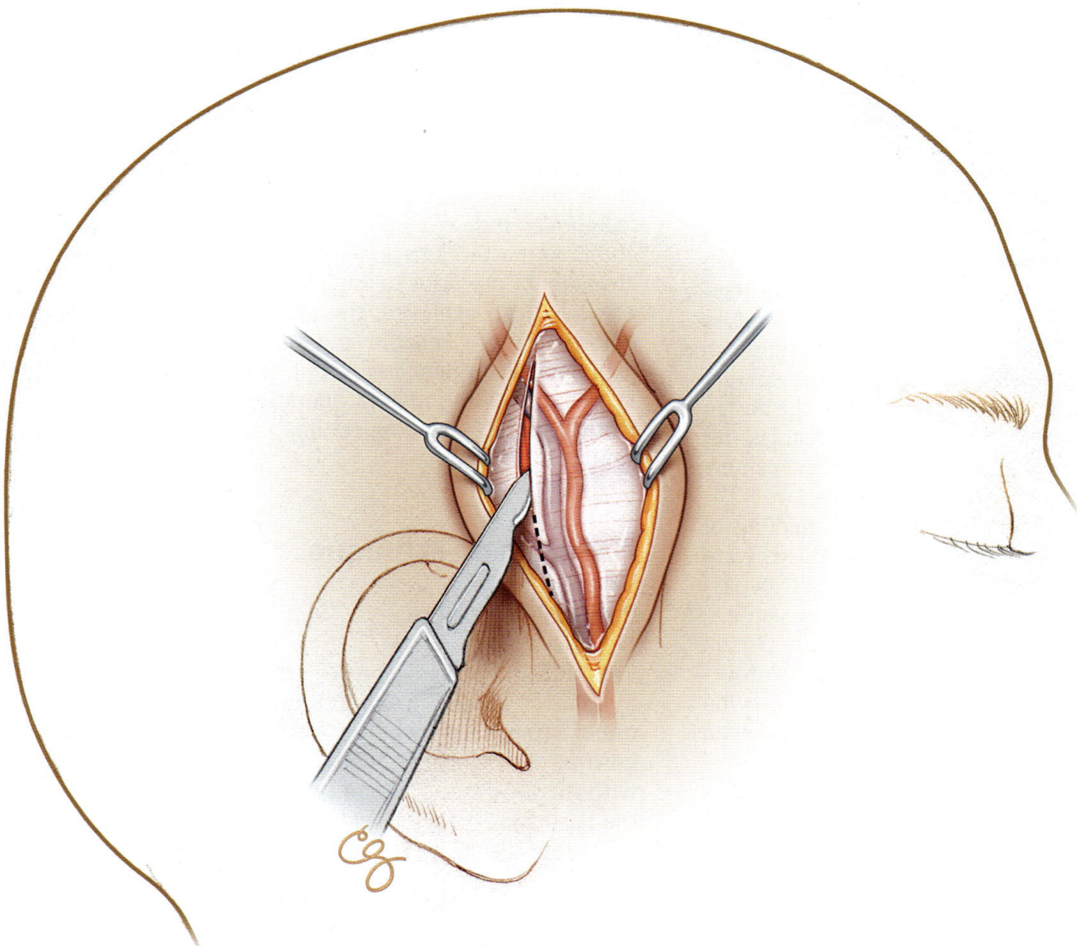

Fig. 5.1 The initial skin incision is made to isolate the superficial temporal artery.

Once, the vessel has been identified, the dissection proceeds superiorly. Sharp dissection in the plane of the artery facilitates exposure while minimizing time and effort. Small side branches are coagulated and divided sharply and the STA is thereby exposed over a long length. Care must be taken to avoid inadvertently injuring the frontal branch, which should be preserved if possible. Often, the accidental division of a branch will produce brisk arterial bleeding that may fill the microscopic field. Rather than blindly coagulating to stop the bleeding, it is critical that the bleeding point be isolated with irrigation, suction, and or tamponade, and then coagulated precisely. It is worth noting that if the STA itself is injured during the dissection, aggressive coagulation may further damage the vessel rendering it unusable as a donor. Instead, we have occasionally applied temporary clips proximal and distal to an area of injury and then utilized 10–0 suture to repair a small rent, or we have even resected a small area to perform an end-to-end reanastomosis of the vessel. In these cases, we have generally utilized intraoperative angiography at the conclusion of the procedure to ensure wide patency of the STA.

If the frontal branch is to be utilized, the incision is started in the same fashion, identifying the root of the STA, and then using sharp microdissection to expose the origin of the frontal branch. The incision is then carried superiorly and then curved anteriorly toward the hairline. At this point, the scalp can be reflected forward, and the artery can be exposed in its plane just above the temporalis fascia. There is often a layer of fat over the artery, and side branches must be carefully identified and divided. It is important to carefully follow the artery, which may suddenly turn superiorly, becoming more superficial within the scalp as this point represents a vulnerable area where the artery can be accidentally injured or even divided. The frontalis branch of the facial nerve may be encountered and should be protected if possible as the dissection proceeds distally along the artery.

In either case, we have favored leaving the STA in continuity at this point rather than dividing the vessel distally. Although others have described a technique of making a large curved incision, identifying the cut end of the STA distally, and then dissecting the vessel out from the undersurface of the scalp, we have not favored such an approach. In our experience, the vessel is more difficult to expose in this fashion, and dissection is greatly facilitated by having the vessel intact and actually carrying normal arterial supply. Injury to the vessel during dissection becomes much more difficult to discern when the artery has been occluded, and there is greater concern for thrombus formation within the vessel when the occlusion time is longer. Nevertheless, alternative techniques such as the one described have been used successfully by some surgeons.

At this point, the artery is dissected free from the underlying temporalis fascia. There may be small branches that require coagulation and division below the vessel. Once free, the artery can be shifted anteriorly or posteriorly while the temporalis fascia and muscle are split. We generally use fishhook retractors to hold the muscle back, leaving the STA free over the exposed bone.

The Craniotomy

The craniotomy is now performed. We have generally placed one or two burr holes and then completed the craniotomy with a high-speed drill. Obviously, great care must be taken to protect the STA during the drilling. The craniotomy is generally circular with a roughly 2.5-cm diameter centered over the squamosal suture, although larger or smaller openings can be made. Ideally, the opening should cover the Sylvian fissure to allow for exposure of a cortical MCA branch emerging from the fissure.

The dura is opened in stellate fashion to maximize exposure of the cortical surface. Often, opening the arachnoid to allow for cerebrospinal fluid (CSF) to drain will relax the brain and facilitate the identification of a suitable recipient vessel that is "hiding" just at the edge of the craniotomy. If no appropriately sized recipient vessel is identified, the craniotomy is enlarged. We typically follow the Sylvian fissure first distally toward the angular gyrus, then proximally. If no vessel is identified, opening the fissure along its superficial aspect may reveal an appropriate MCA branch just below the surface. Care is taken to avoid inadvertent venous injury and to preserve all cortical vessels that may be important in the setting of previous hemodynamic compromise.

At times, a white, flattened artery that has been the victim of an old ischemic injury will be encountered. We have generally avoided the use of these vessels as a recipient.

Dissection of the Recipient

Under high-power magnification, the arachnoid overlying the recipient MCA branch is taken down. This can usually be achieved using jeweler's forceps and a jeweler's microscissors. Several small side branches are coagulated and divided while larger branches can be temporarily tied off or clipped with low-tension clips. A small piece of background material slipped beneath the vessel will greatly facilitate the anastomosis as the opened, thin-walled vessel becomes surprisingly translucent when emptied of blood. The cautery should be turned to a very low setting when coagulating these branches to avoid transmission of current to the main vessel. In addition, the liberal application of topical papaverine will often help reverse narrowing created by iatrogenically induced spasm.

Final Preparation of the Superficial Temporal Artery

At this point, attention is returned to the STA. A small area of the distal artery is then cleared of its adherent fascial cuff. It is critical to be sure there will be enough length on the STA to perform a tension-free anastomosis, so we will often check the length with a piece of suture or a ruler if there is any doubt. The artery is distally clipped or ligated and a temporary clip is applied proximally (**Fig. 5.2**). The artery is opened and a beveled, fishmouth opening is created. The anastomosis will optimally be a nice, long, flat anastomosis to minimize turbulence at the junction of the vessels. Flow

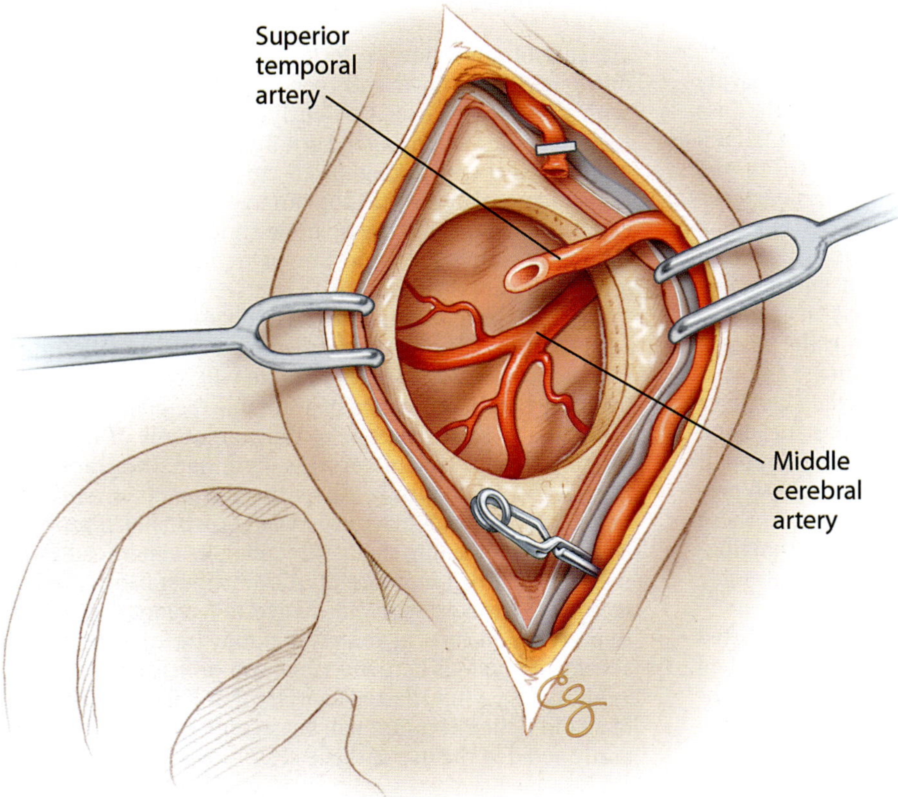

A

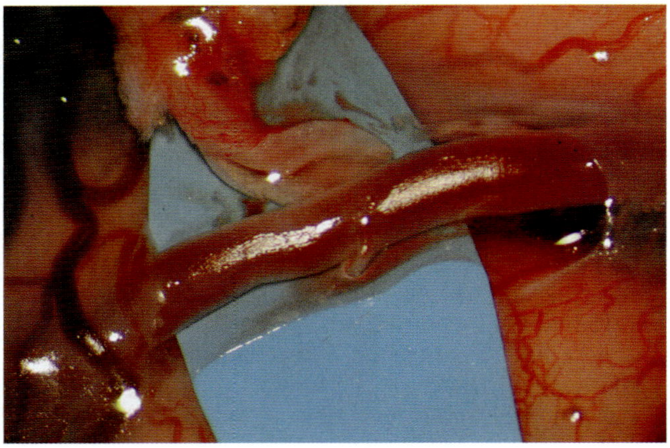

B

Fig. 5.2 (A) Once the superficial temporal artery (STA) has been mobilized, the craniotomy is performed, an appropriate cortical middle cerebral artery (MCA) branch is selected, and the STA is prepared for anastomosis. **(B)** Corresponding operative photomicrograph demonstrating the open distal STA prepared for anastomosis alongside the cortical MCA branch.

within the artery is tested by opening the proximal clip, and the artery is then irrigated with a heparinized saline solution. The vessel is now brought down into the craniotomy to check the length again, and to determine the fashion in which it will comfortably rest to reach the recipient vessel. One should avoid twisting or kinking the donor STA, and an inadequate length of STA at this point will translate into great difficulty during the anastomosis and will decrease the likelihood of achieving a patent bypass.

If after dividing the STA, the length is found to be inadequate, attention should be focused on the root of the STA. Under microscopic visualization, the root should be aggressively dissected, dividing any fascial or soft tissue bands. In addition, further division of the temporalis fascia and muscle may improve the available length. We have often been pleasantly surprised by the additional amount of STA that can be mobilized using these maneuvers. At this point the length of the opening in the STA should be assessed. Again, the longest opening feasible given the length of recipient vessel between large branches is used as a guide to the length of the anastomosis. Typically, a longer anastomosis is favored.

Final Preparation of the MCA Recipient

After infusion of an intravenous neuroprotective agent such as barbiturates or etomidate, the cortical MCA branch is now trapped between low-tension aneurysm clips. The clips should be deliberately applied in a fashion so as to minimize their interference with the bypass. The use of curved or bayoneted clips may be helpful in keeping the working area clear. The MCA branch can be opened with any form of super sharp and fine knife. Beaver eye blades or diamond knives are good options. Next, the opening can be enlarged either in linear or gently curving fashion using the knife or a jeweler's microscissors. The opening is then irrigated with heparin. The length of the opening should be tailored to appropriately match the length of the opening in the STA (**Fig. 5.3**). If a small branch has been missed, there will be arterial inflow, and the branch can be coagulated at this time. Occasionally, there will be a small leak of blood past one of the main clips. In such a case, the clip should be replaced by first positioning a second temporary clip beyond the first and then removing the nonfunctioning clip itself. Under high-power magnification, it is surprising how quickly the field can fill with blood if the clip is simply removed, and this can make proper meticulous replacement difficult. In addition, the use of a microsuction device tucked beneath the dural margin to keep the field clear of CSF may greatly facilitate the procedure from this point forward.

The Anastomosis

There are many optional ways to perform the actual anastomosis. We have generally used 10-0 suture, beginning with interrupted sutures to tack down the apices of the anastomosis. These sutures can then be continued in running fashion, or interrupted sutures can be utilized. We have generally favored interrupted suture when the vessels are small or when the exposure is compromised in any fashion. This allows for more precise suture placement and virtually eliminates the risk of "catching the back wall." Often, we will lay in the last two or three sutures and only tie them at the conclusion to optimize the anastomosis at its corner, where visualization can become difficult (**Fig. 5.4**). If a running anastomosis is used, it is almost impossible to maintain adequate tension on the suture line, and we have generally favored leaving the anastomosis loose, using a technique described by Spetzler, and then tightening the suture line at the conclusion before tying the knot (**Fig. 5.5**). Once the front wall has been completed, the STA can be retracted to allow for inspection of the lumen, looking "into" the open anastomosis to be sure no stitches have caught the back wall inadvertently (**Fig. 5.6**).

Clip Removal

Once the anastomosis has been completed and inspected, clips can be removed, first from the cortical MCA branch and then from the donor STA (**Fig. 5.7**). In general, one should be able to visualize retrograde flow and return of pulsation up into the donor vessel once the clips are removed from the MCA branch and before the proximal STA clip has been opened. Areas of arterial leak can be inspected and tamponaded and will often stop on their own with gentle pressure. Persistent leaks may require an additional 10–0 suture. We prefer to avoid reclamping the vessel, which may promote thrombus formation, and place the suture under direct vision using suction and tamponade to keep the field clear. If there is any question regarding the anastomosis, a Doppler ultrasound can be checked to ensure normal arterial pulsatile flow within the

A
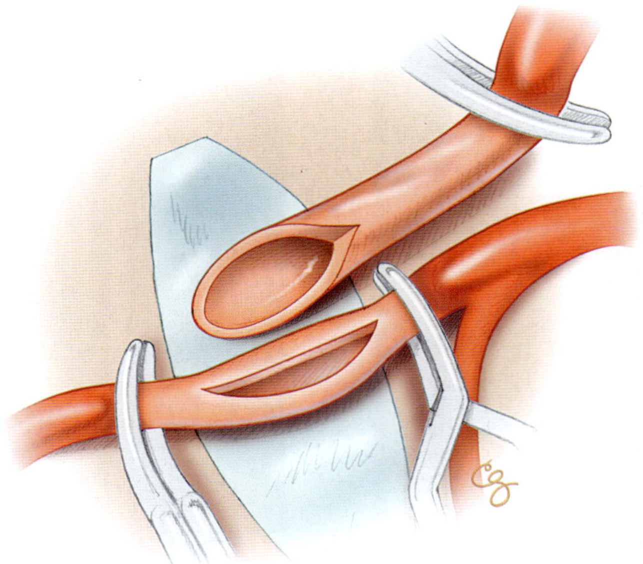

B
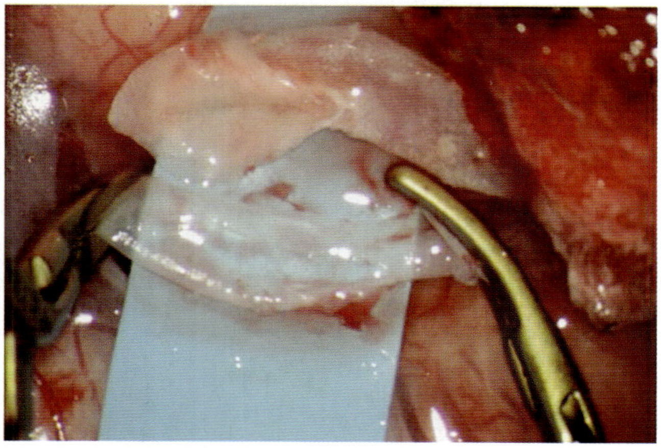

Fig. 5.3 **(A)** The cortical middle cerebral artery (MCA) branch has been trapped and opened to provide an appropriate length match to the STA. **(B)** Corresponding photomicrograph showing the open STA and MCA branch; note the translucent nature of the very thin-walled MCA.

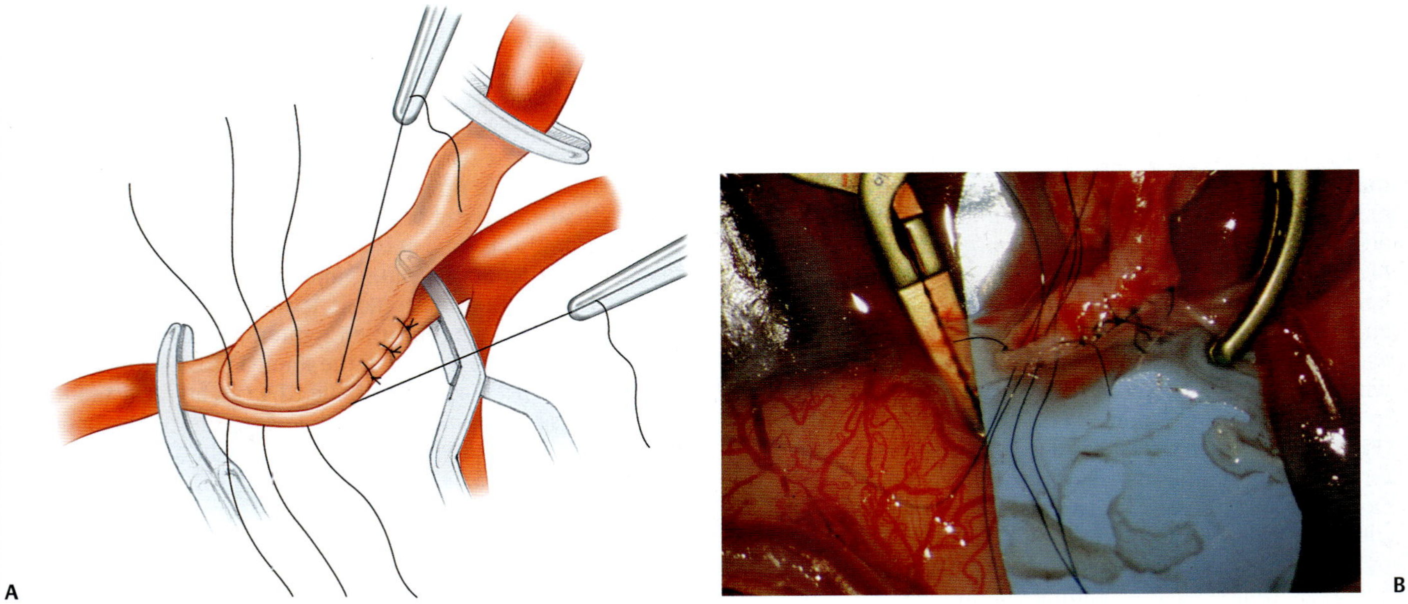

Fig. 5.4 The front wall is being sewn using interrupted 10-0 suture. **(A)** Placing the sutures first and then tying them independently at the end is a useful technique in particularly small vessels or when visualization is difficult. **(B)** Corresponding photo showing the last few interrupted sutures in place before tying, optimizing suture placement in the corner of the anastomosis.

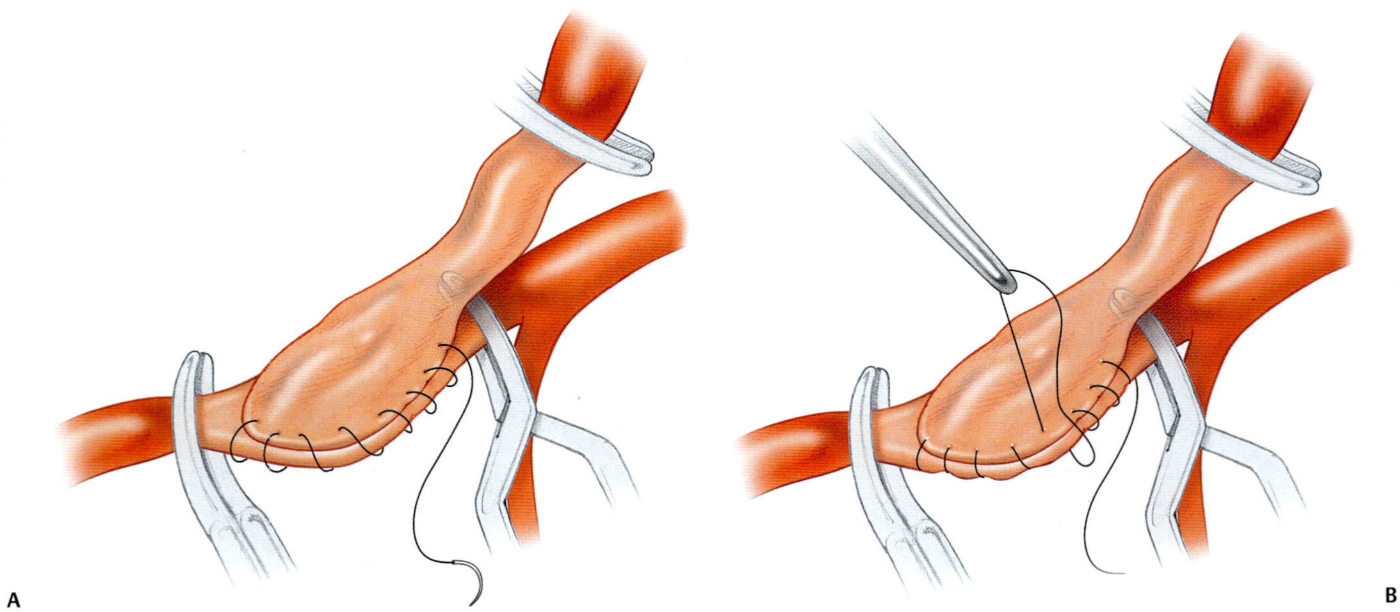

Fig. 5.5 As an alternative, the suture can be placed in a running fashion, left loose initially **(A)**, and then tightened at the conclusion **(B)**. It is extremely difficult to maintain good tension on the suture line because of the fine nature of the suture, so tightening the suture at the end works well. *(continued)*

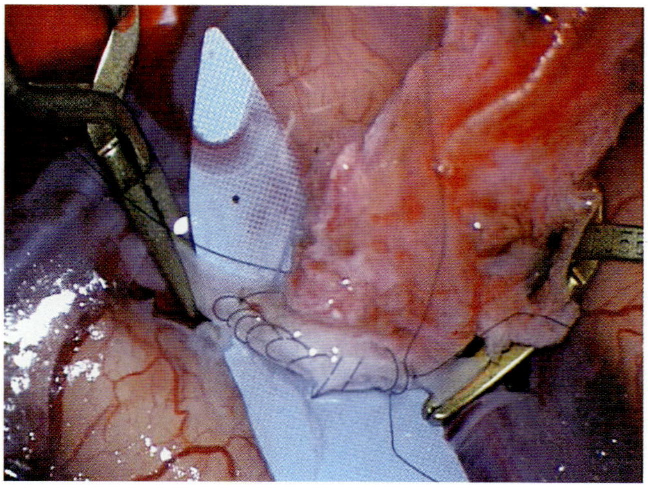

C

Fig. 5.5 *(continued)* **(C)** Illustrative photomicrograph reveals the front wall of the anastomosis left loose initially, ready to be tightened and then tied.

distal aspect of the donor vessel. Alternatively, intraoperative angiography can be performed at this stage. It should be noted that the ability to palpate a pulse within the donor vessel does not guarantee good flow within the bypass (**Fig. 5.8**).

Closure

The dura, bone flap, muscle, and fascia must be closed while leaving adequate room for the donor vessel as it assumes its new resting configuration. When the procedure is performed in the setting of moyamoya disease, we have sometimes discarded the bone flap, covering the defect with a piece of titanium mesh, which can allow for delayed ingrowth of new vascularization from the underside of the temporalis muscle. Otherwise, we have generally resecured the flap with titanium plates and screws. The scalp is closed, with care taken not to injure the underlying donor vessel. Still, one should avoid the natural tendency to take very shallow bites to avoid injuring the STA when closing the skin. This can increase the likelihood of wound dehiscence and superficial skin loss, which can ultimately result in an infection.

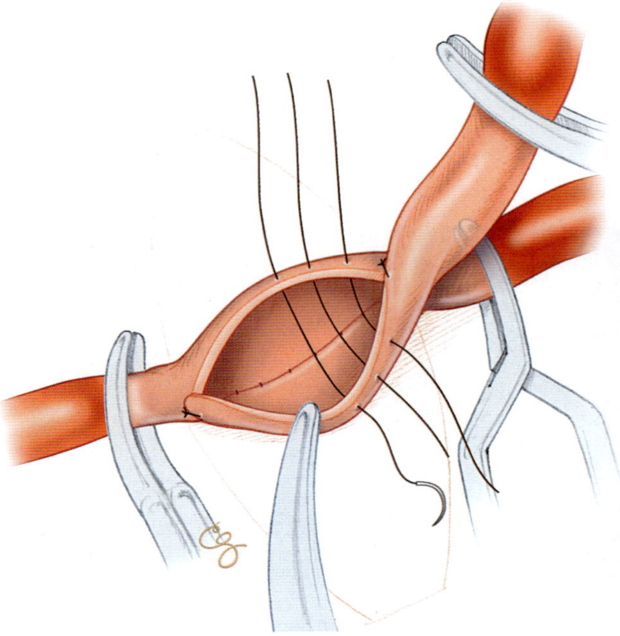

A

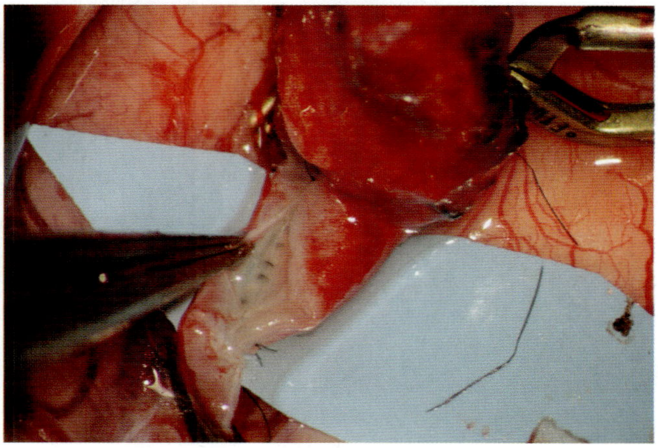

B

Fig. 5.6 **(A)** Once the front wall has been completed, the surgeon can retract the superficial temporal artery to look "into" the open anastomosis, visualize the lumen, and place the back wall sutures.

(B) Corresponding operative photo illustrates inspection of the lumen following completion of the front wall of the anastomosis.

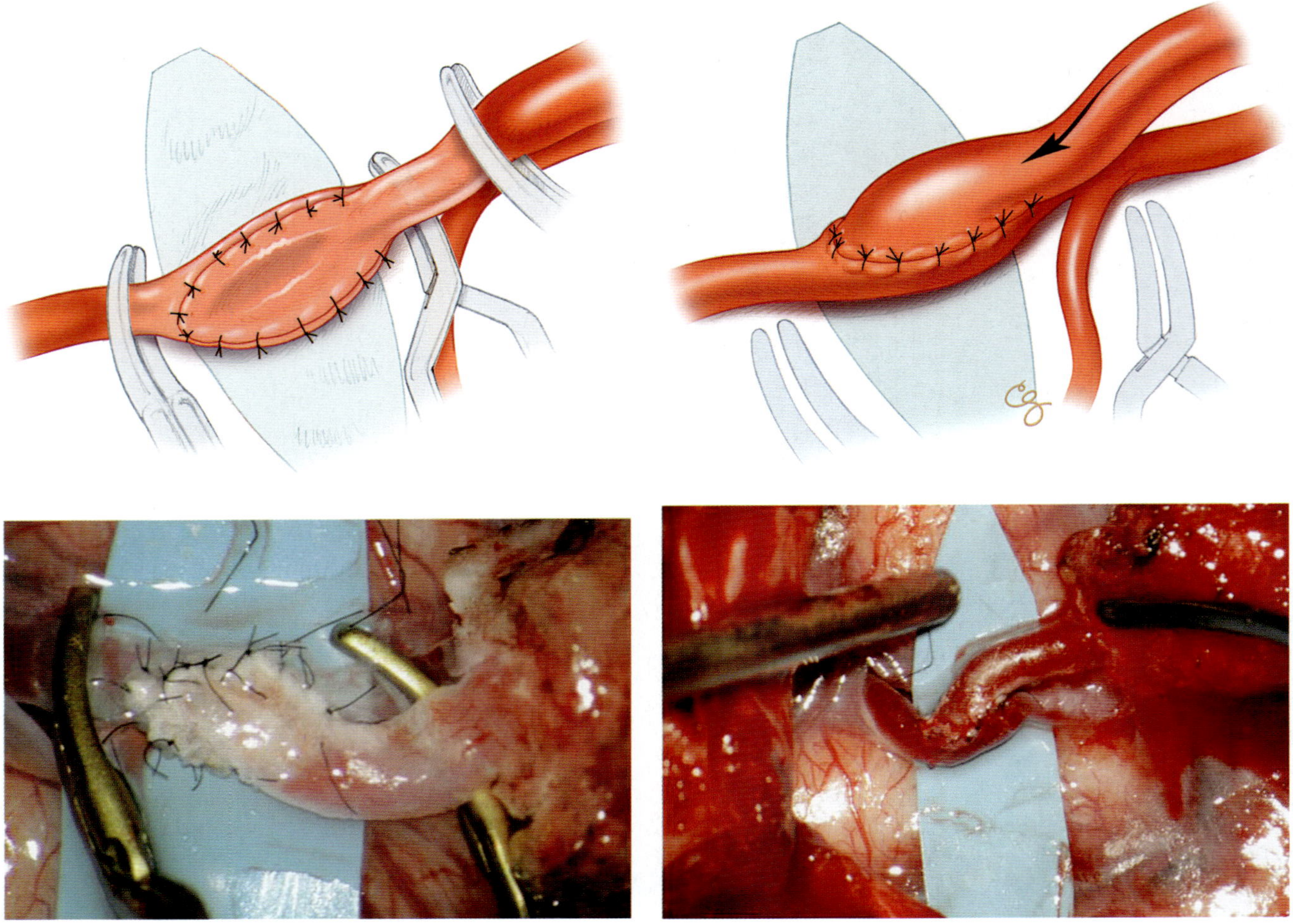

A B C D

Fig. 5.7 After completion of the back wall **(A)**, the clips are removed to reveal the completed anastomosis **(B)**. Corresponding operative photos reveal the completed anastomosis before **(C)** and after **(D)** removal of the clips.

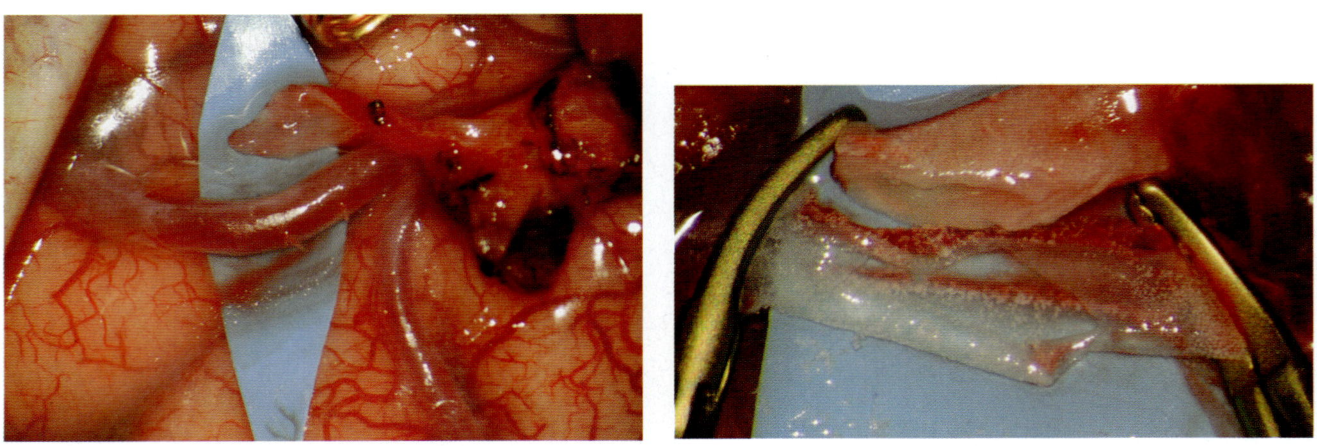

A B

Fig. 5.8 Representative case of superficial temporal artery to middle cerebral artery (STA-MCA) bypass performed with interrupted sutures. **(A)** The recipient cortical MCA branch has been dissected from its arachnoid, two small side branches have been coagulated and divided, and a piece of blue background material has been inserted beneath the artery. The STA has been divided with the distal end beveled and irrigated with heparinized saline. **(B)** The cortical MCA branch has been trapped between low-tension aneurysm clips and opened over a length that roughly matches the opening in the STA. Note the very thin wall of the MCA in comparison with the somewhat thicker-walled STA. *(continued)*

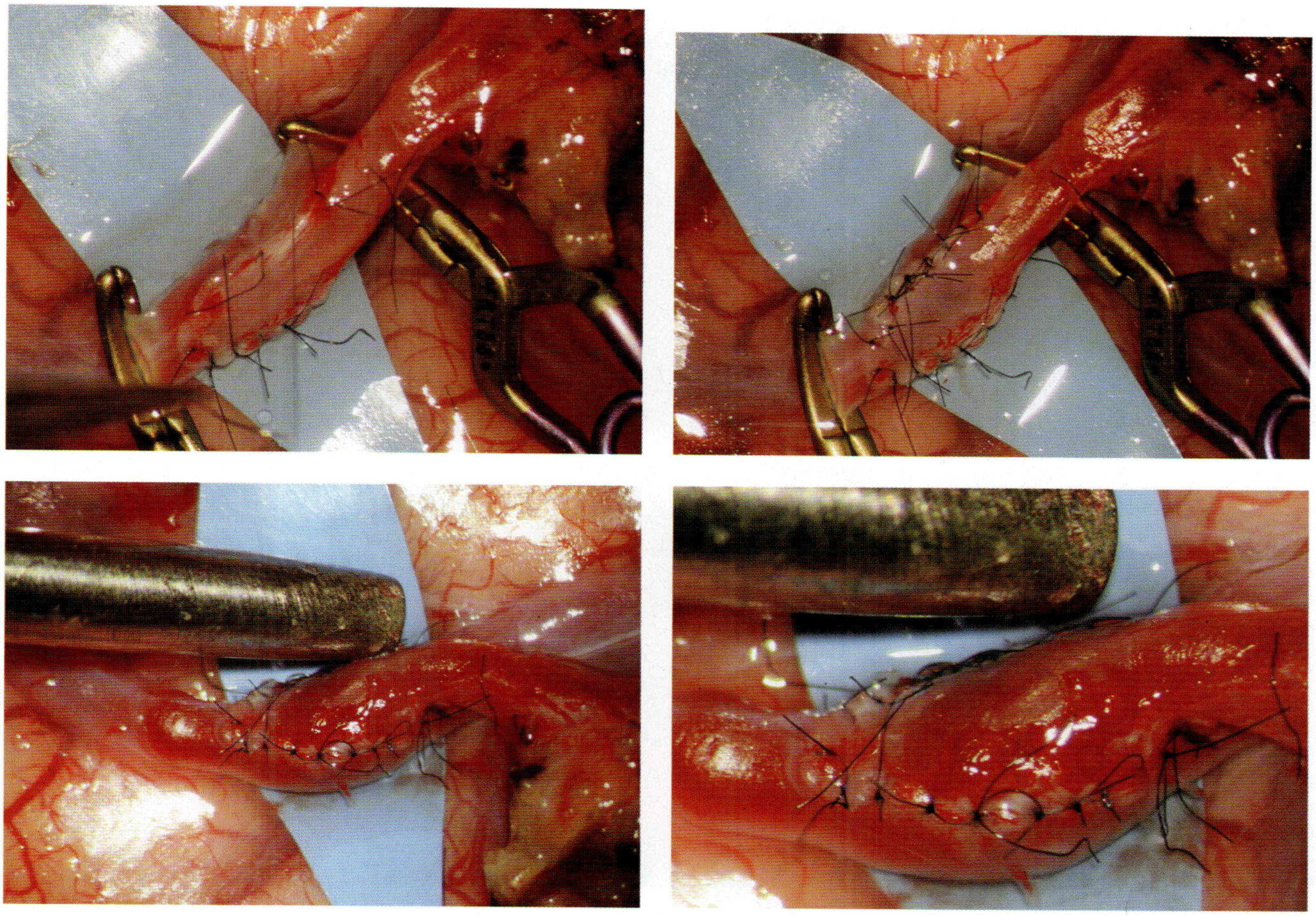

C D E F

Fig. 5.8 *(continued)* **(C)** The front wall anastomosis has been completed using interrupted sutures. **(D)** The back wall has now been completed as well. **(E)** With all clips removed, a nice long, flat anastomosis has been completed. **(F)** Magnified view revealing greater detail.

Pearls and Pitfalls Associated with STA-MCA Anastomosis

Avoid

- Tension on anastomosis
- Unnecessarily large craniotomy
- Overaggressive coagulation to achieve hemostasis
- Overaggressive retraction of STA during drilling of craniotomy
- Bypassing to white, flattened recipient artery
- Working in “wet” or “bloody” field
- Kinking or injuring STA during closure

Do’s

- Practice in microvascular laboratory
- Use high(est) power magnification
- Treat STA and MCA branch gently
- Expose long enough length of STA
- Create elongated, flat anastomosis
- Use interrupted sutures for very small vessels
- Orient STA to assume “comfortable,” natural orientation once bypass completed (**Fig. 5.9**)

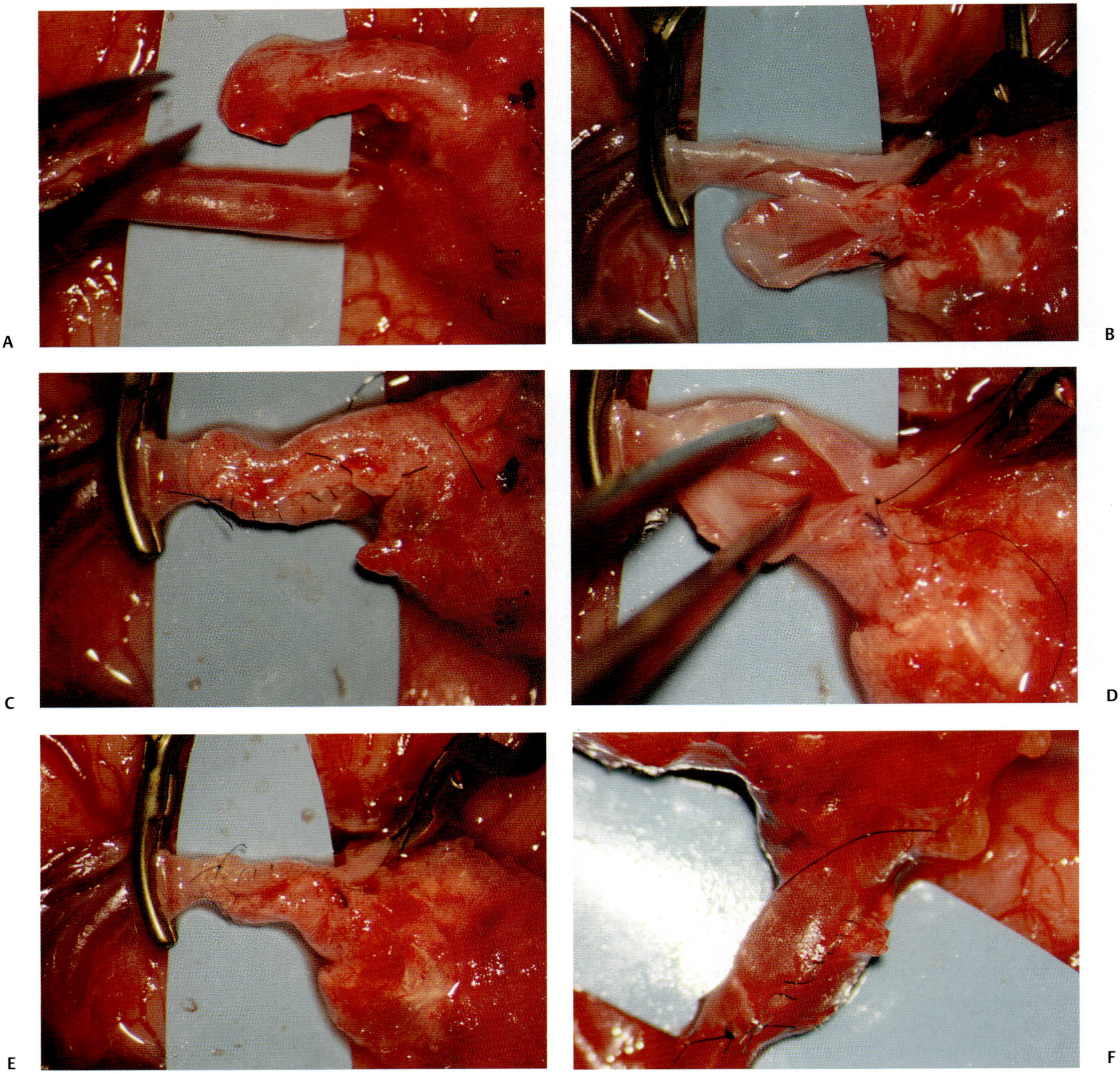

Fig. 5.9 Superficial temporal artery to middle cerebral artery (STA-MCA) anastomosis using running suture technique. **(A)** The cortical MCA branch has been isolated with blue background material beneath, and the STA is shown at the top of the field. **(B)** The MCA has been opened, and the STA is positioned alongside in preparation for anastomosis. **(C)** In this case, the front wall has been completed with a running suture. **(D)** The STA has been reflected to reveal the back wall, allowing us to inspect the interior of the MCA branch and ensure that the back wall was not caught by any of the front wall sutures. **(E)** The back wall anastomosis has now been completed as well. **(F)** The completed anastomosis is seen once all clips have been removed.

◆ Personal Experience

We have used the STA-MCA anastomosis predominantly in the setting of occlusive cerebrovascular disease but also in the management of complex intracranial aneurysms as well as skull base tumors. Although the flow afforded by this bypass is less than what can be expected from a radial artery or saphenous vein graft, a good STA-MCA anastomosis can provide adequate additional blood flow to prevent ischemic injury in many patients undergoing carotid sacrifice, particularly when there is some native collateral supply across the anterior communicating artery or from the posterior circulation via the posterior communicating artery. In addition, a double-barrel bypass can afford additional protection when collateral supply is limited.

We have performed STA-MCA bypass in more than 200 patients with ischemic disease; our earliest cases were published previously.[11] Indications have included carotid occlusion (cervical or intracranial), carotid stenosis not amenable to endarterectomy (typically intracranial), MCA stenosis or occlusion, moyamoya disease, and intracranial or extracranial carotid dissection. We have also used this procedure to treat more than 50 intracranial aneurysms and 10 skull base tumors. Although we have often favored the use of a radial artery or saphenous vein graft in the management of aneurysms and skull base tumors, we have never performed a high-flow bypass in the setting of ischemic disease (**Fig. 5.10**).

A B C D

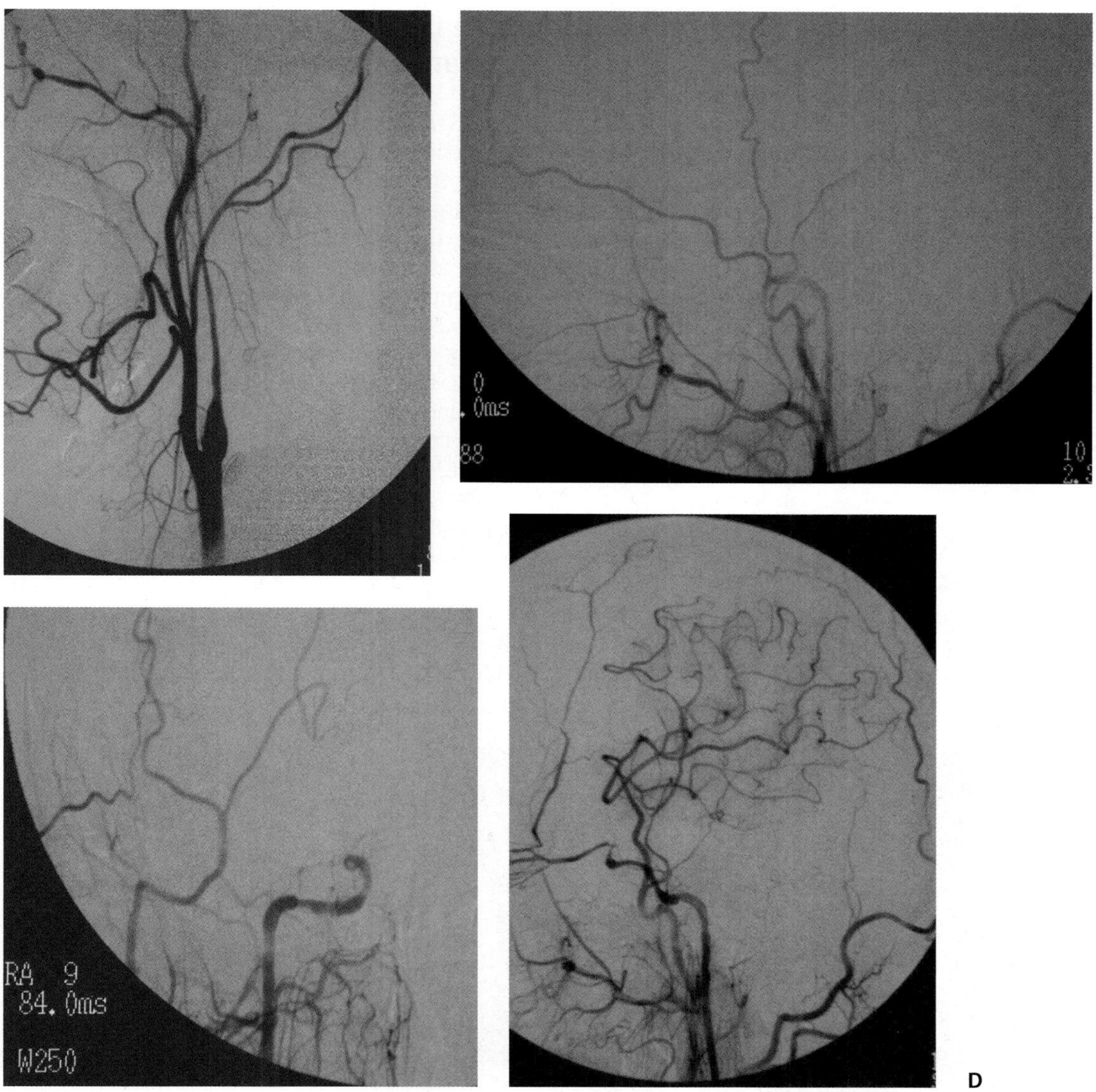

Fig. 5.10 This young woman presented with repeated transient ischemic events. Cervical carotid arteriography reveals a smooth tapering narrowing of the internal carotid artery (ICA; **A**) with limited filling of the intracranial ICA only to the level of the ophthalmic artery **(B,C)**. Postoperative arteriogram **(D)** demonstrates good filling of the middle cerebral artery territory through the anastomosis, *(continued)*

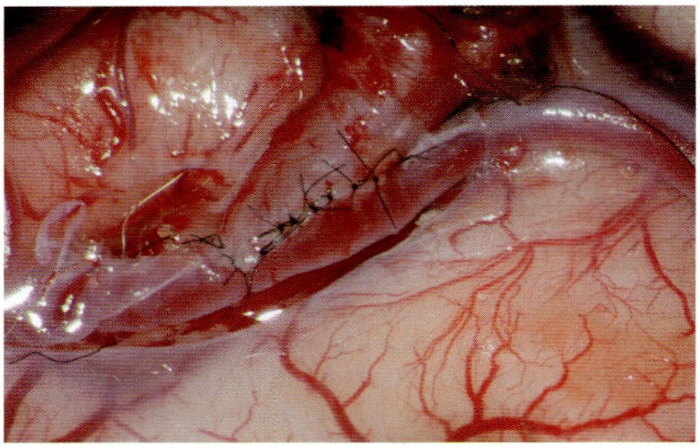

E

Fig. 5.10 *(continued)* which is shown in the operative photomicrograph **(E)**.

◆ Complications

Complications associated with STA-MCA bypass have been limited. Of note, we have performed the operation in an emergency setting for acutely evolving stroke in 15 cases. Our results with this delicate subpopulation have been reported in detail in a recent publication.[12] Excluding these high-risk cases, in a series of ~200 procedures performed for occlusive cerebrovascular disease, three patients experienced an early postoperative TIA, five presented with a TIA more than 3 months after surgery, and four patients suffered a delayed stroke as documented by diffusion-weighted magnetic resonance imaging. Of the patients returning with delayed ischemic events, most had moyamoya disease and developed symptoms in the untreated contralateral or posterior circulation. Several of the patients exhibiting delayed TIAs became symptomatic when a well-intentioned physician increased their antihypertensive medication dosage. These patients all did well when the medication was decreased again.

One very interesting patient did well after surgery and was discharged home on the third postoperative day. He returned one week later with a severe headache and was found to have an unexpectedly large hematoma immediately underlying the site of the anastomosis. Cerebral angiography identified the development of a pseudoaneurysm. At the time of surgical exploration, the pseudoaneurysm was found to have developed at the site of the distal clip that had been placed on the MCA branch. The injured vascular segment required resection and end-to-end reconstruction, the hematoma was removed, and the patient did very well.

Wound dehiscence has been an occasional problem in our patients, most commonly occurring in patients with diabetes mellitus and severe associated atherosclerotic disease. Twelve patients required revision of the wound, with removal of the underlying bone flap in eight patients. No long-term wound complications were noted. In the entire group of patients, only five suffered subsequent ischemic injury in the territory treated by the bypass. Three of these were young women with progressive moyamoya disease that went on to involve multiple vascular territories not addressed by the EC-IC bypass.

◆ Alternate Options and Special Circumstances

In rare cases, the STA may not be suitable for bypass. This may occur on a congenital basis, due to atherosclerotic disease, or as a result of prior surgery. In such cases, several options are available. A large occipital artery can be used in some instances, although the reader is cautioned regarding the increased difficulty associated with dissecting the occipital artery from the surrounding soft tissues in contrast to the much more straightforward STA. If the proximal STA is preserved, we have used short-segment venous grafts or even the contralateral STA, which has been harvested as a free graft at the start of the operation. In one notable case, retrograde filling of the STA was identified on cerebral angiography in the setting of common carotid occlusion. In this case, we were able to dissect out the STA in standard fashion and then anastomose the proximal STA to the MCA branch, allowing the blood flow to come retrograde down the STA to reach the anastomosis. In all such unusual cases, we have used intraoperative angiography to ensure patency of the anastomosis. Rarely, we have encountered a heavily calcified or atherosclerotic STA or MCA necessitating local endarterectomy to allow for anastomosis (**Fig. 5.11**).

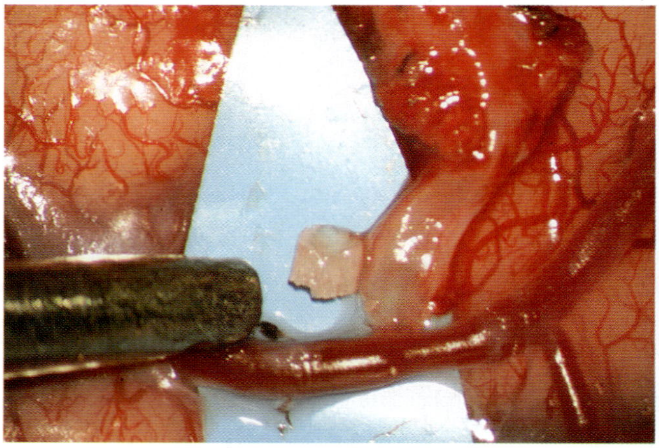

A

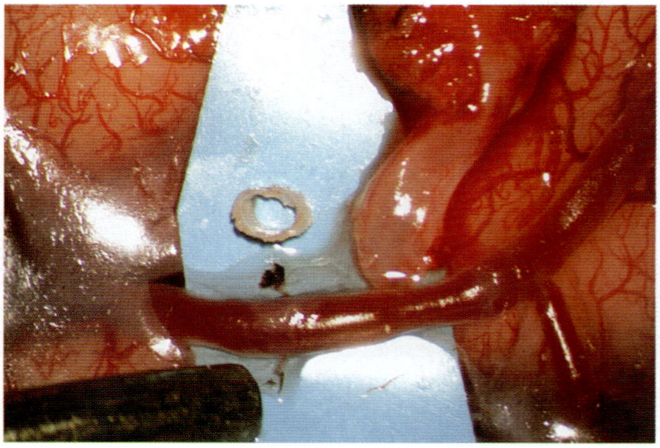

B

Fig. 5.11 **(A)** An unusual case in which the superficial temporal artery (STA) was heavily calcified, necessitating endarterectomy of the distal STA to allow for suturing of the vessels. **(B)** The ring of calcium that has been removed from the distal STA is seen on the blue background material.

◆ Postoperative Management

We have generally treated these patients as we would most other patients undergoing craniotomy, although we have been more liberal with blood pressure limits postoperatively, depending on the specific nature of the underlying disease process. We generally start a full adult aspirin at 325 mg the day of surgery and continue that indefinitely. Patients who cannot tolerate this regimen are switched to 81 mg aspirin per day. We have not used Plavix (Bristol-Myers Squibb, New York, NY) or heparin in our patients unless these agents were recommended for another unrelated issue such as a cardiac valvular disease or atrial fibrillation. Patients are watched overnight in a neurosurgical intensive care unit and then quickly mobilized the next day. We have typically left the skin sutures in place for 10 to 14 days.

◆ Conclusions

The STA-MCA anastomosis represents the most commonly performed EC-IC bypass. The basic microsurgical techniques employed in this operation can be mastered in the laboratory prior to entering the operating room. Because of the very small size of the vessels being anastomosed, continued practice is required to achieve and maintain facility with this operation. In particular, the procedure should be performed on a regular basis to optimize bypass patency rates and to limit complications. The organized microvascular surgeon will establish a methodical and reproducible operative technique that will yield good surgical results in most cases.

References

1. Yasargil MG, Yonekawa Y. Results of microsurgical extra-intracranial arterial bypass in the treatment of cerebral ischemia. Neurosurgery 1977;1(1):22–24
2. Sundt TM Jr, Whisnant JP, Fode NC, Piepgras DG, Houser OW. Results, complications, and follow-up of 415 bypass operations for occlusive disease of the carotid system. Mayo Clin Proc 1985;60(4):230–240
3. Gratzl O, Schmiedek P, Spetzler R, Steinhoff H, Marguth F. Clinical experience with extra-intracranial arterial anastomosis in 65 cases. J Neurosurg 1976;44(3):313–324
4. Chater N. Neurosurgical extracranial-intracranial bypass for stroke: with 400 cases. Neurol Res 1983;5(2):1–9
5. The EC/IC Bypass Study Group. Failure of extracranial-intracranial arterial bypass to reduce the risk of ischemic stroke: results of an international randomized trial. N Engl J Med 1985;313(19):1191–1200
6. EC/IC Bypass Study Group. The International Cooperative Study of Extracranial/Intracranial Arterial Anastomosis (EC/IC Bypass Study): methodology and entry characteristics. Stroke 1985;16(3):397–406
7. Ausman JI, Diaz FG. Critique of the extracranial-intracranial bypass study. Surg Neurol 1986;26(3):218–221
8. Awad IA, Spetzler RF. Extracranial-intracranial bypass surgery: a critical analysis in light of the International Cooperative Study. Neurosurgery 1986;19(4):655–664
9. Day AL, Rhoton AL Jr, Little JR. The extracranial-intracranial bypass study. Surg Neurol 1986;26(3):222–226
10. Amin-Hanjani S, Butler WE, Ogilvy CS, Carter BS, Barker FG II. Extracranial-intracranial bypass in the treatment of occlusive cerebrovascular disease and intracranial aneurysms in the United States between 1992 and 2001: a population-based study. J Neurosurg 2005;103(5):794–804
11. Nussbaum ES, Erickson DL. Extracranial-intracranial bypass for ischemic cerebrovascular disease refractory to maximal medical therapy. Neurosurgery 2000;46(1):37–42
12. Nussbaum ES, Janjua TM, Defillo A, Lowary JL, Nussbaum LA. Emergency extracranial-intracranial bypass surgery for acute ischemic stroke. J Neurosurg 2010;112(3):666–673

Chapter 6

High-Flow Cerebral Revascularization with Radial Artery and Saphenous Vein Grafts

Christopher S. Eddleman, Gregory A. Dumanian, Bernard R. Bendok, and H. Hunt Batjer

Cerebral revascularization—providing additional cerebral blood flow from an alternative source through an in situ or harvested vascular graft—may be required to maintain adequate cerebral perfusion in the treatment of complex intracranial vascular problems.[1–3] Further, challenging vascular cases that will require prolonged temporary occlusion times or risk parent artery sacrifice may require prophylactic augmentation of collateral cerebral blood flow. Several options are available for cerebral revascularization that can involve both in situ or harvested vascular grafts: superficial temporal artery (STA), occipital artery, radial artery, and saphenous vein (SV) are the most common.[1] Careful patient selection has proven to be the most prominent predictor of successful revascularization strategies. Criteria for cerebral revascularization include determining who actively needs flow augmentation, the amount of blood flow required, namely low- or high-flow, and where it should be delivered. Low-flow revascularization is the most common and typically involves either the STA or occipital artery. However, some procedures require the sacrifice of a large parent artery, such as the internal carotid or vertebral artery, and thus may require more cerebral blood flow for adequate revascularization, especially if minimal collateral reserve after parent artery occlusion is demonstrated via a balloon trial occlusion (BTO).[4] In these cases, high-flow revascularization is typically required and either a radial artery or SV graft would be an appropriate choice to provide adequate cerebral perfusion with or without interposition grafting.

◆ Indications for High-Flow Bypass

As endovascular techniques have become more widely available in the treatment of vascular lesions, the types of lesions requiring surgical intervention are likely more complex in nature. Despite the fact that most vascular lesions do not require parent artery sacrifice, many lesions require complex clip reconstruction techniques requiring extended temporary artery occlusion times. For example, large or giant aneurysms of the middle cerebral artery (MCA) bi-/trifurcation may have branches originating from the fundus or close to the neck. In addition, the failure of endovascular techniques for complex vascular lesions can require more complex vascular reconstructions and/or endovascular material extraction at retreatment, necessitating longer occlusion times and possible cerebral revascularization.

Patients with complex vascular lesions are initially evaluated by a multidisciplinary team of neurosurgeons and neuroradiologists. If it is surmised that either long temporary occlusion times or parent artery sacrifice might be necessary, the patient is scheduled to undergo a BTO (**Table 6.1**). After diagnostic angiography is completed, a balloon is placed just proximal to the lesion in question, either in an extracranial or intracranial location. After temporary occlusion, the vascular reserve is determined angiographically, mainly from the leptomeningeal and circle of Willis vessels and subsequently the flow dynamics including venous washout are carefully studied. Although angiographic study of the collateral circulation around a particular lesion is helpful, it does not provide a clinical assessment of the patient's potential cerebral blood flow requirements. To determine clinically significant changes regarding the need for reserve flow, the BTO includes clinical examinations, electroencephalogram (EEG), hypotensive challenges with clinical examinations, and single photon emission computed tomography (SPECT) imaging after performance of the BTO and removal of the balloon. Clinical exams are performed at baseline and every 5 minutes after balloon inflation. If the patient tolerates all forms of clinical testing, then prophylactic bypass grafting is likely unnecessary, and the parent artery in question can be sacrificed with minimal perioperative risk. If the patient tolerates the clinical exams but not the hypotensive challenge

Table 6.1 Bypass Indication from Balloon Trial Occlusion Results

Bypass Procedure Indicated	BTO and SPECT Results
PAO without bypass	No clinical failure to balloon occlusion; no SPECT abnormalities
Low-flow bypass	Failure to tolerate balloon occlusion during hypotensive state with or without EEG changes; no SPECT abnormalities
High-flow bypass	Failure of all clinical exams; SPECT abnormalities

Abbreviations: PAO, parent artery sacrifice; BTO, balloon trial occlusion; EEG, electroencephalogram; SPECT, single photon emission computed tomography.

or demonstrates asymmetric cerebral blood flow on SPECT, then we feel the patient would benefit from a low-flow revascularization procedure. However, if the patient experiences deficits at normotension (120–140 systolic) during the BTO, he or she should undergo a high-flow bypass, usually using a radial artery or SV.[4]

◆ Perioperative Considerations

Patients undergoing revascularization procedures are usually placed on aspirin therapy before or immediately after the revascularization procedure. In cases of hypercholesterolemia, a statin can be administered preoperatively and postoperatively, which has been suggested to affect long-term graft patency.[1,3,5] All patients receive preoperative antibiotics within one hour prior to incision. The utilization of a neuroanesthesia team has several advantages during all phases of the procedure. Throughout the procedure adequate cerebral perfusion is maintained as well as optimal brain relaxation, which reduces the necessity of brain retraction. Postoperatively, controlled emergence from anesthesia is important so that an adequate neurologic exam can be completed without compromise of the bypass graft. Intraoperative neurophysiologic monitoring is also performed, which includes EEG and somatosensory evoked potentials (SSEPs). Other neuromonitoring, such as brainstem evoked potentials or cranial nerve monitoring, may be employed depending on the site of surgery and necessity of cranial nerve manipulation. Intraoperative graft patency monitoring can be done with indocyanine green (ICG) videoangiography, micro-Doppler ultrasound, or intraoperative angiography.

The patient is positioned with regard to the side of the lesion and the anastomosis site. For anterior circulation lesions, the patient is placed supine with the head turned to the opposite side of the lesion. The vascular grafts are often harvested from the opposite side of the lesion. For posterior circulation lesions, the patient is often placed in the lateral position. The radial artery in these cases is taken from the recumbent arm. The choice of the anastomosis site is selected based on the location of the lesion, intended territory of revascularization, and properties of the donor and recipient vessels. Lesions located on the M1 and P1 segments may require prophylactic bypass due to the frequent presence of perforating vessels and low tolerance of temporary occlusion in these territories.

◆ Bypass Graft Selection

For high-flow bypass procedures, the conduits of choice are the radial artery and the SV, both of which can, in most cases, be easily harvested from the patient being treated. Each graft type has advantages and disadvantages and both have significantly different biologic properties that must be accounted for not only during the selection, but also in regard to long-term patency. Each graft is discussed below.

The radial artery has a flow rate ranging between 40 and 150 mL/min and a diameter between 2.5 and 3.5 mm.[1,3] The advantages of the radial artery are that this conduit is normally equipped to handle arterial blood flow. It has a homogeneous intraluminal diameter without valves or varicosities. The smooth laminar blood flow is thought to reduce the incidence of thrombosis that can occur during temporary occlusion or a low-flow state. Furthermore, the luminal diameter more closely matches that of the M2 segment of the MCA and the P2 segment of the posterior carotid artery (PCA) than a vein graft. It has a predictable anatomic location that with training is straightforward to harvest, either with open or endovascular techniques. The main disadvantage of the radial artery is the potential for vasospasm, which often occurs following harvest; however, this can be reduced with preimplantation distension and maintenance of the graft in a solution of calcium channel blockers prior to implantation. There have been reports that the long-term patency of radial artery grafts is threatened by the loss of the vasa vasorum, which is disrupted during dissection. However, preserving the surrounding venous plexus at the time of radial artery harvest has certain technical disadvantages such as the resistance of twisting and kinking. A separate venous anastomosis between the vena comitantes and a neck vein will drain the venous system, allow vascularization of the tissues surrounding the radial artery, and essentially create a miniature free flap out of the radial artery and its surrounding tissue.[6] We believe this technique reduces the incidence of postoperative vasospasm and increases viability.

The SV has a flow rate between 70 and 200 mL/min and an average diameter of ~5 mm.[1,5] The advantages of the SV graft are the ease of harvest, length of graft, absence of atherosclerotic changes, and large caliber. The disadvantages of SV grafts are frequent caliber mismatch, which can lead to intraluminal turbulent flow and thrombosis; the presence of valves; and the potential for kinking at the site of the recipient due to the thick surrounding tissue and vessel wall. Maintenance of the vessel orientation of SV grafts is critical for their functionality and durability as a vascular conduit.

Both vessels require two separate anastomoses (**Fig. 6.1**) and separate incisions for graft harvest, which increases the potential for complications. Long-term patency has not been directly compared between the radial artery and SV

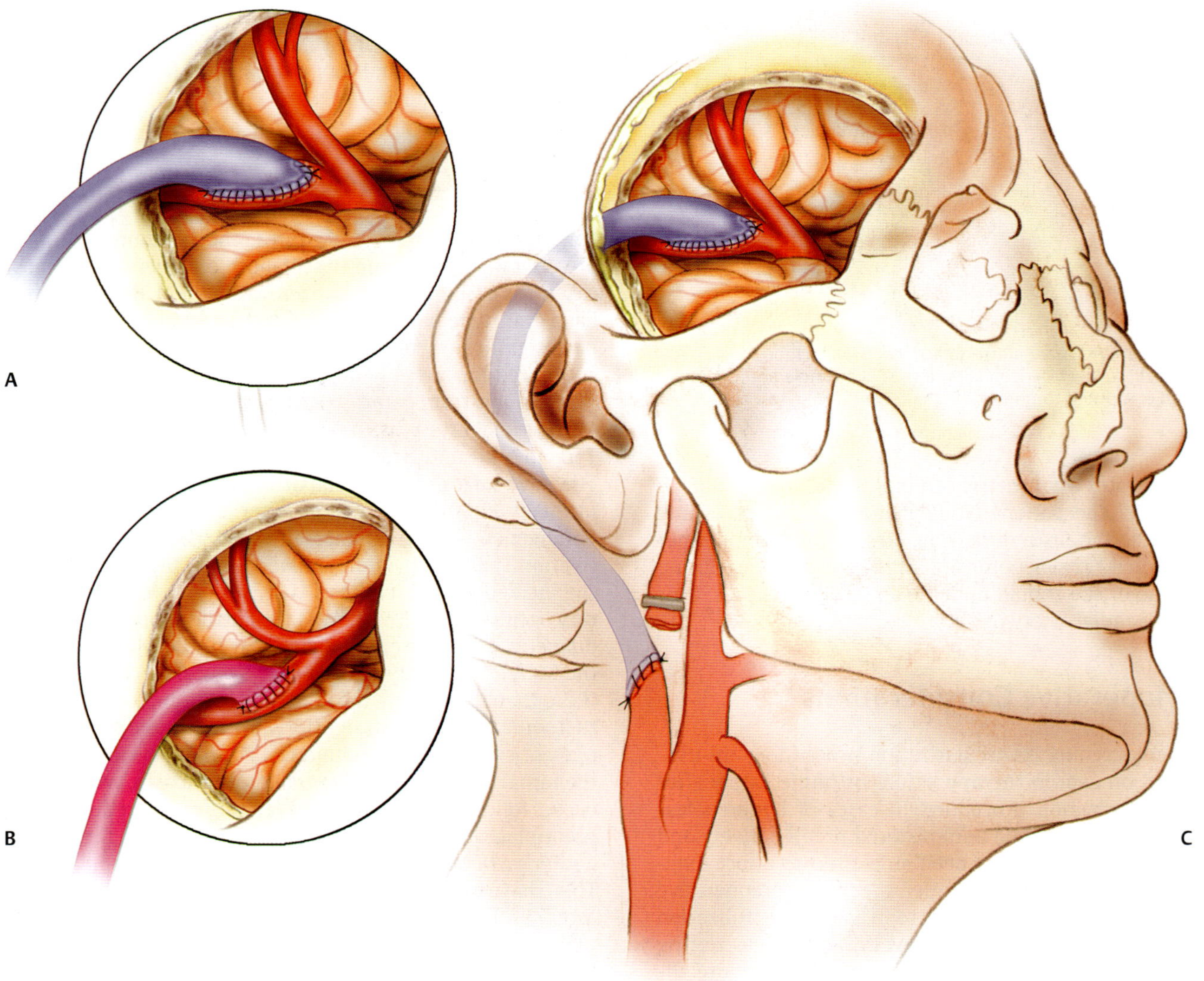

Fig. 6.1 Illustration demonstrating the distal (saphenous vein **[A]** and radial artery **[B]**) and proximal anastomosis **(C)**.

conduits. However, average patency rate at 5 years postimplantation has been reported to be ~90% for radial artery grafts and ~80% for SV grafts. In the coronary literature, radial arteries have been consistently reported to have higher patency rates than SVs.[1,5,7]

◆ Radial Artery Graft

Before harvesting the radial artery, the presence of adequate perfusion of the hand must be confirmed by physical examination. First, the Allen test must show refilling of the hand vasculature with compression of the radial artery at the wrist. Second, filling of the hand capillary bed with compression of the ulnar artery will confirm the patency of the radial system. This is to ensure that a previous radial arterial puncture did not cause injury to the radial artery at the wrist. If there is any uncertainty, the flow within both arteries can be measured in the noninvasive vascular laboratory. It should be remembered that the radial artery is the dominant vessel for hand blood flow, and that this radial artery dominance increases with age.[8]

If both arms have similar physical examinations demonstrating the availability of the radial artery for harvest, typically the nondominant hand is chosen. The harvest begins after the neurosurgeon confirms that the bypass graft is needed and will be used. An incision is made between the brachioradialis and the flexor carpi radialis muscles. The use of a tourniquet facilitates the preservation of small crossing subcutaneous veins, but perhaps increases the chance of a side branch bleeding after revascularization of the brain. Crossing lateral antebrachial cutaneous nerves near the wrist are one source of morbidity of radial artery harvest.[9] The radial artery, vena comitantes, and surrounding fat are harvested as one unit (**Fig. 6.2**). Side branches emerging from this tissue are divided between snaps and ties. Metallic vessel clips are typically added to the ties to ensure that the vessel will remain hemostatic. The dissection proceeds from the palmar cutaneous branch distally to the radial recurrent branch around the elbow proximally. Visualization of the take-off of the ulnar artery and anterior interosseous arteries is helpful to confirm a viable forearm and hand after radial artery harvest.

Once the entire radial artery/venous comitantes system has been dissected free, the artery and veins are divided at the wrist, and a microarterial bulldog clamp is atraumatically applied to the end of the artery. Perfusion against an end-artery tends to break any spasm that develops during

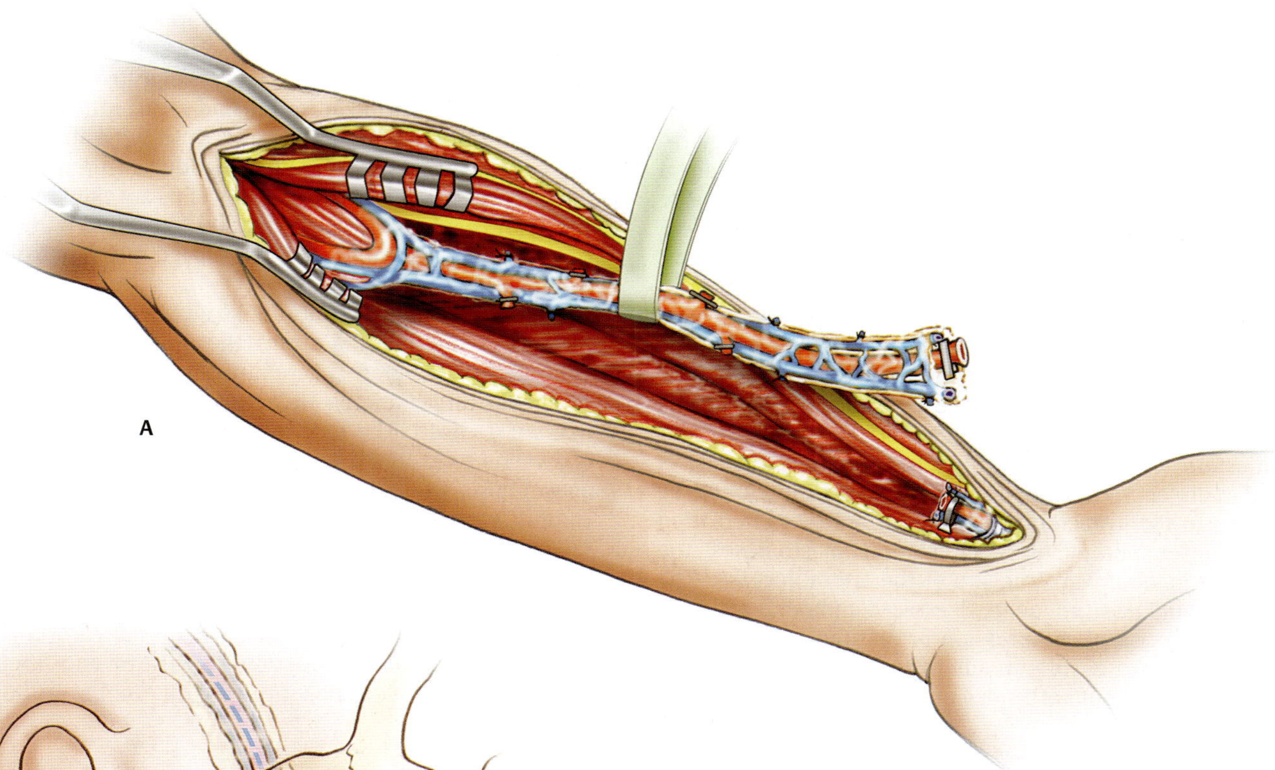

A

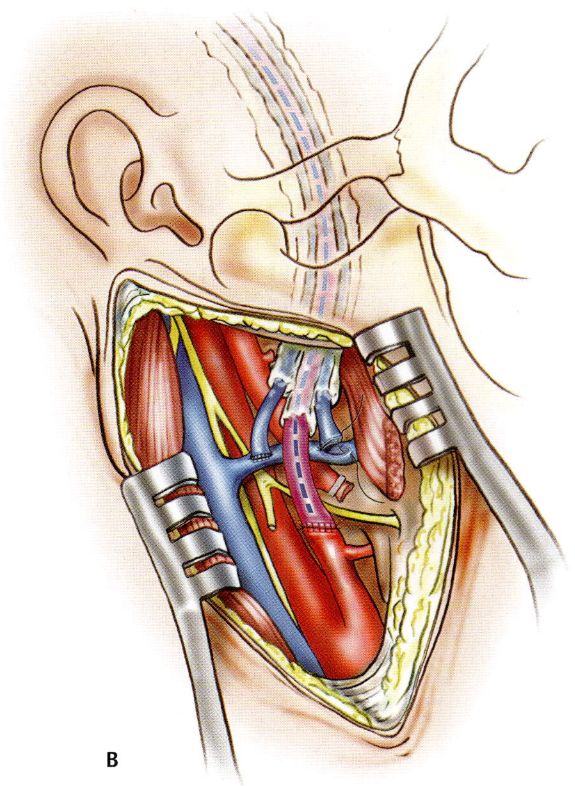

B

Fig. 6.2 Radial artery harvest. **(A)** Radial artery graft unit including the surrounding vena comitantes. **(B)** Proximal anastomosis of radial artery graft including both arterial and venous anastomoses.

dissection. Topical papaverine also tends to break spasm. When the artery visually is dilated, the proximal aspects of the artery and vena comitantes are divided between clips and ties. The radial artery is irrigated with dilute heparinized saline (100 U/mL) and placed in a heparinized sponge.[10] The lumen is flushed with heparinized saline using a small blunt needle tip. The radial artery graft is then distended to test the occlusion of the branches by occluding one end and injected gently with the heparinized saline for distension. We typically mark the artery with blue ink along its entire course to guard against twisting in its subcutaneous tunnel. The arm is closed in one layer over a drain, and a gentle ace bandage applied. Assessment of hand capillary refill must be made after application of the bandage to ensure adequate filling from the ulnar artery. Under the operating room microscope, the ends of the radial artery are prepared by removing the adventitia at both ends for ~10 mm. The distal end is cut at an angle (beveled) and a fishmouth cut is made if the graft is smaller than 3.5 to 4 mm. The radial artery graft is maintained in a basin until use containing calcium-channel blocking agents and heparin.[10]

Both the intracranial and cervical dissections are performed first so that the bypass procedure flows efficiently without delay and unnecessary prolonged occlusion times. Subsequently, we prefer to make the subcutaneous tunnel for the bypass graft. A large Betcher clamp (a long, slender hemostatic clamp with narrow, round-tipped blades) is used to dissect the tunnel from running just superior to the zygoma to the intracranial incision for anterior circulation anastomoses. For posterior circulation anastomoses, the tunnel is made toward the site of the lateral incision. The tunnel should be an adequate size to accommodate the graft without the risk of compression or resistance when passing the graft. To ensure an adequate tunnel size, we pass our fifth digits from both sides until they touch each other. We subsequently pass a Penrose drain in the tunnel space for subsequent use.

We prefer to perform the intradural anastomosis first. The arteriotomy in the recipient vessel should be at least 3 to 4 mm to accommodate the radial artery graft. Anchoring sutures should be placed at the anastomotic ends initially (**Fig. 6.3A**). We like to use 10-0 suture, which is ideal for the recipient vessel. The contralateral side is sutured first (**Fig. 6.3B**). Either a running or interrupted suture technique is acceptable. After the back wall has been completed, the anastomosis is examined to ensure that there has not been suturing of the opposing arterial wall (**Fig. 6.3C**). The ipsilateral wall is then sutured (**Fig. 6.3D**). Before the last sutures are placed, the graft is once again flushed with heparinized saline and redistended. A clip is placed onto the radial artery graft flush with anastomosis site to prevent leakage and blood products from pooling in the graft (**Fig. 6.3E**). The temporary clips are then removed. The graft is again flushed, distended, and filled with heparinized saline. A temporary clip is placed ~10 mm from the proximal end.

The patient is systemically anticoagulated to prevent graft thrombosis and clotting during the proximal anastomosis. The radial artery graft is carefully passed through the subcutaneous tunnel and positioned near the site of the proximal anastomosis. The blue ink line allows the assessment of a vessel twist in the tunnel. The most common proximal anastomosis sites at our institution are the ICA, external carotid artery (ECA), common carotid artery (CCA), or vertebral artery (VA). The arteriotomy in the proximal vessel should be 6 to 8 mm. When anastomosing to the carotid circulation, the site of anastomosis is usually just distal to the superior thyroid artery on the external carotid artery (**Fig. 6.3**). We prefer the anastomosis to be an end-to-end to the ECA using beveled ends sutured with running 6-0 suture.

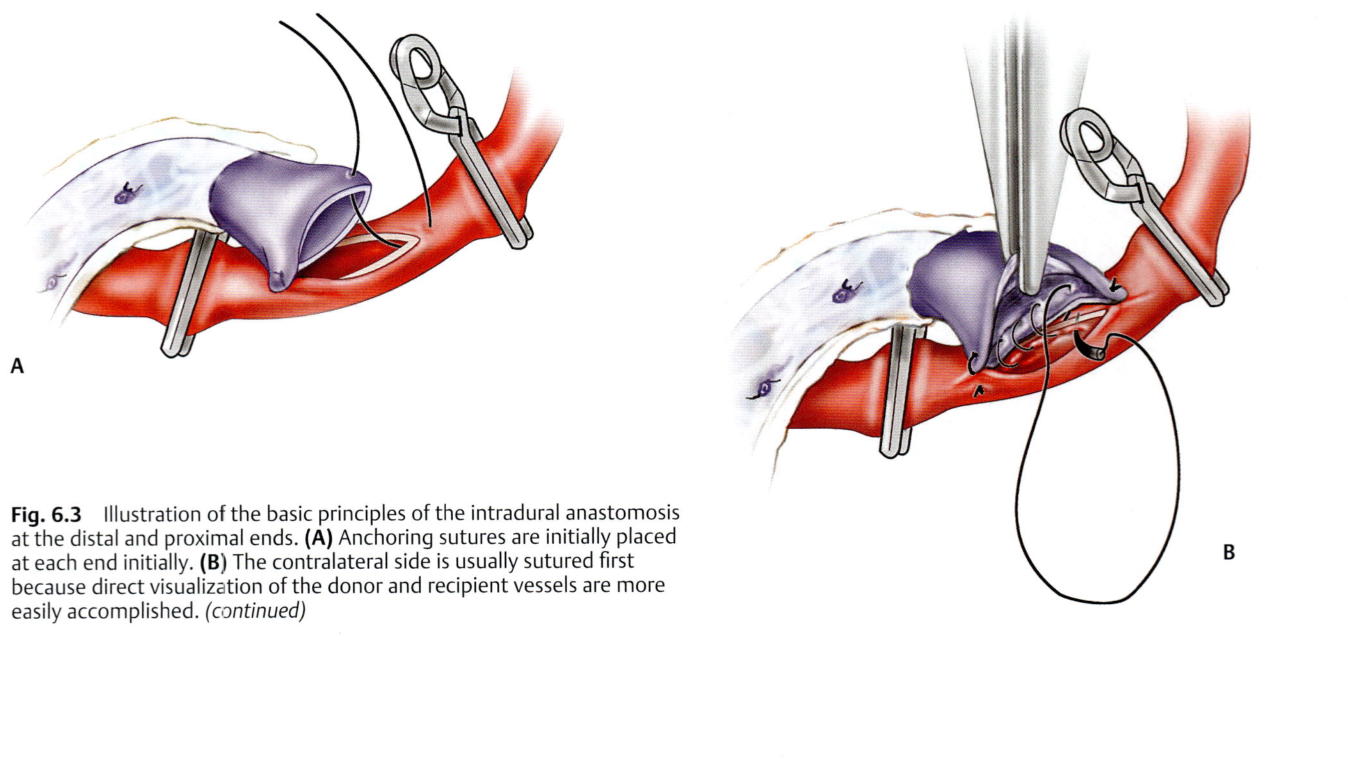

Fig. 6.3 Illustration of the basic principles of the intradural anastomosis at the distal and proximal ends. **(A)** Anchoring sutures are initially placed at each end initially. **(B)** The contralateral side is usually sutured first because direct visualization of the donor and recipient vessels are more easily accomplished. *(continued)*

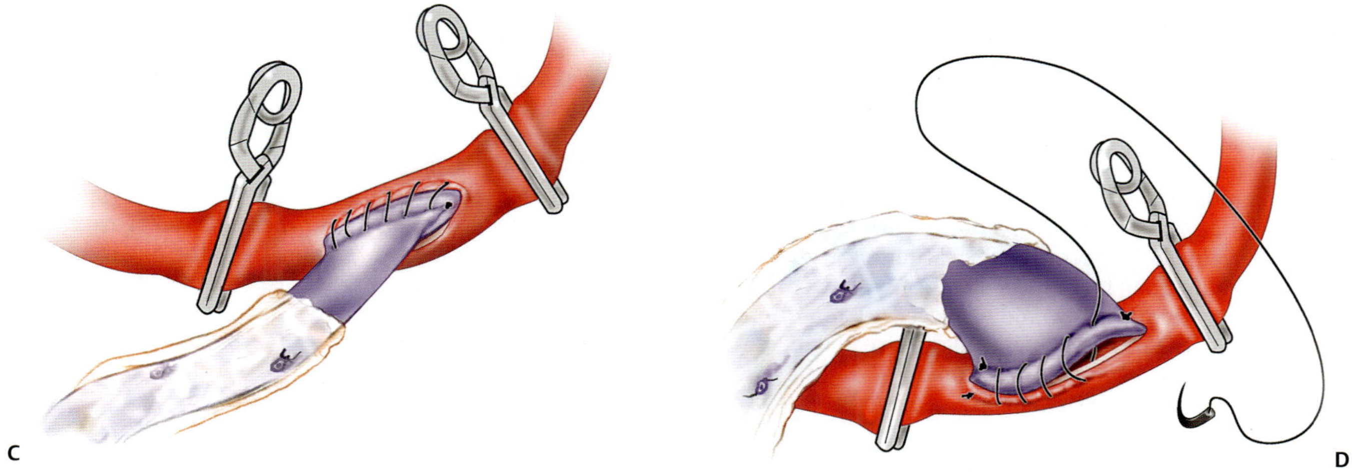

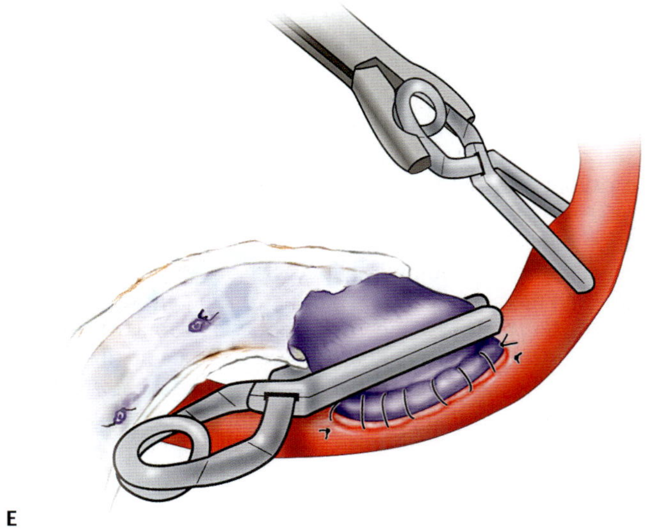

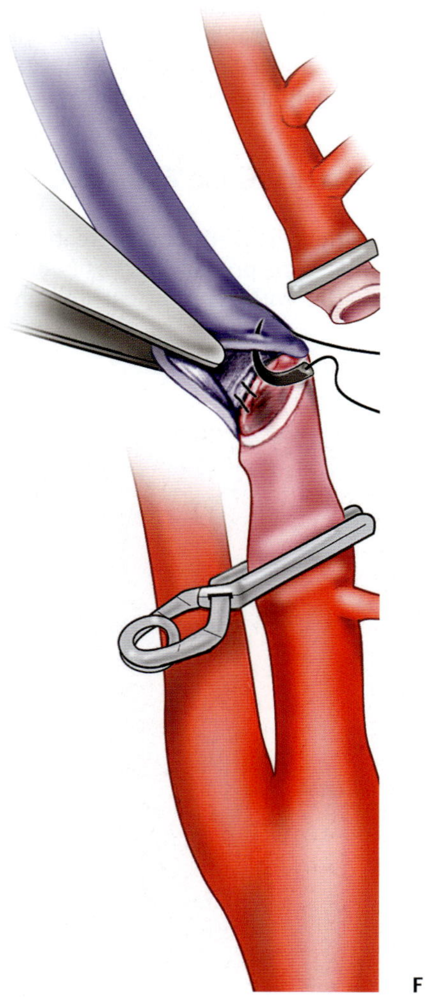

Fig. 6.3 *(continued)* **(C)** After the contralateral side is sutured, the graft is flipped over to ensure that the suture line does not contain gaps or unnecessary tissue. **(D)** The ipsilateral side is then sutured. **(E)** After completion of the anastomosis, a clip is placed near the anastomosis site to ensure that blood products do not enter the graft after the temporary clips are removed. **(F)** Illustration of the extracranial carotid artery anastomosis site, just distal to the origin of the superior thyroid artery.

In the posterior circulation, we prefer an end-to-side sutured with running 10-0 suture to the recipient vessel of choice, most commonly the VA just distal to the origin of PICA.

In some cases, the length of the graft is not sufficient to reach the proximal anastomotic site due to a deep distal anastomosis. In these cases, we prefer to use an interposition graft that can be any of the above grafts discussed. The most common would be the STA. The graft would be harvested and an end-to-end anastomosis with the radial artery graft would be performed using a running 10-0 suture. The graft would again be flushed and filled with heparinized saline and a proximal clip would be placed 10 mm from the proximal end. The proximal end would be treated in a similar fashion with respect to the anastomosis.

Before the distal bypass graft clip is removed, the vena comitantes of the radial artery is further prepared and cleared of fat and adventitia (**Fig. 6.2A**). Any nearby vein in the neck will handle the low flow in the system (**Fig. 6.2B**). We prefer a running end-to-side anastomosis with 10-0 suture, but anastomotic coupling devices can also be used. After completion of the venous anastomosis, the proximal arterial clip is released, thus allowing back bleeding into the graft, which removes most of the residual air in the graft. After inspection of the graft, including evaluation for suture line and kinking, the distal clip is removed. Doppler flow measurements can be used to check pulsation and distal flow.

◆ Radial Artery Case Example

A 54-year-old right-handed man presented to the neurosurgical clinic with the primary complaint of left-sided progressive headache with intermittent episodes of aphasia. Computed tomography angiography (CTA) scan of the head demonstrated a large mass, which partially filled with contrast. A subsequent magnetic resonance imaging (MRI) scan and cerebral angiogram demonstrated a partially thrombosed left MCA aneurysm (**Fig. 6.4**). The patient underwent a BTO, after which he failed to demonstrate adequate collateral flow and also had an asymmetric SPECT scan. A radial artery bypass was chosen. The patient underwent a left modified pterional craniotomy where the radial artery was anastomosed to a distal M2 branch and the aneurysm was trapped. A venous anastomosis was constructed to the facial vein to support the radial artery graft (**Fig. 6.5**).

◆ Saphenous Vein Graft

As with the radial artery, the SV, in the adult leg, can be found with ultrasound prior to the procedure and is normally harvested from the side opposite to the site of revascularization. The greater SV normally runs just anteromedial to the tibia at the ankle and gradually travels more posterior toward the knee and finally posterior to the adductor tubercle in the lower thigh where it then courses proximally along the lateral surface of the femoral artery. The SV is more uniform in caliber and shape in the lower thigh and upper leg. Because the SV is easily identified distally, near the ankle, isolation of the SV is started there. As the SV is dissected, the branches are ligated and divided. It is not recommended to go much further beyond the adductor tubercle as the drainage of the thigh becomes more dependent on the femoral vein. Due to the presence of valves, the distal end of the graft is normally marked with a suture to assure the correct orientation. The graft is removed and placed in a basin filled

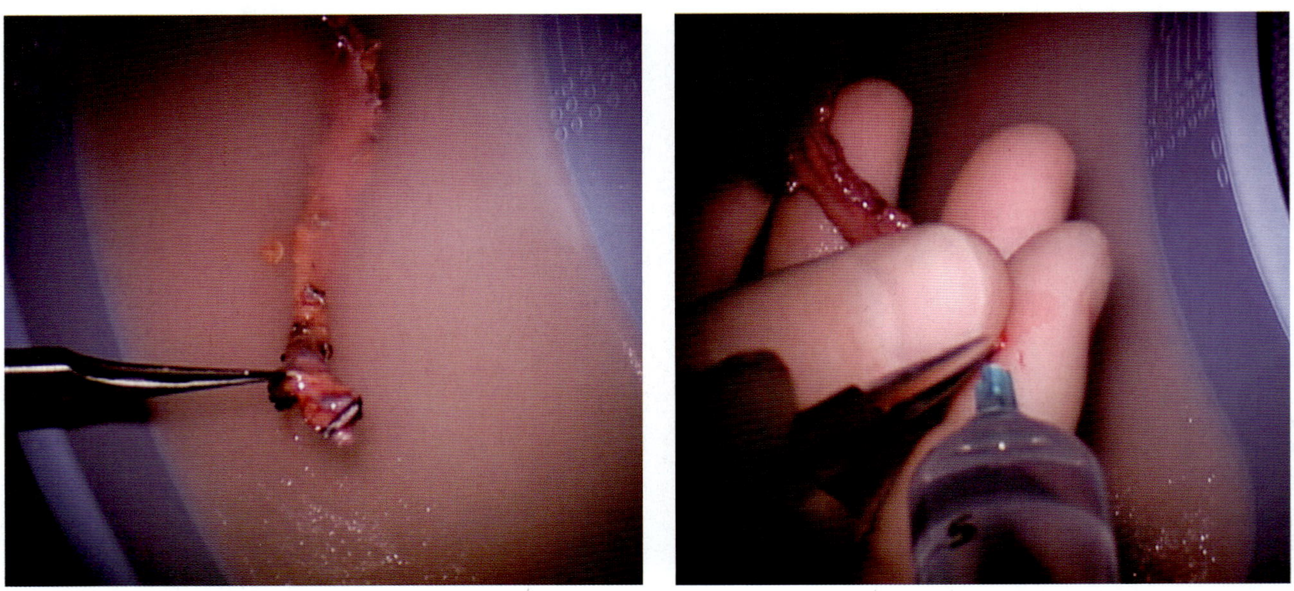

A B

Fig. 6.4 Radial artery bypass graft. **(A)** Harvest radial artery graft in basin. Small clips were used to ligate side branches. Note the presence of surrounding tissue and the vena comitantes around the artery. **(B)** Preimplantation distension using heparinized saline.

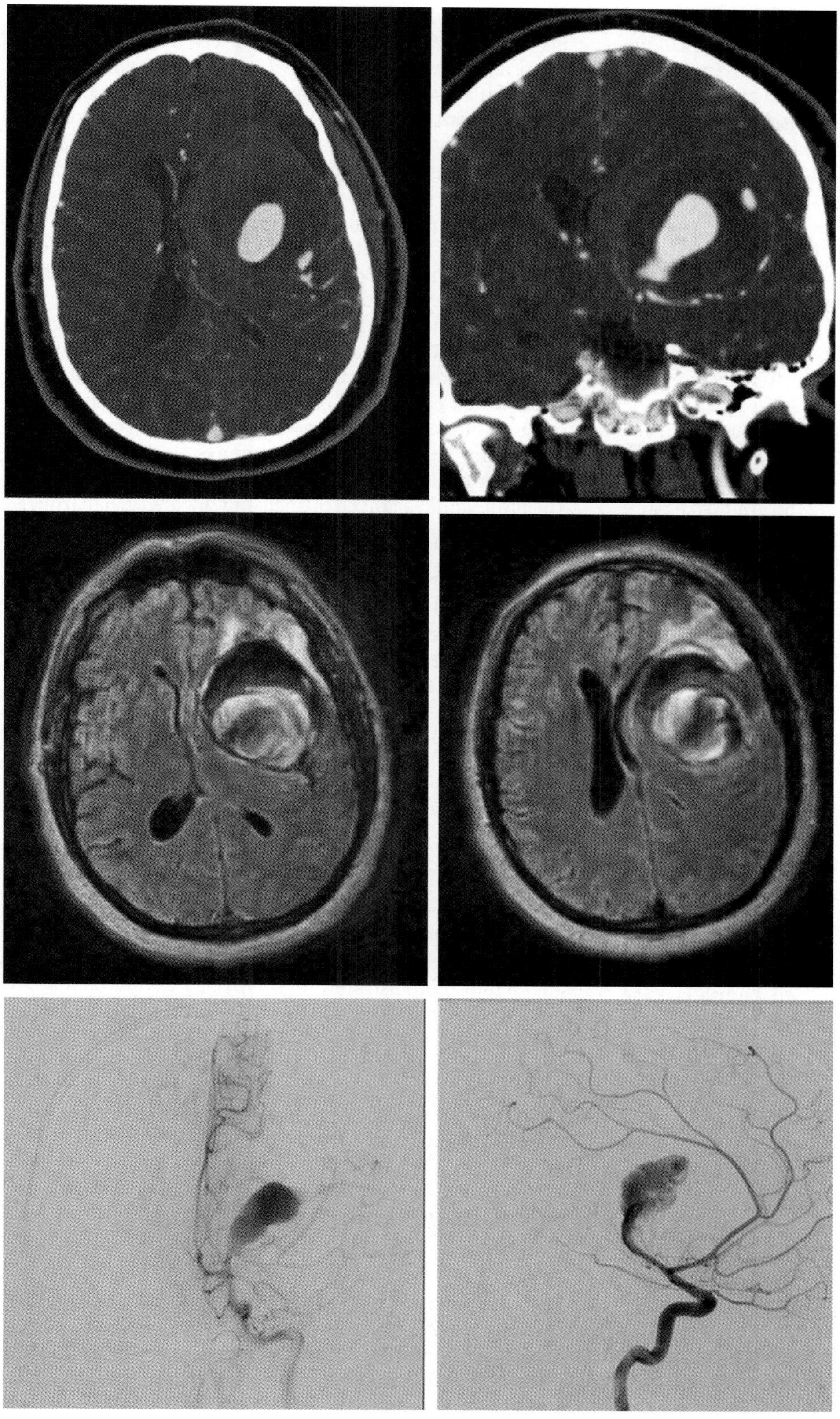

A B C D E F

Fig. 6.5 Preoperative imaging of 54-year-old patient with giant left-sided middle cerebral artery aneurysm. Axial **(A)** and coronal **(B)** planes of the CTA demonstrating partial filling of contrast into the giant partially thrombosed MCA aneurysm. Midline shift and mass effect are also demonstrated. **(C,D)** Axial cuts of the FLAIR MRI demonstrating aneurysmal thrombus as well as focal edema in the surrounding parenchymal tissue. AP **(E)** and lateral **(F)** views of the left internal carotid artery injection digital subtraction angiogram demonstrating the filling characteristics of the giant MCA aneurysm.

with heparinized saline. The adventitia is carefully removed. The tissue is very thick and requires tedious and meticulous care. It is very important for this adventitia to be removed as the suture will become embedded in the surrounding tissue. The orientation of the vein is reconfirmed by flushing saline through the graft and assessing ease of flow. A blue ink line is place on the graft to allow assessment of twisting when passed through the subcutaneous tunnel. The SV graft is maintained in the basin until use.

Both the intracranial and cervical dissections are performed first so that the bypass procedure flows efficiently without delay and unnecessary prolonged occlusion times. Subsequently, we prefer to make the subcutaneous tunnel for the bypass graft first. A large Betcher clamp is used to dissect the tunnel from running just superior to the zygoma to the intracranial incision for anterior circulation anastomoses. For posterior circulation anastomoses, the tunnel is made toward the site of the lateral incision. The tunnel should be an adequate size to accommodate the graft without the risk of compression or resistance when passing the graft. To ensure an adequate tunnel size, we pass our fifth digits from both sides until they touch each other. We subsequently pass a Penrose drain in the tunnel space for future use.

The arteriotomy in the recipient vessel will be greater than that of the radial artery and at least 4 to 5 mm to accommodate the SV graft (**Fig. 6.3**). Anchoring sutures should be placed at the anastomotic ends initially (**Fig. 6.3A**). We like to use a running 10-0 Prolene due the thickness of the graft adventitial tissue and frequent passing of tissue into the suture line with other suture types. The Proline suture passes through the tissue easier and is much better at allowing the needle and suture to be pulled through the vessel with minimal damage to the graft. The contralateral side is sutured first (**Fig. 6.3B**). With the SV graft, the amount of graft tissue will be greater than that of the recipient. As a result, the distance between sutures in the graft will be larger than that of the recipient resulting in an undulated graft. This will ensure a better size-matched anastomotic site. Otherwise, the presence of tissue gaps will lead to leakage at the anastomotic site. After the back wall has been completed, the anastomosis is examined to ensure that there has not been suturing of the opposing arterial wall (**Fig. 6.3C**). Given the large size of the SV graft, it is important to flop the graft so that both sides of the anastomosis are clearly visible. The ipsilateral wall is then sutured (**Fig. 6.3D**). Before the last sutures are placed, the graft is once again flushed with heparinized saline and redistended. A clip is placed onto the SV graft flush with anastomosis site to prevent leakage and blood products from pooling in the graft (**Fig. 6.3E**). The temporary clips are then removed. The graft is again flushed, distended, and filled with heparinized saline. A temporary clip is placed ~10 mm from the proximal end.

With SV grafts, the patient is systemically anticoagulated to prevent graft thrombosis and clotting during the proximal anastomosis. The SV graft is positioned near the site of the estimated proximal anastomosis and trimmed to provide mild tension in the graft, as the graft will expand, sometimes significantly, after restoration of blood flow. This tension should prevent kinking at the distal anastomotic site. The most common proximal anastomosis sites at our institution are the ICA, ECA, CCA, or VA. The arteriotomy in the proximal vessel should be 6 to 8 mm. When anastomosing to the carotid circulation, the site of anastomosis, as with radial artery grafts, is usually just distal to the superior thyroid artery on the external carotid artery (**Fig. 6.3**). We prefer the anastomosis to be an end-to-end to the ECA using beveled ends sutured with running 6-0 Prolene suture. In the posterior circulation, we prefer an end-to-side sutured with running 10-0 suture to the recipient vessel of choice, most commonly the VA just distal to the origin of posterior inferior cerebellar artery (PICA).

In some cases, the length of the graft is not sufficient to reach the proximal anastomotic site due to deep distal anastomoses. In these cases, we prefer to use an interposition graft, which can be any of the grafts discussed above. The most common would be the STA. The graft would be harvested and an end-to-end anastomosis with the radial artery graft would be performed using a running 10-0 suture. The graft would again be flushed and filled with heparinized saline and a proximal clip would be placed 10 mm from the proximal end. The proximal end would be treated in a similar fashion with respect to the anastomosis.

Care should be taken to remove air from within the graft before fully releasing the proximal clips. This can be done with a syringe needle into the vein graft. After inspection of the graft, including evaluation for suture line and kinking, the distal clip is removed. Doppler flow measurements can be used to check pulsation and distal flow.

Saphenous Vein Case Example

A 35-year-old right-handed man presented to the neurosurgery clinic with severe vascular disease that included several cervical aneurysms and previously clipped right ophthalmic aneurysm. The patient complained at the time of presentation of progressive blindness in his right eye. A cerebral angiogram demonstrated regrowth of the ophthalmic aneurysm (**Fig. 6.6**). The patient underwent a BTO and failed all aspects of the clinical exams and required a high-flow bypass. Due to the patient's systemic vascular disease, it was decided to use a SV bypass graft. The aneurysm was trapped surgically after the completion of the SV bypass procedure (**Figs. 6.7** and **6.8**).

◆ Intraoperative Assessment of Bypass Patency

Intraoperative assessment of bypass patency and functionality can avoid complications due to premature graft stenosis or occlusion. Although intraoperative catheter angiograms remain the gold standard, this technique requires additional costs and risks to the patient. At our institution, we prefer bypass assessment using ICG videoangiography, which provides a quick assessment of patency with little to no risk to the patient. We can determine the direction of flow and perform multiple assessments throughout the procedure.

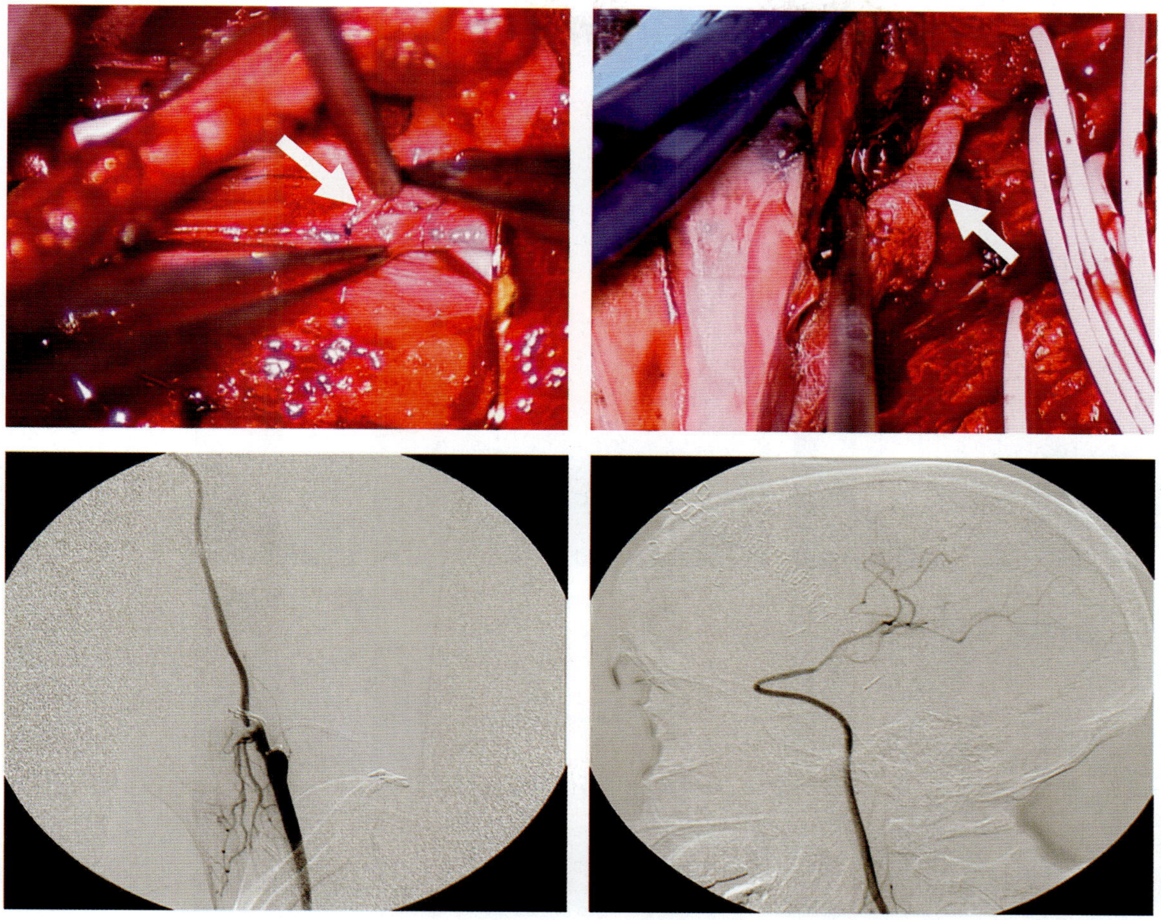

A B C D

Fig. 6.6 Intraoperative and postoperative images of the radial artery bypass procedure. **(A)** Arteriotomy (*arrow*) in the recipient left middle cerebral artery with the anchored radial artery bypass graft. **(B)** Radial artery bypass shown with surrounding tissue and the vena comitantes (*arrow*). Postoperative AP **(C)** and lateral **(D)** left carotid injection digital subtraction angiograms demonstrating patency of the radial artery graft and no residual filling of the aneurysm.

The most common site for stenosis or occlusion is the distal end of the bypass graft likely due to the amount of time of occlusion while the proximal anastomosis is being completed. In the case of stenosis or occlusion, the graft is reopened and flushed and distended with heparinized saline. If successful, the graft is again clipped, filled with saline, and the anastomosis is repeated. If clot or stenosis is still present, a Fogarty balloon may be inserted into the graft and inflated. The balloon can be carefully pulled out of the graft, thus removing any residual clot within the graft. Once the anastomosis is completed, the graft is again checked for stenosis or occlusion. Other technologies exist to assess graft patency, but we have found ICG videoangiography to be useful for patency and functionality assessment intraoperatively.

◆ Complications

Cerebral revascularization with high-flow bypass grafts is more prone to complications than their low-flow counterparts. Radial artery grafts may suffer vasospasm or intimal hyperplasia after implantation and eventually occlude. However, SV grafts can undergo proatherogenic changes after implantation eventually leading to their occlusion as well. Thromboembolic complications are the most common after bypass procedures thought due mainly to the change in intracranial hemodynamics after parent vessel occlusion. Preoperative antiplatelet medications as well as intraoperative anticoagulation can reduce these thromboembolic events. In patients without vascular reserve, prolonged temporary occlusion times can lead to territory infarcts without changes in the cerebral monitoring. It is of paramount importance to minimize occlusion times in these patients or complete the revascularization procedure initially to avoid such ischemic risks. If the perfusion defect had been longstanding, reperfusion hemorrhage may be problematic after revascularization. Although the incidence is low and can mostly be predicted on provocative imaging studies, some regions of infarcted tissue may be fragile to the point of hemorrhage after reperfusion. Other complications involve the site of graft harvest, such as infection, ischemic hand, or hematoma. Although these complications are very low, one

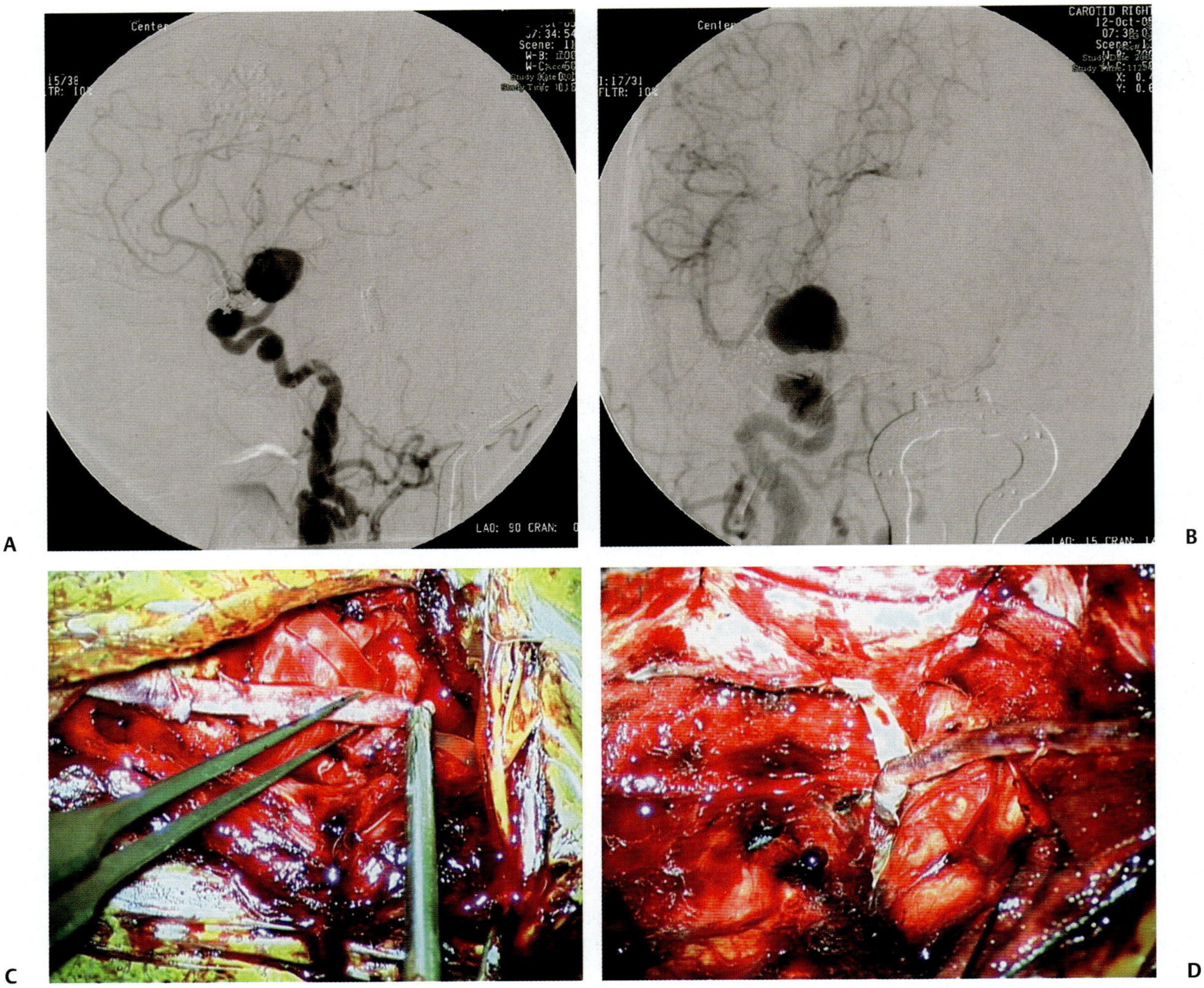

Fig. 6.7 Perioperative imaging of a 35-year-old patient with a recurrent right large ophthalmic aneurysm. Preoperative lateral **(A)** and AP **(B)** right internal carotid artery injection digital subtraction angiograms demonstrating the recurrent ophthalmic artery aneurysm. **(C)** Intraoperative photograph demonstrating the saphenous vein graft with thick associated tissue being sized to the recipient. The graft should be somewhat taut because the vein can expand after the reestablishment of flow, which can lead to kinking. **(D)** Intraoperative photograph demonstrating the final position of the saphenous vein graft.

should pay close attention to the graft harvest site and these can often be overlooked due to the focus on the cerebral manifestations of the revascularization procedure.

◆ Postoperative Considerations

Patients are maintained on aspirin therapy indefinitely and, depending on mobility, on prophylactic doses of heparin beginning 24 to 48 hours postoperatively. Patients are observed in the intensive care unit for at least 48 hours after revascularization. Blood pressure monitoring is strict and maintained at normopressure (120–140 systolic). Graft patency should be monitored closely postoperatively with Doppler evaluation at the bedside every hour for the first 24 hours, then twice a day thereafter. CTA is performed within 48 hours to assess patency. At any point during the immediate postoperative period if there is concern for the patency of the graft, a cerebral angiogram is performed. Follow-up imaging is performed at 3, 6, and 12 months after the procedure.

◆ Other Bypass Procedures

Several other bypass strategies for high-flow bypass grafts have been developed. Frequently, the length of the harvested bypass graft is not adequate for deeper recipient vessels. However, an interposition graft made from the combination of either a radial artery or SV with the STA allows deep bypass procedures to be possible. Further, for patients that cannot tolerate any length of temporary occlusion, even for the performance of a revascularization procedure, the excimer laser-assisted nonocclusive anastomosis (ELANA)

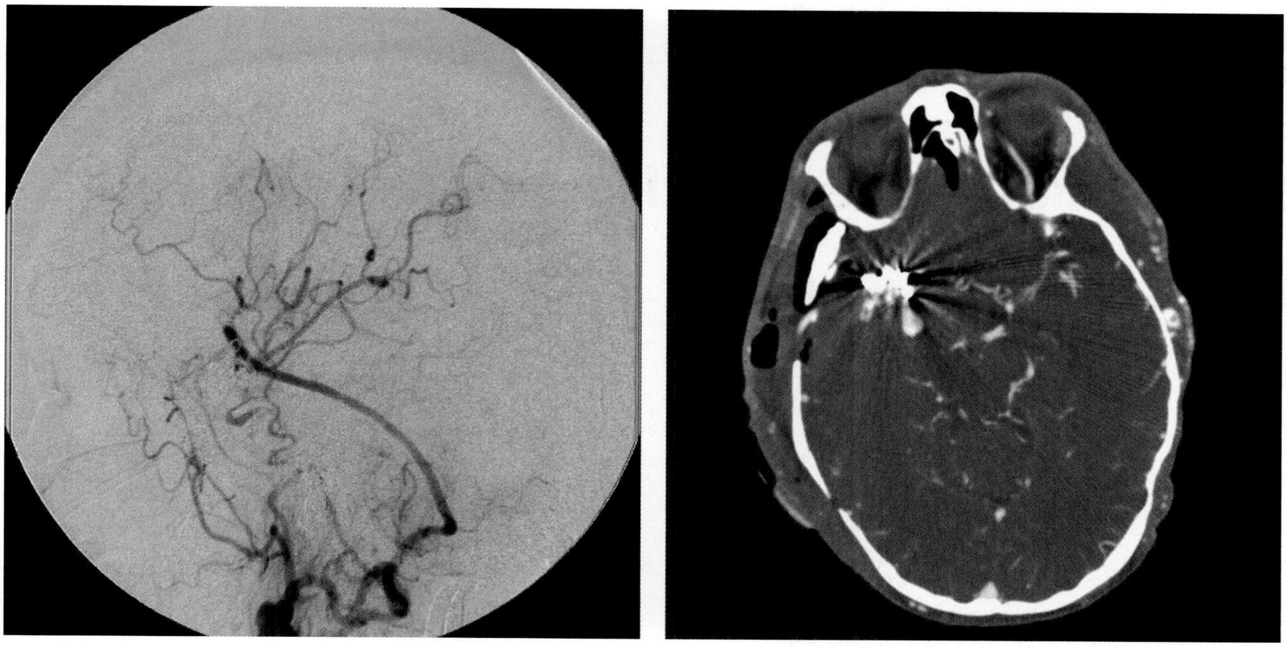

Fig. 6.8 (A) Lateral right carotid injection digital subtraction angiogram demonstrating filling of the saphenous vein bypass graft and no residual filling of the ophthalmic aneurysm. (B) Axial CTA demonstrating filling of the saphenous vein bypass graft at the site of the craniotomy.

technique can be used.[11] This technique allows the completion of a high-flow revascularization procedure using a SV graft without any temporary occlusion. Although this technique is being used more frequently, it still requires a tremendous amount of expertise.

◆ Summary

In the treatment of complex vascular disease, cerebral revascularization is necessary in case of necessary extended temporary occlusion, absence of adequate collateral reserve, and requirement of parent artery sacrifice. High-flow cerebral revascularization can be successfully completed using either harvested radial artery or saphenous vein vascular grafts. Success is dictated by careful patient selection, meticulous surgical technique, thoughtful planning and perioperative care, and mindful knowledge of the potential pitfalls and complications that can accompany cerebral revascularization procedures.

References

1. Surdell DL, Hage ZA, Eddleman CS, Gupta DK, Bendok BR, Batjer HH. Revascularization for complex intracranial aneurysms. Neurosurg Focus 2008;24(2):E21
2. Patel HC, Kirkpatrick PJ. High flow extracranial to intracranial vascular bypass procedure for giant aneurysms: indications, surgical technique, complications and outcome. Adv Tech Stand Neurosurg 2009;34:61–83
3. Kocaeli H, Andaluz N, Choutka O, Zuccarello M. Use of radial artery grafts in extracranial-intracranial revascularization procedures. Neurosurg Focus 2008;24(2):E5
4. Parkinson RJ, Bendok BR, O'Shaughnessy BA, et al. Temporary and permanent occlusion of cervical and cerebral arteries. Neurosurg Clin North Am 2005;16(2):249–256, viii viii
5. Bisson EF, Visioni AJ, Tranmer B, Horgan MA. External carotid artery to middle cerebral artery bypass with the saphenous vein graft. Neurosurgery 2008; 62(3, Suppl 1)134–138
6. Sukkar SM, Daw JA, Chandler J, Dumanian GA. Gracilis muscle free flap transfer using a radial artery/venae comitantes composite vascular pedicle. Plast Reconstr Surg 2001;108(1):156–161
7. Jafar JJ, Russell SM, Woo HH. Treatment of giant intracranial aneurysms with saphenous vein extracranial-to-intracranial bypass grafting: indications, operative technique, and results in 29 patients. Neurosurgery 2002;51:138–144
8. Dumanian GA, Segalman K, Buehner JW, Koontz CL, Hendrickson MF, Wilgis EF. Analysis of digital pulse-volume recordings with radial and ulnar artery compression. Plast Reconstr Surg 1998;102(6):1993–1998
9. Dumanian GA, Segalman K, Mispireta LA, Walsh JA, Hendrickson MF, Wilgis EF. Radial artery use in bypass grafting does not change digital blood flow or hand function. Ann Thorac Surg 1998;65(5):1284–1287
10. He GW, Yang CQ. Use of verapamil and nitroglycerin solution in preparation of radial artery for coronary grafting. Ann Thorac Surg 1996;61(2):610–614
11. Streefkerk HJ, Bremmer JP, Tulleken CA. The ELANA technique: high flow revascularization of the brain. Acta Neurochir Suppl (Wien) 2005;94:143–148

Chapter 7

Extracranial Posterior Circulation Techniques

Maria M. Toledo and Robert F. Spetzler

The surgical management of extracranial occlusive vascular disease of the vertebral artery (VA) is complex, and detailed knowledge of the anatomy of the VA is fundamental for adequate and safe treatment. With advances in the field of endovascular neurosurgery, several extracranial VA pathologic conditions are amenable to this type of treatment. The durability and overall safety of neuroendovascular therapy is still to be determined. Direct surgical approaches are complicated and are not free of risk. Therefore, these patients must be evaluated thoroughly, and the use of medical therapies (anticoagulants and/or antiplatelet therapy) must be maximized before surgery is considered.

◆ Stenosis of Proximal Subclavian Artery and Origin of Vertebral Artery

Hemodynamically, the subclavian steal syndrome is associated with proximal stenosis or occlusion of the subclavian artery and an altered blood flow pattern in the ipsilateral VA. The clinical symptoms are due to vascular insufficiency of the vertebrobasilar artery or rarely ischemia of the upper extremities. The syndrome is an important cause of transient ischemic attacks and acute episodic dizziness. Many patients with a hemodynamic subclavian steal have few or no clinical symptoms and can be treated conservatively. Recent literature indicates that subclavian steal syndrome is often asymptomatic. However, it can be associated with a wide variety of signs and symptoms of vertebrobasilar, carotid artery, or upper extremity ischemia. The manifestation of the condition depends on the collateral supply of the other cranial arteries.

Atherosclerotic disease of the origin of the VA is common. Yet, this condition will only be symptomatic if the contralateral VA is hypoplastic, occluded, ends in posterior inferior cerebellar artery (PICA) or is also severely stenotic and if the posterior communicating arteries are absent or small. Occlusion of the proximal VA is less likely to result in ischemia because of the contralateral VA and the extensive collateral supply to the upper cervical VA from the external carotid artery (ECA) and the thyrocervical and costocervical trunks. Many physicians believe that conservative treatment with antiplatelets or anticoagulation offers the best outcomes with the least risk to patients. When symptoms are refractory to best medical treatment and interfere with the patient's quality of life, endovascular or surgical treatment should be considered. Balloon angioplasty and stenting of extracranial vertebrobasilar arterial stenoses, especially with drug-eluting stents (tacrolimus), appeared to be effective in the treatment of medically resistant vertebrobasilar insufficiency. Yet, early experience suggests that the risk of angiographic and symptomatic recurrence after endovascular treatment is a concern. Long-term randomized studies are needed to establish whether such endovascular treatment will prevent stroke and in-stent restenosis of the subclavian artery and origin of the VA.

Indications for surgery in cases of subclavian steal include embolization to the brain or upper extremity despite best medical treatment, ischemia in the extremities at rest, or recurrent symptoms of vertebrobasilar insufficiency. The principle guiding therapy for this condition should be that of restoration of antegrade flow to the cerebral circulation. Ligation and endovascular occlusion of the origin of the VA are relatively simple procedures that would prevent retrograde flow from the VA to the subclavian artery. Yet, these procedures do not achieve the main goal of treatment, which is to restore antegrade flow in the VA. Proximal occlusion of the VA may be the procedure of choice for patients at high-risk for surgery because of medical conditions.

There are several surgical options for the treatment of subclavian steal, but the two most common and effective procedures are a carotid artery to subclavian artery bypass or a VA-to- common carotid artery (CCA) transposition. The carotid artery to subclavian artery bypass is technically feasible and associated with relatively low morbidity and mortality rates. It also relieves symptoms well. At our center, however, an end-to-side VA-to-CCA anastomosis (VA transposition) is the procedure of choice for treatment of both subclavian steal and stenosis of the origin of the VA and is thus described in detail. VA endarterectomy has been performed to remove plaque from the origin of the VA; however, this procedure is technically difficult to accomplish because the area is restricted and exposure is limited.[1]

A transverse skin incision is made adjacent and parallel to the upper margin of the medial third of the clavicle (**Fig. 7.1**). It begins at the sternoclavicular articulation and extends laterally for 6 cm. The platysma is incised and the anterior head of the sternocleidomastoid muscle is exposed and isolated between suture ligatures. The muscle is then divided between the ligatures, which provide hemostasis and simplify reapproximation of the cut ends during closure (**Fig. 7.2**). Because the contraction produced by the monopolar current can cause the sutures to slip, cauterization should be avoided, if possible, when the muscle is divided. The dissection proceeds deeper and medial to the trachea to expose the CCA and vagus nerve at the base of the neck (**Fig. 7.3**). The carotid sheath is entered; the internal jugular vein is retracted laterally and the CCA medially (**Fig. 7.4**). In approaches to the carotid and subclavian arteries on the left side, the surgeon must always identify the thoracic duct.[2] Multiple branches are often present and must be divided between ligatures to prevent the postoperative complications of lymphocele, cutaneous fistula, or chylothorax.

The transverse process of the C6 vertebra is identified by palpating the carotid tubercle, and the VA is identified by dissecting the space between the insertion of the anterior scalene muscle and the insertion of the longus colli muscle onto the carotid tubercle.[1] The inverted V left by the insertion of these two muscles marks the entry point of the VA into the transverse foramen. Exposure of the anterior scalene muscle and the phrenic nerve indicates that the approach is too far lateral.[2]

A large vein is usually located over the VA. When this vein is carefully moved aside, the VA can be identified. The VA is dissected proximally until its origin from the subclavian artery is reached. Another way of identifying the

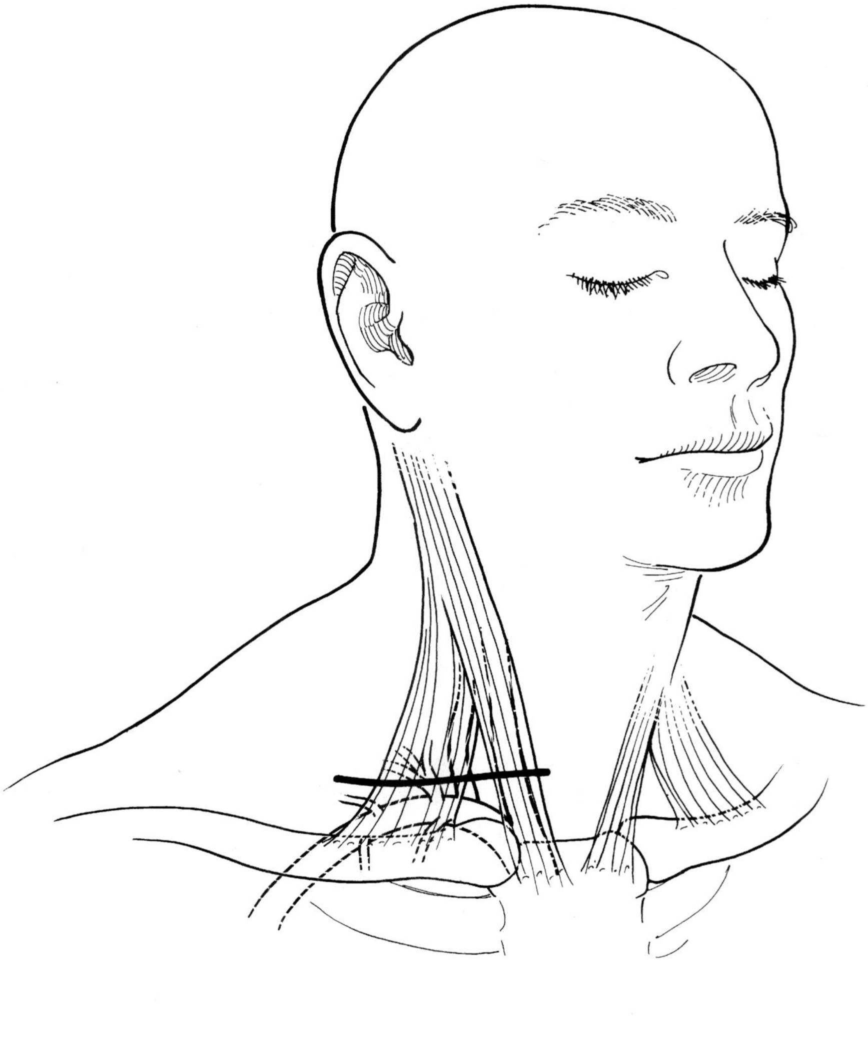

Fig. 7.1 A transverse incision is made 1 cm above and parallel to the upper margin of the medial third of the clavicle. It begins in the sternoclavicular articulation and extends laterally for 6 to 8 cm. (From Spetzler RF, Koos WT, eds. Color Atlas of Microneurosurgery. Vol 3. Intra- and Extracranial Revascularization and Intraspinal Pathology. 2nd ed. New York: Thieme; 2000:153, Case 3-12. Reprinted with permission.)

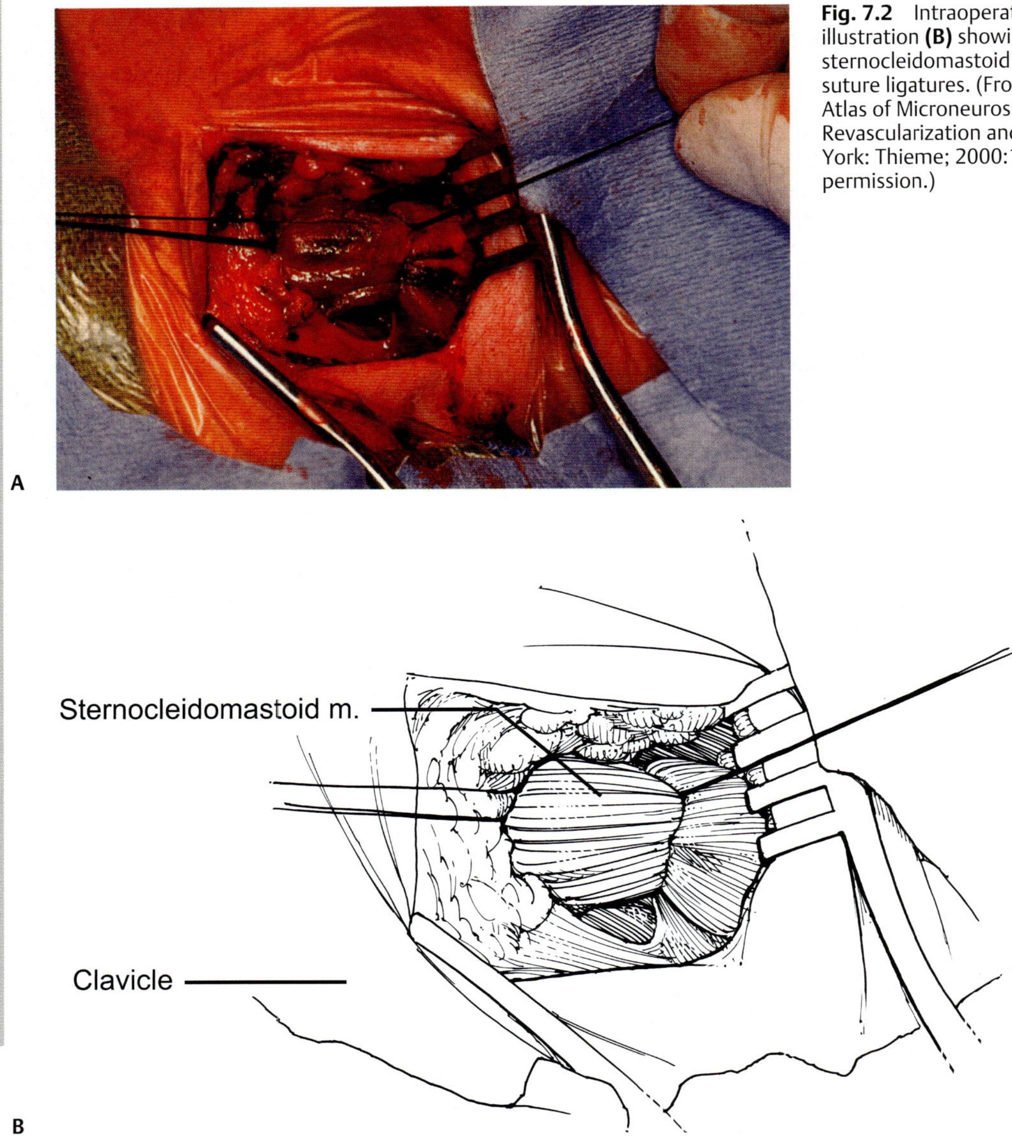

Fig. 7.2 Intraoperative photograph **(A)** and corresponding illustration **(B)** showing the anterior head of the sternocleidomastoid muscle exposed and isolated between suture ligatures. (From Spetzler RF, Koos WT, eds. Color Atlas of Microneurosurgery. Vol 3. Intra- and Extracranial Revascularization and Intraspinal Pathology. 2nd ed. New York: Thieme; 2000:153, Case 3-12b. Reprinted with permission.)

VA is to expose the subclavian artery laterally and follow the vessel until its branches are exposed (**Fig. 7.5**). The VA is the most proximal branch of the subclavian artery and exits from its posterosuperior aspect. The recurrent laryngeal nerve, the cervical sympathetic trunk, and the lower elements of the brachial plexus must be protected during the surgical exposure.

After the CCA and VA have been exposed, the patient is given 5000 units of heparin and is titrated with barbiturates to achieve electroencephalographic burst suppression. During temporary vessel occlusion, mean arterial pressure is maintained 25% above baseline. The VA is occluded with a temporary aneurysm clip as it enters the transverse foramen and doubly ligated with Weck clips as close to the subclavian artery as possible. The VA is transected just above the Weck clips and flushed with heparinized saline. When stenotic plaque is identified, it is excised by gently separating the plaque and everting the VA over the plaque until the plaque is totally removed.[1]

After its division, the VA is held adjacent to the CCA to determine whether sufficient length has been mobilized to allow an end-to-side anastomosis (**Fig. 7.6**). Should more length be required, the VA is mobilized further by opening the bony canal. As the artery enters the transverse foramen, it is surrounded by a plexus of veins that must be carefully cauterized with a bipolar and divided before the artery can be mobilized completely. A short segment of the CCA is then isolated between vascular clamps and rotated medially to expose the posterolateral surface of the vessel wall so that a circular arteriotomy can be made with an aortic punch (4 or 5 mm, tailored to the size of the VA; punches are available in 1-mm increments to match the size of the graft vessel). The

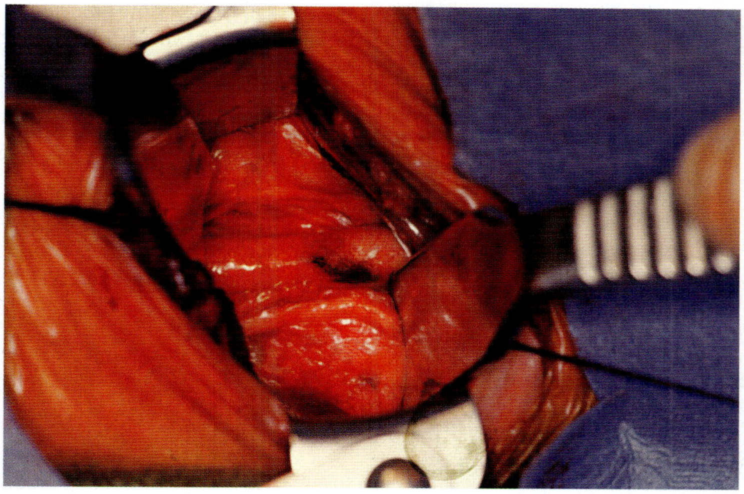

A

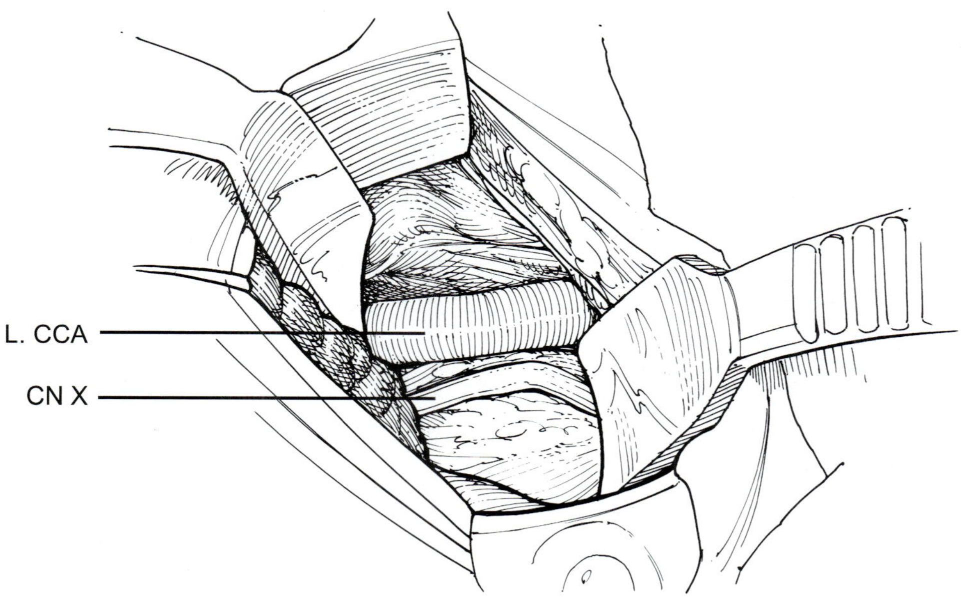

B

Fig. 7.3 Intraoperative photograph **(A)** and corresponding illustration **(B)** showing the dissection carried deeper and medial to the trachea to expose the common carotid artery and vagus nerve at the base of the neck. (From Spetzler RF, Koos WT, eds. Color Atlas of Microneurosurgery. Vol 3. Intra- and Extracranial Revascularization and Intraspinal Pathology. 2nd ed. New York: Thieme; 2000:154, Case 3-12d. Reprinted with permission.)

vagus nerve must be gently retracted medial and superior to the CCA for the anastomosis.

The end of the VA is cut obliquely, a fishmouth opening is created, and the artery is approximated to the CCA using 7-0 monofilament sutures at the superior and inferior ends of the anastomosis. The back wall of the anastomosis is closed first by suturing from the CCA to the VA while viewing the inside of the vessels. After the back wall is closed, the suture is tied to the adjacent tacking stitch. The second suture closes the front wall by inserting the needle from the VA to the CCA while viewing the outer surface of the vessels. Immediately before completing the anastomosis, the lumen is flushed with heparinized saline, and backbleeding is allowed: first from the CCA and then from the VA. The anastomosis is inspected for hemostasis (**Fig. 7.7**). Patency may be corroborated with indocyanine green (ICG) angiography. After the CCA is allowed to rotate back into its normal position, the graft is noted to arise from its posterolateral wall (**Fig. 7.8**). This position minimizes the tension on and angulation of the graft. The wound is closed after the clavicular head of the sternocleidomastoid muscle (SCM) is reapproximated to its origin.

◆ Stenosis of the Cervical Vertebral Artery

The VA, the first and usually the largest branch of the subclavian artery, is divided into four segments. The first segment extends from the origin of the VA to its entry into the intervertebral foramen of the sixth cervical vertebra. The second portion runs through the foramina of C6 through C1.

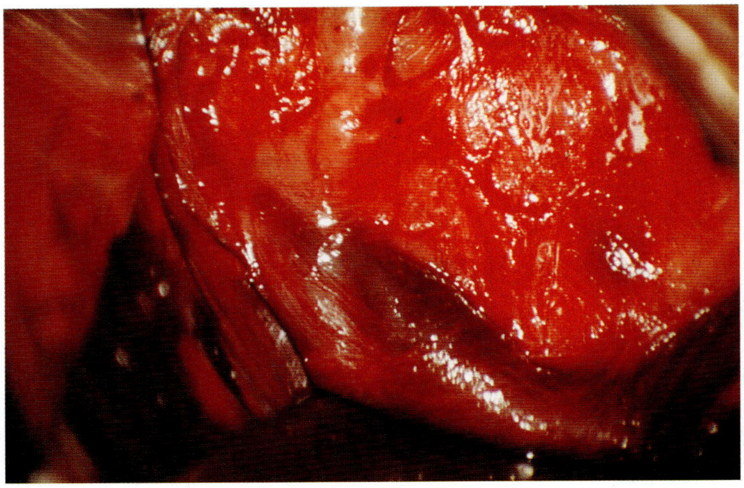

A

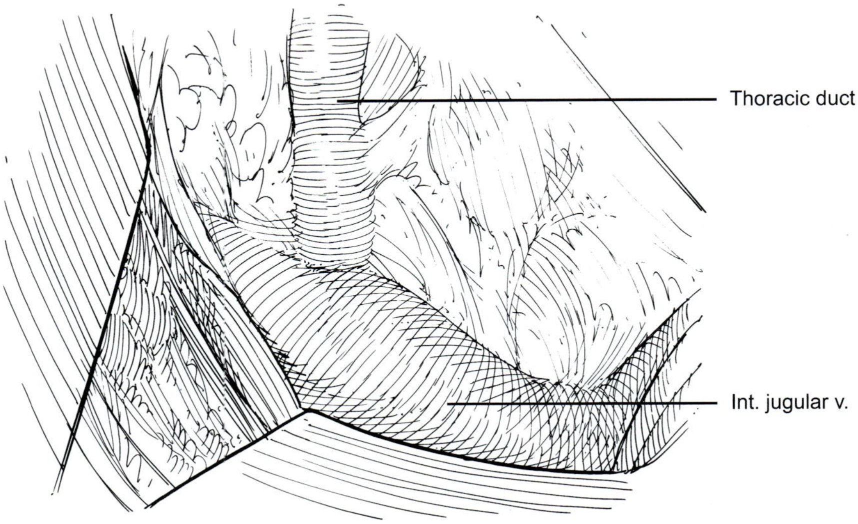

B

Fig. 7.4 Intraoperative photograph **(A)** and corresponding illustration **(B)** showing the internal jugular vein retracted laterally, exposing a branch of the thoracic duct. In approaches to the carotid and subclavian arteries on the left side, the surgeon must always identify the thoracic duct. Multiple branches are often present and must be divided between ligatures to prevent the postoperative complications of lymphocele, cutaneous fistula, or chylothorax. (From Spetzler RF, Koos WT, eds. Color Atlas of Microneurosurgery. Vol 3. Intra- and Extracranial Revascularization and Intraspinal Pathology. 2nd ed. New York: Thieme; 2000:154, Case 3-12e. Reprinted with permission.)

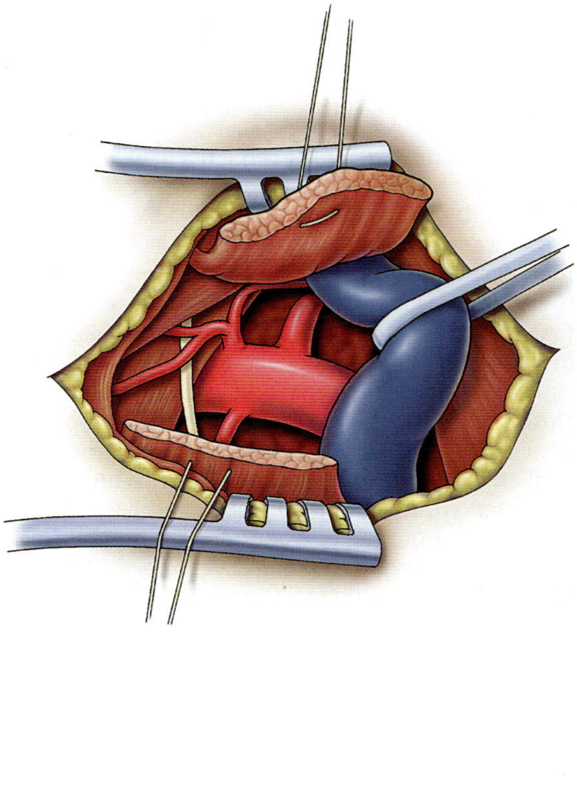

Fig. 7.5 One way of identifying the vertebral artery is to expose the subclavian artery laterally and then follow the vessel until its branches are exposed. The vertebral artery is the first and most proximal branch of the subclavian artery and exits from its posterosuperior aspect. More distally, the thyrocervical and costocervical trunks exit superiorly, while the internal mammary artery exits inferiorly. (Reprinted with permission from Barrow Neurological Institute.)

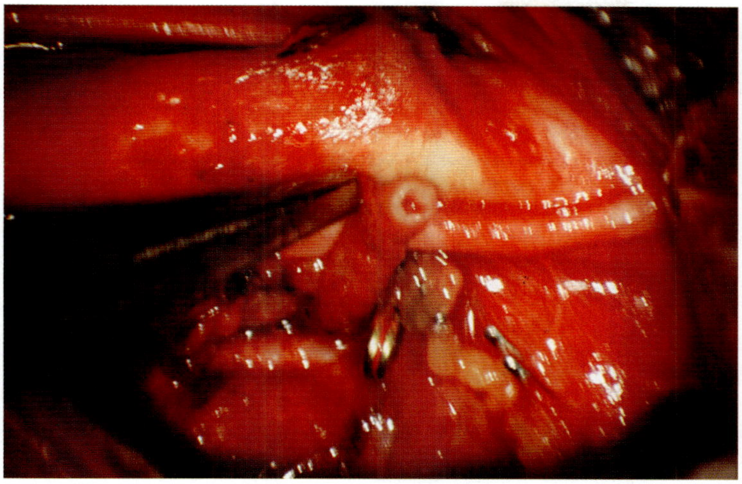

A

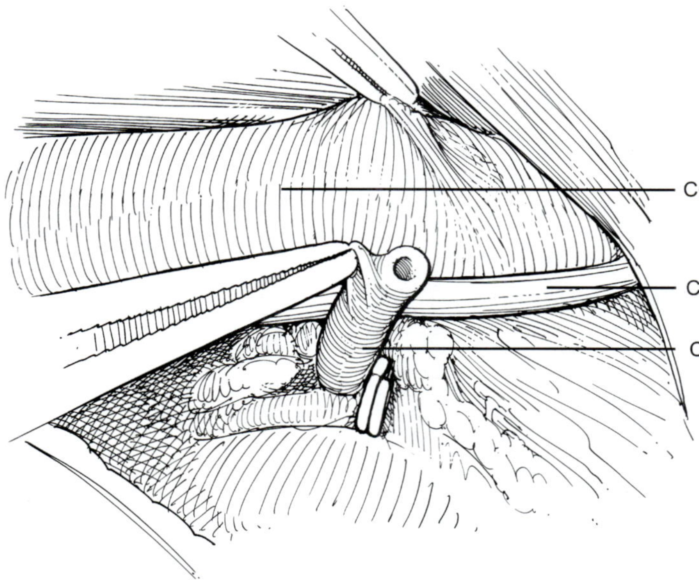

B

Fig. 7.6 Intraoperative photograph **(A)** and corresponding illustration **(B)** showing the vertebral artery divided at its origin from the subclavian artery and held adjacent to the common carotid artery to determine whether sufficient length has been mobilized to allow an end-to-side anastomosis. A temporary aneurysm clip occludes the vertebral artery at its entrance into the C6 transverse foramen. (From Spetzler RF, Koos WT, eds. Color Atlas of Microneurosurgery. Vol 3. Intra- and Extracranial Revascularization and Intraspinal Pathology. 2nd ed. New York: Thieme; 2000:155, Case 3-12g. Reprinted with permission.)

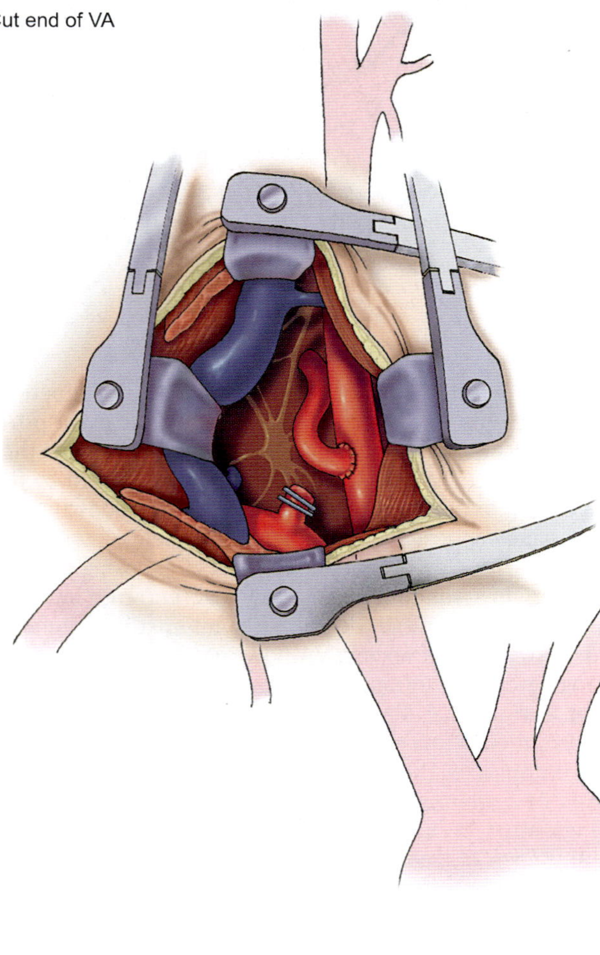

Fig. 7.7 Illustration of the final view after the vertebral artery to common carotid artery end-to-side anastomosis (vertebral artery transposition). (From Spetzler RF, Hadley MN, Martin NA, et al. Vertebrobasilar insufficiency. Part 1: Microsurgical treatment of extracranial vertebrobasilar disease. J Neurosurg 1987;66:648–661. Reprinted with permission.)

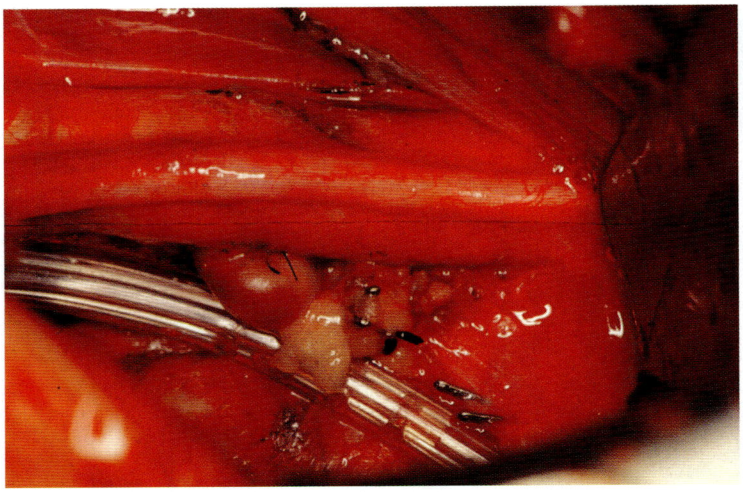

A

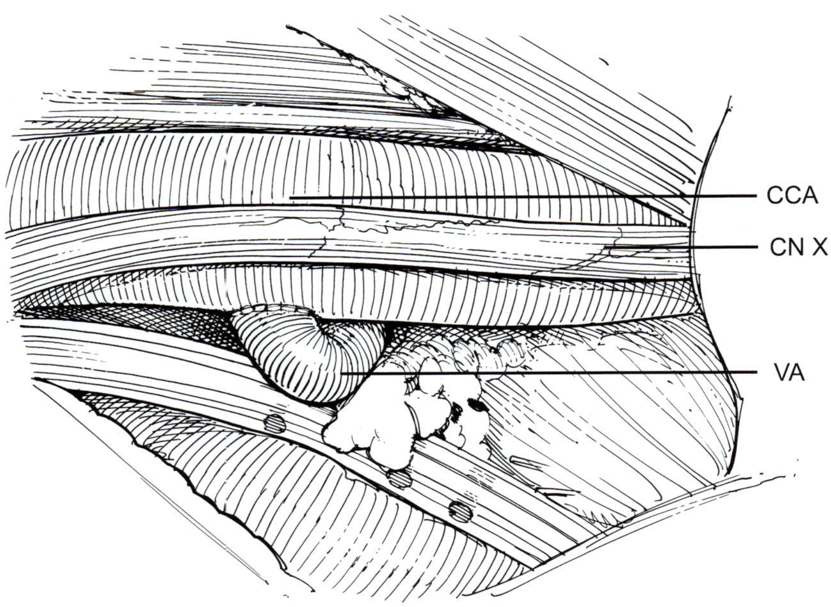

B

Fig. 7.8 Intraoperative photograph **(A)** and corresponding illustration **(B)** showing the final view of the operative site before closure. After the carotid artery is allowed to rotate back into its normal position, the graft arises from its posterolateral wall. This position minimizes tension on and angulation of the graft. CCA., common carotid artery; CN X, cranial nerve X; VA, vertebral artery. (From Spetzler RF, Koos WT, eds. Color Atlas of Microneurosurgery. Vol 3. Intra- and Extracranial Revascularization and Intraspinal Pathology. 2nd ed. New York: Thieme; 2000:156, Case 3-12k. Reprinted with permission.)

It becomes the third segment as it passes over the superior surface of the posterior arch of C1 behind the articular process. It enters the atlantooccipital membrane to become the fourth segment. The first segment can be compressed by fibrous bands[2] or the anterior scalene muscle. The constricting fibrous bands appear to be ligamentous attachments of the longus colli muscles. Treatment consists of exposing the VA from its origin at the subclavian artery to its entrance into the transverse process of C6. The fibrous bands are then carefully lysed. Restoration of normal VA flow may be assessed with ICG angiography or intraoperative angiography.

That extracranial VA disease seldom causes posterior circulation ischemia unless both arteries are compromised emphasizes the importance of flow restriction in the genesis of symptoms.[2] Therefore, abnormal angiographic findings must be correlated with clinical symptoms before any form of treatment is attempted. If symptoms are related to emboli from atherosclerotic plaques or arterial dissection, medical treatment with anticoagulation or antiplatelets is the first choice. Endovascular treatment using balloon angioplasty with intravascular stent placement for symptomatic stenotic lesions causing vertebrobasilar insufficiency unresponsive to medical therapy appears to be of benefit in this high-risk subset of patients with poor collateral flow. Reported data, however, are insufficient to support the primary treatment of extracranial VA stenosis and dissection by stent-supported angioplasty. If symptoms are from hypoperfusion related to intrinsic stenosis of the first or second segment of the VA, flow to the distal VA can be augmented by a bypass from the ECA to the distal VA (end-to-side occipital artery [OA] to third segment of the VA bypass) (**Fig. 7.9**).

Of the many causes of vertebrobasilar insufficiency, extrinsic compression of the VA is relatively uncommon. Hemodynamic compromise from extrinsic compression of the VA most frequently involves the second segment of the VA

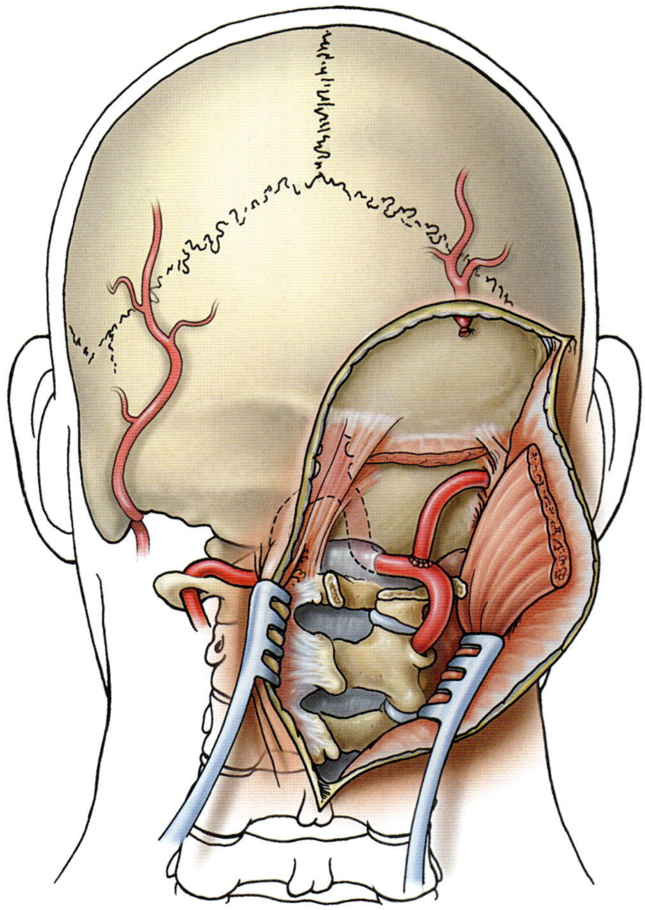

Fig. 7.9 Illustration of an occipital artery–to–vertebral artery (third segment) end-to-side anastomosis. (From Spetzler RF, Hadley MN, Martin NA, et al. Vertebrobasilar insufficiency. Part 1: Microsurgical treatment of extracranial vertebrobasilar disease. J Neurosurg 1987;66:648–661. Reprinted with permission from Journal of Neurosurgery.)

and has been termed positional vertebrobasilar ischemia. It can be caused by osteophytes at the transverse foramina (**Fig. 7.10**), hypertrophy of the uncinate processes or facets, herniation of a cervical disk, subluxation of the apophyseal joint, and hyperrotation of the transverse process. The treatment algorithm depends on the exact location and nature of the pathology. Dynamic angiography is crucial for diagnosis and surgical decompression. Great care must be taken to avoid misdiagnosing the site of occlusion or missing a second occlusive site.[3] The diagnosis of vertebrobasilar ischemia needs to be confirmed by careful exclusion of cardiac or other systemic causes that can mimic this syndrome. Intermittent occlusion of one VA rarely causes ischemic events because of collateral flow from the contralateral VA and the anterior circulation. Therefore, hemodynamic ischemia only occurs when collateral flow is inadequate.

Classically, the term bow hunter's syndrome has been used to describe hemodynamic vertebrobasilar insufficiency caused by mechanical occlusion or stenosis of the VA at C1-C2 when the head is rotated. Treatments include conservative therapies such as verbal warnings or use of a neck brace to limit head and neck rotation. Posterior fusion of C1-C2 has been used to limit atlantoaxial rotational movements. Fusion effectively relieves the symptoms but also markedly reduces the range of head rotation.[4] Decompression of the atlantoaxial portion of the affected VA has also been used because it does not limit physiologic neck movements.

Three approaches have been described for decompression of the VA at the atlantoaxial level: anterior decompression at the transverse foramen of the atlas, anterior decompression at the level of the axis, and posterior decompression at the transverse foramen of the atlas. Fox et al[5] described an anterolateral approach for surgical decompression, through which they untethered the VA at the C1 transverse foramen. The patient's preoperative symptoms resolved, but palsy of the spinal accessory nerve

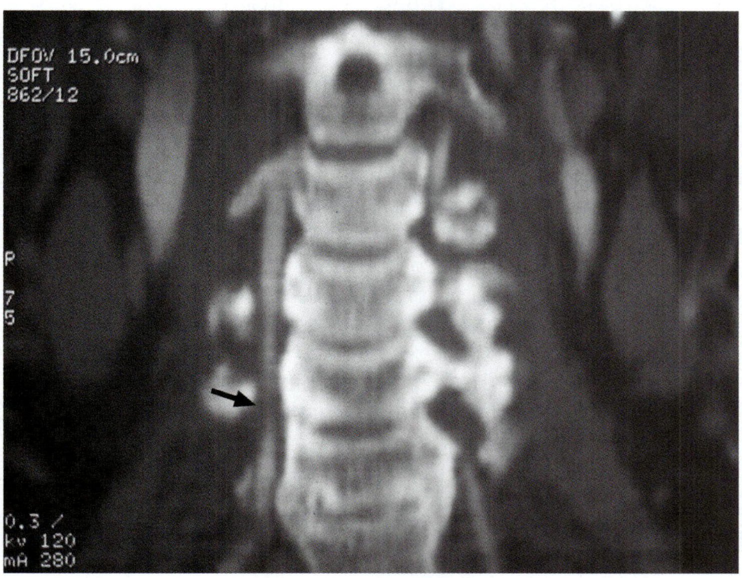

Fig. 7.10 **(A)** MRA demonstrates the almost complete absence of a vestigial left vertebral artery (VA) and stenosis (*arrow*) of the right VA at C5-C6. Unsubtracted *(continued)*

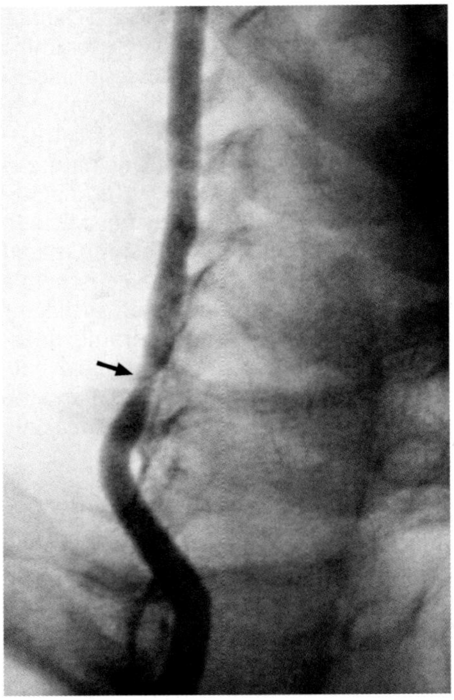

B

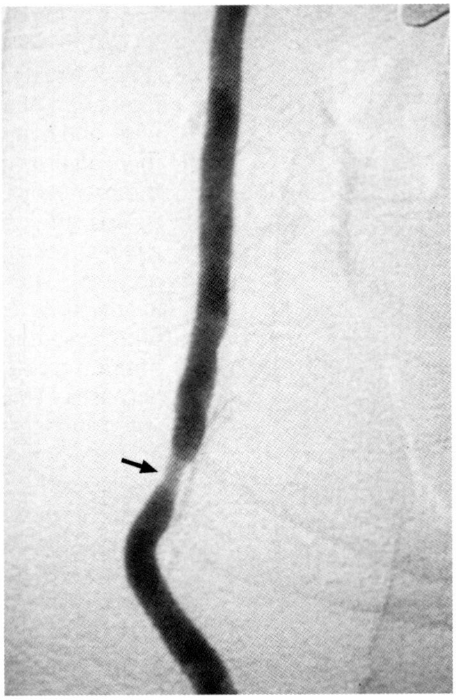

C

Fig. 7.10 *(continued)* **(B)** and subtracted **(C)** selective AP angiograms of the right VA demonstrate stenosis of the VA where it enters the bony canal (arrow). (From Spetzler RF,Koos WT, eds. Color Atlas of Microneurosurgery. Vol 3. Intra- and Extracranial Revascularization and Intraspinal Pathology. 2nd ed. New York: Thieme; 2000:220, Case 4-13a-c. Reprinted with permission.)

complicated the case. Posterior decompression is achieved partly by removing the posterior arch of the atlas and unroofing the transverse foramen of the atlas, thus freeing this segment of the VA. This approach relieves the rate of symptoms without reducing range of motion of the head. However, the rate of reocclusion and restenosis is 33%, making it less effective than C1-C2 posterior fusion in preventing ischemic attacks.[4]

Compression of the VA from spondylotic disease is managed surgically by direct removal of the spurs from the uncinate processes of the vertebral bodies (**Fig. 7.11**). The patient is positioned supine with the head in the neutral position as for an anterior cervical discectomy. Fluoroscopy is useful to identify the correct levels. The skin is incised (transversely for single- or two-level disease, longitudinally for multiple-vessel disease) along the anterior border of the SCM at the level of the VA compression (**Fig. 7.12**). The plane between the strap muscles, thyroid, trachea, and esophagus medially and the carotid sheath laterally is developed until the spine is exposed. The ipsilateral longus colli muscles are dissected from the anterolateral surface of the transverse processes of the cervical vertebrae at the appropriate levels. The sympathetic trunk, which lies on the lateral aspect of the longus colli muscle, must be preserved. The muscle must be dissected carefully when lateral to the anterior tubercle of the transverse process because the cervical nerves are located immediately lateral and posterior.

The transverse foramina above and below the level of stenosis are unroofed under high-power magnification with the operating microscope. The venous plexus that invests the VA and the surrounding fibrotic adventitia must be coagulated and dissected from the artery. If the fibrotic adventitia is not removed entirely, stenosis may persist despite adequate bony decompression. The VA must be mobilized laterally to expose the osteophyte originating from the uncovertebral joint. A high-speed drill and curettes are used to remove the posterior osteophytes. Besides the osteophytes, fibrous adhesions within or between the cervical transverse processes also may constrict the VA. After the foramina have been unroofed, the osteophytes resected, and the adhesions released, the VA should expand to its full size (**Fig. 7.13**). Adequate decompression should be assessed with ICG angiography or intraoperative angiography, with the head in both neutral and rotated position.

If the osteophyte compressing the VA arises from the facet joint, a posterior approach is used. The patient is placed in the prone position. A midline posterior incision allows access to the involved facet. A unilateral subperiosteal dissection is performed. The exposure is more lateral than for a cervical laminectomy because the entire facet complex has to be exposed. The facet is drilled with a high-speed drill under the operative microscope. Once the facet is removed, the VA will be exposed but contained in a fibrous sheath and a perivascular venous plexus. The sheath and plexus must be opened to ensure that the artery is decompressed. ICG

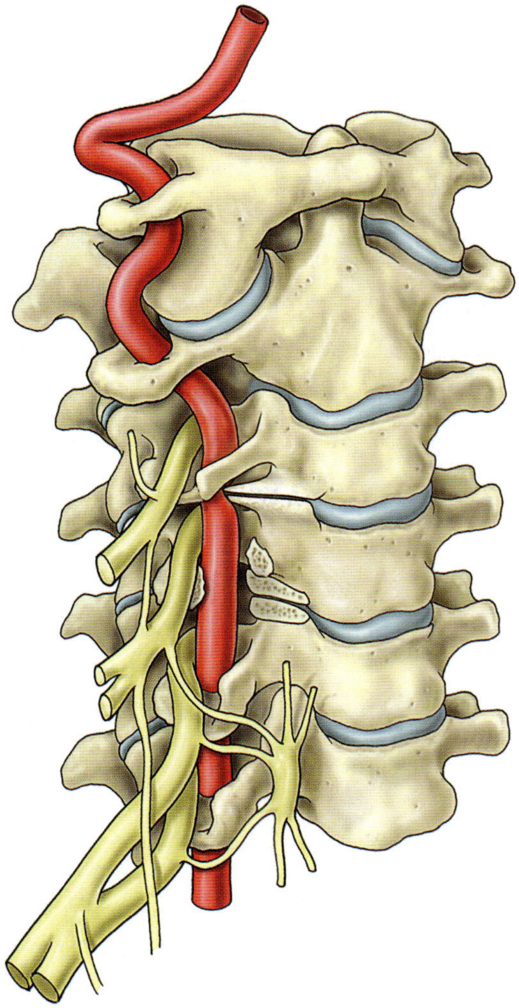

Fig. 7.11 Illustration of anterior decompression of the vertebral artery (VA). The ventral bony surface of the transverse foramen is removed so the VA can be retracted laterally. Then the osteophytes of the hypertrophic uncovertebral that compress the VA are removed with a high-speed drill. (From Spetzler RF, Hadley MN, Martin NA, et al. Vertebrobasilar insufficiency. Part 1: Microsurgical treatment of extracranial vertebrobasilar disease. J Neurosurg 1987;66:648–661. Reprinted with permission from Journal of Neurosurgery.)

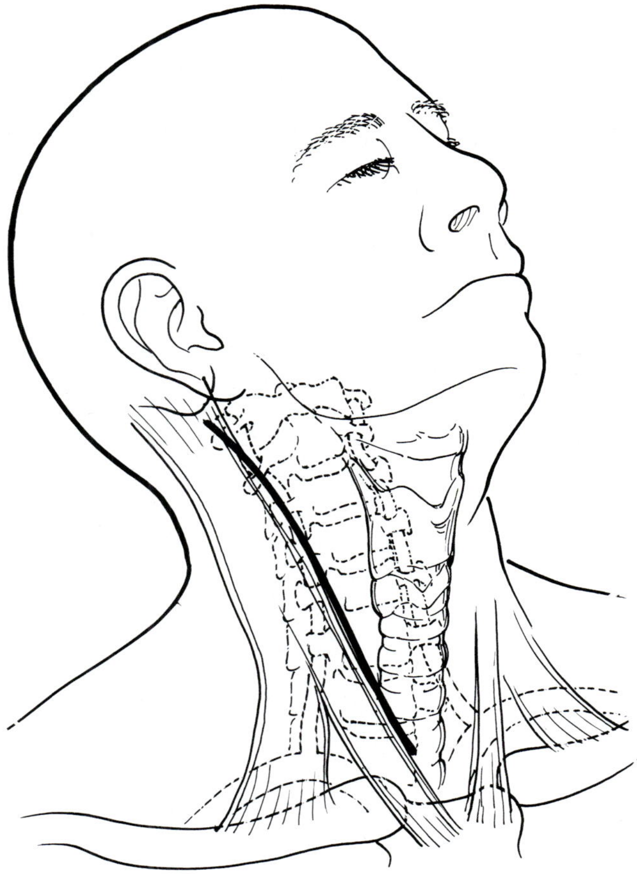

Fig. 7.12 The skin incision is completed along the anterior border of the sternocleidomastoid muscle one level above and one level below the site of vertebral artery compression. (From Spetzler RF, Koos WT, eds. Color Atlas of Microneurosurgery. Vol 3. Intra- and Extracranial Revascularization and Intraspinal Pathology. 2nd ed. New York: Thieme; 2000:220, Case 4-13. Reprinted with permission.)

angiography or intraoperative angiography should be used to assure adequate decompression of the VA. Removal of one facet should not cause instability, and spinal fusion is seldom necessary.

Kawaguchi et al[6] identified hyperrotation of the transverse foramen and subluxation of the apophyseal joint as a mechanism of ipsilateral rotational occlusion of the second segment of the VA. They recommended fusion between the involved vertebrae to prevent hyperrotation and subluxation. Nemececk et al[7] described a case of transient rotational compression of the VA caused by a herniated cervical disk. When the anterior tubercle of the involved level was removed and the VA was identified, a small fragment of disk

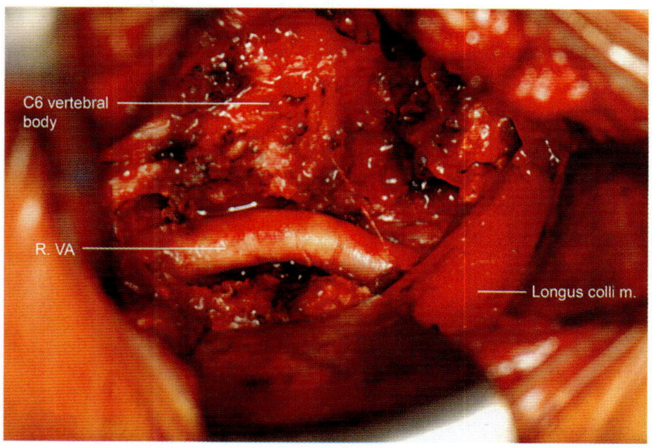

Fig. 7.13 After decompression of the vertebral artery is completed, the vessel should expand to its full size. (From Spetzler RF, Koos WT, eds. Color Atlas of Microneurosurgery. Vol 3. Intra- and Extracranial Revascularization and Intraspinal Pathology. 2nd ed. New York: Thieme; 2000:222, Case 4-13i. Reprinted with permission.)

material was seen to enter the transverse foramen. The fragment was removed, and the disk space was entered laterally to remove additional disk material. The patient had no further episodes. Akar et al[8] described a case of rotational compression of the fourth segment of the VA at the point of dural penetration, which is located above the atlantooccipital membrane.

References

1. Diaz FG, Ausman JI, de los Reyes RA, et al. Surgical reconstruction of the proximal vertebral artery. J Neurosurg 1984;61(5):874–881
2. Spetzler RF, Hadley MN, Martin NA, Hopkins LN, Carter LP, Budny J. Vertebrobasilar insufficiency. Part 1: Microsurgical treatment of extracranial vertebrobasilar disease. J Neurosurg 1987;66(5):648–661
3. Kuether TA, Nesbit GM, Clark WM, Barnwell SL. Rotational vertebral artery occlusion: a mechanism of vertebrobasilar insufficiency. Neurosurgery 1997;41(2):427–432
4. Matsuyama T, Morimoto T, Sakaki T. Comparison of C1-2 posterior fusion and decompression of the vertebral artery in the treatment of bow hunter's stroke. J Neurosurg 1997;86(4):619–623
5. Fox MW, Piepgras DG, Bartleson JD. Anterolateral decompression of the atlantoaxial vertebral artery for symptomatic positional occlusion of the vertebral artery. Case report. J Neurosurg 1995;83(4): 737–740
6. Kawaguchi T, Fujita S, Hosoda K, Shibata Y, Iwakura M, Tamaki N. Rotational occlusion of the vertebral artery caused by transverse process hyperrotation and unilateral apophyseal joint subluxation: case report. J Neurosurg 1997;86(6):1031–1035
7. Nemecek AN, Newell DW, Goodkin R. Transient rotational compression of the vertebral artery caused by herniated cervical disc: case report. J Neurosurg 2003; **98**(1, Suppl)80–83
8. Akar Z, Kafadar AM, Tanriover N, et al. Rotational compression of the vertebral artery at the point of dural penetration: case report. J Neurosurg 2000; 93(2, Suppl)300–303

Chapter 8

Intracranial Posterior Circulation Techniques

Maria M. Toledo and Robert F. Spetzler

Although the usefulness of cerebral revascularization for intracranial atherosclerotic disease in the anterior circulation was questioned in the Cooperative Study of Extracranial-Intracranial Arterial Anastomosis,[1] investigators made no reference to the use of cerebral revascularization for intracranial atherosclerotic disease in the posterior circulation. No prospective randomized trial has been performed to assess the efficacy of cerebral revascularization to treat stenoocclusive disease in the posterior circulation. Therefore, the use of cerebral revascularization for treatment of intracranial atherosclerotic disease in the posterior circulation has yet to be determined.

Symptomatic intracranial arterial stenosis is associated with a high rate of recurrent stroke when treated medically, but because of the high incidence of in-stent stenosis, the widespread use of the self-expanding nitinol Wingspan stent (Boston Scientific, Natick, MA) for intracranial disease is controversial.[2] Endovascular treatment of intracranial atherosclerotic disease either by angioplasty or combined angioplasty and stenting are being investigated in randomized trials to evaluate their efficacy in treating intracranial vascular occlusive disease and stroke prevention.

Yet, microsurgical revascularization is an important and essential component in the treatment of complex skull base tumors and in complex and giant aneurysms that involve dominant vessels in the posterior circulation. When such aneurysms are not amenable to direct clipping, parent vessel occlusion or trapping may be necessary to exclude the lesions from the circulation. If the patient's collateral circulation is insufficient to supply vascular territories distal to the occlusion, cerebral revascularization must be considered to augment blood flow.[3] At present, endovascular techniques, with or without bypass surgery, offer an alternative therapy for the treatment of patients with complex and giant posterior circulation aneurysms.[4] Nevertheless, there are contraindications and limitations to endovascular treatment, including partially thrombosed and wide-necked aneurysms, dissecting aneurysms, or aneurysms causing symptoms due to mass effect.

The choice of bypass option depends on multiple factors, including the goals of the procedure, the availability and accessibility of donor and recipient vessel, and the patient's particular pathology and anatomy. Extracranial-to-intracranial bypass surgery typically involves the anastomosis of branches from the external carotid artery (ECA), usually the superficial temporal artery (STA) or occipital artery (OA) to an intracranial artery directly, but it also may use saphenous vein, radial artery, OA, or STA grafts connected to the donor arteries more proximally.[5]

The STA is the artery most commonly used as a donor vessel for posterior cerebral artery (PCA) and superior cerebellar artery (SCA) revascularization. The STA also may be used for anterior inferior cerebellar artery (AICA) and posterior inferior cerebellar artery (PICA) bypasses. Frequently, the OA rather than the STA is used as the extracranial vascular conduit for revascularization of the AICA or PICA distributions. Indocyanine green videoangiography provides a reliable and rapid intraoperative assessment of bypass patency and adequacy.[6] During surgery, somatosensory evoked potentials and electroencephalography are monitored at all times. Barbiturates are titrated to maintain encephalographic burst suppression for cerebral protection during the time the anastomosis is being performed and the parent artery is temporarily occluded. During temporary vessel occlusion, mean arterial blood pressure is increased with pressors, with the goal of achieving values 25% above baseline.

◆ Donor Vessels

The STA, the smaller of the two terminal branches of the ECA, appears, from its direction, to be a continuation of that vessel.[4] It begins in the substance of the parotid gland, behind the neck of the mandible where it is crossed by the temporal and zygomatic branches of the facial nerve. It ascends over the posterior root of the zygoma and divides into anterior and posterior branches that run with the superficial temporal vein and the auriculotemporal nerve over the superficial temporalis fascia.[7] The STA divides into two main branches: the frontal and parietal. The parietal branch is most frequently used as donor vessel. Catheter angiography performed for evaluation of the primary offending vascular lesion should include selective ECA injections to evaluate the caliber and course of the STA branches on the affected side. If there is concern regarding the adequacy of the STA, alternative strategies, like an interposition graft or an in situ bypass, could be entertained.

The STA trunk is palpated just anterior to the tragus in the region of the zygoma, and Doppler ultrasonography is used to map the vessel from the trunk to the anterior and posterior branches. Minimal shaving is performed over the marked area, and dissection is performed under the operative microscope. A superficial skin incision is made near, but distal to, the main trunk, through the epidermis and dermis, with great care to avoid transecting or damaging the vessel. Once the subcutaneous tissue is reached, small curved scissors are used to dissect down to the STA. Once the artery is visualized, it is dissected in the areolar plane distally and further proximally to the main trunk. All bleeding vessels in the skin are coagulated with the bipolar forceps. The main goal is to obtain a long enough length of the vessel to be able to mobilize the artery freely into the anastomotic site without applying any tension. Once the vessel is dissected, its surrounding tissue is freed and divided with the Bovie, and the dissected STA and its surrounding tissue are wrapped in a wet Telfa.

The OA arises from the posterior wall of the ECA, usually proximal to the origin of the facial artery. From its origin, the OA runs in a posterosuperior direction along the medial surface of the digastric muscle (posterior belly) to reach the cranial base a few millimeters posterior to the styloid process and medial to the mastoid in the occipital groove.[8] This vessel is covered by the sternocleidomastoid, splenius capitis, longissimus capitis, and digastric muscles and rests over the rectus capitis lateralis, superior oblique, and semispinalis capitis muscles while it passes horizontally backward in the occipital groove.[4] After the OA emerges from the occipital groove, it turns medially and slightly superiorly first passing posterior to the superior oblique muscle and then to the semispinalis capitis muscle. When the OA reaches the superior nuchal line, it pierces the insertion of the splenium capitis.[8] Catheter angiography performed for evaluation of the primary offending vascular lesion should include selective ECA injections to evaluate the caliber and course of the OA branches on the affected side. If there is concern regarding the adequacy of the OA, alternative strategies, such as an interposition graft or an in situ bypass, could be entertained.

For the purpose of bypass surgery, the artery is usually palpated or localized with Doppler ultrasonography and identified as it exits the mastoid groove posterior and medially to the mastoid process; it is then followed medially.[8] It is also mapped with Doppler ultrasonography and dissected from the subcutaneous tissues and muscles with curved scissors. Freeing the distal segment of the OA is much more difficult than dissecting the STA, mainly because unlike the STA, it lies deep to or within the fascia of the muscles.[8] It is important to dissect and follow the vessel as far medially and superiorly as possible to obtain an adequate mobilizable segment for the anastomosis.[8] The main goal is to obtain an adequate vessel length to be able to mobilize the artery freely into the anastomotic site without applying any tension. Once the vessel is dissected, its surrounding tissue is freed and divided with the Bovie, and the dissected OA and its surrounding tissue are wrapped in a wet Telfa.

◆ Posterior Cerebral Artery and Superior Cerebellar Artery Revascularization

The STA-SCA anastomosis has most commonly been used to treat rostral brainstem ischemia.[9] STA-PCA anastomosis may be used to treat significant stenosis of the PCA or fusiform and dissecting aneurysms of the PCA, or those rare cases amenable only to trapping or excision. For both anastomoses, the recipient vessel is exposed via a subtemporal approach. The temporal fossa is exposed through a subtemporal craniotomy (**Fig. 8.1**). Care should be taken to assure that the lateral wall of the temporal fossa and root of the zygoma are drilled flat in relation to the temporal fossa (**Fig. 8.2**). This flat approach minimizes the retraction

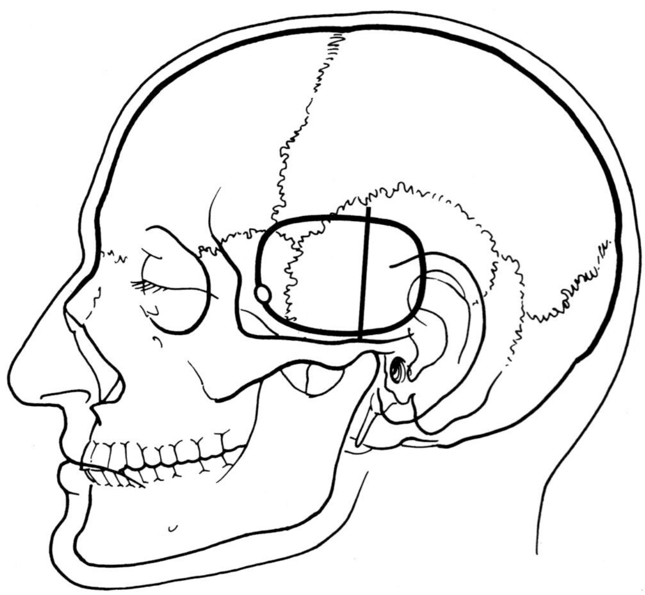

Fig. 8.1 The patient's head is rotated to the contralateral side until the zygomatic arch is in the horizontal position. To facilitate this position, the ipsilateral shoulder may be elevated with a cushion. Then, the head is laterally flexed to support gravity-related self-retraction of the temporal lobe. The skin incision is performed at a right angle to the zygomatic arch, ~1 cm anterior to the external auditory meatus. (From Spetzler RF, Koos WT, eds. Color Atlas of Microneurosurgery. Vol 3. Intra- and Extracranial Revascularization and Intraspinal Pathology. 2nd ed. New York: Thieme; 2000:164, Case 3-14. Reprinted with permission.)

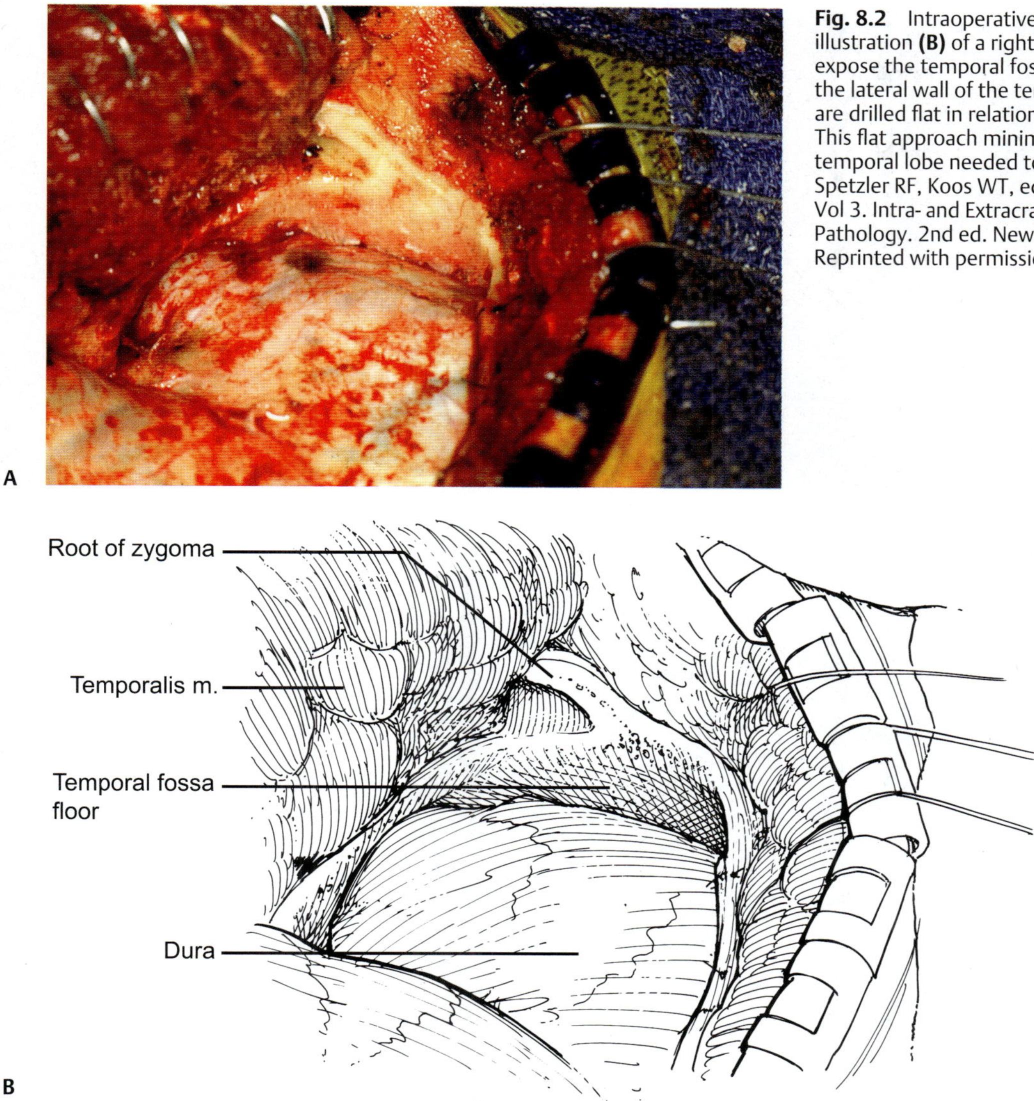

Fig. 8.2 Intraoperative photograph **(A)** and corresponding illustration **(B)** of a right temporal craniotomy performed to expose the temporal fossa. Care must be taken to assure that the lateral wall of the temporal fossa and root of the zygoma are drilled flat in relation to the floor of the temporal fossa. This flat approach minimizes the amount of retraction on the temporal lobe needed to expose the basal cisterns. (From Spetzler RF, Koos WT, eds. Color Atlas of Microneurosurgery. Vol 3. Intra- and Extracranial Revascularization and Intraspinal Pathology. 2nd ed. New York: Thieme;2000:164, Case 3-14. Reprinted with permission.)

of the temporal lobe needed to expose the basal cisterns. Care should be taken not to injure the vein of Labbé or the posterior cerebral veins as they enter the transverse sinus. The exposure can be enhanced, if necessary, with an orbitozygomatic approach.

The dura is then opened (**Fig. 8.3**). The temporal lobe is exposed and gently elevated until the edge of the tentorium is identified (**Fig. 8.4**). The basal cisterns are opened sharply. The edge of the tentorium may be cut to expose the SCA and trochlear nerve. For pathology involving more distal PCA or SCA segments (ambient or quadrigeminal cisterns), aneurysm trapping, excision, or proximal occlusion of a diseased vessel followed by revascularization may be performed via a lateral supracerebellar infratentorial approach.

If the PCA is targeted as a recipient vessel, the microscope is angled anteriorly and the PCA is exposed as it passes over the oculomotor nerve (**Fig. 8.5**). The SCA can be identified passing beneath the oculomotor nerve. The PCA is dissected free from the arachnoid as the vessel courses around the cerebral peduncle. A portion of the P2 segment, ~1.5 cm in length and having no perforating vessels, is isolated for the anastomosis. A small latex dam is placed beneath the artery and a no. 3 MicroVac suction tubing is placed on the surgical field to improve visualization.

After the PCA has been exposed, the cut end of the STA is stripped from its fascial layer and a 7- to 8-mm portion of that vessel is exposed.[4] The tip of the STA is cut into a shape that is suitable for the anastomotic site. The recipient artery is prepared by placing temporary clips on both sides of the exposed vessel and performing a small arteriotomy.[4] After two stay sutures have been placed on both ends of the arteriotomy, a loose running 10-0 suture is placed along one wall. Tightening the sutures after they have all been placed helps the surgeon visualize the vessel walls for these deep anastomoses. Furthermore, tightening assures uniform suture tension and improves hemostasis. Next, the suture on the other wall is placed to complete

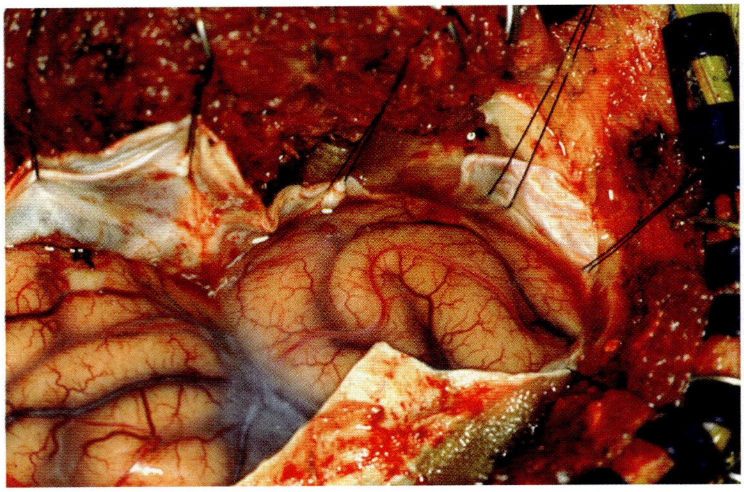

A

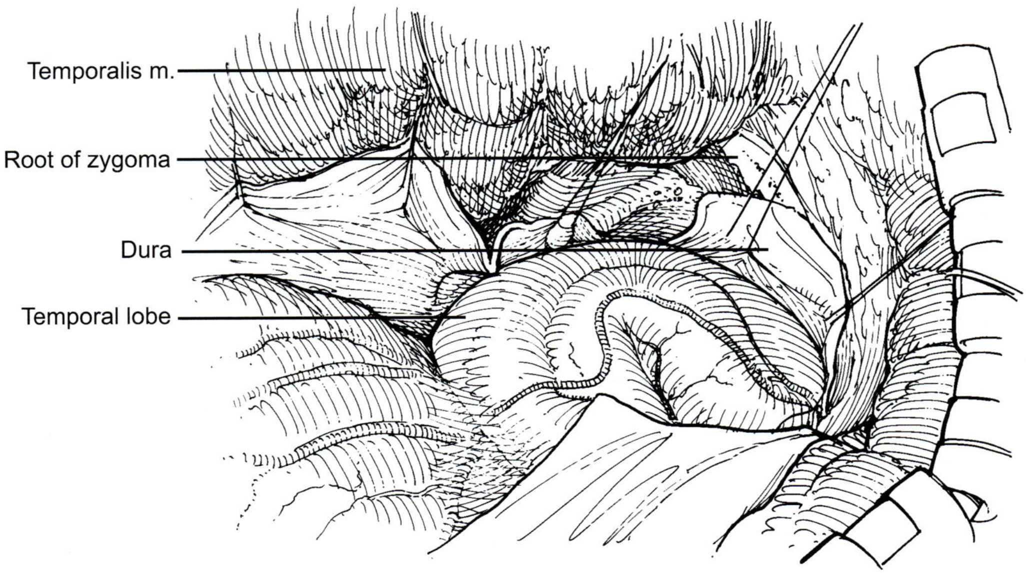

B

Fig. 8.3 Intraoperative photograph **(A)** and corresponding illustration **(B)** showing the dura opened in a semicircular shape with its base toward the temporal base. The dural flap is tacked downward with sutures. The temporal lobe is exposed. (From Spetzler RF, Koos WT, eds. Color Atlas of Microneurosurgery. Vol 3. Intra- and Extracranial Revascularization and Intraspinal Pathology. 2nd ed. New York: Thieme; 2000:165, Case 3-14. Reprinted with permission.)

an end-to-side anastomosis (**Fig. 8.6**). When the bone flap is replaced, the surgeon must be careful to avoid twisting, damaging, or compromising the donor vessel. When the galea is reapproximated for skin closure, the surgeon must visualize the STA at all times to avoid injuring the artery or compromising the anastomosis. **Figure 8.7** demonstrates a case of severe VA stenosis treated with an STA-PCA bypass.

If the STA cannot be exposed sufficiently to reach the anastomotic site comfortably, either a saphenous vein or a radial artery graft may be used to perform an ECA-PCA bypass. The distal end of the anastomosis between the P2 segment and the graft is performed in an end-to-side fashion with 8-0 nylon suture.[4] Then, the graft is pulled down through a subcutaneous tunnel. The cervical ECA is occluded proximally and distally. An arteriotomy is performed, and the proximal end of the graft is anastomosed in an end-to-side fashion using 6-0 nylon sutures.

Ulku et al[10] described a proximal STA to proximal PCA bypass using a radial artery graft. They concluded that using a short radial artery graft can provide sufficient blood flow and may be a reasonable alternative to an ECA-PCA bypass using long venous or arterial grafts. Nagasawa et al[9] proposed the inferior temporal branch of the PCA as a possible recipient artery for the STA for the treatment of rostral brainstem ischemia. They concluded that by using a cortical artery as the recipient vessel for the STA, it is possible to ensure a shorter bypass and less complicated surgery than would be involved in anastomosis to the main trunk of the PCA or the SCA at a deeper level. Touho et al[11] described the use of an OA-PCA anastomosis with interposition of an STA graft using an occipital interhemispheric transtentorial approach as an alternative for treatment of stenosis or occlusion of the rostral portion of the basilar artery. This approach places the visual cortex at risk from retraction, and the deep venous system makes visualization more difficult.

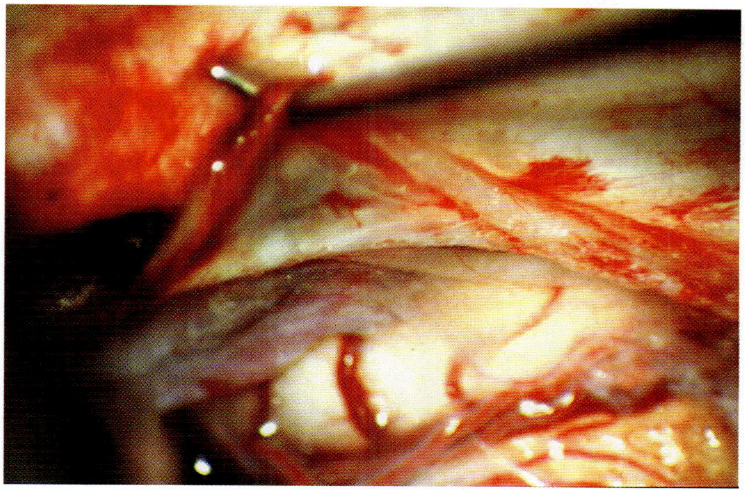

A

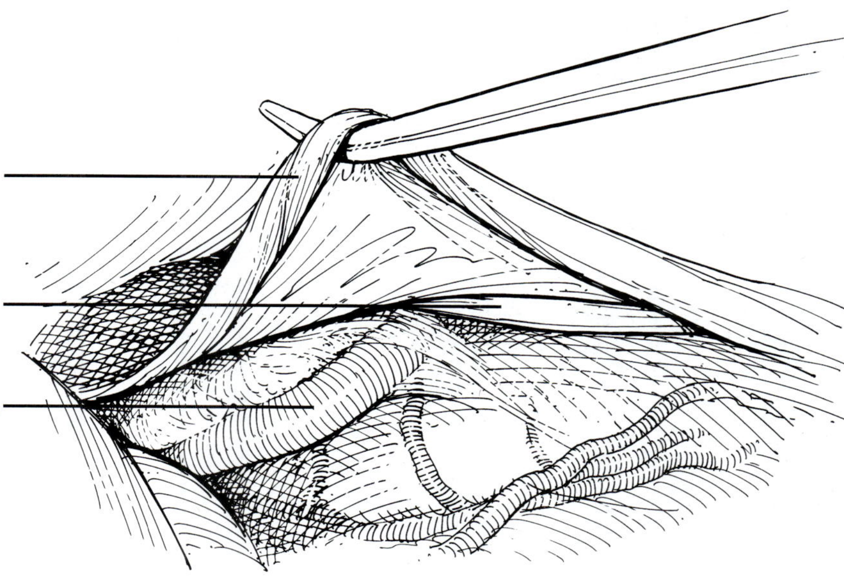

B

Fig. 8.4 Intraoperative photograph **(A)** and corresponding illustration **(B)** showing the temporal lobe carefully retracted until the ambient cistern can be opened and cerebrospinal fluid drained. A blunt hook retracts the edge of the tentorium exposing the superior cerebellar artery and trochlear nerve. CN IV, cranial nerve IV. (From Spetzler RF, Koos WT, eds. Color Atlas of Microneurosurgery. Vol 3. Intra- and Extracranial Revascularization and Intraspinal Pathology. 2nd ed. New York: Thieme; 2000:165, Case 3-14. Reprinted with permission.)

After a subtemporal approach is performed in cases of STA-SCA anastomosis, the tentorial edge is identified, cut, and coagulated to increase exposure (**Fig. 8.8**). During this maneuver, care must be taken not to damage the fourth cranial nerve, which courses below the edge of the tentorium. The fourth nerve must be visualized before the tentorial edge is cut and coagulated. The SCA is identified in the lateral pontomesencephalic segment.[4] If branches to the brainstem are visualized, a portion of the SCA distal to those branches is selected for the anastomosis.[4] Because the SCA frequently divides into rostral and caudal branches in this segment, the larger of the two branches is used for the anastomosis.[4] A short segment of the SCA is then isolated between temporary clips (**Fig. 8.9**). After the distal end of the cut STA is stripped from its fascial layer and cut into a shape that is suitable for the anastomotic site, it is tacked to the SCA at two points. A loose running 10-0 suture is placed along one wall (**Fig. 8.10**). Tightening the sutures after they have all been placed helps the surgeon visualize the vessel walls for these deep anastomoses. Tightening ensures uniform suture tension and improves hemostasis. Then the suture on the front wall is placed to complete an end-to-side anastomosis (**Figs. 8.11** and **8.12**). **Figure 8.13** demonstrates a case of symptomatic midbasilar stenosis treated with an STA-SCA bypass.

◆ PICA and AICA Revascularization

Unclippable aneurysms of the PICA and vertebral artery (VA) are typically dissecting or fusiform in nature. Some VA dissecting aneurysms and partially thrombosed aneurysms involve the origin of PICA and may be treated only with aneurysm trapping or parent vessel occlusion. If there is a high probability of disturbing PICA blood flow after surgical or endovascular treatment for a local aneurysm, PICA

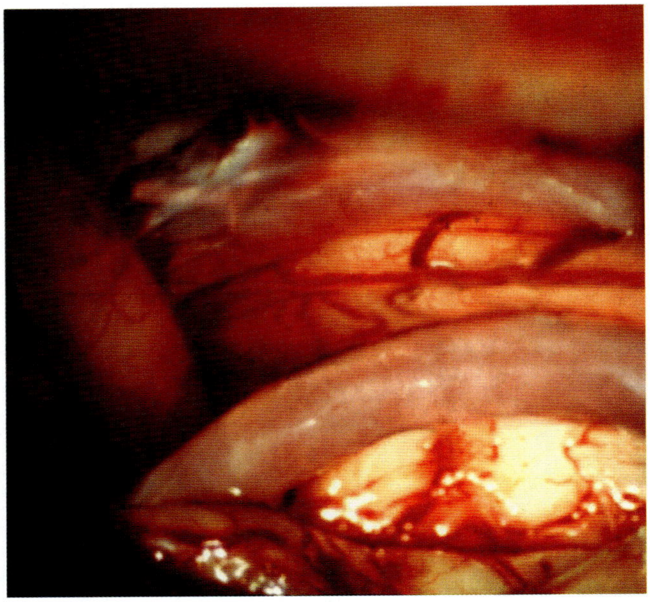

A

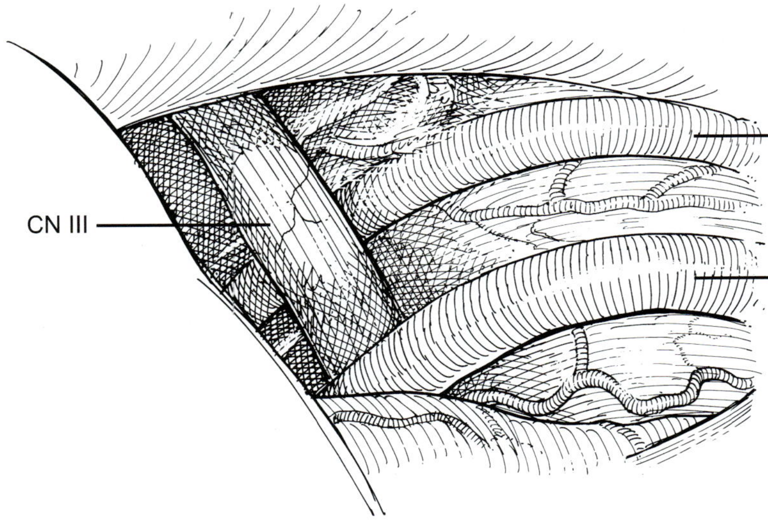

B

Fig. 8.5 Intraoperative photograph **(A)** and corresponding illustration **(B)** showing the posterior inferior cerebral artery (PCA) exposed as it passes over the oculomotor nerve. The microscope has been angled anteriorly. The superior cerebellar artery can be identified under the oculomotor nerve. CN III, cranial nerve III. (From Spetzler RF, Koos WT, eds. Color Atlas of Microneurosurgery. Vol 3. Intra- and Extracranial Revascularization and Intraspinal Pathology. 2nd ed. New York: Thieme; 2000:165, Case 3-14. Reprinted with permission.)

revascularization should be considered to prevent cerebellar infarction and lateral medullary syndrome. Options include an OA-PICA anastomosis,[12] VA-PICA anastomosis using an interposition graft (STA or radial artery graft),[13] an end-to-side or end-to-end reimplantation of the PICA into the VA, or a side-to-side PICA-PICA in situ bypass.[3] Depending the caliber of the arteries, either an end-to-end or an end-to-side VA-PICA anastomosis (PICA transposition) may be completed.[14] The diseased PICA segment that is involved with aneurysm or tumor can be excised, and the remaining portions of the vessel can be directly reattached in an end-to-end fashion. For this end-to-end anastomosis to be technically and functionally feasible, there needs to be enough redundancy in the arterial ends to reapproximate them without tension.

The choice of revascularization procedure used for PICA is determined by several factors: degree of collateral blood flow, aneurysm location, availability of ECA branches, and the surgeon's preference. The OA is more cumbersome to dissect and is more prone to occlusion than the STA.[5] Thus, some surgeons prefer a PICA-PICA bypass over an OA-PICA bypass. Yet, a PICA-PICA bypass requires temporary occlusion of two major vessels to perform the side-to-side anastomosis instead of just temporarily occluding one recipient artery.[5] Thus, using the extracranial OA as a donor graft pedicle may represent a safe primary option when feasible.

The patient is placed in the prone position. A hockey stick incision is made, with the long arm extending down the midline plane of the neck and the short arm over the mastoid tip (**Fig. 8.14**). The OA is dissected and mobilized as described above (**Fig. 8.15**). The OA is gently retracted from the surgical field, and the craniotomy is performed. If necessary, the arch of C1 is removed. Most VA-PICA junction aneurysms are approached through a far-lateral approach, with partial drilling of the occipital condyle and jugular tubercle.

A
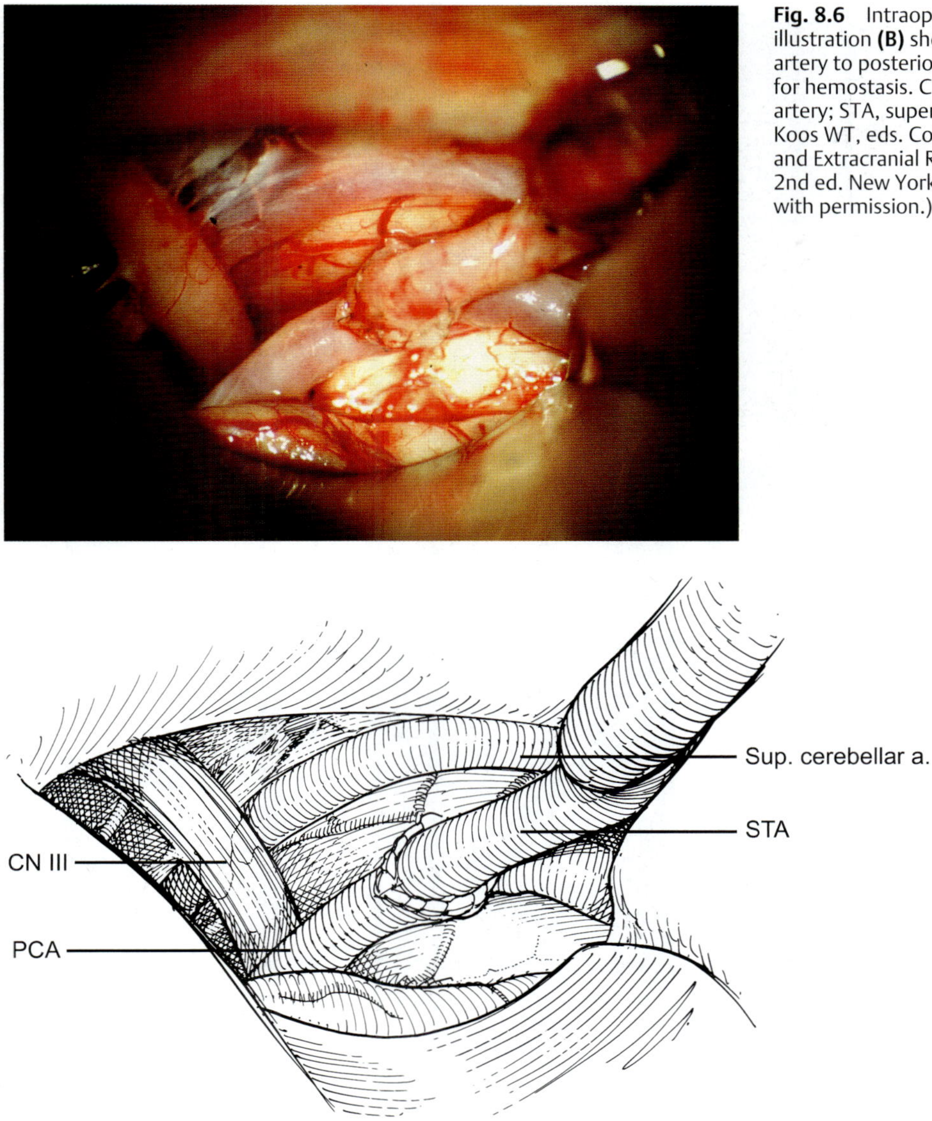

B

Fig. 8.6 Intraoperative photograph **(A)** and corresponding illustration **(B)** showing the completed superficial temporal artery to posterior cerebral artery bypass ready for inspection for hemostasis. CN III, cranial nerve III; PCA, posterior cerebral artery; STA, superficial temporal artery. (From Spetzler RF, Koos WT, eds. Color Atlas of Microneurosurgery. Vol 3. Intra- and Extracranial Revascularization and Intraspinal Pathology. 2nd ed. New York: Thieme; 2000:166, Case 3-14. Reprinted with permission.)

This craniotomy is used in most cases for management of the aneurysm per se. The decision to perform the bypass often is made after inspection of the aneurysm and awareness that preservation of the parent artery is not feasible for complete treatment. When an aneurysm is treated with endovascular means (with trapping or proximal vessel occlusion), a simple midline suboccipital craniotomy is performed solely for the bypass procedure.

The dura mater is opened, and the cerebellar tonsils and lower medulla are exposed (**Fig. 8.16**). The caudal loop of the PICA is exposed, and the vessel is freed from the arachnoid. The severed end of the OA is stripped of its fascial layer, sectioned at an angle, and fishmouthed to produce a long anastomosis two to three times the diameter of the recipient vessel (**Fig. 8.17**). A short segment of the PICA, isolated between temporary clips, lies open over a latex dam as the first suture is placed. After anchoring sutures are placed at the apices of the incision, the back wall of the anastomosis is completed first with a loose running 10-0 suture. Tightening the sutures after they have all been placed helps the surgeon visualize the vessel walls for these deep anastomoses. Tightening ensures uniform suture tension and improves hemostasis. Next, the front wall of the anastomosis is performed to complete an end-to-side anastomosis (**Fig. 8.18**). Care must be taken when the bone flap is replaced to avoid twisting, damaging, or compromising the donor vessel. When the galea is reapproximated for skin closure, the surgeon must visualize the OA at all times to avoid injuring the artery or compromising the anastomosis. **Figure 8.19** demonstrates a case of symptomatic occlusion of a dominant VA treated with an OA-PICA bypass.

Side-to-side in situ anastomosis of the PICA is used mainly for cerebral revascularization of the distal portion of the PICA after occlusion of its proximal portion. A far-lateral approach is performed initially for inspection and evaluation of the aneurysm or tumor and the involved PICA. When the aneurysm

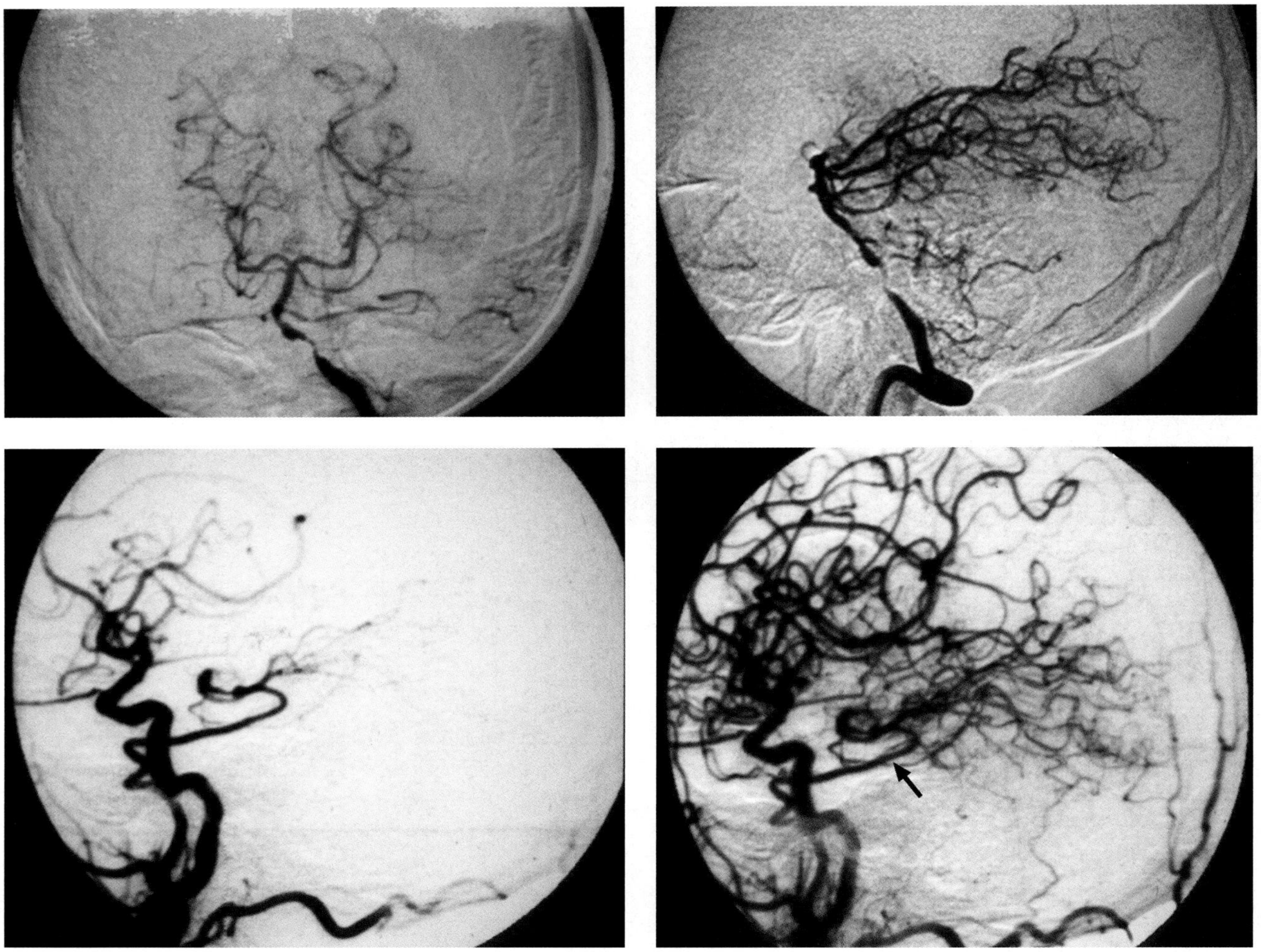

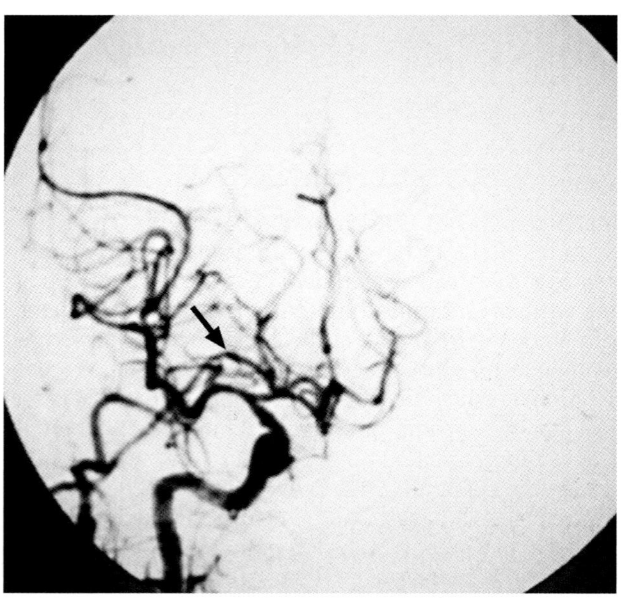

Fig. 8.7 AP **(A)** and lateral **(B)** angiograms of the left vertebral artery (VA) demonstrating severe stenosis of the most distal segment of the VA at its junction with the basilar artery. The right VA was occluded at its origin, and the posterior communicating arteries were vestigial. Early **(C)** and late **(D)** postoperative lateral angiograms of the right carotid artery demonstrate rapid filling of the posterior cerebral arteries and upper basilar artery via the patent bypass (*arrow*). **(E)** AP angiogram of the right internal carotid artery confirms the extent of the filling provided by the bypass. (From Spetzler RF, Koos WT, eds. Color Atlas of Microneurosurgery. Vol 3. Intra- and Extracranial Revascularization and Intraspinal Pathology. 2nd ed. New York: Thieme; 2000:164167, Case 3-14a,b,h–j. Reprinted with permission.)

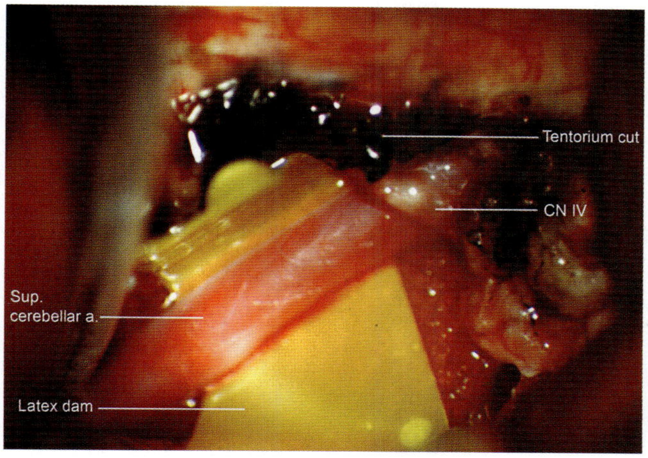

Fig. 8.8 The right superior cerebellar artery is exposed through a subtemporal approach. The edge of the tentorium has been cut and coagulated, and a small latex dam has been placed beneath the artery to enhance visualization. CN IV, cranial nerve IV. (From Spetzler RF, Koos WT, eds. Color Atlas of Microneurosurgery. Vol 3. Intra- and Extracranial Revascularization and Intraspinal Pathology. 2nd ed. New York: Thieme; 2000:169, Case 3-15d. Reprinted with permission.)

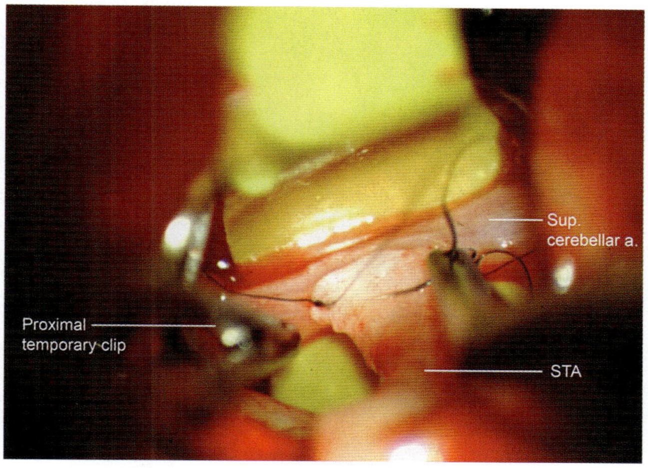

Fig. 8.9 A short segment of the superior cerebellar artery is isolated between temporary aneurysm clips. The distal end of the superficial temporal artery is tacked at two points to the superior cerebellar artery in preparation for the end-to-side anastomosis. STA, superficial temporal artery. (From Spetzler RF, Koos WT, eds. Color Atlas of Microneurosurgery. Vol 3. Intra- and Extracranial Revascularization and Intraspinal Pathology. 2nd ed. New York: Thieme; 2000:169, Case 3-15e. Reprinted with permission.)

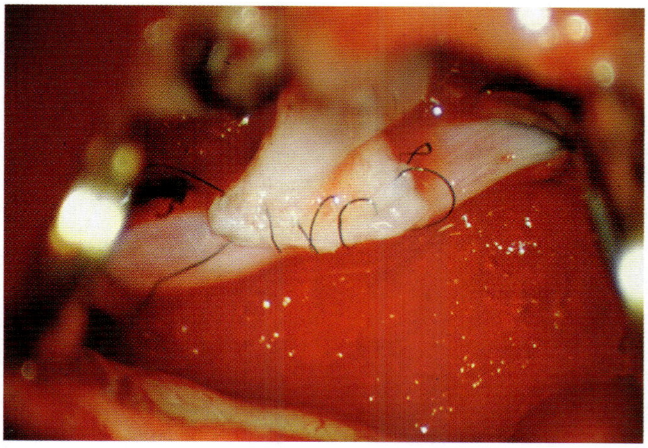

Fig. 8.10 A loose running 10-0 suture is placed along one wall. Tightening the sutures after they have all been placed helps the surgeon to visualize the vessel walls for these deep anastomoses. Additionally, tightening assures uniform suture tension and improves hemostasis. (From Spetzler RF, Koos WT, eds. Color Atlas of Microneurosurgery. Vol 3. Intra- and Extracranial Revascularization and Intraspinal Pathology. 2nd ed. New York: Thieme; 2000:169, Case 3-15f. Reprinted with permission.)

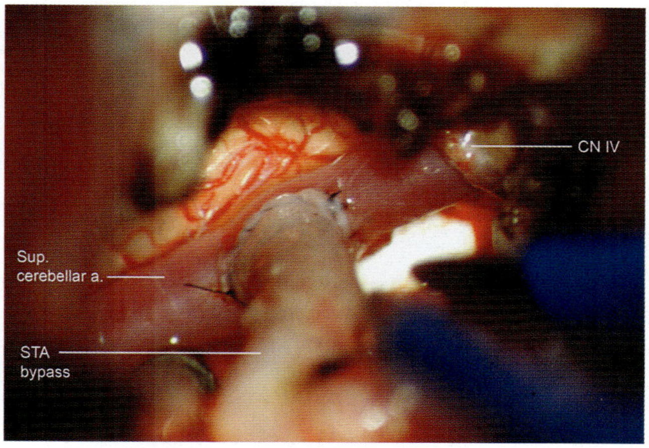

Fig. 8.11 The superficial temporal artery-to-superior cerebellar artery anastomosis is completed and inspected for hemostasis. CN IV, cranial nerve IV; STA, superficial temporal artery. (From Spetzler RF, Koos WT, eds. Color Atlas of Microneurosurgery. Vol 3. Intra- and Extracranial Revascularization and Intraspinal Pathology. 2nd ed. New York: Thieme; 2000:170, Case 3-15g. Reprinted with permission.)

is addressed via endovascular means (with trapping or proximal vessel occlusion), a simple midline suboccipital craniotomy is performed solely for the bypass procedure. During surgical treatment, once the decision is made that primary clipping is not possible, and that parent artery occlusion and revascularization of the distal PICA are necessary, the PICA-PICA bypass is performed. The proximity and parallel courses of the tonsillomedullary and telovelotonsillar segments of the PICA permit side-to-side anastomosis (**Fig. 8.20**).[4] The most difficult part of the procedure is making a tight suture on the back wall. The first bite after approximating the two arteries requires passing the needle from outside to inside the lumen.[5] The next sutures are placed in a continuous fashion to the opposite ends of the arteriotomies, where the needle is passed from inside to outside the lumen.[5] Once these sutures are loosely placed along the entire line, they are

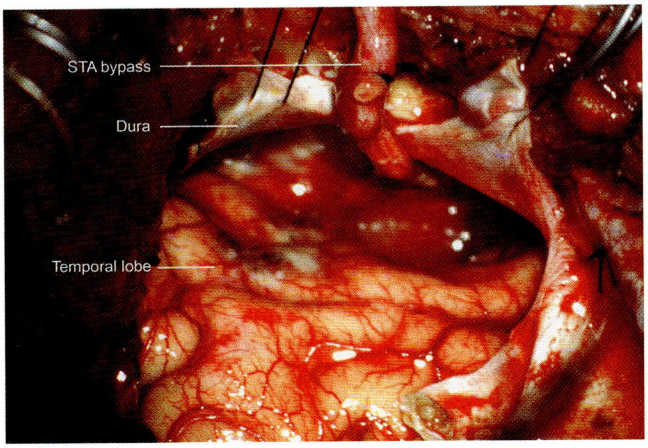

Fig. 8.12 Overview of operative field shows the superficial temporal artery (STA) coursing over the floor of the middle cranial fossa. When the dura is closed and the bone flap is replaced, the surgeon must be careful to avoid twisting, damaging, or compromising the donor vessel. When the galea is reapproximated for skin closure, the surgeon must visualize the superficial temporal artery at all times to avoid injuring the artery or compromising the anastomosis. (From Spetzler RF, Koos WT, eds. Color Atlas of Microneurosurgery. Vol 3. Intra- and Extracranial Revascularization and Intraspinal Pathology. 2nd ed. New York: Thieme; 2000:170, Case 3-15h. Reprinted with permission.)

A

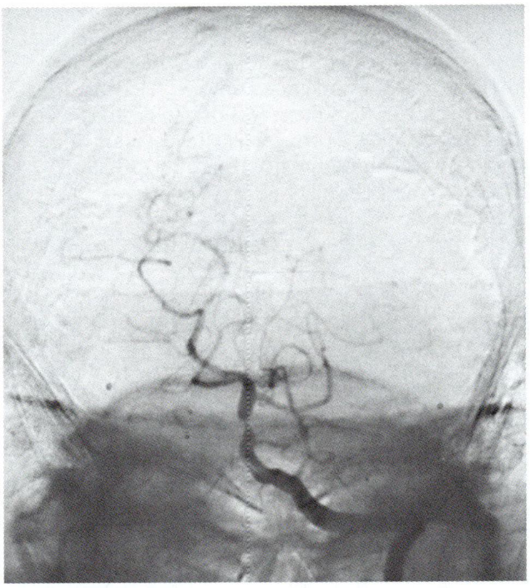

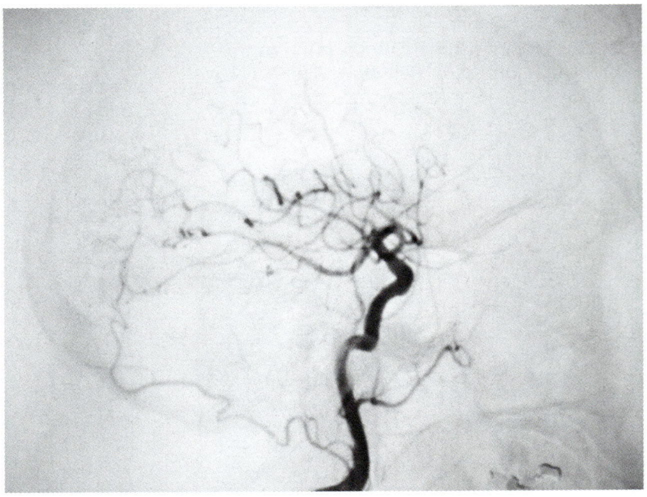

B

C

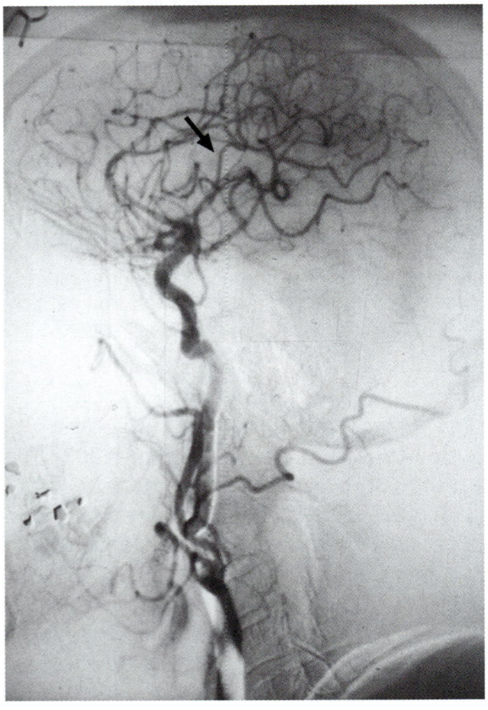

Fig. 8.13 **(A)** AP angiogram of the left vertebral artery demonstrates severe stenosis of the midportion of the basilar artery. **(B)** Lateral angiogram of the left carotid artery reveals the fetal origin of the left posterior cerebral artery with no evidence of collateral supply to the upper portion of the basilar artery. **(C)** Lateral angiogram of the right carotid artery shows normal anterior circulation with no apparent collateral supply to the posterior circulation. Note the large branch of the superficial temporal artery (*arrow*). *(continued)*

D 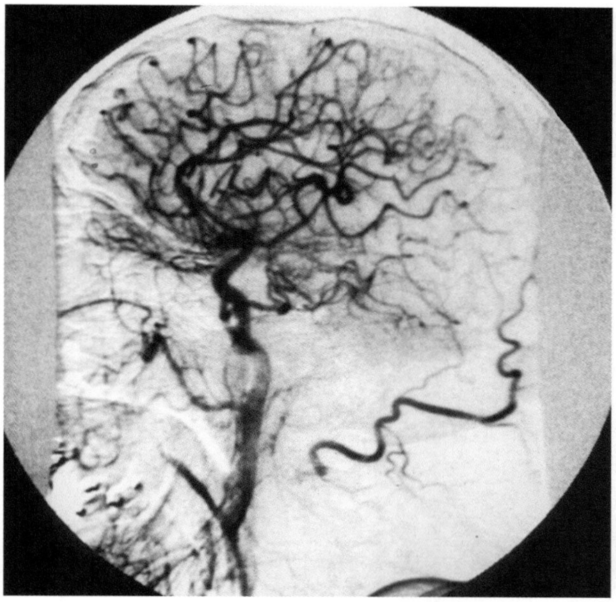 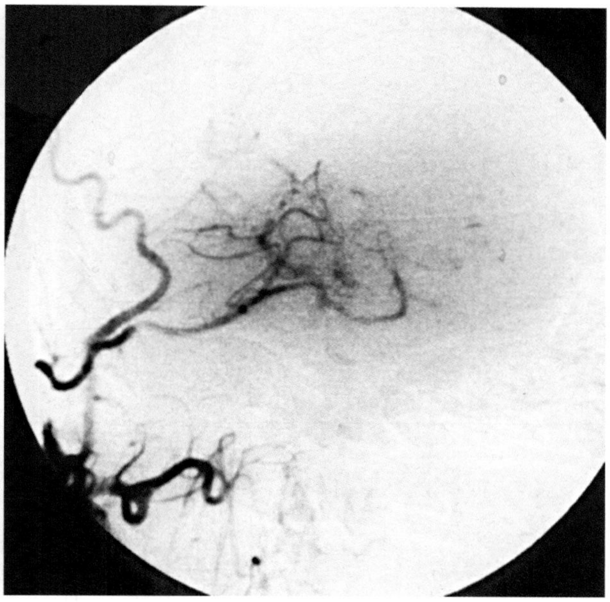 E

Fig. 8.13 *(continued)* **(D)** Postoperative lateral angiogram of the right common carotid artery demonstrates rapid filling of the superior cerebellar arteries and right posterior cerebral artery through the patent bypass. A magnified postoperative selective angiogram of the right external carotid artery. **(E)** The superficial temporal artery to superior cerebellar artery bypass. (From Spetzler RF, Koos WT, eds. Color Atlas of Microneurosurgery. Vol 3. Intra- and Extracranial Revascularization and Intraspinal Pathology. 2nd ed. New York: Thieme; 2000:168–171, Case 3-15a–c,i,j. Reprinted with permission.)

tightened and tied to a second suture at the other end of the arteriotomy.[5] The front wall of the anastomosis is performed with a simple continuous suture from outside the lumen.[5] A no. 3 MicroVac suction tubing is placed on the surgical field to keep it clear of blood and cerebral spinal fluid at all times, thus optimizing visualization. Lemole et al[3] described an end-to-side PICA-PICA bypass with aneurysmal trapping in a patient whose PICA aneurysm could not be occluded by direct clipping. The PICA stump was reimplanted into the contralateral PICA (**Fig. 8.21**).

Sometimes a PICA-to-PICA anastomosis is not feasible because the contralateral PICA is either hypoplastic or because it courses far away from the ipsilateral PICA and cannot be mobilized. If in addition to any of those limitations, the OAs are hypoplastic, other alternatives exist. The PICA may be reconstructed by transposition directly into the VA. A far-lateral craniotomy is necessary for this procedure. The cerebellar tonsil ipsilateral to the aneurysm or tumor is elevated to reveal both the VA and lesion. Sometimes, the PICA will originate from the aneurysm itself, and the aneurysm may be trapped by occluding the VA just proximal and distal to the lesion and PICA.[14] The VA proximal to the aneurysm and the proximal portion of the PICA are dissected, and the two arteries are mobilized. The VA and PICA are cut just proximal and distal to the aneurysm, respectively.[14]

If there is no significant discrepancy in the calibers of the two arteries, they may be anastomosed in an end-to-end fashion. If a discrepancy exists, they are anastomosed in an end-to-side fashion. Bertalanffy et al[15] described that despite a mismatch in the calibers of the VA and PICA, a direct end-to-end anastomosis could be completed. They did so by using microscissors to cut the VA in a straight manner and the PICA in an oblique 45-degree angle to enlarge the diameter of the vascular end.

Nevertheless, the VA-PICA transposition technique has several limitations.[14] Because of the depth and space constraints of the operative field, the procedure is more technically challenging than an OA-PICA or PICA-PICA anastomosis.[14] The lower cranial nerves can be injured. The proximal segment of the PICA gives rise to several perforating vessels that supply the brainstem, further complicating mobilization of PICA. Forced mobilization may injure the perforating vessels, resulting in lateral medullary syndrome.[14] Thus, when the proximal PICA cannot be mobilized easily, an interposition graft using either the STA or radial artery may be a useful alternative. Hamada et al[13] described nine cases where a VA-PICA bypass with an STA graft was used to treat VA aneurysms involving the PICA.

An OA-AICA anastomosis is rarely performed. It is one of the alternatives for treatment of rostral brainstem ischemia, but an STA-SCA anastomosis is better tolerated and is less technically demanding.[16] After the OA is dissected, the artery is gently retracted from the field. A retrosigmoid craniotomy is performed from the foramen magnum to the transverse sinus and from the edge of the mastoid process to midline. Spinal fluid is drained both by preoperative placement of a spinal drain and by opening the arachnoid in the cistern magna to relax the cerebellum. The cerebellum is carefully retracted, and the AICA on the petrous surface is visualized. Anastomosis of the proximal portion of

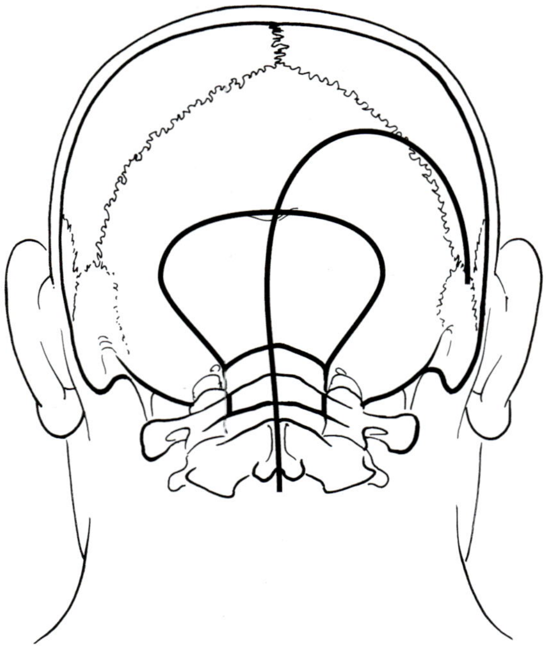

Fig. 8.14 For an occipital artery to posterior inferior cerebellar artery bypass, a hockey stick incision is made, with the long arm extending down the midline plane of the neck and the short arm over the mastoid tip. After the occipital artery has been harvested, a midline suboccipital craniotomy is performed. (From Spetzler RF, Koos WT, eds. Color Atlas of Microneurosurgery. Vol 3. Intra- and Extracranial Revascularization and Intraspinal Pathology. 2nd ed. New York: Thieme; 2000:172, Case 3-16. Reprinted with permission.)

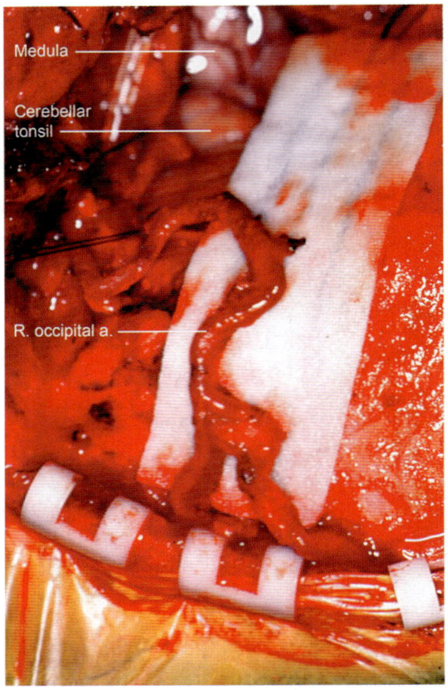

Fig. 8.15 Intraoperative photograph showing the right occipital artery dissected free and mobilized. (From Spetzler RF, Koos WT, eds. Color Atlas of Microneurosurgery. Vol 3. Intra- and Extracranial Revascularization and Intraspinal Pathology. 2nd ed. New York: Thieme; 2000: Case 3-16d, p. 173. Reprinted with permission.)

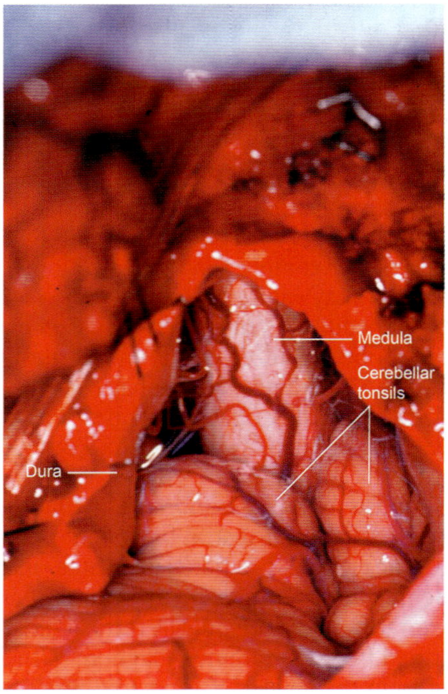

Fig. 8.16 Intraoperative photograph showing the cerebellar tonsils and lower medulla exposed through a midline suboccipital craniotomy. (From Spetzler RF, Koos WT, eds. Color Atlas of Microneurosurgery. Vol 3. Intra- and Extracranial Revascularization and Intraspinal Pathology. 2nd ed. New York: Thieme; 2000:173, Case 3-16c. Reprinted with permission.)

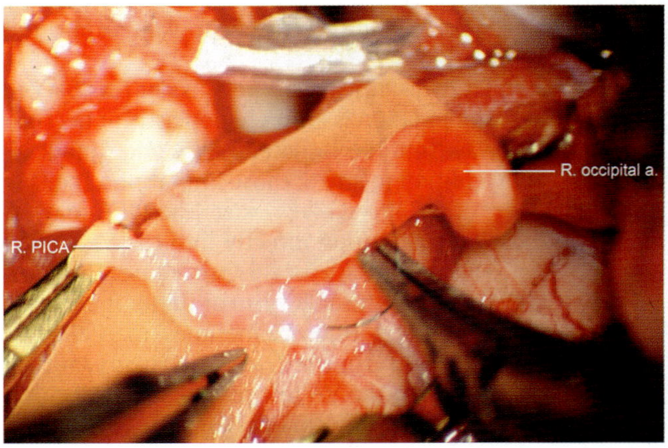

Fig. 8.17 The distal end of the occipital artery is sectioned at an angle and fishmouthed to produce a long anastomosis two two three times the diameter of the recipient vessel. A short segment of the posterior inferior cerebellar artery (PICA), isolated between temporary aneurysm clips, lies open over a latex dam as the first suture is placed. (From Spetzler RF, Koos WT, eds. Color Atlas of Microneurosurgery. Vol 3. Intra- and Extracranial Revascularization and Intraspinal Pathology. 2nd ed. New York: Thieme; 2000:174, Case 3-16e. Reprinted with permission.)

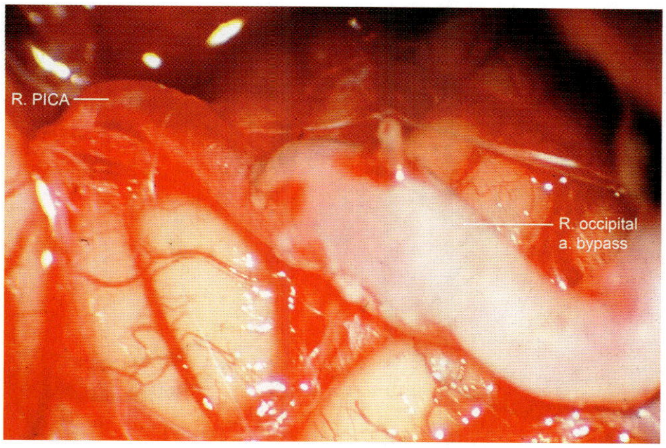

Fig. 8.18 The anastomosis is completed and inspected for hemostasis. PICA, posterior inferior cerebellar artery. (From Spetzler RF, Koos WT, eds. Color Atlas of Microneurosurgery. Vol 3. Intra- and Extracranial Revascularization and Intraspinal Pathology. 2nd ed. New York: Thieme; 2000:174, Case 3-16f. Reprinted with permission.)

the AICA near the basilar artery would require continuous compression of the cerebellum, compromising the collateral branches between the AICA and PICA and between the AICA and SCA.[4,17] Therefore, the flocculonodular or cortical segment of the AICA, distal to the facial-vestibulocochlear nerve complex, is selected for the anastomosis.[4] The vessel is freed from the petrous cortex of the cerebellum and placed over a small latex dam.[17] The distal end of the OA is cleaned of adventitia, fishmouthed, and brought to the site of the anastomosis. The recipient artery is prepared by placing temporary clips on both sides of the exposed vessel and performing a small arteriotomy. After two stay sutures have been placed on both ends of the arteriotomy, a loose running 10-0 suture is placed along one wall. Tightening the sutures after they have all been placed helps the surgeon visualize the vessel walls for these deep anastomoses. Tightening also assures uniform suture tension and improves hemostasis. The suture on the other wall is placed to complete an end-to-side anastomosis. The anastomosis procedure for the AICA is usually more difficult than for PICA because of the depth of the operative field and the smaller diameter of the recipient vessel.[4]

Dissection of a sufficiently long segment of OA for anastomosis with the cerebellar arteries is difficult and time consuming. When an appropriate length of OA cannot be dissected to reach the cerebellar arteries, the anastomosis can be completed using an interposition graft of the radial artery or STA. Touho et al[18] described an anastomosis of the OA to the AICA with interposition of the STA.

◆ In Situ Bypass

Sometimes, ECA branches either have a small caliber or are unavailable or occluded. When donor and recipient arteries lie parallel and in proximity to each other, another option is the in situ bypass. In the posterior circulation, an in situ bypass has a few indications. Basilar terminus aneurysms in which clipping cannot preserve flow in the ipsilateral P1 of the PCA and the posterior communicating artery is small or occluded and cases of fusiform or dissecting aneurysms of the P2 segment unamenable to direct clipping[19] might benefit from a

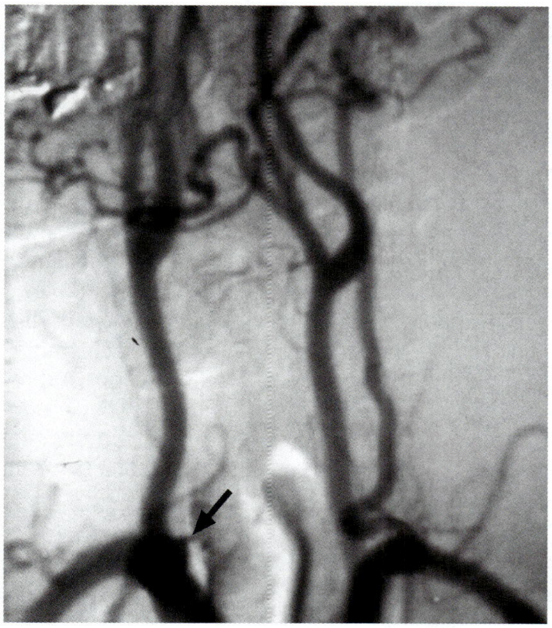

A

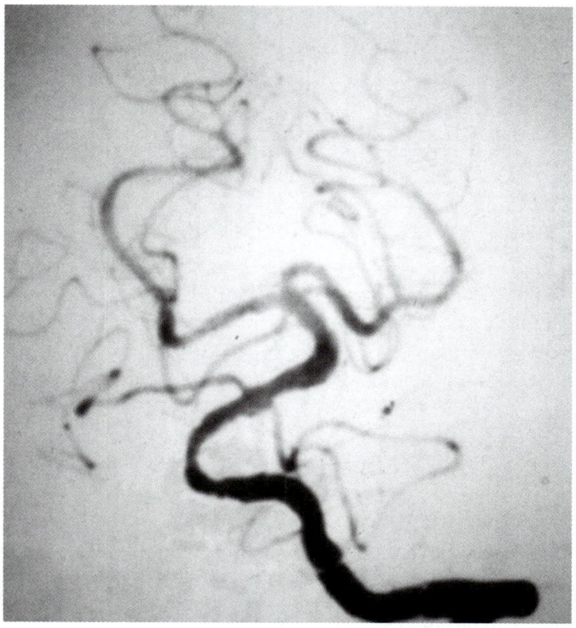

B

Fig. 8.19 A 6-year-old boy presented with a history of repeated attacks of dizziness and right facial numbness. **(A)** Angiogram of the aortic arch demonstrates occlusion of the right vertebral artery (VA) at its origin (*arrow*). **(B)** AP view of the left VA reveals moderate atherosclerotic changes of the distal intracranial VA. There is no evidence of retrograde filling of the right VA or the right posterior inferior cerebellar artery. *(continued)*

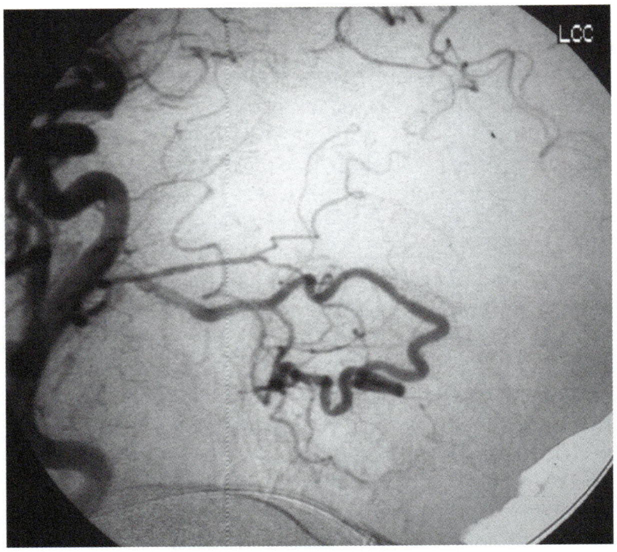

C

Fig. 8.19 *(continued)* **(C)** Postoperative lateral right carotid artery angiogram demonstrates patent bypass. (From Spetzler RF, Koos WT, eds. Color Atlas of Microneurosurgery. Vol 3. Intra- and Extracranial Revascularization and Intraspinal Pathology. 2nd ed. New York: Thieme; 2000:172–174, Case 3-16a,b,g. Reprinted with permission.)

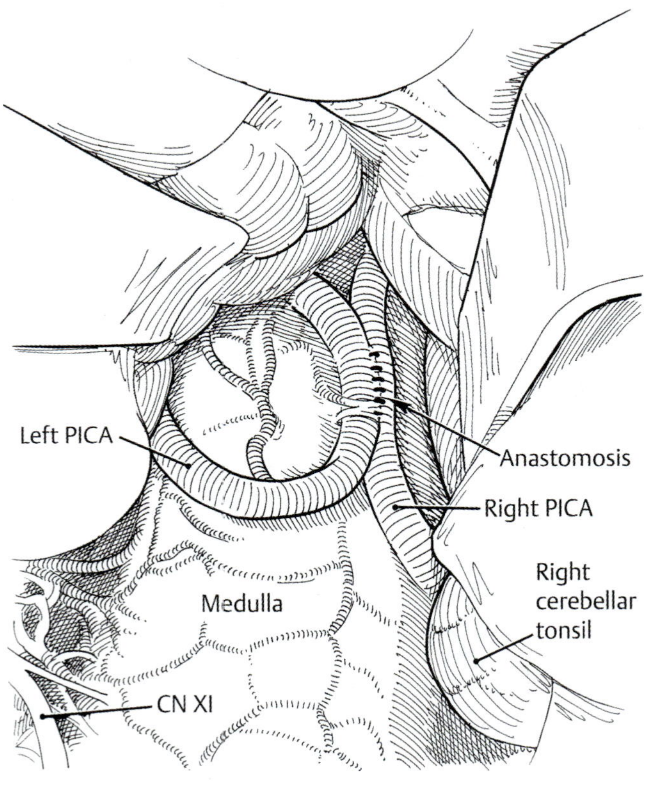

Fig. 8.20 Illustration of a completed side-to-side posterior inferior cerebellar artery (PICA) to PICA in situ anastomosis. The proximity and parallel courses of the tonsillomedullary and telovelotonsillar segments of the posterior inferior cerebellar artery make them ideal for this type of revascularization technique. (From Lemole GM, Henn J, Javedan S, Deshmukh V, Spetzler RF. Cerebral revascularization performed using posterior inferior cerebellar artery–posterior inferior cerebellar artery bypass: Report of four cases and literature review. J Neurosurg 2002;97:219–223. Reprinted with permission from Journal of Neurosurgery.)

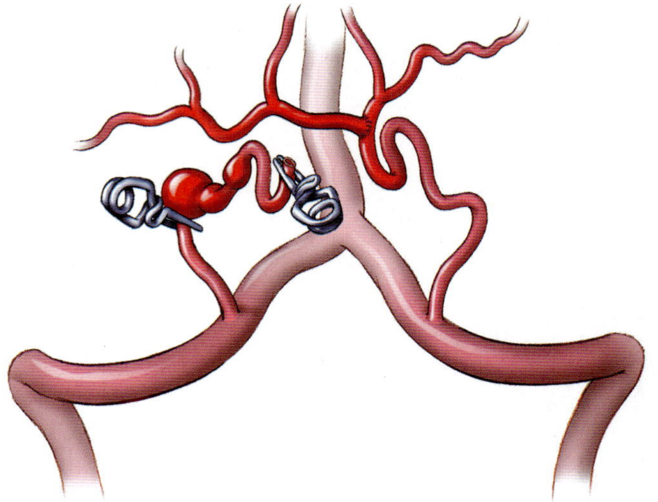

Fig. 8.21 Illustration of an end-to-side posterior inferior cerebellar artery (PICA) to PICA bypass with aneurysmal trapping in a patient whose PICA aneurysm could not be occluded by direct clipping. The stump of the PICA was reimplanted into the contralateral posterior inferior cerebellar artery. (From Lemole GM, Henn J, Javedan S, Deshmukh V, Spetzler RF. Cerebral revascularization performed using posterior inferior cerebellar artery–posterior inferior cerebellar artery bypass. J Neurosurg 2002;97:219–223. Reprinted with permission from Journal of Neurosurgery.)

PCA-SCA bypass. A proximal diseased PICA that is involved with tumor or aneurysm may be treated by trapping or excision and a PICA-PICA in situ anastomosis. The side-to-side in situ anastomosis is not as familiar to neurosurgeons as the end-to-end or end-to-side anastomosis.[5] It requires suturing the back wall of the anastomosis from inside the lumen.

Aneurysm excision and end-to-end anastomosis is another variant of an in situ bypass that can be performed, if there is enough redundancy in the arterial ends to reapproximate them without tension.[5] Excision and reanastomosis is particularly useful for distally located mycotic or fusiform aneurysms. These in situ bypasses have several advantages. They eliminate the need to harvest a donor artery extracranially. They also allow a close match in caliber between donor and recipient vessel. There is one suture line and the length of the bypass is short. The bypasses are less vulnerable to injury or occlusion. These bypasses are all associated with high patency rates. The bypasses are entirely intracranial, allowing a watertight dural closure. Yet, both donor and recipient territories are at risk in the rare event of bypass occlusion or extended crossclamping. Thus, using extracranial ECA branches as a donor graft pedicle may represent a safe primary option when feasible.

References

1. The EC/IC Bypass Study Group. Failure of extracranial-intracranial arterial bypass to reduce the risk of ischemic stroke. Results of an international randomized trial. N Engl J Med 1985;313(19):1191–1200
2. Albuquerque FC, Levy EI, Turk AS, et al. Angiographic patterns of Wingspan in-stent restenosis. Neurosurgery 2008;63(1):23–27

3. Lemole GM Jr, Henn J, Javedan S, Deshmukh V, Spetzler RF. Cerebral revascularization performed using posterior inferior cerebellar artery-posterior inferior cerebellar artery bypass: report of four cases and literature review. J Neurosurg 2002;97(1):219–223
4. Kawashima M, Rhoton AL Jr, Tanriover N, Ulm AJ, Yasuda A, Fujii K. Microsurgical anatomy of cerebral revascularization. Part II: Posterior circulation. J Neurosurg 2005;102(1):132–147
5. Quiñones-Hinojosa A, Lawton MT. In situ bypass in the management of complex intracranial aneurysms: technique application in 13 patients. Neurosurgery 2005; **57**(1, Suppl)140–145, discussion 140–145
6. Rhoton AL Jr. The temporal bone and transtemporal approaches. In: Cranial Anatomy and Surgical Approaches. 8th ed. Philadelphia: Lippincott Williams & Wilkins; 2003:667
7. Woitzik J, Horn P, Vajkoczy P, Schmiedek P. Intraoperative control of extracranial-intracranial bypass patency by near-infrared indocyanine green videoangiography. J Neurosurg 2005;102(4):692–698
8. Alvernia JE, Fraser K, Lanzino G. The occipital artery: a microanatomical study. Neurosurgery 2006; 58(1, Suppl)ONS114–ONS122
9. Nagasawa S, Sakaguchi I, Ohta T. The posterior temporal artery as the recipient in superficial temporal artery to posterior cerebral artery bypass: technical note. Surg Neurol 1999;52(1):73–77
10. Ulku CH, Cicekcibasi AE, Cengiz SL, Ustun ME, Buyukmumcu M. Proximal STA to proximal PCA bypass using a radial artery graft by posterior oblique transzygomatic subtemporal approach. Neurosurg Rev 2009;32(1):95–99, discussion 99
11. Touho H, Karasawa J, Ohnishi H, Kobitsu K. Anastomosis of occipital artery to posterior cerebral artery with interposition of superficial temporal artery using occipital interhemispheric transtentorial approach: case report. Surg Neurol 1995;44(3):245–249, discussion 249–250
12. Khodadad G. Occipital artery-posterior inferior cerebellar artery anastomosis. Surg Neurol 1976;5(4):225–227
13. Hamada J, Todaka T, Yano S, Kai Y, Morioka M, Ushio Y. Vertebral artery-posterior inferior cerebellar artery bypass with a superficial temporal artery graft to treat aneurysms involving the posterior inferior cerebellar artery. J Neurosurg 2002;96(5):867–871
14. Ogasawara K, Kubo Y, Tomitsuka N, et al. Treatment of vertebral artery aneurysms with transposition of the posterior inferior cerebellar artery to the vertebral artery combined with parent artery occlusion: technical note. J Neurosurg 2006;105(5):781–784
15. Benes L, Kappus C, Sure U, Bertalanffy H. Treatment of a partially thrombosed giant aneurysm of the vertebral artery by aneurysm trapping and direct vertebral artery-posterior inferior cerebellar artery end-to-end anastomosis: technical case report. Neurosurgery 2006;59(1, Suppl 1) E166–E167
16. Ausman JI, Diaz FG, Vacca DF, Sadasivan B. Superficial temporal and occipital artery bypass pedicles to superior, anterior inferior, and posterior inferior cerebellar arteries for vertebrobasilar insufficiency. J Neurosurg 1990;72(4):554–558
17. Ausman JI, Diaz FG, de los Reyes RA, Pak H, Patel S, Boulos R. Anastomosis of occipital artery to anterior inferior cerebellar artery for vertebrobasilar junction stenosis. Surg Neurol 1981;16(2):99–102
18. Touho H, Karasawa J, Ohnishi H, et al. Anastomosis of occipital artery to anterior inferior cerebellar artery with interposition of superficial temporal artery: case report. Surg Neurol 1993;40(2):164–170
19. Saito H, Ogasawara K, Kubo Y, Tomitsuka N, Ogawa A. Treatment of ruptured fusiform aneurysm in the posterior cerebral artery with posterior cerebral artery-superior cerebellar artery anastomosis combined with parent artery occlusion: case report. Surg Neurol 2006;65(6):621–624

Chapter 9

In Situ Revascularization Options

Nader Sanai and Michael T. Lawton

Revascularization of a territory distal to an unclippable, giant, dolichoectatic, or thrombotic aneurysm enables the aneurysm to be occluded without risk of ischemic complications, or the parent artery's blood flow to be reversed or reduced safely. Superficial temporal artery to middle cerebral artery (STA-MCA) bypass was the prototype,[1] and subsequently an array of bypasses was developed with the same concept of redirecting extracranial blood flow from scalp arteries or cervical carotid arteries to the brain,[2–17] either directly with one anastomosis or with interposition grafts and two anastomoses. In recent years, innovative bypasses have been introduced anecdotally that revascularize intracranial arteries with other intracranial arteries, without extracranial donor arteries.[8,9,18–22] These intracranial to intracranial (IC-IC) bypasses are simple, elegant, and more anatomic than their EC-IC counterparts. IC-IC bypasses require no harvest of extracranial donors, spare patients a neck incision, shorten any interposition grafts, are protected within the cranium, and use caliber-matched donor and recipient arteries. These advantages of IC-IC bypasses appeal to experienced bypass surgeons, and their use has increased noticeably.

◆ Indications

IC-IC bypasses are generally performed only when conventional clipping fails, due to complex anatomy, large or giant size, dolichoectatic morphology, intraluminal thrombus, or atherosclerotic tissue at the neck. Balloon test occlusion (BTO) can be used to identify candidates who fail the test with balloon inflation alone or with additional hypotensive challenge (lowering mean arterial pressure with nitroprusside drip by 20 mm Hg, or 25% of mean arterial pressure, whichever was greater). In general, high-flow bypass is used in patients who fail BTO immediately, and low-flow bypass is used in patients who fail BTO after hypotensive challenge. Imaging of cerebral blood flow during the BTO with perfusion computed tomography (CT) scans, xenon CT scans, single photon emission CT, or positron emission tomography, can also be used instead of a provocative test such as the hypotensive challenge. Other factors to be considered include the aneurysm's unclippability and patient's angiographic anatomy (presence or absence of collateral circulation from the circle of Willis or leptomeningeal connections).

◆ Surgical Technique

The microsurgical corridor depends on aneurysm location. Internal carotid artery (ICA) aneurysms are approached through a pterional craniotomy, with an orbitozygomatic craniotomy used for additional exposure with giant aneurysms. Similarly, a pterional craniotomy is adequate for MCA aneurysms, with an orbitozygomatic craniotomy used with giant aneurysms. Anterior cerebral artery (ACA) aneurysms are exposed through bifrontal craniotomies, with the midline of the head positioned parallel to the floor and angled up 45 degrees to allow gravity to retract the dependent hemisphere. All bypasses for basilar apex aneurysms can be performed through orbitozygomatic craniotomies. For vertebral artery to superior cerebellar artery (VA-SCA) bypasses of basilar trunk aneurysms, a combined far lateral-subtemporal craniotomy is often necessary. Some occipital artery to posterior cerebral artery (OA-PCA) bypasses require a torcular craniotomy, while most posterior inferior cerebellar artery (PICA) bypasses are performed through far lateral craniotomies.

Brain relaxation is achieved with mannitol (1 g/kg) and cerebrospinal fluid drainage through a ventriculostomy, fenestration in the lamina terminalis, or dissection into a subarachnoid cistern. During the anastomosis when parent arteries are temporarily occluded, mild hypothermia and barbiturate-induced electroencephalographic burst suppression will increase tolerance to ischemia. In our experience, the average intracranial cross-clamp time for an EC-IC bypass was 46 minutes (range 32–63 minutes), and for an IC-IC bypass it was also 46 minutes (range 26–76 minutes). Changes in somatosensory evoked potentials or the electroencephalogram are rare, but can be managed by increasing blood pressure with pressor agents. Heparin irrigation should be used liberally in the surgical field during the anastomosis, but systemic heparin is not needed.

In the context of complex aneurysm treatment, in situ revascularization is generally a part of several surgical strategies. Aneurysm occlusion is usually performed during surgery, typically consisting of aneurysm trapping, proximal occlusion, distal occlusion, or direct aneurysm clipping. The remaining patients typically undergo staged endovascular aneurysm occlusion. Endovascular staging is typically performed 2 or 3 days after the bypass procedure. Patients should be started on aspirin (350 mg daily) immediately after surgery.

Table 9.1 Standard Intracranial-Intracranial Bypasses

Technique	Patients	Graft	Flow	Anastomosis	Technique
In situ bypass					
ATA-MCA	1	No	Low	1	S-S
MCA-MCA	1	No	Low	1	S-S
ACA-ACA	2	No	Low	1	S-S
PCA-SCA	0	No	Low	1	S-S
PICA-PICA	5	No	Low	1	S-S
Reimplantation					
MCA-MCA	1	No	Low	1	E-S
PC-CM	1	No	Low	1	E-S
ATA-SCA	1	No	Low	1	E-S
PICA-VA	3	No	Low	1	E-S
Reanastomosis					
MCA	5	No	Low	1	E-E
ACA	1	No	Low	1	E-E
PICA	5	No	Low	1	E-E
IC bypass graft					
Petrous-supraclinoid ICA	2	Yes	High	2	E-S
ICA-MCA	0	Yes	High	2	E-S
ACA-MCA	1	Yes	High	2	E-S
MCA-ACA	1	Yes	High	2	E-S
ACA-ACA	1	Yes	High	2	E-S
MCA-PCA	2	Yes	High	2	E-S
VA-SCA	2	Yes	High	2	E-S

Abbreviations: ICA, internal carotid artery; ATA, anterior temporal artery; ACA, anterior cerebral artery; MCA, middle cerebral artery; PCA, posterior cerebral artery; SCA, superior cerebellar artery; AICA, anterior inferior cerebellar artery; PICA, posterior inferior cerebellar artery; VA, vertebral artery; PC, pericallosal artery; CM, callosomarginal artery; S-S, side-to-side; E-S, end-to-side; E-E, end-to-end.

Table 9.2 Mixed and Complex Bypasses

	EC-IC Bypass	IC-IC Bypass
Double reimplantation		
ECA-MCA-MCA	1	0
ACA-MCA-MCA	0	1
ACA-PC-CM	0	1
IC-IC plus EC-IC		
MCA-MCA reanastomosis + STA-MCA	0	1
ATA-MCA + STA-MCA	0	1
Reanastomosis with interposition STA		
MCA-STA-MCA	0	1
Double EC-IC		
STA-MCA, double barrel	1	0

Abbreviations: EC, extracranial; IC, intracranial; ECA, external carotid artery; ACA, anterior cerebral artery; MCA, middle cerebral artery; PC, pericallosal artery; CM, callosomarginal artery; ATA, anterior temporal artery; STA, superficial temporal artery.

Four categories of IC-IC bypass exist. In our experience, they can be used individually (**Table 9.1**), or in combination with one another (**Table 9.2**). Each approach has its own set of anatomic requirements, and therefore every aneurysm must be considered within this context (See Bypass Selection section below).

In Situ Bypass

In situ bypass requires donor and recipient arteries that lie parallel and in close proximity to one another. Four sites have this anatomy: MCA branches (M2 and M3 segments) and anterior temporal artery (ATA) as they course through Sylvian fissure (**Fig. 9.1**); bilateral ACAs as they course through interhemispheric fissure over corpus callosum (A3 and A4 segments) (**Fig. 9.2**); PCA (P2 and P3 segments) and SCA as they course through ambient cistern around cerebral peduncle (**Fig. 9.3**); and bilateral PICAs as they course through cisterna magna to meet behind medulla underneath cerebellar tonsils (**Fig. 9.4**). In situ bypasses require one side-to-side anastomosis.

Reimplantation

Complex aneurysms with branches that originate from the aneurysm base can often be reconstructed with tandem clipping techniques that preserve branch arteries (a fenestrated clip encircling the branch origin and a stacked straight clip

(text continued on page 104)

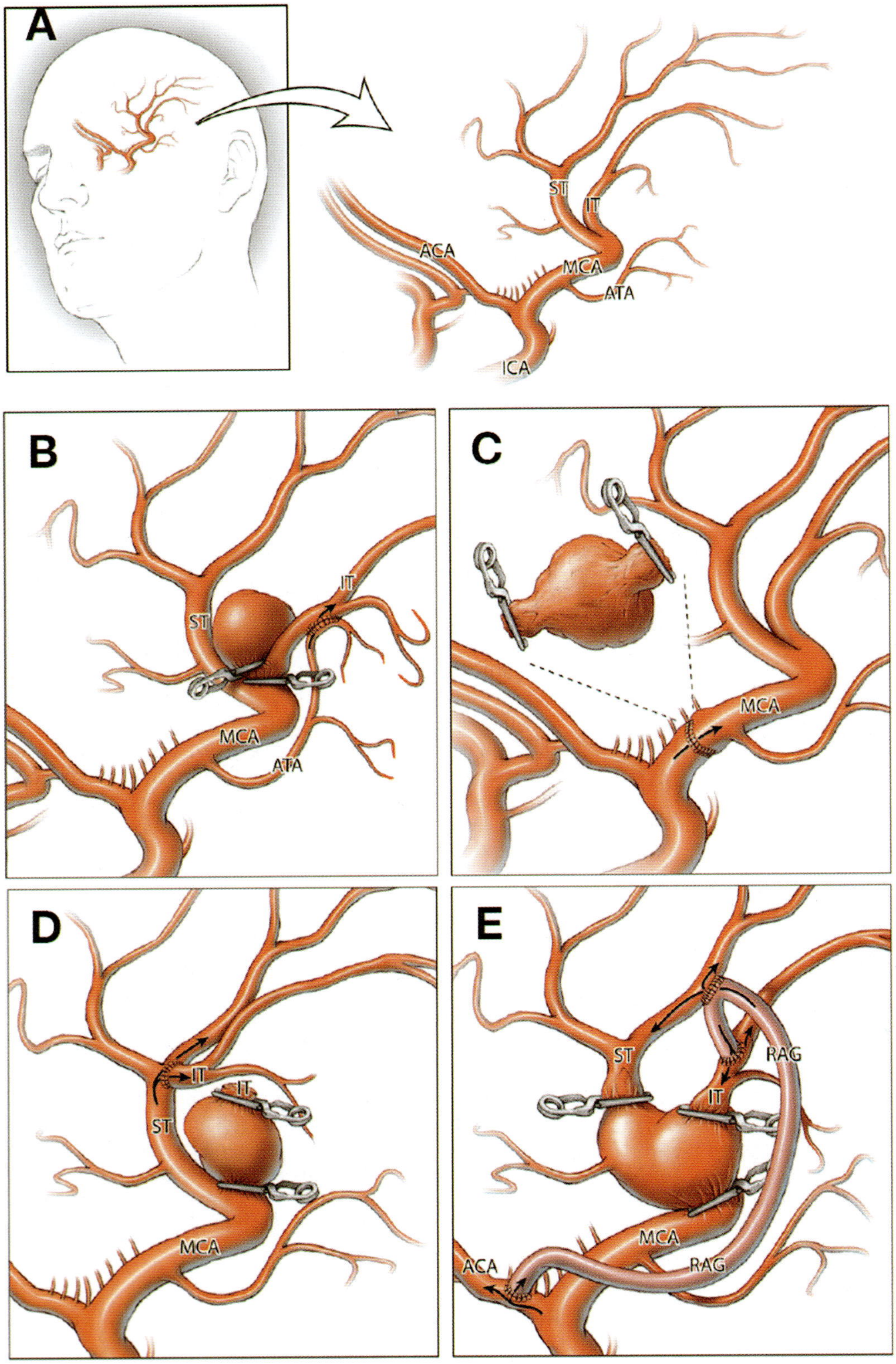

Fig. 9.1 (A–E) Intracranial-intracranial bypass techniques for middle cerebral artery aneurysms. ICA, internal carotid artery; ATA, anterior temporal artery; ACA, anterior cerebral artery; MCA, middle cerebral artery; ST, superior trunk; IT, inferior trunk. (From Sanai N, Zador Z, Lawton MT. Bypass surgery for complex brain aneurysms: an assessment of intracranial-intracranial bypass. Neurosurgery 2009;65(4):670–683. Reprinted with permission.)

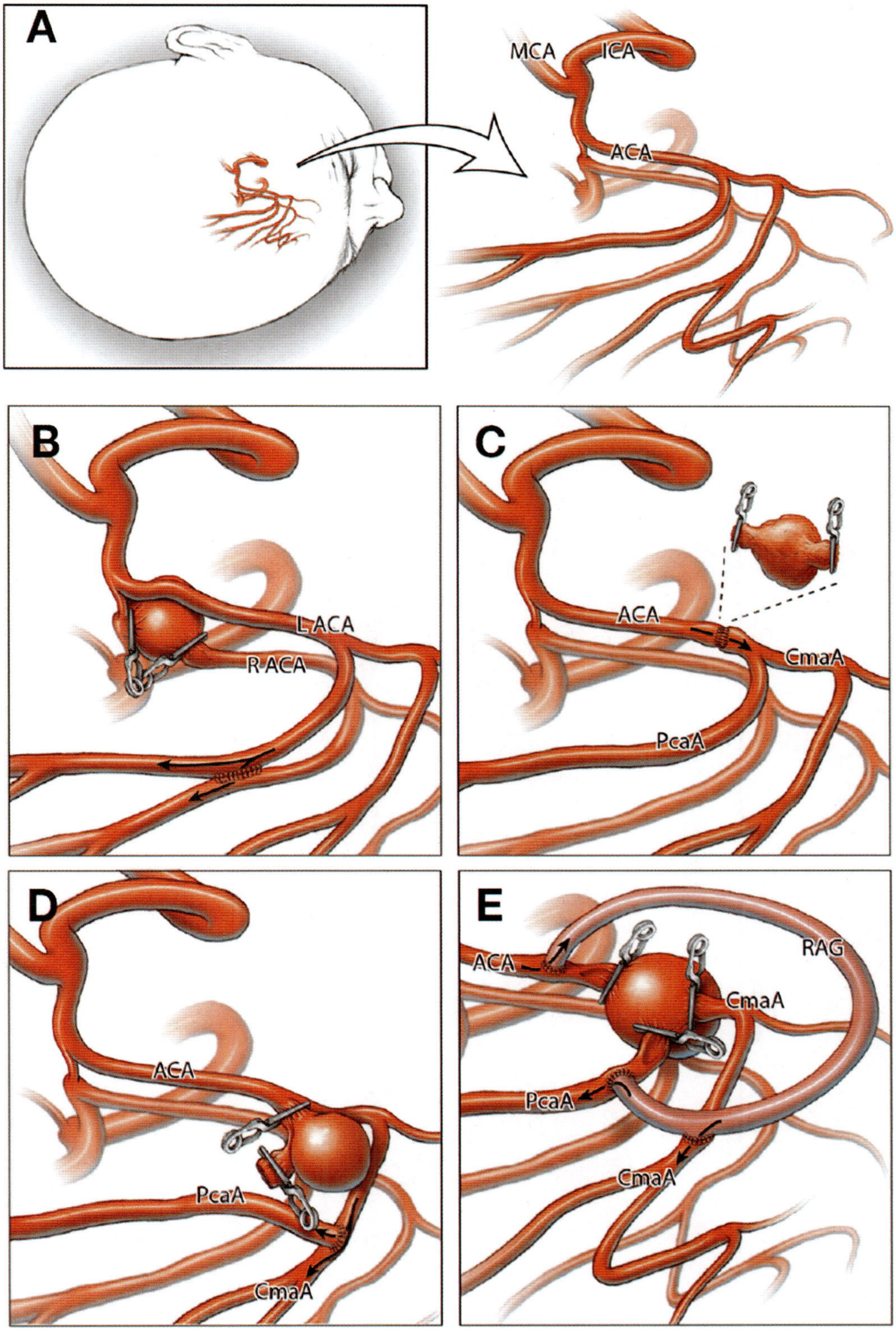

Fig. 9.2 (A–E) Intracrania -intracranial bypass techniques for anterior cerebral artery aneurysms. ICA, internal carotid artery; ACA, anterior cerebral artery; MCA, midd e cerebral artery; PcaA, pericallosal artery; CmaA, callosomarginal artery; L, left; R, right. (From Sanai N, Zador Z, Lawton MT. Bypass surgery for complex brain aneurysms: an assessment of intracranial-intracranial bypass. Neurosurgery 2009;65(4):670–683. Reprinted with permission.)

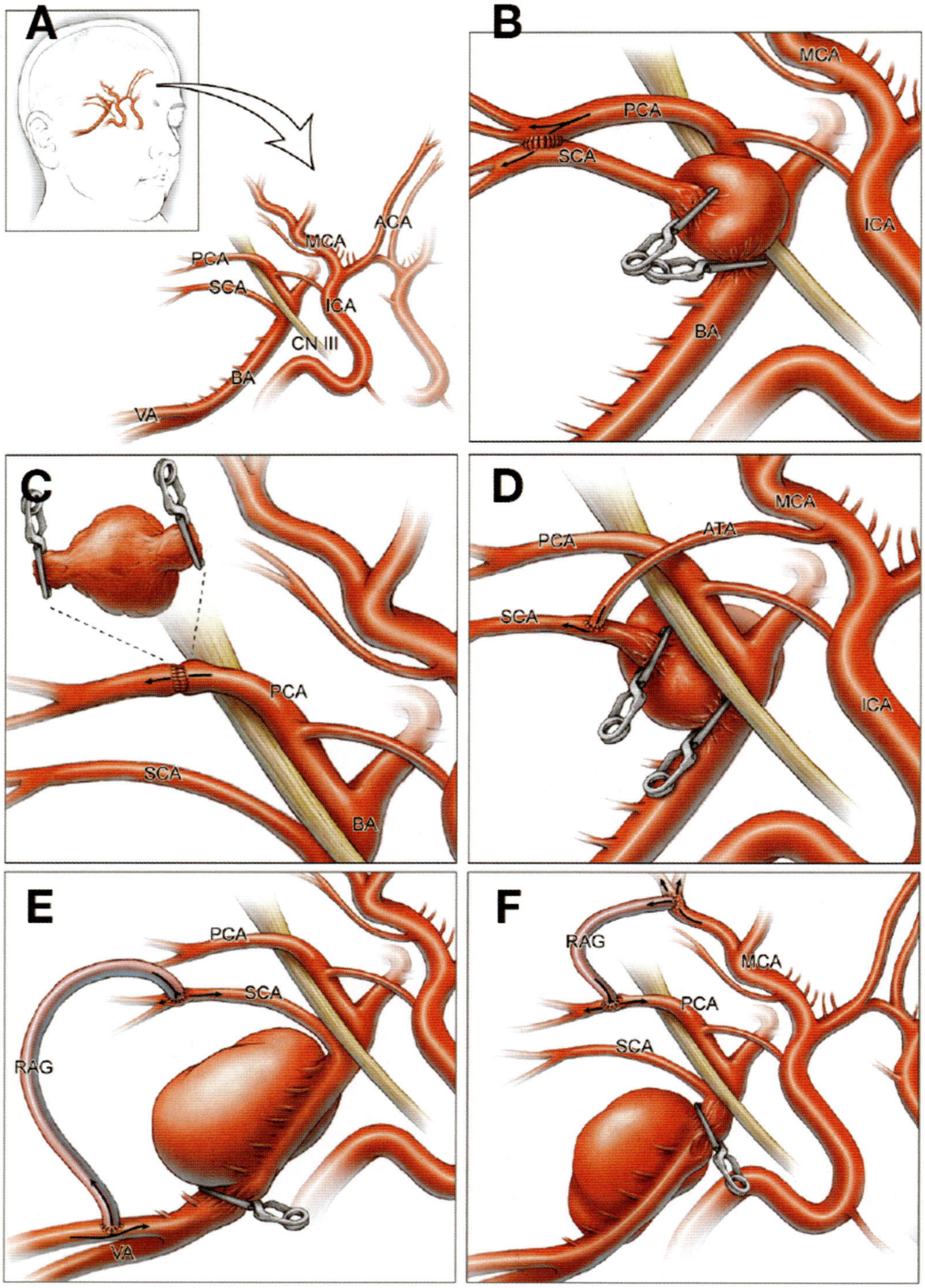

Fig. 9.3 (A–F) Intracranial-intracranial bypass techniques for basilar artery apex aneurysms. ICA, internal carotid artery; ATA, anterior temporal artery; ACA, anterior cerebral artery; MCA, middle cerebral artery; PCA, posterior cerebral artery; SCA, superior cerebellar artery; BA, basilar artery; VA, vertebral artery; CNIII, oculomotor nerve. (From Sanai N, Zador Z, Lawton MT. Bypass surgery for complex brain aneurysms: an assessment of intracranial-intracranial bypass. Neurosurgery 2009;65(4):670–683. Reprinted with permission.)

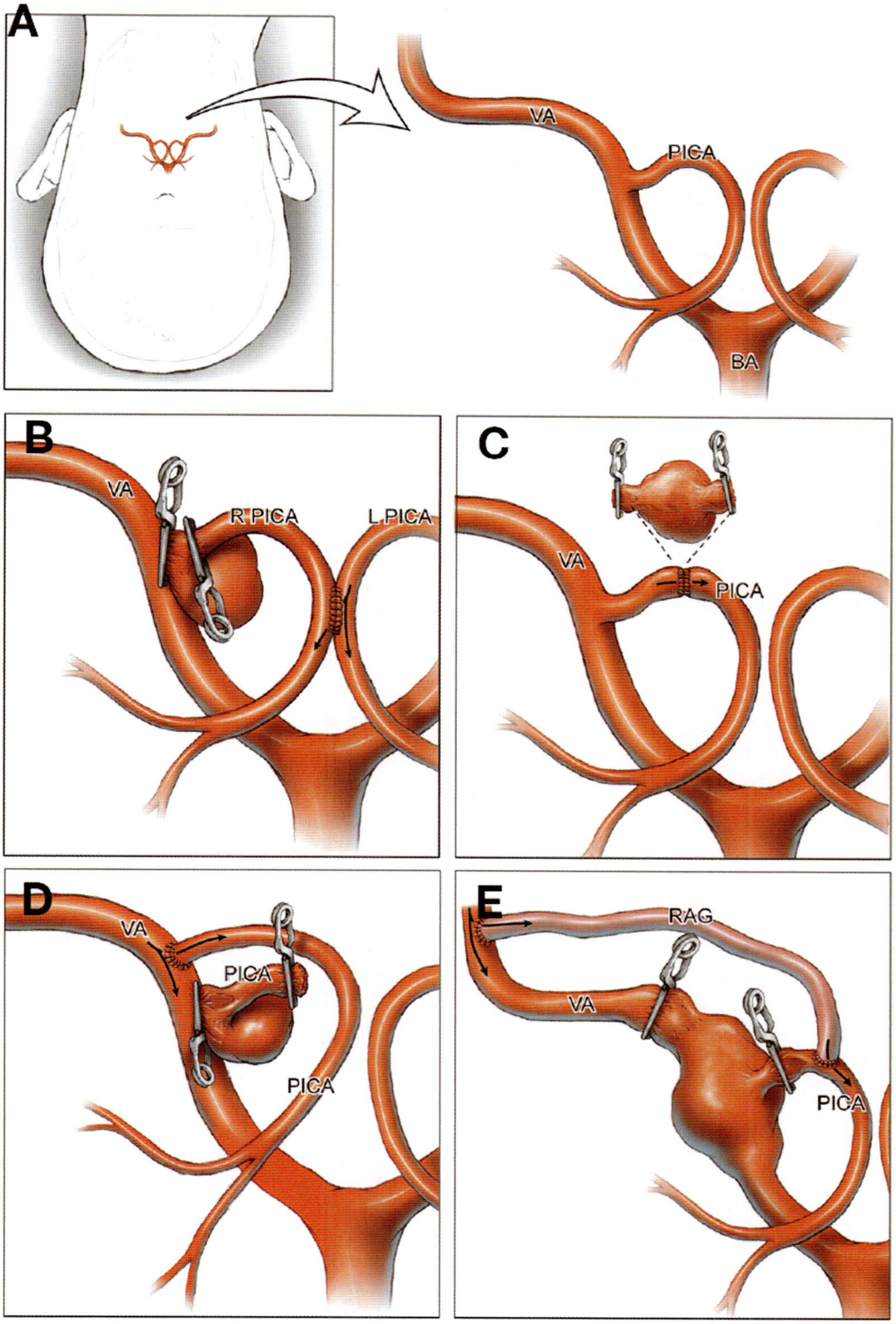

Fig. 9.4 (A–E) Intracranial-intracranial bypass techniques for posterior inferior cerebellar artery aneurysms. PICA, posterior inferior cerebellar artery; VA, vertebral artery; BA, basilar artery; L, left; R, right; RAG, radial artery graft. (From Sanai N, Zador Z, Lawton MT. Bypass surgery for complex brain aneurysms: an assessment of intracranial-intracranial bypass. Neurosurgery 2009;65(4):670–683. Reprinted with permission.)

closing the fenestration). In cases in which clip reconstruction fails, the neck can be clipped to exclude the aneurysm, preserve parent artery, and sacrifice the branch artery. The occluded branch artery can then be reconstituted with reimplantation onto the parent artery. Alternatively, the branch artery can be reimplanted to an adjacent donor artery that is not the parent artery, as long as that donor artery lies near the branch. Like in situ bypasses, this favorable anatomy occurs with MCA, ACA, and PICA aneurysms. Reimplantation requires one end-to-side anastomosis.

Reanastomosis

Reanastomosis requires trapping the aneurysm, completely detaching afferent and efferent arteries, and reconnecting cut ends with an end-to-end anastomosis. This technique works well with fusiform aneurysms that are small or medium in size. Saccular aneurysms at bifurcations are difficult to reconstruct with primary reanastomosis because the second efferent branch must either be reimplanted or bypassed with an extracranial donor artery. Large and giant aneurysms may be difficult to reanastomose because ends of parent artery are separated after excising an aneurysm. Mobilizing the ends of afferent and efferent arteries may enable the first stitch to pull them together with minimal tension. If the gap in the parent artery is too long and the tension too great, suture will tear through artery wall as it is tightened and ruin the repair. Some large aneurysms in PICA and MCA territories have a redundant parent artery that will allow primary reanastomosis despite their size. Reanastomosis requires one end-to-end anastomosis.

Intracranial Bypass with Grafts

Bypasses with interposition grafts connect donor and recipient arteries that are entirely intracranial, differentiating them from EC-IC bypasses that use extracranial donors. In contrast to EC-IC bypasses with saphenous vein grafts spanning from the neck to Sylvian fissure, intracranial bypass grafts are shorter and radial artery grafts are sufficiently long. Radial artery grafts are preferred over saphenous vein grafts because they are composed of arterial tissue, have higher long-term patency rates, and match the caliber of intracranial arteries. A preoperative Allen test with Doppler ultrasound ensures adequate perfusion of the hand with ulnar artery and a competent palmar arch. Intraoperatively, the forearm is accessed for harvest more easily than the thigh, particularly when the patient is positioned laterally or prone for posterior circulation aneurysms. Vasospasm in radial artery grafts has been described but can be avoided by using pressure distension to dilate the graft before implantation, and by bathing the graft in a mixture of nitroprusside and heparin. Unlike other IC-IC techniques, intracranial bypass grafts require at least two anastomoses, which may be end-to-side, end-to-end, or side-to-side. Anastomoses are planned to minimize brain ischemia during the time that intracranial arteries are temporarily occluded and sutured.

◆ Bypass Selection

Most current EC-IC bypasses convert to an IC-IC bypass. ACA and PICA territories were particularly amenable to intracranial reconstruction, and even though MCA and basilar apex territories were divided between EC-IC and IC-IC techniques in our cohort of bypass patients, growing experience with A1 ACA-MCA and MCA-PCA bypasses have made them preferred choices.

Selecting a bypass from among the four IC-IC techniques depends on aneurysm anatomy, suitability of the donor artery, depth of the surgical field, and type of anastomosis. Fusiform aneurysms lend themselves to reanastomosis because they are often distally located away from bifurcations, with one afferent and one efferent artery. End-to-end repair requires aneurysm excision back to healthy arterial tissue on both ends, and joining ends without tension. Mobilizing redundant artery and resecting aneurysm can bring the arteries together. End-to-end anastomosis is the easiest anastomosis: forceps tips in the lumen visualize translucent arterial walls and guide the needle through its bites; the number of bites needed to complete the anastomosis is less; and arteries rotate to visualize both suture lines.

In contrast to fusiform aneurysms, saccular aneurysms with multiple efferent arteries require other reconstructive techniques. In situ bypass and reimplantation revascularize one efferent artery when the other can be preserved with clipping. For example, the ACA-ACA bypass works when clipping or coiling an ACoA aneurysm sacrifices one A2 ACA. The other patent A2 ACA supplies the distal bypass and restores flow to the opposite ACA. Side-to-side anastomosis is probably the most difficult anastomosis because the deep suture line is sewn inside the lumen. After approximating the two arteries with sutures at each end of the arteriotomies, the first bite transitions the needle from outside the lumen where the knot is tied, to inside the lumen where running bites are taken. Bites are taken between two outer layers of arterial wall, keeping track of four translucent layers. The last bite transitions the needle again from inside to outside the lumen to tie the knot. The second suture line is performed from outside the lumen and is much easier. The arteriotomy length should be three times the diameter of the arteries to communicate generously between arteries. Consequently, side-to-side anastomoses require more bites than other anastomoses. This difficult anastomosis should be avoided in deep, narrow surgical corridors, but can be performed in the Sylvian fissure, cisterna magna, and interhemispheric fissure.

Reimplantation also salvages a branch artery compromised by aneurysm clipping with an end-to-side anastomosis to the parent artery, the other efferent artery, or an uninvolved bystander. PICA-VA reimplantation was the most frequent location for this technique, but it works well in MCA and ACA territories (pericallosal to callosomarginal reimplantation; **Fig. 9.5**). These recipient reimplantations connect the proximal end of a branch to the side of a donor, but donor reimplantations can also connect the distal end of a branch to a recipient artery to rededicate the branch artery to supplying a new vascular territory. For example, ATA supplies a silent vascular territory and, when reimplanted onto SCA, can supply SCA or basilar apex (**Fig. 9.6**). Reimplanted arteries can therefore donate or receive blood flow. The end-to-side anastomosis is identical to STA-MCA bypass, with a generous arteriotomy in the donor (at least twice the diameter of the artery) and a spatulated end of the reimplanted recipient to cover the arteriotomy. Simple continuous sutures are placed loosely and tightened after all bites have been taken. The site of reimplantation is selected to slacken the reimplanted artery and allow it to be shifted from side to side to visualize both suture lines.

Complex reconstructions are required when multiple efferent arteries are compromised by clipping. For example, the double reimplantation technique rebuilds a bifurcation with three anastomoses (**Fig. 9.7**). A radial artery graft is first connected proximally to a donor artery to ready the bypass graft. The first efferent artery is reimplanted on the live graft and blood flow is restored immediately. The second efferent artery is reimplanted distally on the graft, allowing the graft to supply the first reimplanted artery during this second reimplantation. Placement of a temporary clip distal to the first and proximal to the second anastomosis redirects blood flow to the reimplanted trunk while keeping the other surgical site dry. This successive reimplantation of branch arteries minimizes ischemia, with temporary occlusion times for each of the efferent arteries equal to the time needed to complete one anastomosis. Double reimplantation technique adapts to triple reimplantation for trifurcated anatomy. Other intracranial bypass grafts replenish cerebral blood flow with fewer anastomoses (**Fig. 9.8**). For example, MCA-PCA bypass revascularizes quadrifurcated anatomy of the basilar apex with a single deep anastomosis to the P2 PCA and a superficial anastomosis to an MCA trunk that is already exposed en route to the PCA site. Intracranial bypass grafts like the MCA-PCA bypass do not fully reconstruct arterial anatomy and may not enable complete exclusion of the aneurysm, but may

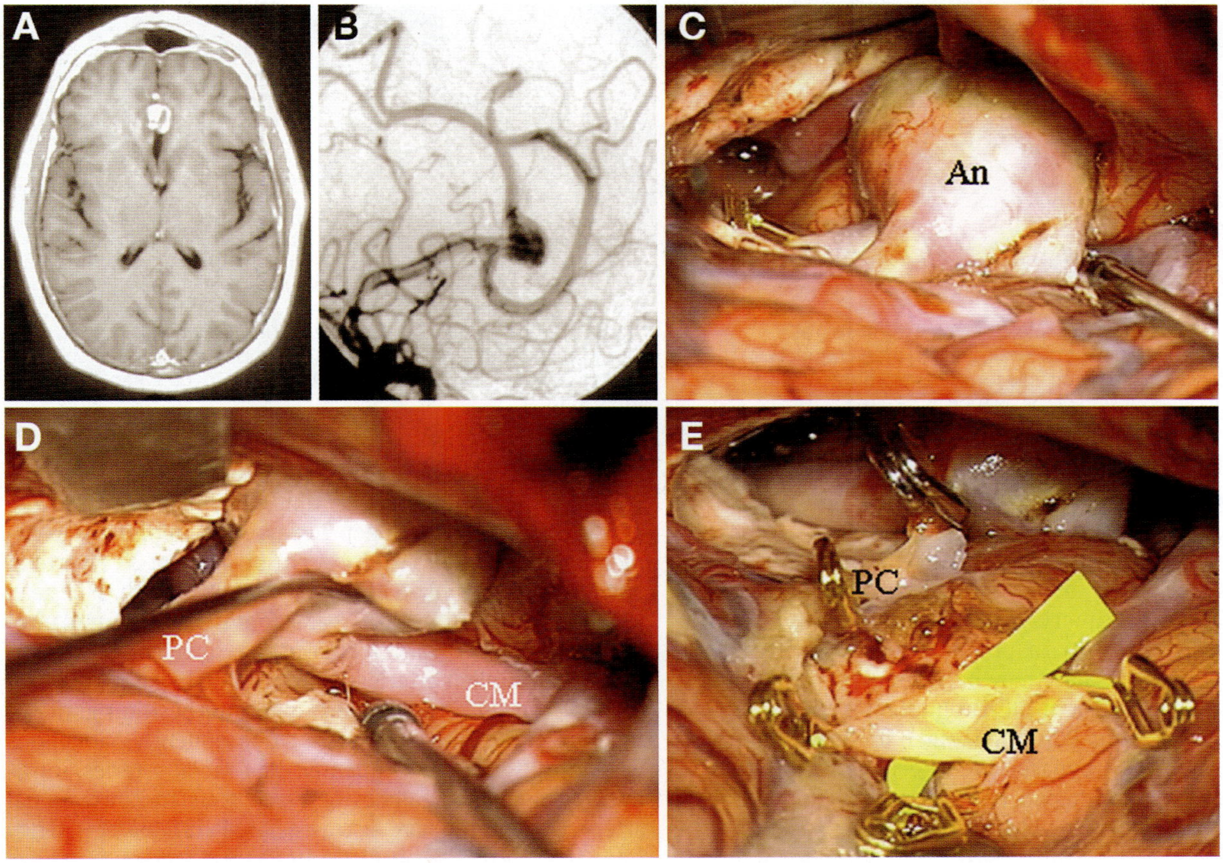

Fig. 9.5 Recipient reimplantation. This thrombotic anterior cerebral artery (ACA) aneurysm, seen on axial T1-weighted MRI **(A)**, originated at the bifurcation of the pericallosal (PC) and callosomarginal (CM) arteries, and on right internal carotid artery angiogram, lateral view **(B)**. **(C,D)** The aneurysm (An) was exposed in the interhemispheric fissure through a bifrontal craniotomy, using gravity to retract the right hemisphere (right hemisphere down; left hemisphere up; nose facing to the right). Attempts to clip reconstruct the neck were unsuccessful; intraluminal thrombus caused the clips to occlude the pericallosal artery. **(E)** Rather than opening the aneurysm, removing thrombus, and attempting to reconstruct a neck, the pericallosal artery was clip occluded, transected, and mobilized to the callosomarginal artery. *(continued)*

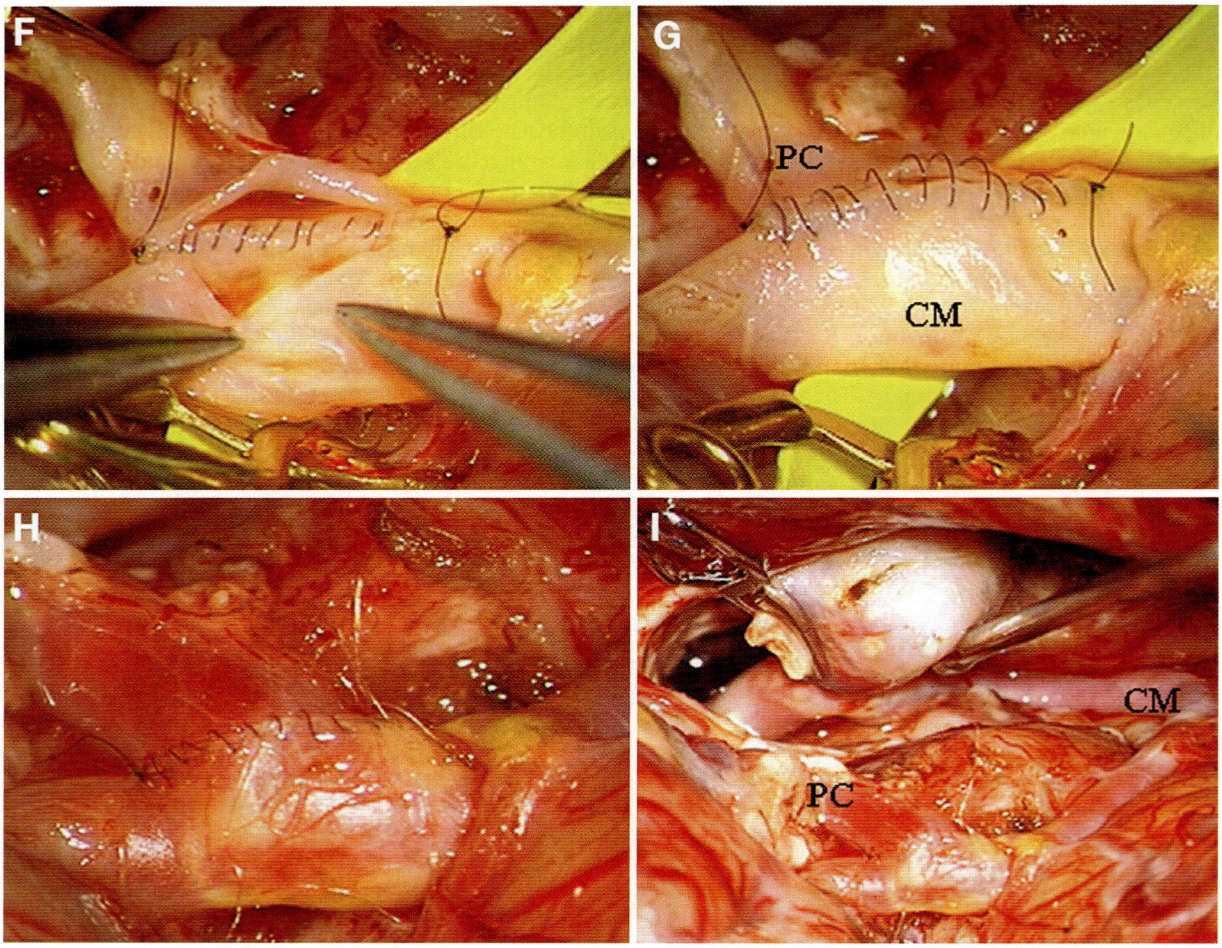

Fig. 9.5 *(continued)* An end-to-side PC-CM anastomosis was performed (**[F]** back wall, **[G]** front wall, and **[H]** after completion). **(I)** The CM artery supplied blood flow for the entire distal ACA territory. Distal clip occlusion of the aneurysm resulted in its complete thrombosis. (From Sanai N, Zador Z, Lawton MT. Bypass surgery for complex brain aneurysms: an assessment of intracranial-intracranial bypass. Neurosurgery 2009;65(4):670–683. Reprinted with permission.)

reverse flow or create more benign hemodynamics inside the aneurysm.

Bypass selection ultimately depends on an intraoperative assessment of the aneurysm and surrounding anatomy. We devise a primary bypass strategy and several contingency strategies, with preparations for each (like prepping a graft site). There may be several viable options (e.g., PICA-PICA bypass and PICA reimplantation), no options (e.g., P3 segment PCA aneurysm), or serendipitous options (e.g., ATA-SCA bypass). We select the bypass that facilitates aneurysm occlusion, restores normal blood flow, and is technically most feasible.

◆ Conclusions

Although it is more technically challenging to perform, the IC-IC bypass offers certain advantages that justifies its use. First, the caliber of scalp arteries is variable and sometimes too diminutive to revascularize an efferent artery. Although scalp arteries can dilate over time, they may not meet the demand immediately. Deep bypasses to midline or paramedian arteries can require 8 cm or more of scalp artery, and it may be too small at the anastomotic depth to be safe. In contrast, in situ bypass, reanastomosis, and reimplantation techniques use donor arteries that match or exceed the caliber of recipient arteries. Second, EC-IC bypasses that use cervical carotid artery require long interposition grafts at the limit of the radial artery graft. Consequently, saphenous veins are used more frequently than radial arteries, introducing caliber mismatches between graft and intracranial artery. Longer grafts are also associated with lower patency rates long term. In contrast, intracranial bypass grafts are shorter and enable frequent use of radial artery grafts. Their smaller caliber closely resembles that of intracranial arteries and enhances the anastomosis. Third, IC-IC bypasses eliminate neck incisions, reduce invasiveness, and improve cosmesis. Intracranial bypasses are less vulnerable than EC-IC bypasses to neck torsion, injury, and occlusion with external compression. Fourth, IC-IC bypasses eliminate the harvest of

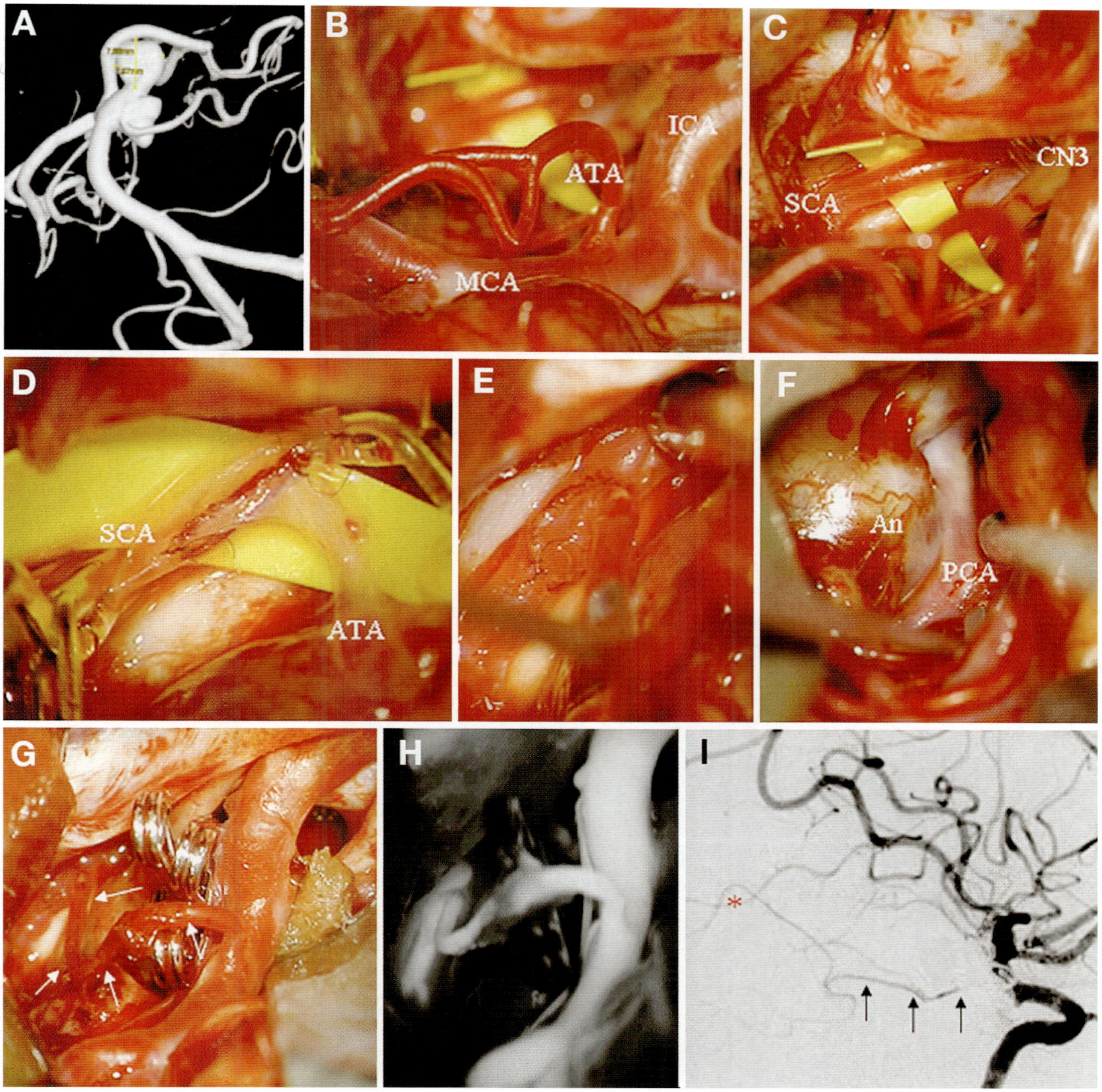

Fig. 9.6 Donor reimplantation. **(A)** A 55-year-old woman presented with a subarachnoid hemorrhage from this multilobulated left superior cerebellar artery (SCA) aneurysm, seen on rotational angiogram with three-dimensional reconstruction. Only the superior lobule could be coiled, leaving residual neck to preserve the SCA origin. She was referred for surgery to protect her from rehemorrhage. After inspecting the anatomy intraoperatively, it seemed unlikely that the aneurysm could be clipped without occluding SCA and likely that a bypass would be needed to preserve it. A prominent anterior temporal artery (ATA) was found in the Sylvian fissure **(B)**, and it had sufficient length to reach the SCA **(C)**. **(D)** ATA was transected distally and reimplanted onto SCA with an end-to-side anastomosis. After bypass patency was confirmed **(E)**, the aneurysm (An) was neck was dissected **(F)** and clipped **(G)**. Indocyanine green videography confirmed good flow in the ATA-SCA bypass **(H)**, as did the postoperative angiogram (left ICA injection, lateral view, with opacification of the left SCA (*arrows* in **I**). Note the course of the SCA over the cerebellar vermis (*red asterisk*)). The patient tolerated ATA sacrifice without neurologic sequela. MCA, middle cerebral artery; ICA, internal carotid artery; PCA, posterior cerebral artery; CN3, oculomotor nerve. (From Sanai N, Zador Z, Lawton MT. Bypass surgery for complex brain aneurysms: an assessment of intracranial-intracranial bypass. Neurosurgery 2009;65(4):670–683. Reprinted with permission.)

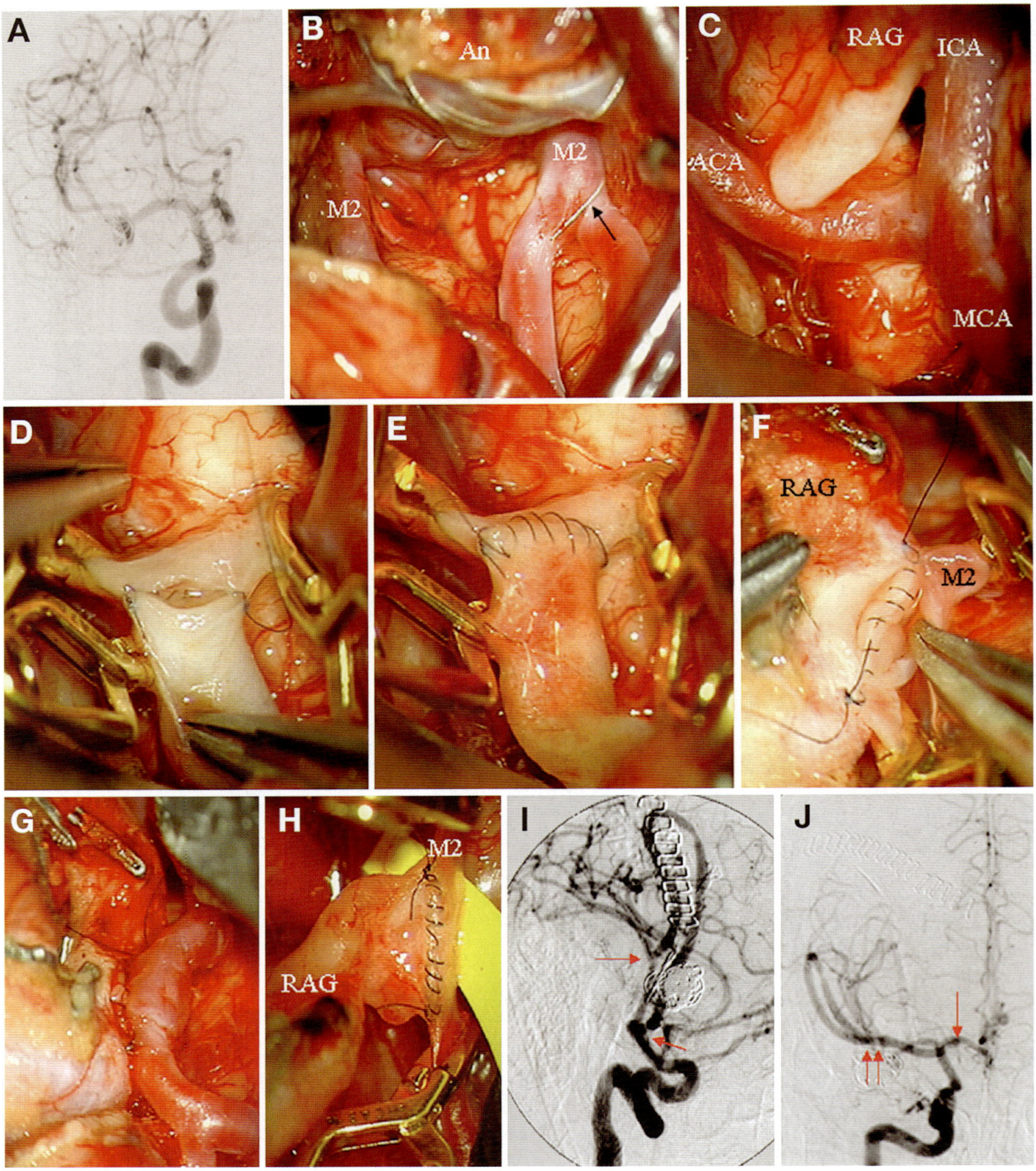

Fig. 9.7 Intracranial bypass graft with double reimplantation. **(A)** This ruptured right middle cerebral artery (MCA) aneurysm was coiled and recurred 6 months later (right internal carotid artery [ICA] angiogram, anterior oblique view). **(B)** Intraoperatively, the two M2 MCA trunks originated from the aneurysm (An) base and could not be kept open with direct clipping. Note the strand of coil in the lumen of the temporal M2 trunk (*black arrow*). The A1 segment of the anterior cerebral artery (ACA) was used as the donor for a radial artery graft (RAG; **C**) that was sutured with an end-to-side anastomosis **(D,E)**. The frontal M2 trunk was reimplanted onto the RAG with a side-to-side anastomosis, shown after suturing the deep suture line intraluminally **(F)** and after completing the superficial suture line **(G)**. **(H)** The end of the RAG was looped to the temporal M2 trunk and sewn with an end-to-side anastomosis. Postoperative angiography (right ICA injection, lateral **[I]** and AP **[J]** views) confirmed patency of the bypass and filling of both MCA trunks (*red arrows* indicate anastomoses). (From Sanai N, Zador Z, Lawton MT. Bypass surgery for complex brain aneurysms: an assessment of intracranial-intracranial bypass. Neurosurgery 2009;65(4):670–83. Reprinted with permission.)

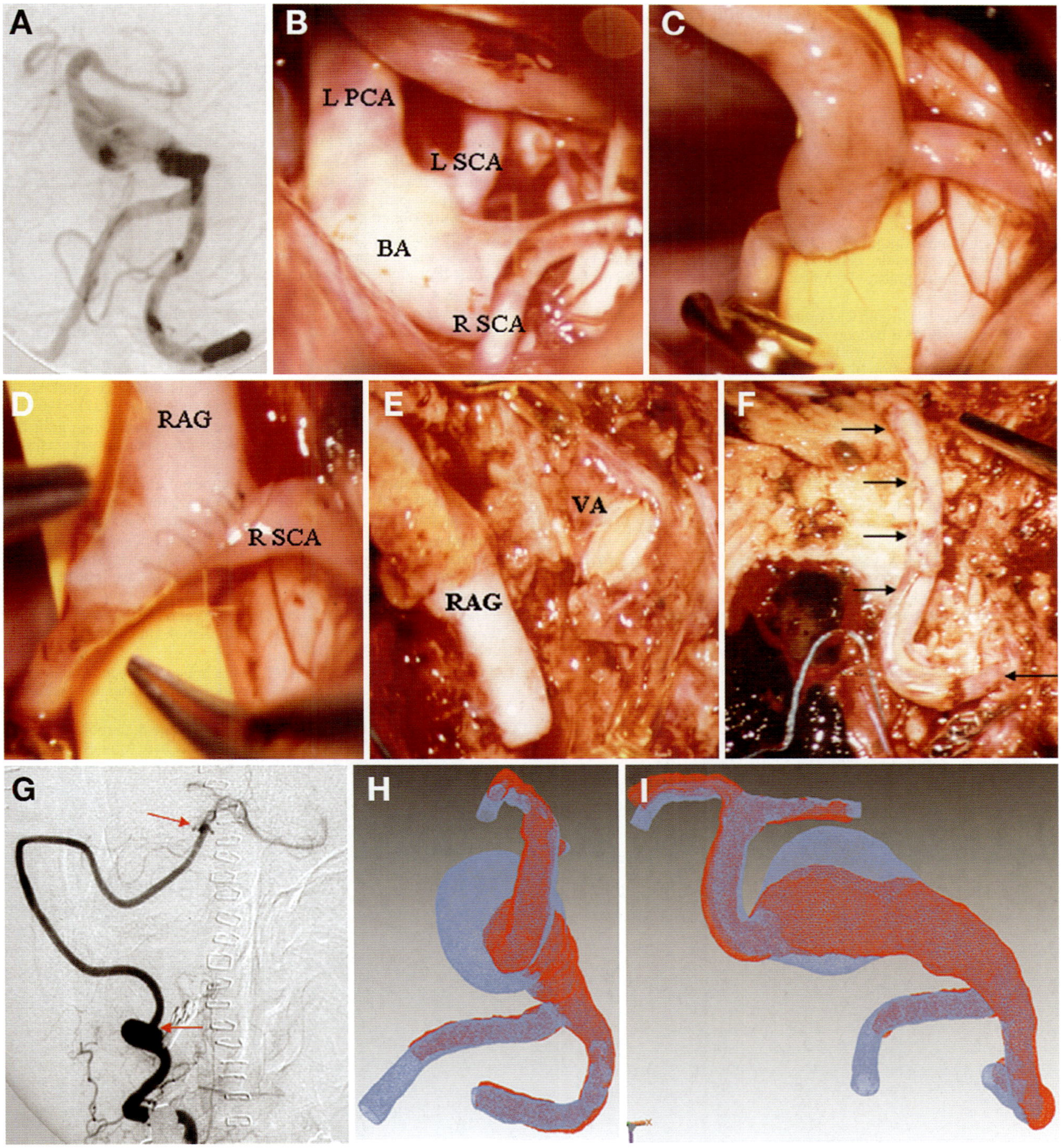

Fig. 9.8 Intracranial bypass graft. **(A)** This fusiform, giant basilar trunk aneurysm (left vertebral artery [VA] angiogram, anterior oblique view) enlarged rapidly over a 2-year period, changing from a small, asymptomatic bump in the basilar trunk to a compressive mass with new hemiparesis, dysarthria, and gait instability. It was treated with a VA-to-superior cerebellar artery (SCA) bypass. **(B)** A combined far lateral-temporal craniotomy provided a subtemporal view of the basilar artery (BA) apex. **(C,D)** A radial artery graft (RAG) was anastomosed to the right SCA. **(E)** The proximal end of the graft was connected to the side of extradural VA at the foramen magnum. The course of the VA-SCA bypass is shown intraoperatively (*arrows* in **F**) and angiographically (**G;** right VA injection, AP view, with anastomoses indicated by the *red arrows*). VA-SCA bypass and clip occlusion of the right VA resulted in thrombosis of the aneurysm lumen, shown preoperatively in *blue* and postoperatively in *red* on overlaid volumetric images generated from contrast-enhanced MRA (lateral **[H]** and AP **[I]** views). (From Sanai N, Zador Z, Lawton MT. Bypass surgery for complex brain aneurysms: an assessment of intracranial-intracranial bypass. Neurosurgery 2009;65(4):670–683. Reprinted with permission.)

an extracranial donor artery, saving time and tedious effort. Intracranial donor arteries reside in the surgical field and require minimal preparation.

References

1. Yasargil M. Anastomosis between Superficial Temporal Artery and a Branch of the Middle Cerebral Artery. Stuttgart: Georg Thieme Verlag; 1969
2. Auguste KI, Quiñones-Hinojosa A, Lawton MT. The tandem bypass: subclavian artery-to-middle cerebral artery bypass with Dacron and saphenous vein grafts. Technical case report. Surg Neurol 2001;56(3):164–169
3. Barnett DW, Barrow DL, Joseph GJ. Combined extracranial-intracranial bypass and intraoperative balloon occlusion for the treatment of intracavernous and proximal carotid artery aneurysms. Neurosurgery 1994;35(1):92–97, discussion 97–98
4. Başkaya MK, Kiehn MW, Ahmed AS, Ateş O, Niemann DB. Alternative vascular graft for extracranial-intracranial bypass surgery: descending branch of the lateral circumflex femoral artery. Neurosurg Focus 2008;24(2):E8
5. Friedman JA, Piepgras DG. Current neurosurgical indications for saphenous vein graft bypass. Neurosurg Focus 2003;14(3):e1
6. Kato Y, Sano H, Imizu S, et al. Surgical strategies for treatment of giant or large intracranial aneurysms: our experience with 139 cases. Minim Invasive Neurosurg 2003;46(6):339–343
7. Langer DJ, Van Der Zwan A, Vajkoczy P, Kivipelto L, Van Doormaal TP, Tulleken CA. Excimer laser-assisted nonocclusive anastomosis: an emerging technology for use in the creation of intracranial-intracranial and extracranial-intracranial cerebral bypass. Neurosurg Focus 2008;24(2):E6
8. Lawton MT, Hamilton MG, Morcos JJ, Spetzler RF. Revascularization and aneurysm surgery: current techniques, indications, and outcome. Neurosurgery 1996;38(1):83–92
9. Lemole GM Jr, Henn J, Javedan S, Deshmukh V, Spetzler RF. Cerebral revascularization performed using posterior inferior cerebellar artery-posterior inferior cerebellar artery bypass: report of four cases and literature review. J Neurosurg 2002;97(1):219–223
10. Mohit AA, Sekhar LN, Natarajan SK, Britz GW, Ghodke B. High-flow bypass grafts in the management of complex intracranial aneurysms. Neurosurgery 2007;60(2, Suppl 1)ONS105–ONS122
11. Morgan MK, Sekhon LH. Extracranial-intracranial saphenous vein bypass for carotid or vertebral artery dissections: a report of six cases. J Neurosurg 1994;80(2):237–246
12. Quiñones-Hinojosa A, Du R, Lawton MT. Revascularization with saphenous vein bypasses for complex intracranial aneurysms. Skull Base 2005;15(2):119–132
13. Regli L, Piepgras DG, Hansen KK. Late patency of long saphenous vein bypass grafts to the anterior and posterior cerebral circulation. J Neurosurg 1995;83(5):806–811
14. Rivet DJ, Wanebo JE, Roberts GA, Dacey RG Jr. Use of a side branch in a saphenous vein interposition graft for high-flow extracranial-intracranial bypass procedures: technical note. J Neurosurg 2005;103(1):186–187
15. Santoro A, Guidetti G, Dazzi M, Cantore G. Long saphenous-vein grafts for extracranial and intracranial internal carotid aneurysms amenable neither to clipping nor to endovascular treatment. J Neurosurg Sci 1999;43(4):237–250
16. Ustün ME, Büyükmumcu M, Ulku CH, Cicekcibasi AE, Arbag H. Radial artery graft for bypass of the maxillary to proximal middle cerebral artery: an anatomic and technical study. Neurosurgery 2004;54(3):667–670
17. Zhang YJ, Barrow DL, Day AL. Extracranial-intracranial vein graft bypass for giant intracranial aneurysm surgery for pediatric patients: two technical case reports. Neurosurgery 2002;50(3):663–668
18. Bederson JB, Spetzler RF. Anastomosis of the anterior temporal artery to a secondary trunk of the middle cerebral artery for treatment of a giant M1 segment aneurysm: case report. J Neurosurg 1992;76(5):863–866
19. Candon E, Marty-Ane C, Pieuchot P, Frerebeau P. Cervical-to-petrous internal carotid artery saphenous vein in situ bypass for the treatment of a high cervical dissecting aneurysm: technical case report. Neurosurgery 1996;39(4):863–866
20. Evans JJ, Sekhar LN, Rak R, Stimac D. Bypass grafting and revascularization in the management of posterior circulation aneurysms. Neurosurgery 2004;55(5):1036–1049
21. Quiñones-Hinojosa A, Lawton MT. In situ bypass in the management of complex intracranial aneurysms: technique application in 13 patients. Neurosurgery 2005;57(1, Suppl)140–145
22. Sekhar LN, Natarajan SK, Ellenbogen RG, Ghodke B. Cerebral revascularization for ischemia, aneurysms, and cranial base tumors. Neurosurgery 2008;62(6, Suppl 3)1373–1408

Chapter 10

Indirect Revascularization for Moyamoya Syndrome

E. R. Smith and R. Michael Scott

Moyamoya syndrome is an increasingly recognized cause of stroke characterized by progressive stenosis of the intracranial internal carotid arteries (ICAs) and their proximal branches. As these vessels narrow, a network of collateral vessels develops near the carotid bifurcation, on the cortical surface, and also from branches of the external carotid artery (ECA). In rare cases, this process may involve the posterior circulation, including the basilar and posterior cerebral arteries. Some authors have distinguished between *moyamoya disease*—the idiopathic form of moyamoya—and *moyamoya syndrome*—defined as the vasculopathy found in association with other conditions. These conditions include, but are not limited to, prior radiotherapy to the head or neck for tumors, Down syndrome, neurofibromatosis type I, large facial hemangiomas, sickle cell disease; autoimmune disorders such as Graves disease, congenital cardiac disease, and renal artery stenosis.

Most patients present with ischemic symptoms; recurrent transient ischemic attacks (TIAs) or strokes. Adults also commonly present with intraparenchymal hemorrhage. Seizures and headaches have been described as presenting symptoms in a minority of patients.

The natural history of moyamoya is not well known. Disease progression can be slow with rare, intermittent strokes, or fulminant, with rapid neurologic decline.[1,2] However, moyamoya inevitably progresses in the majority of patients—including asymptomatic individuals—and medical therapy alone does not halt the process.[3–5] Two-thirds of patients with moyamoya have symptomatic progression over a 5-year period with poor outcomes if left untreated.[6–8] This number contrasts strikingly with an estimated rate of only 2.6% of symptomatic progression following surgical treatment in a meta-analysis of over 1100 patients.[9]

The workup of a patient in whom the diagnosis of moyamoya syndrome is suspected typically begins with either a magnetic resonance imaging (MRI) study or computed tomography (CT) of the brain. Findings include narrowed ICAs, middle cerebral arteries (MCAs), and anterior cerebral arteries (ACAs) in association with moyamoya collaterals in the basal ganglia and frequently evidence of previous infarcts. Sometimes reduced cerebral blood flow can be inferred from fluid-attenuated inversion recovery (FLAIR) images with the so-called ivy sign, a bright signal in cortical sulci. Definitive diagnosis is based on a distinct arteriographic appearance characterized by bilateral stenosis of the distal intracranial ICA extending to the proximal ACA and MCA (**Fig. 10.1**). Disease severity is frequently classified into one of six progressive stages originally defined by Suzuki et al.[3] Development of an extensive collateral network at the base of the brain along with the classic "puff of smoke" appearance on angiography is seen during the intermediate stages of the Suzuki grading system. External carotid imaging is essential to identify preexisting collateral vessels so that surgery, if performed, will not disrupt them. Aneurysms or arteriovenous malformations, known to be associated with some cases of moyamoya, can also be best detected by conventional angiography.

Once diagnosed, patients should be referred to a specialized center experienced with the treatment of moyamoya. In general, neurologic status at time of treatment, more so than the age of the patient, predicts long-term outcome.[1] As such, early diagnosis of moyamoya is of paramount importance and needs to be coupled with expeditious institution of therapy. The curious fact that the arteriopathy of moyamoya involves the ICA, while sparing the ECA provides the foundation underlying surgical treatment of moyamoya, which is predicated on

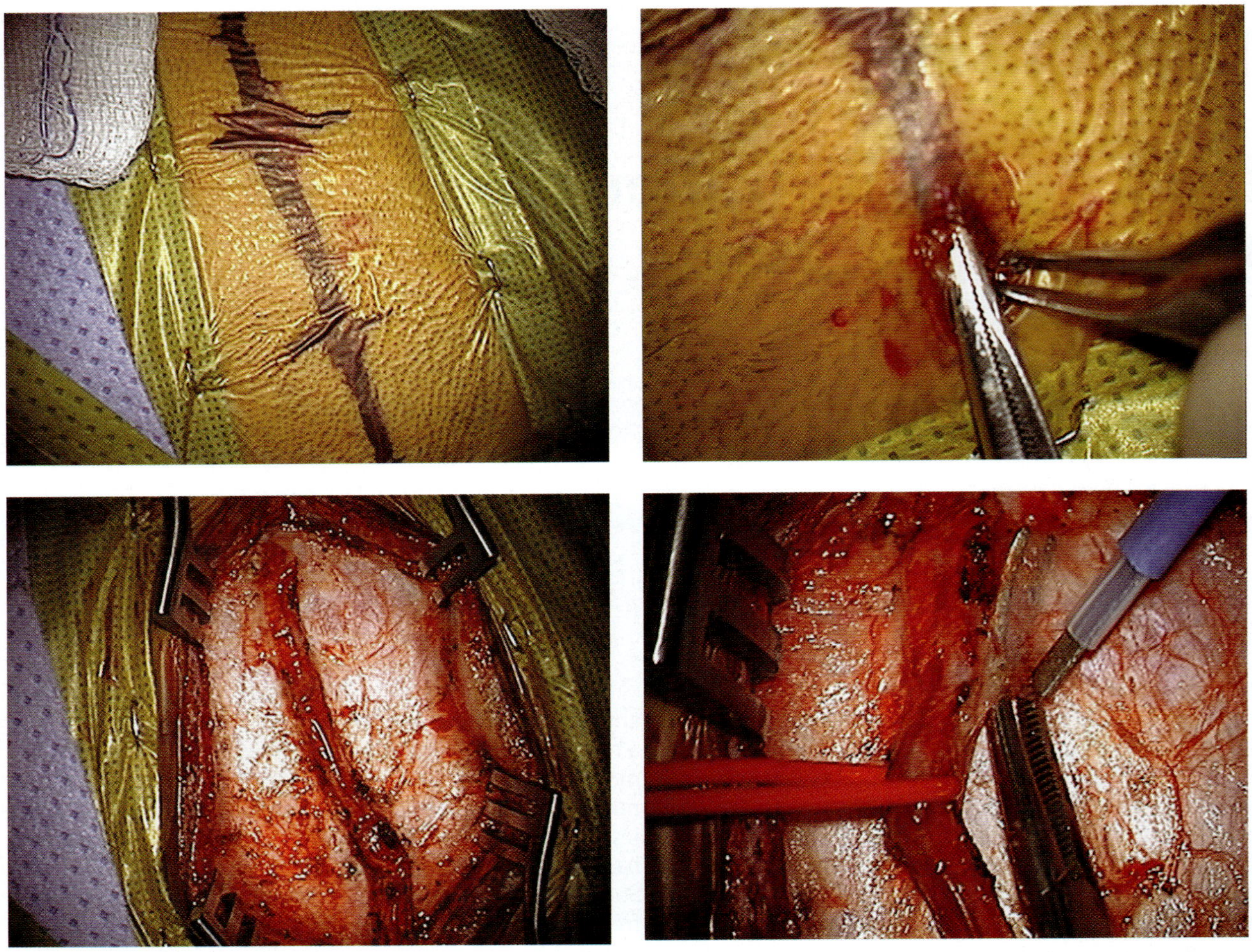

Fig. 10.1 The initial steps in performing a pial synangiosis. **(A)** Course of the parietal branch of the superficial temporal artery (STA) marked out following Doppler mapping. **(B)** Distal incision with subcutaneous dissection using fine S-curved snap. **(C)** Completed dissection of the STA branch prior to freeing up an adventitial cuff. **(D)** Elevation of the STA with an associated adventitial cuff, using the monopolar cautery. Note that all of the surgery occurs under the microscope.

utilizing the ECA to provide arterial supply to the ischemic hemisphere. Two general methods are employed: direct and indirect.

In direct revascularization, a branch of the ECA (usually the superficial temporal artery [STA]) is divided and anastomosed to a cortical artery (usually a distal branch of the MCA)—an STA-MCA bypass. In contrast, indirect techniques involve mobilizing vascularized tissue supplied by the ECA (dura, muscle, pedicles of the STA) and placing it in contact with the brain; facilitating ingrowth of new vessels to the cortex.

Historically, direct procedures have been used in adults, with immediate increase of blood flow to the ischemic brain cited as a major benefit. Augmentation of cerebral blood flow usually does not occur for several weeks with indirect techniques. However, direct bypass is often technically difficult to perform in children because of the small size of donor and recipient vessels, making indirect techniques appealing. Nonetheless, direct operations have been successful in children as have indirect procedures in adults.[10–12] Considerable debate exists regarding the relative merits and shortcomings of the two approaches with some centers advocating combinations of both.[12–14] Here we review a variant of the indirect approach, pial synangiosis used successfully in both children and adults first described by the senior author, including indications, perioperative management, surgical technique, and strategies for complication avoidance.[1]

◆ Pial Synangiosis

We have recently published a specific perioperative protocol for sickle cell patients with moyamoya (**Table 10.1**).[15] This protocol—absent the hematology-related interventions—has been adapted from our practice for all patients with moyamoya and highlights general strategies we have found useful in the surgical management of this condition.

Table 10.1 Perioperative Management Protocol Used for Patients with Moyamoya

One day before surgery
Continue aspirin therapy (usually 81 mg once a day orally if <70 kg, 325 mg once a day orally if 70 kg or more)
Admit patient to hospital for overnight intravenous hydration (isotonic fluids 1.25–1.5 times maintenance)
At induction of anesthesia
Institute EEG monitoring
Maintain normotension during induction; also normothermia (especially with smaller children), normocarbia (avoid hyperventilation to minimize cerebral vasoconstriction, pCO_2 >35 mm Hg), and normal pH
Place additional intravenous lines, arterial line, Foley catheter, and pulse oximeter
Place precordial Doppler to monitor for venous air emboli (relevant with thicker bone resulting from extramedullary hematopoiesis).
During surgery
Maintain normotension, normocarbia, normal pH, adequate oxygenation, normothermia, and adequate hydration
EEG slowing may respond to incremental blood pressure increases or other maneuvers to improve cerebral blood flow.
Postoperatively
Avoid hyperventilation (relevant in crying children); pain control is important
Maintain aspirin therapy on postoperative day 1
Maintain intravenous hydration at 1.25–1.5 times maintenance until child is fully recovered and drinking well (usually 48–72 hours)

Source: Revised from Smith ER, McClain CD, Heeney M, Scott RM. Pial synangiosis in patients with moyamoya syndrome and sickle cell anemia: perioperative management and surgical outcome. Neurosurg Focus 2009;26(4):E10.

◆ Indications for Surgery

In the setting of patients with radiographically confirmed moyamoya syndrome, surgery is indicated in the cases with the following:

- History of neurologic symptoms due to apparent cerebral ischemia
- Cerebral circulation and metabolism studies indicating deficiencies in regional cerebral blood flow, vascular response, and/or perfusion reserve (helpful but not mandatory)

Surgery is relatively contraindicated in patients who are a poor operative risk (severe cardiac disease, advanced debilitation from stroke burden, or other severe comorbidities). In addition, patients with an unclear diagnosis or who have individual hemispheres with a low Suzuki grade (I or—rarely—II) are sometimes observed closely with serial imaging before committing to surgery.

◆ Preoperative Strategy and Imaging

Preoperative management of moyamoya patients is critical to the success of surgery. Strategy is based on the use of appropriate imaging for planning and the maintenance of hypervolemia, normocarbia, and prevention of thrombosis. A full six-vessel (both ICAs, both ECAs, and both vertebrals) diagnostic angiogram is critical to the planning of the procedure for

- Accurate identification of disease status
- Identification of transdural collaterals so that they may be preserved during surgery
- Confirmation of the presence of a suitable donor scalp vessel (usually the parietal branch of the STA)

Once the decision to operate has been made, we follow a standardized perioperative protocol. Dehydration is a significant risk given the hypoperfused intracranial circulation. To minimize shifts in blood pressure during the induction of anesthesia, we routinely admit patients to the hospital on the evening prior to surgery for intravenous hydration. If there are no underlying cardiac or renal limitations, isotonic fluids are run at 1.5 times maintenance rate. Barring medical contraindication, patients are treated with daily aspirin therapy from the time of their diagnosis of moyamoya to minimize the risk of thrombosis in the slow-flowing cortical vessels. Dosing is continued up to and including the day prior to surgery (and restarted the day after surgery). Pain and anxiety must be aggressively managed, especially with children because hyperventilation, as occurs with crying, can induce cerebral vasoconstriction—leading to stroke. Steroids, cerebral dehydrating agents such as mannitol, and anticonvulsants are not administered on a routine basis.

◆ Anesthetic Issues and Monitoring

An experienced team of anesthesiologists is critical to the success of the operation. Generally, premedication is useful to minimize crying in children to prevent cerebral vasoconstriction and possible ischemic events. Hypotension, hyperthermia, and hypercarbia are to be avoided at all times, especially during induction. Muscular blockade is established by a nondepolarizing muscle relaxant prior to intubation. Anesthesia is maintained with low-dose isoflurane (a cerebral vasodilator) and a balanced nitrous oxide/oxygen mixture with fentanyl. End-tidal CO_2 is usually kept on the high-normal side (35–40 mm Hg) to minimize cerebral vasoconstriction. Normotension is maintained. Diuretics [mannitol and Lasix (Aventis Pharmaceuticals, Parsippany, NJ)] are usually avoided due to the possibility of hypotension.

We routinely supplement routine anesthetic monitoring with the use of intraoperative electroencephalography (EEG). EEG is employed during surgery to identify focal slowing, which is indicative of compromised cerebral blood flow so that immediate compensatory measures can be instituted by the operative team. EEG technicians must communicate changes in the EEG to allow the team to respond immediately with appropriate changes in blood pressure, pCO_2, and anesthetic agents.

◆ Operative Technique and Setup

In patients with bilateral disease, we will commonly treat both sides in a single operative sitting. We will usually treat the most affected side first, as determined either by clinical history or radiographic studies. If both sides are comparable in Suzuki grade and clinical status, we will often treat the dominant (usually left) hemisphere first.

The technique involves the following steps:

1. A scalp donor artery (most commonly, the posterior branch of the superficial temporal artery) is identified by Doppler then dissected from distal to proximal along with a cuff of galea and surrounding soft tissue.
2. A large craniotomy is turned in the region that is subjacent to the artery.
3. The dura is opened into at least six flaps to increase the surface area of dura exposed to the pial surface and thereby enhance formation of collateral vessels from the dural vascular supply.
4. The arachnoid is opened widely over the surface of brain exposed by the dural opening.
5. The intact donor artery is sutured directly to the pial surface using four to six interrupted 10-0 nylon sutures placed through the donor vessel adventitia and the underlying pia.
6. The bone flap is replaced over a Gelfoam (Pfizer Pharmaceuticals, New York, NY) cover of the dura, which is left widely open and carefully secured to avoid compression of the donor artery.
7. The temporal muscle and skin edges are carefully closed with absorbable sutures to similarly avoid compression of the donor vessel.

The rationale behind this procedure is that opening the arachnoid removes a barrier to the ingrowth of new blood vessels into the brain and provides greater access of growth factors from the spinal fluid and brain to the donor vessel. The donor vessel's adventitia is then sutured to the pial surface to maintain its contact with the brain in areas where the arachnoid has been cleared to keep stable contact between the donor vessel and the brain; making in-growth easier.

Prior to surgery, a list of specific equipment is needed. This list includes

- ◆ Hand-held "pencil" Doppler probes—necessary for mapping the STA
- ◆ Intraoperative microscope
- ◆ Powered drill (including footplate attachment)
- ◆ Microdissection instruments (including jeweler's forceps, microtying instruments, Vanass ophthalmic scissors, and a disposable arachnoid knife)
- ◆ Colorado tip electrocautery (a very fine tip for the monopolar cautery)
- ◆ Multiple no. 15 blades (for STA dissection)
- ◆ Papaverine

The operating room is then set up in a standardized fashion. The EEG tech is in the room with EEG monitors available for viewing. The microscope set for an assistant on the right side of the surgeon (assuming a right-handed surgeon) and is draped and ready from the onset of the case. The scrub is also on the surgeon's right. Immediate equipment is placed on Mayo stands over the patient's torso. The microscope is positioned with the base to the left of the surgeon. The anesthesia team is to the surgeon's left or at the foot of the table.

The patient is then positioned. EEG electrodes are affixed in a standard array, and the scalp is shaved over the expected course of the STA based on the angiogram. The parietal branch of the STA is mapped out using the Doppler probe and the skin is carefully marked with fine scratches from a sterile 22-gauge needle to outline its course from the distal end near the vertex to the root of the zygoma. The head is placed in pin fixation and the patient is positioned supine with the head turned parallel to the floor such that the STA site is level. Rolls are used as needed to reduce tension on the neck and the head is translated superior to the torso to facilitate venous drainage. The STA site is prepped, usually leaving the ear and face out of the field.

◆ Operative Approach

Prior to incision, intravenous antibiotics are given. The microscope is employed from the onset of the case.

Vessel Dissection

Using high magnification, a no. 15 blade is used to score the dermis at the distal end of the STA. A thin, curved pediatric hemostat and toothed Adson pickups are used by the surgeon (with suction and a second pickups by the assistant) to identify the STA under the skin. Using a repeated technique of subcutaneous dissection with the hemostat over the STA followed by elevation of the skin by the hemostat and an incision over the hemostat by the assistant, the STA is dissected along its length down to the root of the zygoma. Care must be taken to avoid tearing the vessel, particularly at tortuous bends or side branches. Irrigating bipolar (usually set at 25 with fine tips) is employed for hemostasis of small scalp vessels. A 0.50 × 3-cm cottonoid is often useful to cover the distal opening as proximal dissection continues. A longer length of STA dissection is preferable (10 cm is optimal, although not always possible, especially in smaller children; **Fig. 10.1**).

Following dissection of the STA branch, an electrocautery device with a Colorado needle tip (at low settings—usually half to one third of the standard skin setting) is used in conjunction with the bipolar and microscissors to divide the galea and soft tissue on either side of the STA down to the temporalis fascia; leaving a 1- to 2-mm of cuff on either side of the vessel. Two self-retaining retractors are then placed: one proximal and one distal. Dissection often terminates at the takeoff of the frontal branch, which should be preserved, if possible. However, if the bifurcation is high enough to

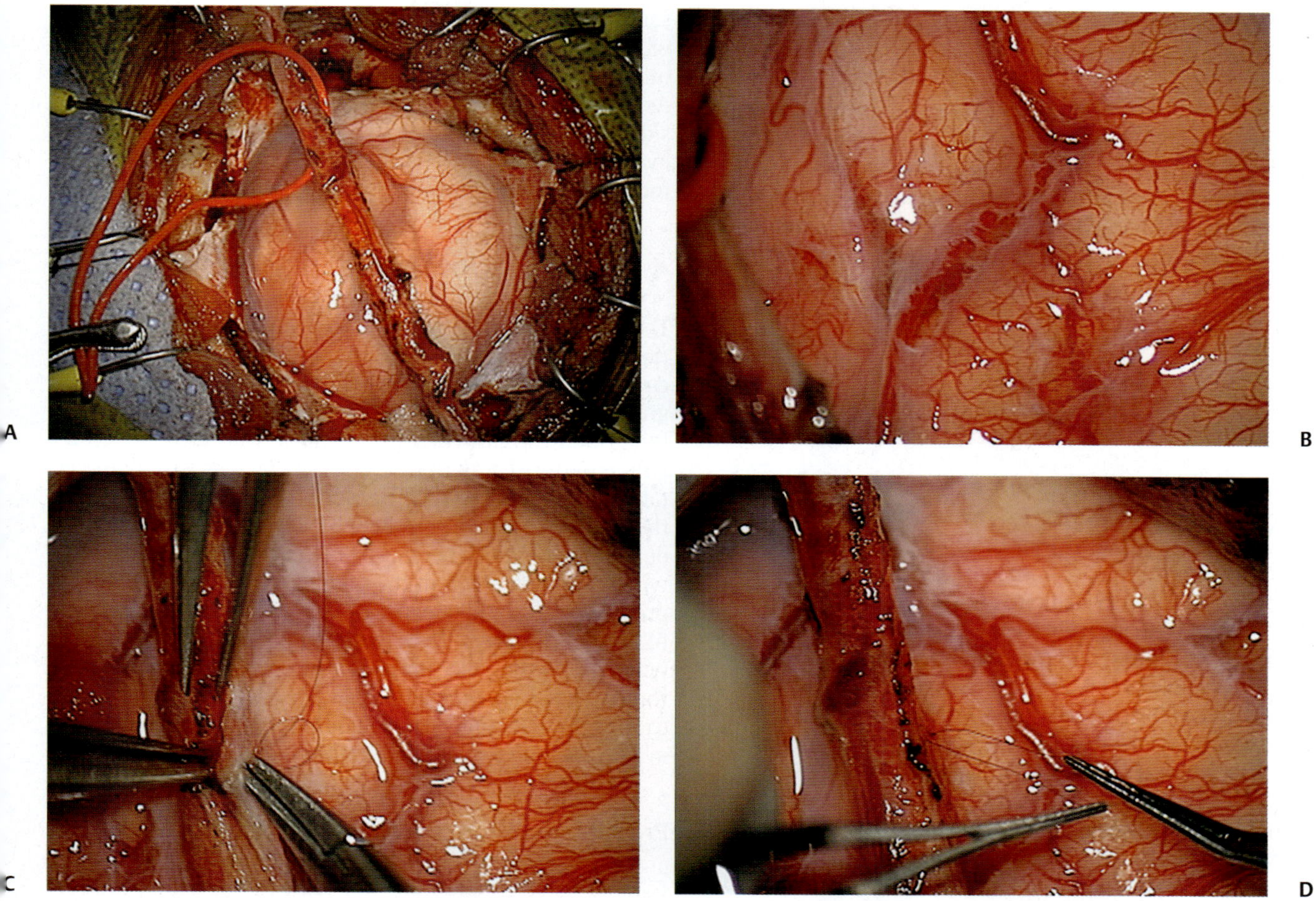

Fig. 10.2 Intraoperative photographs documenting the steps of the craniotomy for pial synangiosis. **(A)** Initial dural opening with stellate flaps and course of the superficial temporal artery (STA). **(B)** Arachnoidal opening, usually performed over vessels first, followed by subsequent opening over the cortex, if possible. **(C)** Technique for placing 10–0 nylon stitch through pia and STA adventitial cuff. **(D)** Completed suture, demonstrating good pial apposition to the vessel.

prohibit mobilization of the STA then it can be divided. The preoperative arteriogram will indicate whether the frontal branch provides any significant intracerebral collaterals, which can be relevant to the decision to potentially sacrifice the branch. Following the dissection of the vessel, a vessel loop is placed under the distal end of the STA and used to elevate the dissected portion of the vessel from the temporalis muscle. Monopolar electrocautery is then used to free up connective tissue around and beneath the vascular pedicle.

Craniotomy

Once the STA is freed, the microscope is removed and scalp flaps are developed using the electrocautery to minimize bleeding, creating a subgaleal dissection plane anteriorly and posteriorly. The temporalis is then divided into quadrants with the electrocautery. The muscle is reflected from the bone (with use of the electrocautery) and held back with multiple Lone Star (CooperSurgical, Inc., Trumbull, CT) retractors (fishhooks). Two burr holes are made: one inferior and one superior in the bony exposure at the proximal and distal sites of the STA over the exposed bone. Following dural dissection with a no. 3 Penfield, the footplate is then used to turn the widest possible craniotomy flap. Care must be taken to avoid injury to the vessel. This is usually best performed by the assistant protecting the vessel with a retractor (**Fig. 10.2**).

Dural Opening

Review of the angiogram is helpful to attempt to avoid disrupting preexisting dural collaterals. The dura is opened with a no. 15 blade, with the initial incision line along the axis of the donor vessel. A stellate opening is made with a total of six leaves of dura, three per side, retracted with 4-0 sutures. Small pieces of Gelfoam are placed between the retracted dura and craniotomy edge for hemostasis. Care is taken to minimize use of the bipolar on the dura to maximize collateral vessel development; although, hemostasis is paramount in these patients.

Microsurgical Arachnoid Opening and Pial Synangiosis

Under the microscope, the arachnoid is opened widely using the arachnoid knife, van Ness scissors, and jeweler's forceps. Bleeding is controlled with irrigation or small dots of Gelfoam. The donor vessel is laid on the brain surface in apposition to areas of open arachnoid. The adventitia of the donor vessel is sutured to the superficial pia of the subjacent cortex, using 10-0 nylon suture on a BV-75 needle using three knots per suture. Generally, at least three sutures are placed. Vasospasm, if seen, is treated with topical papaverine.

Closure

After synangiosis, the microscope is removed. The dura flaps are repositioned on the brain surface but not sutured. The entire craniotomy exposure is then covered with a large piece of Gelfoam, soaked in saline (not thrombin, as thrombin appears to increase the risk of vasospasm). Burr holes are enlarged on the bone flap to facilitate entry and exit of the vessel (**Fig. 10.3**). The bone flap is replaced with small titanium plates (not over the burr holes) and the temporalis muscle is closed vertically only to prevent pressure on the entering and exiting STA. Galea is closed with interrupted 3-0 Vicryl sutures (4-0 in smaller patients), taking care to avoid injuring the STA. Finally, the skin is closed with a running 4-0 Rapide (Ethicon, Somerville, NJ) or other absorbable suture. Occasionally, EEG slowing will be noted with replacement of the bone flap. These usually resolve with removal of the flap and a brief delay, followed by successful replacement of the bone.

Contralateral Side

If the EEG is stable and the contralateral side is affected, then the wound is dressed. The patient is repositioned and the same operation is performed on the contralateral side. Loss of cerebrospinal fluid (CSF) from the first operation may make arachnoid opening more difficult on the second side. As previously discussed, the dominant or most symptomatic side is generally done first so that if there are intraoperative events that preclude continuing with the second side, the most important hemisphere has been treated.

◆ Complication Avoidance

The most significant postoperative complication in our series has been stroke, which in a series of 143 patients occurred at ~4% per operated hemisphere. Patients at the greatest risk appear to be those with neurologic instability around the time of surgery, those who have suffered a stroke within 1 month of the operation, or those with certain angiographic risk factors such as moyamoya disease in the posterior circulation. There have been two perioperative deaths related to ischemic stroke: one in a 5-year-old child who was operated on in the midst of a crescendo of strokes preoperatively, and one in a 15-year-old boy with unusually fulminant disease with preexisting basilar artery occlusion whose ICA—the sole supply of his posterior circulation—thrombosed following a unilateral operation. Other complications have included four subdural hematomas requiring evacuation and two spinal fluid leaks.

Preoperative

Careful management of moyamoya patients before they get to the operating room can have a significant influence on complication avoidance. Patients, ideally, should be neurologically stable prior to surgery and at least 1 month out from any significant stroke. Patients must be medically optimized for surgery including prehydration, as described in

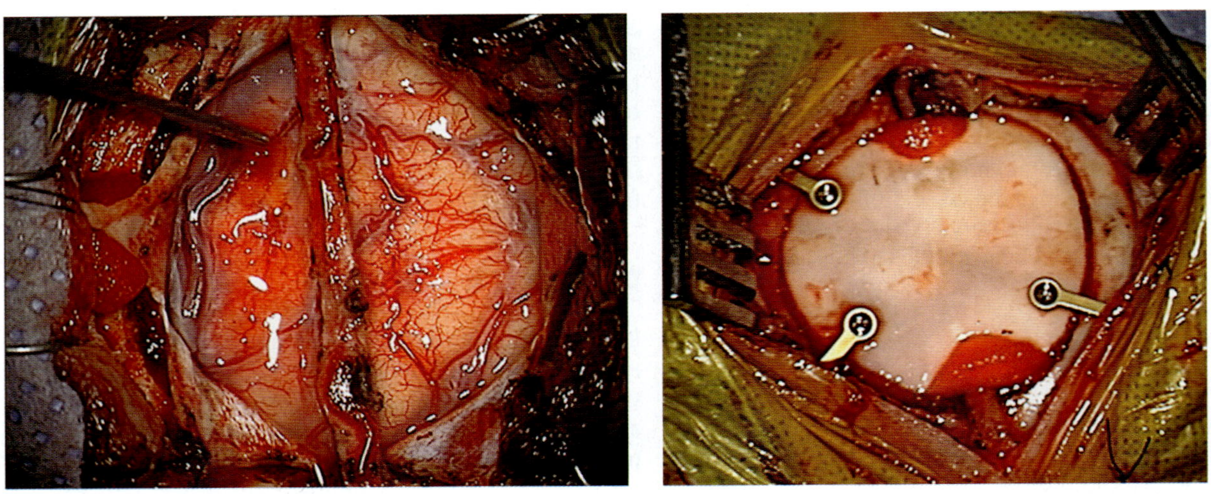
A B

Fig. 10.3 Images taken at the conclusion of pial synangiosis. **(A)** Final view of synangiosis prior to folding dural flaps down and placing Gelfoam (Pfizer Pharmaceuticals, New York, NY) on site. Note the course of the artery, wide arachnoidal opening, and significant area of the brain exposed to facilitate collateral development. **(B)** View following replacement of the craniotomy flap. It is important to leave tension-free entry and exit sites for the superficial temporal artery at the base and apex of the craniotomy.

our protocol (**Table 10.1**). Preoperative imaging is critical to planning vessel selection (the parietal branch of the STA may be small or absent, necessitating utilization of a frontal or retroauricular branch).

Intraoperative

Patient hyperventilation and hypotension should be avoided at all times. There should be awareness of EEG slowing. Anesthetic efforts to restore normal physiology often improve EEG changes. Throughout the case, meticulous hemostasis is vital to prevent postoperative hemorrhage in the setting of acetylsalicylic acid (aspirin) therapy. Careful dissection of the STA is critical to avoid tears or avulsion of side branches. Cautery of side branches further out from the donor vessel helps to minimize risk of inadvertently injuring the graft. Attentive detail to the closure reduces the likelihood of a CSF leak.

Postoperative

Continue IV fluids at 1.5 times maintenance for 48 to 72 hours until the patient is clearly taking enough liquids orally. Aggressive pain control is important to minimize blood pressure fluctuations and hyperventilation. Frequent and detailed neurologic examinations by nursing staff and physicians are critical to identify possible postoperative ischemia so that interventions can be instituted in an attempt to avoid progressing to a completed stroke.

◆ Follow-Up

Careful follow-up of patients with moyamoya is warranted to monitor for disease progression and for response to therapy.[9,16] Postoperative angiograms are usually obtained 12 months after surgery and typically demonstrate excellent MCA collateralization from both the donor STA and the meningeal arteries. For high-risk patients, MRI or MRAd may be undertaken in lieu of angiography if contrast from the angiogram presents a substantial risk to the kidneys. Generally, annual MRI scans are obtained in all patients for 3 to 5 years after the initial 1-year angiogram and then spaced out subsequent to the 5-year time point. Particular attention must be paid to patients with unilateral moyamoya as the opposite side can progress in up to 33% of patients, especially in children.[17] Patients are maintained on lifelong ASA therapy.

A review of 143 children with moyamoya syndrome treated with pial synangiosis showed marked reductions in their stroke frequency after surgery, especially after the first year postoperatively. In this group, 67% had strokes preoperatively and only 3.2% had strokes after at least 1 year of follow-up. The long-term results are excellent, with a stroke rate of 4.3% (2 patients in a group of 46) in patients with a minimum of 5 years of follow-up.[1] This work supports the premise that pial synangiosis provides a significant protective effect against new strokes in this patient population.

◆ Conclusions

Moyamoya syndrome is an increasingly recognized entity that is associated with cerebral ischemia. Diagnosis is made on the basis of clinical and radiographic findings, including a characteristic stenosis of the internal carotid arteries in conjunction with abundant collateral vessel development. Treatment is predicated on revascularization of the ischemic brain which can be direct (STA-MCA bypass) or indirect (including pial synangiosis). The use of pial synangiosis is a safe, effective, and durable method of cerebral revascularization in moyamoya syndrome and should be considered as a primary treatment for moyamoya, especially in the pediatric population.

References

1. Scott RM, Smith JL, Robertson RL, et al. Long-term outcome in children with moyamoya syndrome after cranial revascularization by pial synangiosis. J Neurosurg 2004; 100(2, Suppl)142–149
2. Ohaegbulam C, Scott RM. In: American Society of Pediatric Neurosurgeons, Section of Pediatric Neurosurgeons of the AANS, eds. Pediatric Neurosurgery: Surgery of the Developing Nervous System. 4th ed. Philadelphia: WB Saunders; 2001:1077–1092
3. Suzuki J, Takaku A. Cerebrovascular "moyamoya" disease: disease showing abnormal net-like vessels in base of brain. Arch Neurol 1969;20(3):288–299
4. Imaizumi T, Hayashi K, Saito K, Osawa M, Fukuyama Y. Long-term outcomes of pediatric moyamoya disease monitored to adulthood. Pediatr Neurol 1998;18(4):321–325
5. Kuroda S, Ishikawa T, Houkin K, Nanba R, Hokari M, Iwasaki Y. Incidence and clinical features of disease progression in adult moyamoya disease. Stroke 2005;36(10):2148–2153
6. Choi JU, Kim DS, Kim EY, Lee KC. Natural history of moyamoya disease: comparison of activity of daily living in surgery and non surgery groups. Clin Neurol Neurosurg 1997;99(Suppl 2):S11–S18
7. Kurokawa T, Chen YJ, Tomita S, Kishikawa T, Kitamura K. Cerebrovascular occlusive disease with and without the moyamoya vascular network in children. Neuropediatrics 1985;16(1):29–32
8. Ezura M, Takahashi A, Yoshimoto T. Successful treatment of an arteriovenous malformation by chemical embolization with estrogen followed by conventional radiotherapy. Neurosurgery 1992;31(6):1105–1107, discussion 1107
9. Fung LW, Thompson D, Ganesan V. Revascularisation surgery for paediatric moyamoya: a review of the literature. Childs Nerv Syst 2005;21(5):358–364
10. Isono M, Ishii K, Kobayashi H, Kaga A, Kamida T, Fujiki M. Effects of indirect bypass surgery for occlusive cerebrovascular diseases in adults. J Clin Neurosci 2002;9(6):644–647
11. Smith ER, Scott RM. Surgical management of moyamoya syndrome. Skull Base 2005;15(1):15–26
12. Veeravagu A, Guzman R, Patil CG, Hou LC, Lee M, Steinberg GK. Moyamoya disease in pediatric patients: outcomes of neurosurgical interventions. Neurosurg Focus 2008;24(2):E16
13. Ikezaki K. Rational approach to treatment of moyamoya disease in childhood. J Child Neurol 2000;15(5):350–356
14. Matsushima T, Inoue T, Ikezaki K, et al. Multiple combined indirect procedure for the surgical treatment of children with moyamoya disease: a comparison with single indirect anastomosis and direct anastomosis. Neurosurg Focus 1998;5(5):e4
15. Smith ER, McClain CD, Heeney M, Scott RM. Pial synangiosis in patients with moyamoya syndrome and sickle cell anemia: perioperative management and surgical outcome. Neurosurg Focus 2009;26(4):E10
16. Fukui M. Guidelines for the diagnosis and treatment of spontaneous occlusion of the circle of Willis ("moyamoya" disease). Research Committee on Spontaneous Occlusion of the Circle of Willis (Moyamoya Disease) of the Ministry of Health and Welfare, Japan. Clin Neurol Neurosurg 1997;99(Suppl 2):S238–S240
17. Smith ER, Scott RM. Progression of disease in unilateral moyamoya syndrome. Neurosurg Focus 2008;24(2):E17

III

Endovascular Revascularization Techniques

Chapter 11

Carotid Artery Stenting

Paul T. L. Chiam and Gary S. Roubin

Carotid stenting (CS) has evolved to become a widely utilized method of carotid artery revascularization. Improved periprocedural outcomes have been achieved through technical and procedural innovations including improved devices, increased operator experience, and a better understanding of optimal technique, as well as the importance of patient selection.

◆ Historical Perspective

Results of several randomized trials showed that carotid endarterectomy (CEA) was more effective than medical therapy in reducing the risk of stroke.[1–5] Thus, the American Heart Association (AHA) guidelines recommend CEA for symptomatic carotid stenosis >50%, and for asymptomatic carotid stenosis >60% if these asymptomatic patients also have an expected life expectancy of 5 years, provided the periprocedural complication rates are less than 6% and 3%, respectively.[6,7]

During the late 1980s, several investigators began to apply the percutaneous approach to carotid revascularization.[8,9] Early results by Roubin and others[10,11] showed that CS was feasible and had acceptable complication rates despite the novel experience with this technique, use of primitive equipment, and lack of distal embolic protection devices (EPDs). Subsequently, long-term (up to 5 years) follow-up demonstrated that CS could be accomplished with acceptable complication rates and with durable results.[12]

◆ Multicenter Clinical Trials

Several studies have demonstrated equivalence of CS versus CEA. The first was the Carotid and Vertebral Artery Transluminal Angioplasty Study (CAVATAS), randomizing mostly symptomatic patients (90%) who were at standard surgical risk. The 30-day stroke or death rate (10% CS vs 9.9% CEA) and 3-year ipsilateral stroke rate were not different.[13]

The Stenting and Angioplasty with Protection in Patients at High Risk for Endarterectomy (SAPPHIRE) Trial[14] – a multicenter randomized trial of high surgical risk patients with either symptomatic >50% carotid stenosis or asymptomatic >80% carotid stenosis – demonstrated that CS was noninferior to CEA with myocardial infarction (MI)/stroke/death rates of 12.2% vs 20.1%, respectively, at 1 year, with clinical equipoise maintained at 3 years.[15]

The Clopidogrel and Aspirin for Reduction of Emboli in Symptomatic Carotid Stenosis (CaRESS) Trial, a multicenter, nonrandomized prospective comparative study of symptomatic and asymptomatic patients at high or low surgical risk, revealed no significant differences in the 30-day and 1-year stroke or death rates between CS and CEA (2.1% vs 3.6% and 10.0% vs 13.6%, respectively).[16]

Recently, the Endarterectomy versus Angioplasty in Patients with Symptomatic Severe Carotid Stenosis (EVA-3S) and Stent-Protected Angioplasty versus Carotid Endarterectomy (SPACE) Trials randomizing symptomatic patients at normal surgical-risk however, showed that CS did not achieve parity with CEA.[17,18] Although 30-day ipsilateral stroke or death rates in the SPACE Trial were similar (CS 6.84% vs CEA 6.34%), CS was not proved noninferior.[17] In the EVA-3S study, not only was noninferiority not reached, CS performed worse, with a higher 30-day stroke or death rate (9.6% vs 3.9%, $p = 0.01$).[18]

◆ Indications and Contraindications of Carotid Stenting

The indications for carotid stenting are similar to those for CEA if the procedure can be accomplished with event rates within the American Heart Association (AHA) guidelines. Patients with increased surgical risk due to comorbidities such as severe cardiac or pulmonary disease or anatomic factors such as high lesions behind the mandible (C2 and above), low lesions (necessitating thoracic exposure), restenosis after previous CEA, contralateral internal carotid artery (ICA) occlusion and prior neck dissection/irradiation may be ideal candidates for CS.

With present-day devices and technologies, almost any carotid lesion can be stented. It is not a question, however, of an operator being able to access the lesion or eliminate the stenosis by placing a stent, but is absolutely related to the ability to perform these tasks safely with a low stroke/death rate. Thus, several situations increase the likelihood of adverse events during CS (i.e., relative contraindications):

- Inability of the patient to tolerate the dual antiplatelet agents that are mandatory for at least 1 month after CS
- Inability to advance the EPD distal to the lesion and its deployment in a safe "landing" zone (**Fig. 11.1**)
- Inability to safely access the common carotid artery (CCA; such as with severe CCA bifurcation stenosis or external carotid artery [ECA] occlusion with a type III arch)
- Recent (<14 days) moderate to large cerebral infarction
- Large thrombus burden
- Unfavorable arch anatomy
- Severe carotid artery tortuosity
- Heavy concentric lesion calcification
- The "string sign"

These patients may be more safely treated with CEA or medical therapy.

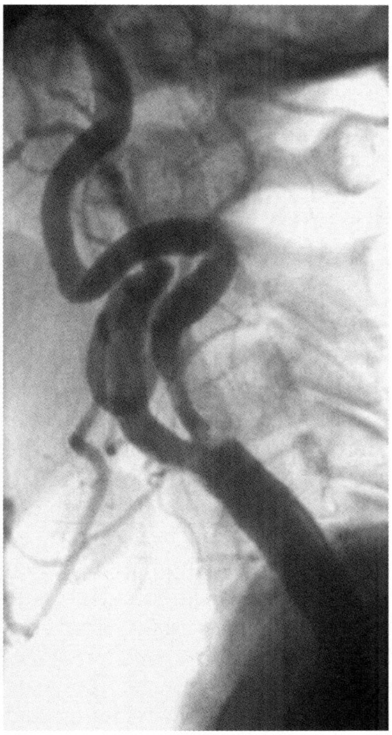

Fig. 11.1 Angiogram demonstrating severe distal tortuosity, increasing the difficulty of placing a distal filter in a "safe landing zone."

◆ Preprocedural Imaging

Similar to guideline recommendations,[19] we advocate that experienced operators study both carotid arteries, with optional angiographic imaging of a vertebral artery if that can be safely performed. One of the most important points to note is that the final decision to proceed with CS should be made after adequate carotid/cerebral angiograms have been performed, and the sheath placed in the CCA. Often, certain anatomic findings (e.g., vascular tortuosity, heavy concentric lesion calcification) that significantly increase stent risk are first detected during angiography, especially after sheath or guide placement. Depending on these findings, the decision to proceed with CS should be carefully reconsidered and the procedure terminated, if appropriate.

◆ Patient Selection

As experience with CS has accumulated, we have identified clinical and anatomic markers for increased stroke risk during CS (high stent risk).[20] These are age, reduced cerebral reserve, excessive vascular tortuosity, and heavy concentric lesion calcification (**Table 11.1**). Patients with any two or more of the four risk markers should be excluded from CS because the risk of periprocedural stroke will be excessive. Alternative therapies, either medical or surgical, are recommended for these patients.

Table 11.1 Markers of Increased Risk during Carotid Stenting

	Risk Factor	Features
Clinical	Age ≥80 years	
	Decreased cerebral reserve	Prior (remote) large stroke (>1/3 middle cerebral artery territory infarction on CT brain)
		Multiple lacunar infarcts (diffuse lacunes associated with encephalomalacia and/or cerebral atrophy on CT brain)
		Intracranial microangiopathy (CT or MRI brain changes most prominent in the periventricular region)
		Dementia
Angiographic	Excessive tortuosity	≥2 90-degree bends within 5 cm of the lesion (including the takeoff of the ICA from the CCA)
	Heavy calcification	Concentric calcification; width ≥3 mm

Abbreviations: CT, computed tomography; MRI, magnetic resonance imaging; CCA, common carotid artery; ICA, internal carotid artery.

Excessive vascular tortuosity (**Fig. 11.2**) and heavy concentric lesion calcification (**Fig. 11.3**) increase stroke risk through increased manipulation and procedural time,[21,22] whereas reduced cerebral reserve decreases brain tolerance to further potential ischemic insult. It must be emphasized that even moderate vascular tortuosity can increase the complexity of the procedure, and presents a hazard for less-experienced operators. Assessing vascular tortuosity in multiple views is essential to fully appreciate the challenge.

Age was demonstrated to be a predictor of adverse outcomes before[12] and even after the advent of EPDs.[23,24] The ongoing Carotid Revascularization Endarterectomy vs Stent Trial (CREST) lead-in phase showed that octogenarians had a significantly increased risk of adverse events (12.1% vs 3.2% in nonoctogenarians) not accounted for by other factors, and recruitment of these patients was stopped in the lead-in phase.[23] The SPACE Trial documented a twofold increase in ipsilateral stroke or death among those >75 years vs ≤75 years (11% vs 5.9%).[17] Possible reasons are that increased vascular tortuosity and vessel calcification are more common in elderly patients,[25,26] and they are also more likely to have reduced cerebral reserve compared with a younger population.

Recently, however, several investigators have demonstrated that CS can be performed in well-selected elderly patients (≥80 years) with low adverse event rates.[25,27,28] In the largest single-center series of CS in selected elderly patients with independent neurologic assessment, it was demonstrated that CS can be performed with 30-day periprocedural event rates of 5.1% and 2.6% in the symptomatic and asymptomatic groups, respectively,[29,30] consistent with the AHA guidelines.

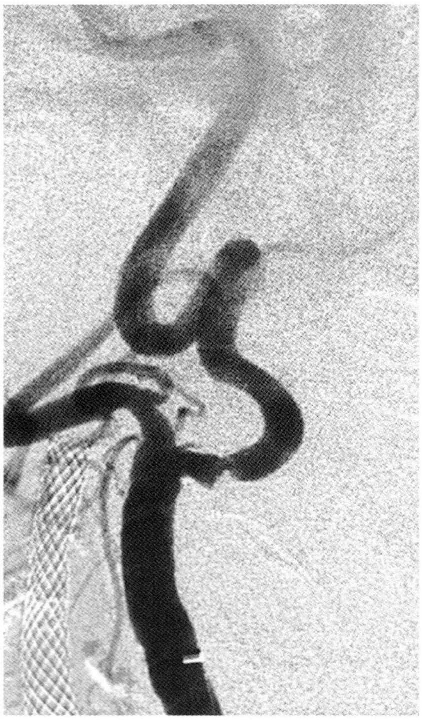

Fig. 11.2 Angiogram demonstrating excessive vascular tortuosity.

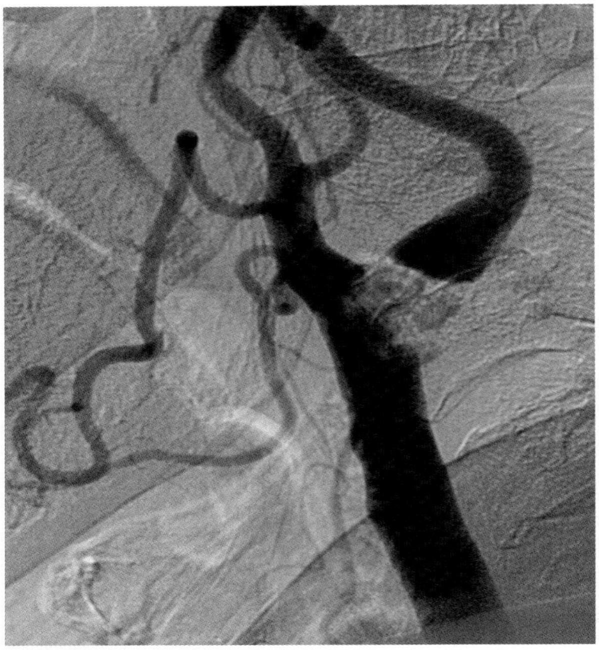

Fig. 11.3 Angiogram demonstrating heavy concentric lesion calcification.

Therefore, CS and CEA should be viewed as complementary and not competitive revascularization options. There will be patients who are at high surgical risk and more suitable for CS; conversely, there will be patients who are at increased stent risk and will be more suitable for CEA. Patients at increased risk for both procedures may be better and more safely treated with optimal medical therapy.

◆ Expected Results with Experienced Operators and Appropriate Patient Selection

As with any interventional procedure, particularly with CS, there is a steep learning curve. Increased operator experience leads to reduced complication rates,[12] emphasizing the importance of thorough operator training on the technical and cognitive (patient selection) aspects of CS. It can be expected that events rates will meet the guidelines in ideal patient subsets performed by experienced operators. For example, the CREST lead-in phase reported 1.7% and 1.3% stroke or death rates for patients <60 years and 60–69 years, respectively. Initial data from the Asymptomatic Carotid Trial (ACT I) also showed a remarkably low 1.7% stroke or death rate for patients <80 years (unpublished data). Guidelines on operator training and credentialing have been detailed in a recent consensus statement of several societies.[19]

◆ Technique

Access for the procedure is usually via the femoral artery. Occasionally, in patients with severe peripheral vascular disease (PVD), the brachial or radial route can be used. Diagnostic cerebral angiography is routinely performed to confirm lesion severity, assess vascular tortuosity, vessel calcification, and intracranial collateral circulation. Dedicated neurovascular catheters are used. Arch aortograms are not routinely performed in some experienced centers, although for operators with lesser experience these are certainly useful to help guide decision making and choice of equipment.

All patients should be on dual antiplatelet therapy with aspirin and clopidogrel or ticlopidine. Strict adherence to this regimen has contributed toward the improved results seen with CS. Control of blood pressure (BP) must be meticulous. Antihypertensive medications are usually omitted on the morning of the procedure, as mild hypotension and bradycardia usually occur with balloon dilation and stenting of the carotid bifurcation. Should BP remain >160–180 systolic after stent implantation, rapidly performing postdilation usually reduces BP expeditiously. Less commonly, control of BP with medication is required if it is still >160–180 mm Hg systolic after postdilation. Strict BP control ≤140/90 mm Hg reduces the risk of hyperperfusion syndrome or cerebral hemorrhage.[31] Intravenous or intraarterial nitroglycerin or IV labetalol can be used.

Sheaths are preferred over guide catheters as they have a less traumatic tip design and also require a smaller arteriotomy in the vascular access site. Usually, 6F sheaths are adequate for CS procedures. Occasionally, for adverse arch anatomy or tortuous vessels, a 7F sheath may be required, or an 8F guide with the appropriate curve can be used. The standard technique of placing the sheath in the CCA is most often used. This entails manipulating the diagnostic neurocatheter into the ECA over a 0.038-inch Glidewire (Terumo, Tokyo, Japan) and then exchanging it for a sheath over a stiff wire such as the Supracore wire (Abbott Vascular, Santa Clara, CA). Alternatively, if the lesion involves the bifurcation of the CCA (**Fig. 11.4**) or if the ECA is occluded, the more advanced "telescopic" technique is employed. The 6F sheath is first placed in the descending thoracic aorta. A 125-cm 5F Vitek catheter with a 0.038-inch Glidewire or 0.035-inch Amplatz J stiff wire within are advanced through the sheath and positioned in the CCA below the lesion. The sheath is then advanced to the CCA over the Vitek catheter and Glidewire/Amplatz wire. After sheath or guide placement, vascular tortuosity is reassessed. Occasionally, the vascular tortuosity significantly worsens and careful reconsideration is required to determine whether CS should still proceed, as the risk-benefit ratio may have altered.

Once the sheath is in place anticoagulation is undertaken with either weight-adjusted heparin or bivalirudin. Irrespective of the regimen used, care must be taken to avoid over-anticoagulation to reduce the risk of cerebral hemorrhage. Atropine is administered before balloon predilation to reduce the incidence of severe bradycardia and hypotension, unless an elevated heart rate is present at the beginning of the procedure or if the lesion is a post-CEA restenosis.

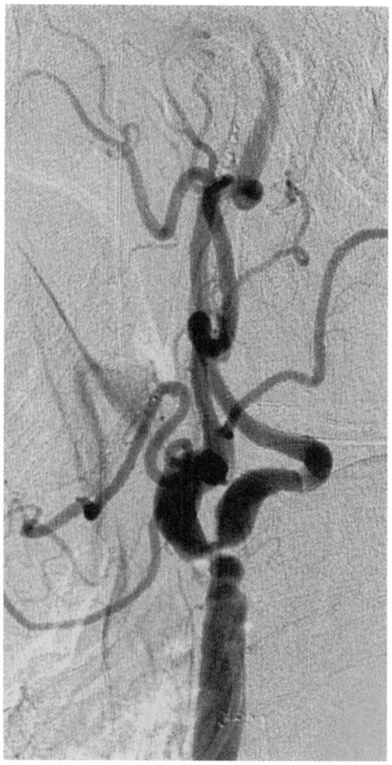

Fig. 11.4 Angiogram demonstrating severe common carotid artery disease. This increases technical difficulty of the procedure as external carotid artery access for wire support is not possible.

After crossing the lesion with an EPD – a separated wire/filter system, is preferred – the filter is deployed well distal to the lesion in a straight segment of the ICA. Deploying the filter around a bend may reduce its efficacy due to suboptimal apposition of the filter against the vessel wall. In the presence of a severe angulation distal to the filter, the risk of ICA dissection is increased as the filter may move during the procedure. In such situations, the procedure may be more safely performed with a proximal occlusion device or the patient considered for CEA.

In very severe stenosis, in which difficulty crossing with the filter is anticipated, the "pre-predilation" technique is used. Any 0.014-inch wire, usually a hydrophilic wire such as the PT2 (Boston Scientific, Natick, MA) is first advanced across the severe lesion and pre-predilation is performed with a small 2.0 to 2.5 mm balloon to facilitate advancement of the filter beyond the stenosis. This unprotected but controlled dilation with a small balloon is preferable to multiple and prolonged attempts at passing the filter across the stenosis. Once the filter is deployed, gentle predilation is performed using a small balloon (3.0–3.5 mm) with a single inflation. The intent is to create a controlled dissection and "plastering" of plaque to facilitate stent placement and yet minimize plaque disruption from stent delivery.

Self-expandable nitinol stents are used almost exclusively, with stent design falling into two broad groups. The open cell design (e.g., Acculink; Abbott Vacular, Santa Clara, CA) is more flexible and trackable and conforms better to the vascular anatomy especially if tortuous. Conversely, the closed cell design (e.g., Xact stent; Abbott Vascular, Santa Clara, CA) is less flexible, but theoretically would "entrap" atheromatous debris better and also cause less "hang-up" when retrieving the distal filter with the retrieval catheter. Cases in which closed cell stents cannot be placed because of tortuosity are exceedingly uncommon. In vitro experimental work by Ohki and colleagues showed that plaque prolapse through the stent struts was significantly less for closed cell stents.[32] Clinical studies examining superiority of stent cell designs have yielded conflicting results although it appears that symptomatic patients experience lower adverse event rates with the use of closed cell stents.[33] Oversized stents should be used to maximize plaque coverage by metal and usually includes stenting a segment of the distal CCA. It is advisable not to skimp on stent length because restenosis rates are low and stenting across the ECA usually results in no sequelae. A 30- or 40-mm stent length is thus recommended for most cases. When positioning the stent, it is important not to underestimate the "landing zone" length needing proximal to the filter. This is particularly critical if there is a sharp bend in the ICA distal to the filter as inadvertent pushing and pulling on the filter may occur while attempting to position the stent, leading to dissection of the distal ICA (with possible catastrophic consequences). The stent should also be positioned well below a sharp bend, otherwise severe distal kinking of the ICA may result.

Postdilation is performed with an undersized balloon (usually 5.0-mm diameter) with a single inflation. The intention is to gently layer the stent onto the plaque, leaving the stent to slowly expand outward against the arterial wall. Our experience and that of others[34] indicates that this is the step most likely to cause clinically significant emboli. Aggressive postdilation must be avoided to minimize dislodging of plaque fragments that have prolapsed through the stent struts. Angioplasty in this setting should be used only to facilitate stent placement and not as a treatment in itself. Therefore, the previous term carotid angioplasty and stenting (CAS) is better termed carotid stenting (CS) in light of this new understanding, emphasizing that stenting is the primary focus with balloon dilation only facilitating the process.

Contrast injections are kept to a minimum throughout the intervention. This reduces risk of injecting microbubbles or microthrombi into the brain, and reduces risk of contrast-induced nephropathy in patients with chronic renal impairment. Balloon dilation and stent placement can be performed accurately using bony landmarks. Residual stenoses up to 30%, residual ulcers, and mild to moderate distal vessel spasm are best left alone (**Fig. 11.5**).

CS is now performed routinely with EPDs as studies have documented reduction in adverse clinical events although no randomized data are available. The Clinical Trial of Reviparin and Metabolic Modulation in Acute Myocardial Infarction Treatment Evaluation (CREATE) registry showed that filter deployment duration was a predictor for adverse events. Likely reasons are that increased filter deployment time is a surrogate for case complexity and that the longer the filter is deployed, the more the accumulation of fibrin and the filter itself may become a source of embolism. Distal balloon occlusion protection with the PercuSurge GuardWire system (Medtronic, Santa Rosa, CA) has the advantages of a lower profile, better trackability, and more complete emboli protection, although it is suitable only in patients with sufficient intracranial collateral circulation. With all distal protection devices, the initial wiring of the lesion is unprotected and has been shown to cause small

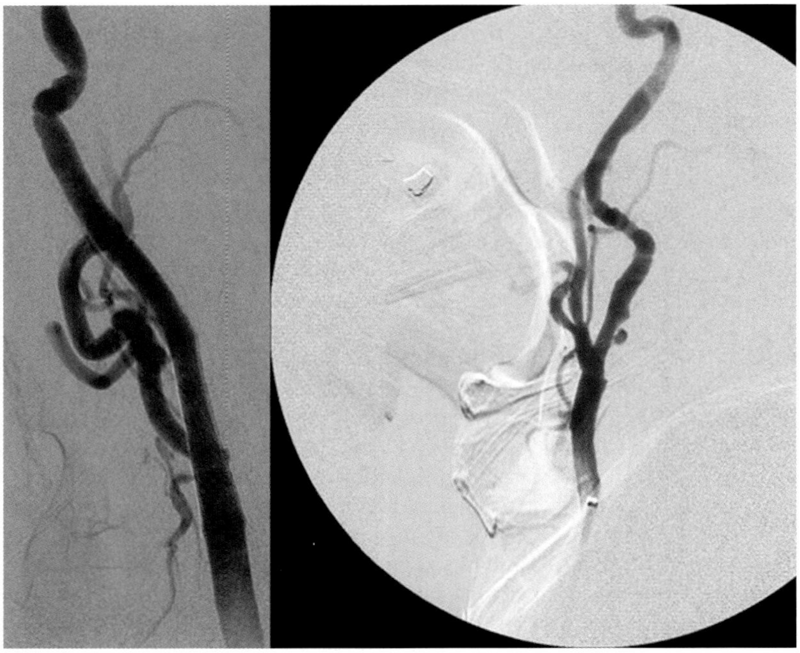

Fig. 11.5 Poststent angiograms demonstrating residual kinks and ulcer. These should be left alone.

amounts of microemboli. Proximal protection devices, such as the Parodi Anti-Emboli System (W.L. Gore and Associates, Flagstaff, AZ) and Moma device (Moma Therapeutics, Inc., Brighton, MA) have been developed to overcome this limitation. Both systems work using balloon occlusion of proximal flow in the CCA and a second balloon occluding flow from the ECA before the lesion is crossed. An added advantage is that any 0.014-inch wire can be used. The Parodi system has an extra feature of creating a shunt and reversing blood flow in the ICA. These systems are however, more cumbersome to use, require a 9F sheath, and like the distal balloon occlusion system, are not suitable for patients with contralateral ICA occlusion or "isolated hemisphere." To date they have not gained widespread usage. Regardless of the system used, the procedure should be performed relatively fast by an operator facile in the technique. An average time of filter deployment of <9 minutes can be achieved even in the octogenarian population.[29]

◆ Postprocedure Management

Patients are usually monitored closely in a dedicated unit for 4 to 6 hours. BP control is essential since either excessively low or elevated BP can have deleterious consequences. Simple hydration should not be overlooked as this not only reduces the risk of contrast-induced nephropathy but is also beneficial for the relative hypotension that most patients experience post-CS. Frequent neurologic assessments should be performed during the initial 24 hours, and patients are usually discharged the day after uncomplicated procedures. Dual antiplatelet therapy is continued for at least 4 weeks, and thereafter aspirin or clopidogrel is maintained lifelong. Doppler ultrasound should be performed at 1 month, serving as a baseline reference value for future follow-up.

◆ Management of Hemodynamics

Hypotension and bradycardia usually occur after stenting and postdilation as a result of stretching of the baroreceptors, especially if the procedure involved the bulbous carotid. It is usually transient and resolves with fluid bolus. More persistent or severe cases of hypotension can be rapidly reversed with small boluses of intravenous phenylephrine. Prophylactic atropine administration before balloon dilation and stenting reduces bradycardia or hypotension.[35] Rarely, hypotension and bradycardia can persist for several days and intravenous pressors such as dopamine may be required. Early ambulation may reduce the frequency and severity of this phenomenon, and groin closure devices may provide an advantage in this aspect.

Hyperperfusion syndrome can occur after relief of a very severe stenosis especially if the periprocedural BP was elevated. Treatment includes BP reduction with intravenous agents, withholding antiplatelet agents until symptom resolution, and close monitoring of neurologic status. Stringent BP control pre- and post-CS has been shown to reduce this complication.[31]

◆ Complication Avoidance

Several factors are known to increase risk of periprocedural stroke before treatment of the lesion. Excessive manipulation in the aortic arch, particularly with 8F guides, inadvertent placement of the 0.035-inch Supracore or Amplatz wire across the stenosis while attempting to access the CCA, and allowing the sheath to "snowplow" into a lesion extending into the CCA can occur even with experienced operators. Minimizing manipulations in the arch and paying careful attention to the wire and sheath tips can help to reduce or eliminate these complications.

In cases with very tortuous vascular anatomy, the use of larger sheaths or guides may help provide extra support. An extra 0.014-inch wire can also be placed in the ECA as a "buddy wire" to provide stability of the system. These maneuvers may increase the risk of periprocedural adverse events, however.

Crossing a lesion in tortuous anatomy may be further aided by maneuvers such as neck extension by removing the head restraint and getting the patient to turn the head from side to side. Use of separated wire filter systems such as the Emboshield filter (Abbott Vascular, Santa Clara, CA) or Spider filter (ev3 Endovascular, Inc., Plymouth, MN) may be helpful. Other options include using a hydrophilic 0.014-inch wire to cross the lesion to reduce tortuosity (buddy wire) and then passing the filter wire. In very severely stenotic lesions, prepredilation with a small balloon may facilitate crossing of the filter.

Infrequently, the ICA take-off is severely angulated and the 0.014-inch filter wire does not negotiate the bend due to wire prolapse. A useful technique is to advance a 125-cm 5F JR4 or IMA catheter through the sheath or guide, positioning and directing the JR4 or IMA catheter toward the ICA ostium. This then facilitates passage of the 0.014-inch wire into the ICA and across the stenosis.

References

1. Beneficial effect of carotid endarterectomy in symptomatic patients with high-grade carotid stenosis. North American Symptomatic Carotid Endarterectomy Trial Collaborators. N Engl J Med 1991;325(7):445–453
2. Barnett HJ, Taylor DW, Eliasziw M, et al. Benefit of carotid endarterectomy in patients with symptomatic moderate or severe stenosis. North American Symptomatic Carotid Endarterectomy Trial Collaborators. N Engl J Med 1998;339(20):1415–1425
3. Randomised trial of endarterectomy for recently symptomatic carotid stenosis: final results of the MRC European Carotid Surgery Trial (ECST). Lancet 1998;351(9113):1379–1387
4. Endarterectomy for asymptomatic carotid artery stenosis. Executive Committee for the Asymptomatic Carotid Atherosclerosis Study. JAMA 1995;273(18):1421–1428
5. Halliday A, Mansfield A, Marro J, et al; MRC Asymptomatic Carotid Surgery Trial (ACST) Collaborative Group. Prevention of disabling and fatal strokes by successful carotid endarterectomy in patients without recent neurological symptoms: randomised controlled trial. Lancet 2004;363(9420):1491–1502
6. Biller J, Feinberg WM, Castaldo JE, et al. Guidelines for carotid endarterectomy: a statement for healthcare professionals from a Special Writing Group of the Stroke Council, American Heart Association. Circulation 1998;97(5):501–509

7. Sacco RL, Adams R, Albers G, et al; American Heart Association; American Stroke Association Council on Stroke; Council on Cardiovascular Radiology and Intervention; American Academy of Neurology. Guidelines for prevention of stroke in patients with ischemic stroke or transient ischemic attack: a statement for healthcare professionals from the American Heart Association/American Stroke Association Council on Stroke: co-sponsored by the Council on Cardiovascular Radiology and Intervention: the American Academy of Neurology affirms the value of this guideline. Stroke 2006;37(2):577–617
8. Bockenheimer SA, Mathias K. Percutaneous transluminal angioplasty in arteriosclerotic internal carotid artery stenosis. AJNR Am J Neuroradiol 1983;4(3):791–792
9. Théron J, Raymond J, Casasco A, Courtheoux F. Percutaneous angioplasty of atherosclerotic and postsurgical stenosis of carotid arteries. AJNR Am J Neuroradiol 1987;8(3):495–500
10. Roubin GS, Yadav S, Iyer SS, Vitek J. Carotid stent-supported angioplasty: a neurovascular intervention to prevent stroke. Am J Cardiol 1996;78(3A):8–12
11. Diethrich EB, Ndiaye M, Reid DB. Stenting in the carotid artery: initial experience in 110 patients. J Endovasc Surg 1996;3(1):42–62
12. Roubin GS, New G, Iyer SS, et al. Immediate and late clinical outcomes of carotid artery stenting in patients with symptomatic and asymptomatic carotid artery stenosis: a 5-year prospective analysis. Circulation 2001;103(4):532–537
13. Endovascular versus surgical treatment in patients with carotid stenosis in the Carotid and Vertebral Artery Transluminal Angioplasty Study (CAVATAS): a randomised trial. Lancet 2001;357(9270):1729–1737
14. Yadav JS, Wholey MH, Kuntz RE, et al; Stenting and Angioplasty with Protection in Patients at High Risk for Endarterectomy Investigators. Protected carotid-artery stenting versus endarterectomy in high-risk patients. N Engl J Med 2004;351(15):1493–1501
15. Gurm HS, Yadav JS, Fayad P, et al; SAPPHIRE Investigators. Long-term results of carotid stenting versus endarterectomy in high-risk patients. N Engl J Med 2008;358(15):1572–1579
16. CaRESS Steering Committee. Carotid Revascularization Using Endarterectomy or Stenting Systems (CaRESS) phase I clinical trial: 1-year results. J Vasc Surg 2005;42(2):213–219
17. Ringleb PA, Allenberg J, Brückmann H, et al; SPACE Collaborative Group. 30 day results from the SPACE trial of stent-protected angioplasty versus carotid endarterectomy in symptomatic patients: a randomised non-inferiority trial. Lancet 2006;368(9543):1239–1247
18. Mas JL, Chatellier G, Beyssen B, et al; EVA-3S Investigators. Endarterectomy versus stenting in patients with symptomatic severe carotid stenosis. N Engl J Med 2006;355(16):1660–1671
19. Bates ER, Babb JD, Casey DE Jr, et al; American College of Cardiology Foundation; American Society of Interventional & Therapeutic Neuroradiology; Society for Cardiovascular Angiography and Interventions; Society for Vascular Medicine and Biology; Society of Interventional Radiology. ACCF/SCAI/SVMB/SIR/ASITN 2007 clinical expert consensus document on carotid stenting: a report of the American College of Cardiology Foundation Task Force on Clinical Expert Consensus Documents (ACCF/SCAI/SVMB/SIR/ASITN Clinical Expert Consensus Document Committee on Carotid Stenting). J Am Coll Cardiol 2007;49(1):126–170
20. Roubin GS, Iyer S, Halkin A, Vitek J, Brennan C. Realizing the potential of carotid artery stenting: proposed paradigms for patient selection and procedural technique. Circulation 2006;113(16):2021–2030
21. Segal AZ, Abernethy WB, Palacios IF, BeLue R, Rordorf G. Stroke as a complication of cardiac catheterization: risk factors and clinical features. Neurology 2001;56(7):975–977
22. Al-Mubarak N, Roubin GS, Vitek JJ, Iyer SS, New G, Leon MB. Effect of the distal-balloon protection system on microembolization duringcarotid stenting. Circulation 2001;104(17):1999–2002
23. Hobson RW II, Howard VJ, Roubin GS, et al; CREST Investigators. Carotid artery stenting is associated with increased complications in octogenarians: 30-day stroke and death rates in the CREST lead-in phase. J Vasc Surg 2004;40(6):1106–1111
24. Gray WA, Yadav JS, Verta P, et al; CAPTURE Trial Collaborators. The CAPTURE registry: predictors of outcomes in carotid artery stenting with embolic protection for high surgical risk patients in the early post-approval setting. Catheter Cardiovasc Interv 2007;70(7): 1025–1033
25. Setacci C, de Donato G, Chisci E, et al. Is carotid artery stenting in octogenarians really dangerous? J Endovasc Ther 2006;13(3):302–309
26. Lam RC, Lin SC, DeRubertis B, Hynecek R, Kent KC, Faries PL. The impact of increasing age on anatomic factors affecting carotid angioplasty and stenting. J Vasc Surg 2007;45(5):875–880
27. Velez CA, White CJ, Reilly JP, et al. Carotid artery stent placement is safe in the very elderly (> or =80 years). Catheter Cardiovasc Interv 2008;72(3):303–308
28. Henry M, Henry I, Polydorou A, Hugel M. Carotid angioplasty and stenting in octogenarians: is it safe? Catheter Cardiovasc Interv 2008;72(3):309–317
29. Chiam PT, Roubin GS, Iyer SS, et al. Carotid artery stenting in elderly patients: importance of case selection. Catheter Cardiovasc Interv 72(3): 318–324
30. Chiam PT, Roubin GS, Panagopoulos G, et al. One-year clinical outcomes, midterm survival, and predictors of mortality after carotid stenting in elderly patients. Circulation 2009;119(17):2343–2348
31. Abou-Chebl A, Reginelli J, Bajzer CT, Yadav JS. Intensive treatment of hypertension decreases the risk of hyperperfusion and intracerebral hemorrhage following carotid artery stenting. Catheter Cardiovasc Interv 2007;69(5):690–696
32. Ohki TV, Veith FJ. In-vitro models to analyse embolization during carotid stenting. In: Amor M, Bergeron P, Mathias K, Raithel D, eds. Carotid Artery Angioplasty and Stenting. Turin, Italy: Edizioni Minerva Medica; 2002:178–186
33. Bosiers M, de Donato G, Deloose K, et al. Does free cell area influence the outcome in carotid artery stenting? Eur J Vasc Endovasc Surg 2007;33(2):135–141, discussion 142–143
34. Théron J. My history of carotid angioplasty and stenting. J Invasive Cardiol 2008;20(4):E102–E108
35. Cayne NS, Faries PL, Trocciola SM, et al. Carotid angioplasty and stent-induced bradycardia and hypotension: Impact of prophylactic atropine administration and prior carotid endarterectomy. J Vasc Surg 2005;41(6):956–961

Chapter 12

Technical Aspects of Intracranial Angioplasty and Stenting

David Fiorella, Thomas J. Masaryk, and Aquilla S. Turk

The endovascular techniques used for the revascularization of intracranial stenosis have evolved over the past two decades. Initially, the procedure was limited to angioplasty alone using devices designed for the coronary circulation. As coronary interventions transitioned from angioplasty alone to angioplasty and stenting using balloon-expandable coronary stents, intracranial interventions followed suit. Although balloon-expandable coronary stents provided better luminal gain than angioplasty alone, these results were achieved at the expense of higher rates of procedural complications. In 2005, the Gateway-Wingspan system was granted Food and Drug Administration (FDA) approval under a humanitarian device exemption (HDE) for intracranial angioplasty and stenting. The Gateway-Wingspan system (Boston Scientific, Natick, MA) represents a hybrid technique that combines aspects of traditional angioplasty and primary stenting. The technique was designed to maximize safety but at the same time optimize the luminal gain achieved during the procedure. The present review will focus on the technical aspects of intracranial angioplasty and stenting using the Gateway-Wingspan system.

◆ Clinical Decision Making in Angioplasty and Stenting

The Warfarin and Aspirin in Symptomatic Intracranial atherosclerotic Disease (WASID) Study and the subsequent subset analyses served to identify those patients with symptomatic intracranial atherosclerotic disease (ICAD) who were at the highest risk for recurrent stroke on medical therapy.[1,2] Similarly, these data serve to guide the interventionist with respect to the selection of those patients who stand to benefit the most from endovascular treatments.

On the basis of these data, we can outline several important considerations for patient selection for intracranial percutaneous transluminal angioplasty and stenting (PTAS):

- *High-grade (70–99%) intracranial stenosis:* Patients presenting with 70 to 99% stenosis had a markedly higher ipsilateral stroke risk while on medical therapy than those with less severe stenosis (50–69%). For patients presenting with a qualifying event of stroke, the ipsilateral recurrent stroke rate was 24.6% over 2 years (in comparison with only 11.2% in those patients with lower-grade stenosis).[1,3] Thus, with the existing endovascular technology, it is very feasible that intracranial PTAS (if added to standard medical therapy) could provide a better secondary prevention of ipsilateral stroke in patients with high-grade stenosis. It is much less likely that a significant benefit would be provided to those with lower grades of stenosis.
- *Early treatment (within days to weeks) after the qualifying event (QE):* Similar to symptomatic cervical carotid stenosis, in symptomatic ICAD, most of the risk for recurrent stroke after a qualifying event (either transient ischemic attack [TIA] or stroke) is incurred over the first few weeks after presentation. When patients with symptomatic high-grade stenosis were enrolled in WASID within 30 days of their QE, the stroke risk over the next year was 22.9%, with most of these events occurring within the first few weeks after enrollment. When patients were enrolled after 30 days, their stroke risk was only 9%.[2] Therefore, endovascular revascularization, if performed, needs to be undertaken soon after the patient presents with symptoms. Although the labeled indication for Wingspan specifies that it is for use only in patients with symptomatic intracranial atherosclerotic stenosis, which is "refractory to medical therapy," the WASID results suggest that waiting for a second event to develop may be ill-advised.

In WASID, patients who presented with a QE while on antithrombotic therapy (e.g., aspirin, clopidogrel, warfarin) were at no higher risk to reach primary endpoint than those who were not on antithrombotic therapy at the time of their QE.[4] Thus, in waiting for a second event to occur, it is entirely possible that the "time window" for the greatest potential benefit of revascularization could be missed altogether in most patients.

◆ Premedication

Intracranial angioplasty and stenting must be performed with adequate platelet inhibition, which is typically achieved using two oral agents (aspirin and clopidogrel) administered prior to the procedure.[5]

Aspirin

Aspirin has a very fast onset of action and if administered even a few hours prior to the procedure in standard doses (325 mg by mouth per day) will yield adequate platelet inhibition. We typically start aspirin at least 24 hours prior to the procedure and continue it indefinitely after treatment. The effects of aspirin can be considered to be irreversible for the lifespan of the affected platelet, requiring the endogenous generation of new platelets or the administration of exogenous platelets to reverse its activity.[5]

Clopidogrel

Clopidogrel (Plavix; Bristol-Myers Squibb, New York, NY) is a prodrug, which requires hepatic metabolism to become active. As such, the onset of platelet inhibition with clopidogrel is considerably slower and to some extent more variable than with aspirin. Given that symptomatic intracranial atherosclerosis represents a disease that should be addressed very shortly after the patient comes to clinical attention, it is important to be able to achieve adequate platelet inhibition quickly so that revascularization can be undertaken promptly. A growing body of literature from interventional cardiology has indicated that this is best achieved using a one-time 600-mg loading dose of clopidogrel. In comparison to other clopidogrel dosing regimens, this loading dose is associated with lower rates of resistance, lower rates of clinical events, and no greater incidence of bleeding complications in patients undergoing percutaneous coronary interventions (PCI). We typically give patients this 600-mg loading dose the day before the anticipated intervention. Similar to aspirin, the effects of clopidogrel can be considered, for all intents and purposes, to be irreversible for the life span of the affected platelet.[6–9]

IIb/IIIa Receptor Antagonists

In some instances, patients have not been adequately pretreated with aspirin and/or clopidogrel, or preoperative testing has shown them to be nonresponsive or suboptimally responsive to these medications. In these cases, platelet inhibition can be rapidly and adequately achieved with the IIb/IIIa receptor antagonists (abciximab; Reopro, Centocor Ortho Biotech, Inc., Horsham, PA), eptifibatide (Integrilin, Schering-Plough Corp., Memphis, TN) or tirofiban (Aggrastat, MGI Pharma, Inc., Bloomington, MN) administered either intravenously or intraarterially. There are no neuroendovascular studies to support the use of these agents as adjuncts in intracranial stenting. Correspondingly, the dosing and route of administration of these agents is based primarily on extrapolations from the cardiology literature and clinical experience. We have typically administered these agents in divided doses (3–5 mg) intraarterially during the case through the guiding catheter. Serial measurements of the level of IIb/IIIa receptor inhibition can be obtained with the goal of achieving 70% receptor inhibition by the end of the case.[5]

Assays designed for the verification of the efficacy of the administered antiplatelet medications, although controversial, have been increasingly incorporated into the practice of interventional cardiology and more recently, interventional neuroradiology. Although there are a myriad of available tests to assess the level of platelet inhibition, the most widely used is probably the commercially available VerifyNow system (Accumetrics, San Diego, CA), which is a point-of-care test that can be used to measure responsivity to aspirin, clopidogrel, and the IIb/IIIa antagonists.[10,11]

◆ Procedure

To perform intracranial angioplasty and stenting successfully, each step of the procedure must be performed without complication. As with any procedure, this is best accomplished by proceeding in a protocolized manner, which is performed the same way each time. The institution of a systematic approach allows the operator (and the ancillary staff) to develop a routine approach to the case and apply a more focused concentration to the critical aspects of the case.

Access

Access Technique

Most intracranial stenting cases are performed through a common femoral artery access. Femoral access is best achieved for these cases with a micropuncture kit (e.g., Cook Medical, Indianapolis, IN) using a careful single-wall puncture technique. The dual antiplatelet agents and procedural heparinization create an unforgiving scenario for any femoral access complications. Multiple arterial punctures during attempted access or a "double-wall" arterial puncture can create significant bleeding complications.

Evaluation of Femoral Access

Immediately after groin access is secured and a sheath is in place, we evaluate the puncture site with an angiogram

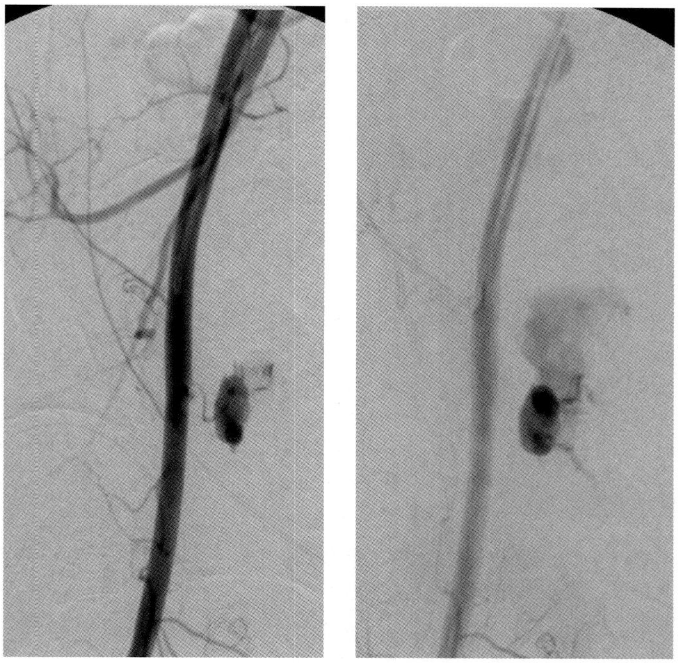

.B

Fig. 12.1 Puncture site evaluation. Early **(A)** and late **(B)** angiographic images over a right femoral puncture site demonstrate active extravasation from a right femoral pseudoaneurysm. The patient had had several previous angiograms and had developed a large right femoral pseudoaneurysm that extended into the retroperitoneum. The aneurysm was inadvertently perforated during femoral access for intracranial stenting. The patient had been on aspirin and clopidogrel and was loaded with heparin during the procedure. An abrupt drop in blood pressure during the procedure prompted imaging of the femoral puncture site. The procedure was aborted, and the femoral pseudoaneurysm was ultimately secured through a combination of open surgical exploration and placement of an endovascular stent graft from a contralateral access.

performed in the ipsilateral oblique projection. This projection demonstrates the arterial entry site of the sheath into the femoral artery to best advantage. This information allows the operator to know immediately that it is safe to heparinize the patient and that at the conclusion of the case it will be safe to use an arterial closure device. Performing this simple step prior to proceeding with intracranial stenting can reduce the chances of fully heparinizing the patient while there is active bleeding at the groin puncture site (**Fig. 12.1**).

Immediate Heparinization

As soon as femoral access is secured and the puncture site has been demonstrated to be intact, we fully load the patient with heparin (70–80 U/kg, targeting a procedural activated clotting time [ACT] of 250–300 s). Loading the patient with heparin as soon as access is secure allows the operator to perform the entire diagnostic portion of the procedure under full heparinization. In addition, this avoids having to wait to achieve a therapeutic level of heparinization later in the procedure. If the initial bolus does not achieve a therapeutic ACT, the operator can then use the time that elapses during the diagnostic angiography to administer additional boluses to achieve the level that is ultimately required to proceed with the intervention.

Diagnostic Angiography

Catheter Selection

Diagnostic angiography is performed using a standard 5F catheter. When the patient has had complete vascular imaging, the catheter can be selected specifically for the catheterization of the targeted cervical vessel. When the right carotid circulation is the target, we prefer the H1 catheter (Cook Medical). When the left carotid or left vertebral circulations are targeted, we typically start with the Vertebral (VER; Cordis Corp., Warren, NJ). When the left carotid is backward facing, often the Davis (DAV, Cook Medical) can be useful for direct catheterization prior to moving onto a Simmons-2 (Cordis Corp.).

Cervical Artery Evaluation

Once the proximal cervical segment of the target artery is catheterized, we perform cervical angiography before proceeding with intracranial runs. An evaluation of the cervical anatomy allows the operator to select the guiding catheter platform, which will be used to complete the case. Also, the size and tortuosity of the cervical artery may allow the operator to preemptively prepare and administer an antispasmodic medication (e.g., nicardipine, verapamil, nitroglycerin) to avoid flow-limiting vasospasm and an iatrogenic arterial injury. The guiding catheter should be positioned at the level of the skull base whenever possible.

Cerebral Angiography

After the cervical anatomy is interrogated, the catheter is positioned within the proximal internal carotid or vertebral artery so that selective intracranial angiography can be performed. A standard posteroanterior (PA) and lateral branch vessel arteriogram must be done initially such that the operator will be able to exclude procedural thromboembolic complications at the conclusion of the procedure (**Fig. 12.2**). Next, high-magnification images of the target lesion demonstrating the stenosis to best advantage should be obtained (**Fig. 12.2**). The goal of the operator should be to optimally show the patent, stenotic residual lumen so that it can be successfully navigated with the microcatheter and microwire. The most stenotic view of the lesion provides the "truest" measurement of the actual stenosis. Once defined, these views will represent the working angles for intracranial angioplasty and stenting. After the working angles have been defined, all measurements of the intracranial vessel should be performed. The most critical measurements are the vessel diameter (proximal and distal to the lesion) and the length of the lesion. These measurements will determine the selection of the angioplasty balloon and stent.

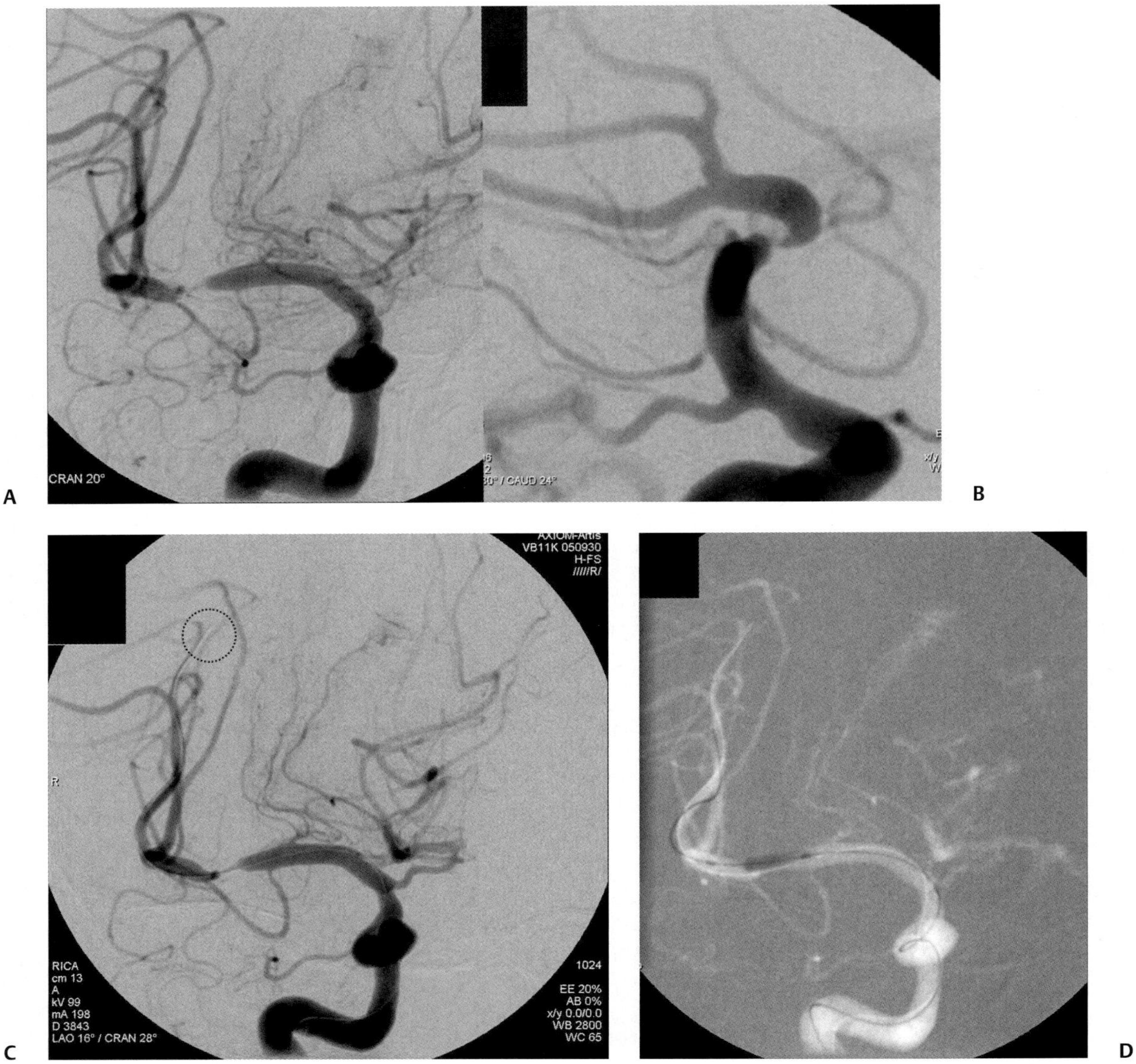

Fig. 12.2 Wingspan procedure overview. Patient with a high-grade M1 segment, right middle cerebral artery (MCA) stenosis symptomatic with minor stroke. Preprocedural angiogram shows flow limitation to the right cerebral hemisphere. **(A,B)** High-magnification views in the working angle for stenting demonstrate the stenosis to best advantage. The optimal A-plane working views are typically a cranial angulation with a slight contralateral oblique projection, which elongates the MCA. The optimal B-plane working views are achieved with an "uphill" view, which tends to elongate the M1 segment and separate the M2 branches at the bifurcation. After guiding catheter access is established, a microcatheter and microwire are manipulated across the lesion. After distal access is established, the microcatheter is exchanged over a 300-cm exchange length microwire. **(C)** A control angiogram is made to assess the distal wire position and evaluate for any perforations or iatrogenic issues created during the exchange (and prior to stenting). In this case, the angiogram showed that the microwire tip was within a small branch. For this reason, the wire was retracted slightly and repositioned prior to proceeding. **(D)** Next, the Gateway angioplasty balloon (Boston Scientific, Natick, MA) is manipulated across the lesion and inflated under fluoroscopic roadmap control. *(continued)*

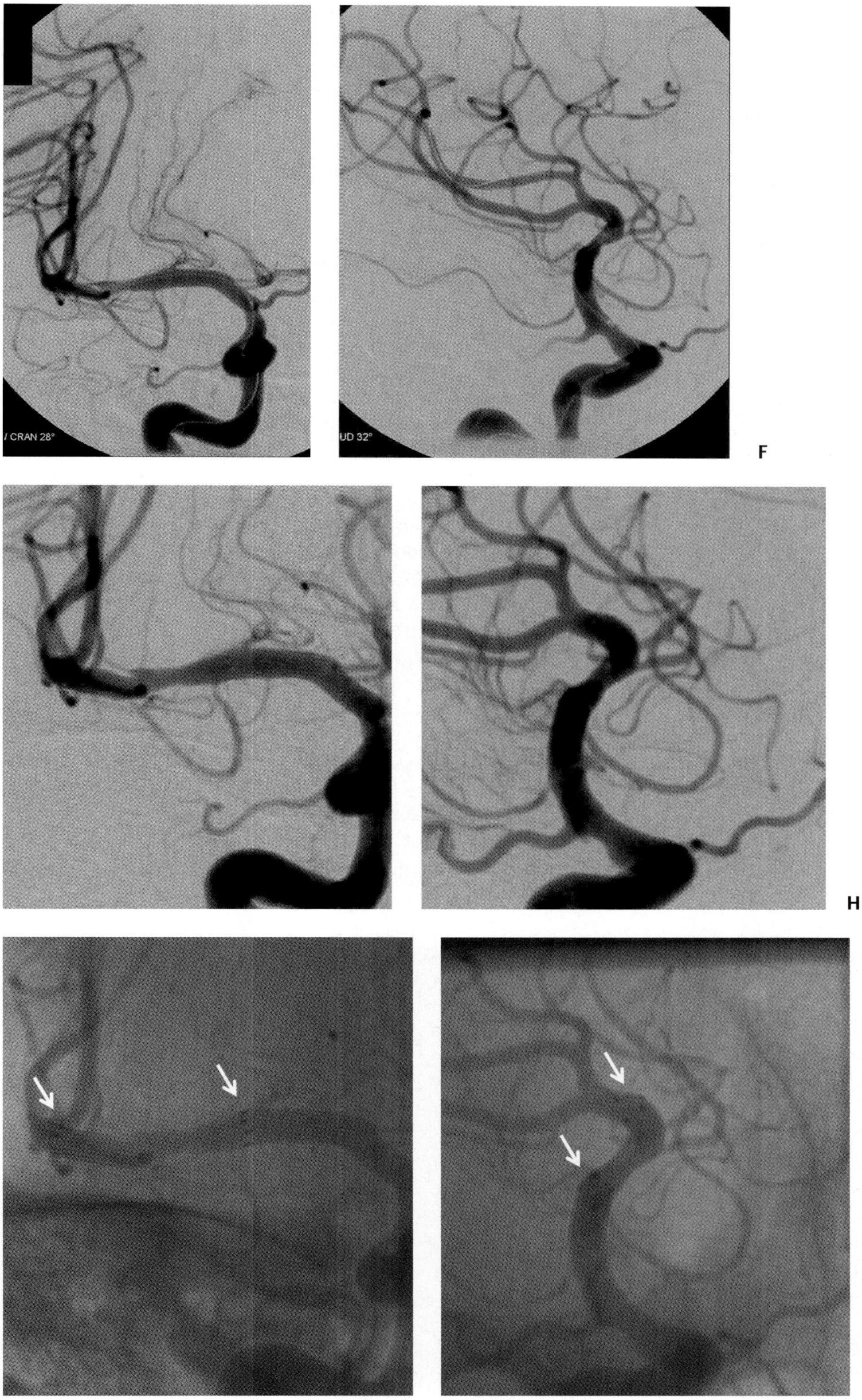

E F G H J

Fig. 12.2 *(continued)* **(E,F)** Following angioplasty, control angiograms in the working projections show a satisfactory degree of luminal gain, sufficient to proceed with stenting. The Wingspan delivery system (Boston Scientific) can then be manipulated across the lesion into position and deployed. Completion angiography shows marked improvement in the luminal diameter after angioplasty and stenting with a commensurate improvement in flow and transit time over the right hemisphere. **(G,H)** Final high-magnification angiography in the working angle for stenting demonstrates only minimal residual stenosis and no local thrombus formation. **(I,J)** The native projection images show the Wingspan in position across the lesion. The proximal and distal ends of the device are demarcated by four grouped radiopaque markers (*arrows*). The body of the device is radiolucent.

Equipment Preparation

Prior to exchanging for the guiding catheter, we select and prepare all of the equipment that will be necessary for the procedure. This limits the time that the larger profile guiding catheter is in place within the cervical vessel. In many cases, these patients with symptomatic intracranial atherosclerosis also have severe extracranial atheromatous disease. In these patients, the guiding catheter may be flow limiting or preocclusive in the targeted cervical vessel. As such, it is critical to reduce, to the extent possible, the total time that the guiding catheter is limiting intracranial flow during the intervention.

Guiding Catheter Selection

There are several different options for guiding catheter selection. If the cervical vessels are relatively straight, standard guiding catheters can be used. For the anterior circulation, a 6F MPD-shaped catheter (MPD Cordis Envoy, Cordis Corp.; MPD Neuropath, Micrus Endovascular, San Jose, CA) often fits best within the distal cervical carotid artery with the tip sitting optimally at the junction between the vertical and horizontal petrous segments at the skull base. For the vertebral arteries, a 6F straight guiding (Cordis STR Envoy; STR Neuropath) catheter often works well to achieve a position just proximal to the horizontal V2 segment at the level of the C2 vertebral body. For more tortuous anatomy, secure distal access can often be atraumatically achieved with a coaxial platform consisting of a 6F KSAW Shuttle select (Cook Medical) fitted with a Check-Flo performer (Cook Medical) and an internal 6F 105 cm 0.070-inch internal diameter (ID) Neuron catheter (Penumbra Inc, Mountain View, CA). The Shuttle sheath provides stable proximal cervical access. When fitted with the Check-Flo performer, the Neuron provides an additional 15 cm of length beyond the tip of the Shuttle. The Neuron can then be manipulated into the distal carotid, often extending intracranially to the level of the cavernous segment.

Microcatheter-Microwire Selection

The most hazardous portion of the intervention is typically the initial crossing of the stenosis with a microcatheter and microwire. A mistake during this portion of the intervention could lead to an occlusive dissection or catastrophic perforation. In addition, it is critical to carefully achieve the stable distal access after the stenosis is crossed. This is best achieved with a standard 0.0165-inch ID microcatheter and steerable 0.014-inch microwire. Some operators have tried to eliminate a step by primarily crossing the stenosis with the angioplasty balloon and an exchange length 0.014-inch microwire. Although this procedure may eliminate the need for a single catheter exchange, it comes at the expense of navigability and often stable distal microwire position, which can be hazardous (**Fig. 12.3**).

Microcatheter

Any standard low-profile microcatheter (SL-10, Boston Scientific; Echelon-10, ev3 Endovascular, Inc., Plymouth, MN; Prowler-10, Cordis Corp.) can be used.

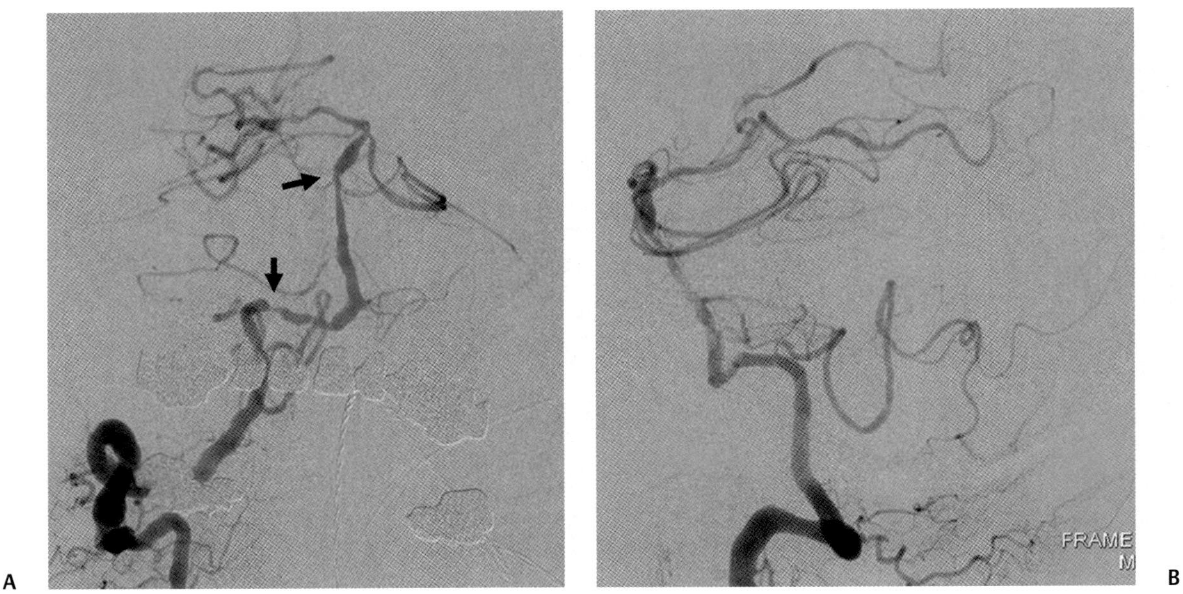

Fig. 12.3 Hazards of proximal exchange wire position. Patient with symptomatic severe multifocal vertebrobasilar atherosclerotic stenoses. Initial angiographic images in the PA **(A)** and lateral **(B)** projections show a diffusely diseased basilar artery with two particularly high-grade stenoses involving the distal right vertebral artery and distal basilar (*arrows*). Rather than traversing the lesion with a microcatheter and microwire, the Gateway balloon (Boston Scientific, Natick, MA) was primarily navigated across the lesion over an exchange microwire. *(continued)*

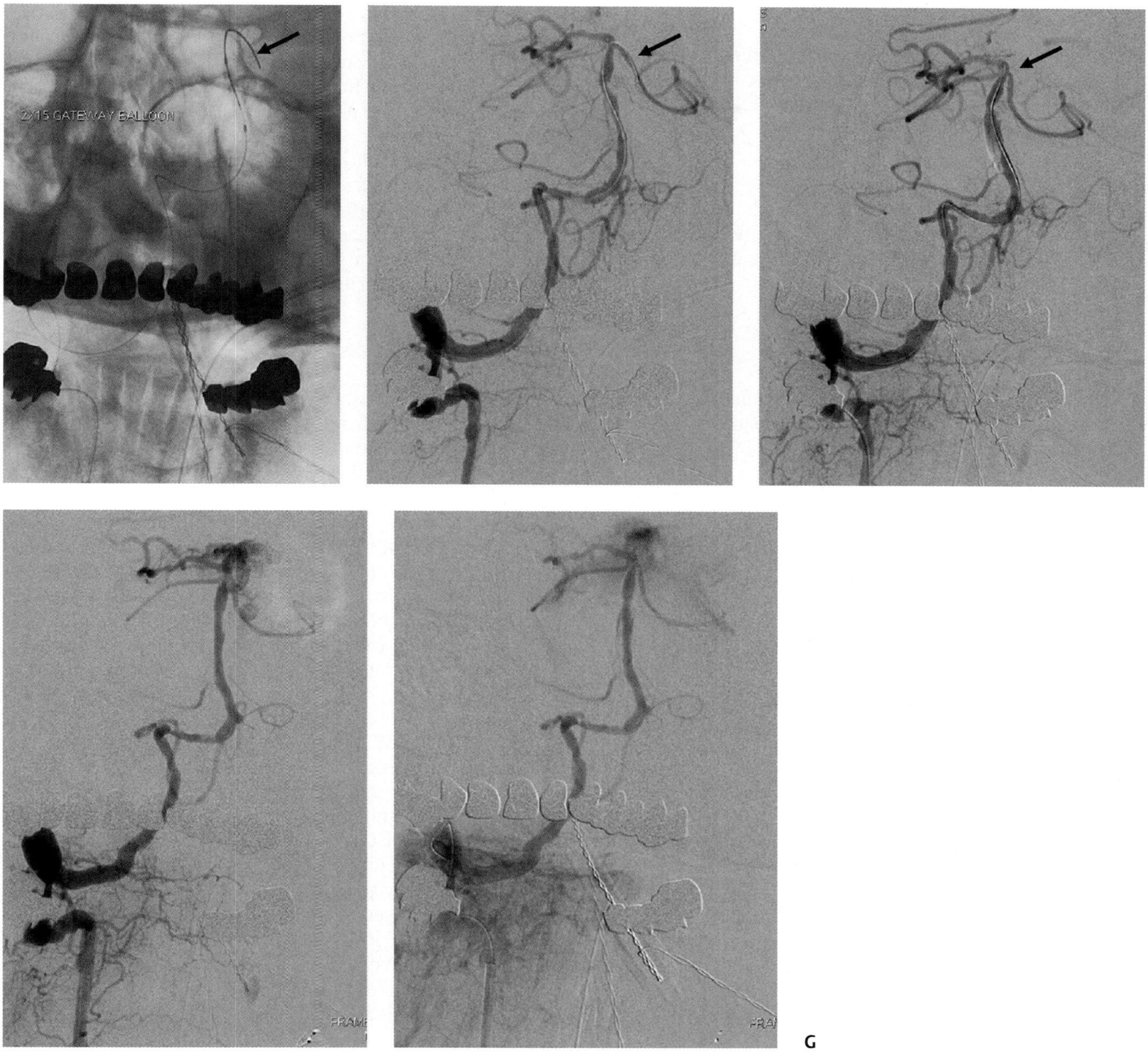

C–E

F

G

Fig. 12.3 *(continued)* Because of the severely diseased nature of the vertebrobasilar system, native **(C)** and subtracted **(D)** images in the working angle for percutaneous transluminal angioplasty and stenting (PTAS) show that secure distal wire access into the left posterior cerebral artery was never secured (*arrows*). **(***E, arrow***)** Although this access was sufficient to perform the angioplasty, the wire came back during the attempted placement of the Wingspan delivery system, ultimately terminating in the region of the basilar apex. Some resistance was encountered when the Wingspan system was navigated over the wire. **(F,G)** When the forward pressure on the delivery system ultimately released, the entire system and microwire moved forward, resulting in perforation of the basilar apex.

Standard Microwire

The 0.014-inch Synchro-2 (Boston Scientific) microwire is often very steerable and provides superior navigability and control for crossing these highly stenotic lesions, particularly within tortuous vascular segments.

Exchange Microwire

The exchanges are performed with a floppy exchange length (300 cm) wire (0.014-inch Transcend floppy [Boston Scientific].

Gateway Balloon Selection

We have typically followed the recommended instructions for use when using the Gateway–Wingspan system to perform angioplasty.

Balloon Diameter

The balloon is chosen to approximate 80% of the diameter of the "normal" proximal parent artery.

Balloon Length

The balloon should equal or slightly exceed the length of the diseased segment.

Wingspan Stent Selection

Stent Diameter

The Wingspan stent is chosen to equal or slightly exceed the diameter of the normal parent artery. Typically if the size just larger than the diameter of the vessel is selected, the stent will be appropriately sized. When possible we avoid oversizing the stent, as this does not reliably provide additional luminal gain after angioplasty.

Stent Length

The stent should equal or exceed the length of the angioplasty balloon used and should extend at least 3 mm both proximal and distal to the ends of the stenotic lesion to be treated.

Once the microcatheter, microwire, exchange wire, balloon, stent, and guiding catheter are all prepared, the operator is ready to go forward with the intervention.

Guiding Catheter Placement

After a therapeutic ACT has been achieved and all of the equipment has been prepared, the operator can proceed to exchange the diagnostic catheter for the guiding catheter. This is best accomplished on a biplane road map with the A-plane demagnified to demonstrate the aortic arch and as much of the distal catheter as possible and the B-plane positioned over the cervical segment of the parent artery and slightly magnified to allow visualization of the exchange wire. The B-plane should demonstrate the distal tip of the diagnostic catheter as well as the targeted distal cervical segment for placement of the guiding catheter. Once the roadmap image has been obtained, the diagnostic catheter can be exchanged for the guiding catheter. When a standard 6F guiding catheter is used, an internal (coaxial) 110-cm 4F UCSF-3 (Cordis Corp.) extends distally out the guiding catheter and provides a more tapered interface between the guiding catheter and the 0.035-inch exchange wire, thus facilitating guide catheter placement.

Crossing the Lesion

Once the guiding catheter is in position, the microwire and microcatheter are manipulated beyond the stenotic lesion and positioned within a large, straight vascular segment distal to the stenosis. The selection of this branch vessel is critical as it represents the location where the distal tip of the exchange wire will lie for all of the exchanges that will occur throughout the case. It is not uncommon for the distal wire to move forward and backward slightly during the exchanges (particularly in tortuous anatomy). As such the larger and straighter the recipient branch is, the more forgiving it will be to such movement. If the distal exchange wire position is tenuous (e.g., within a tortuous, small, or diseased branch), even small amounts of movement can have catastrophic consequences (**Fig. 12.3**).

Once distal position is secured with the microcatheter and microwire, the microcatheter can be removed over a 0.014-inch exchange microwire. After removal of the microcatheter, an angiographic run should be performed to assess the position of the distal microwire and the status of the lesion. If any extravasation is visualized at this point (distally at the tip of the microwire or in the region of the lesion), the heparin can be reversed immediately with fewer consequences than if the stent has already been placed. In addition, the exchange wire may distort the anatomy of the target vessel, thus altering the expected location and orientation of the stenosis on the roadmap image. As such, the angiographic run will verify that there is adequate flow beyond the lesion and will allow the operator to determine whether a new working roadmap image can and should be obtained. If the target vessel is distorted by the wire, it is possible that the angioplasty balloon could be suboptimally positioned for the procedure if this is not appreciated by the operator.

Angioplasty

Once the balloon is in position across the lesion, the angioplasty is performed using a slow inflation technique as advocated by Wojak, Connors, and Marks.[12–15] Typically, we inflate to the nominal inflation pressure (usually 6 atmospheres [ATM]) over 2 to 3 minutes. It is thought that this slow inflation technique can limit the rates of dissection, vessel rupture, and thromboembolic complications.

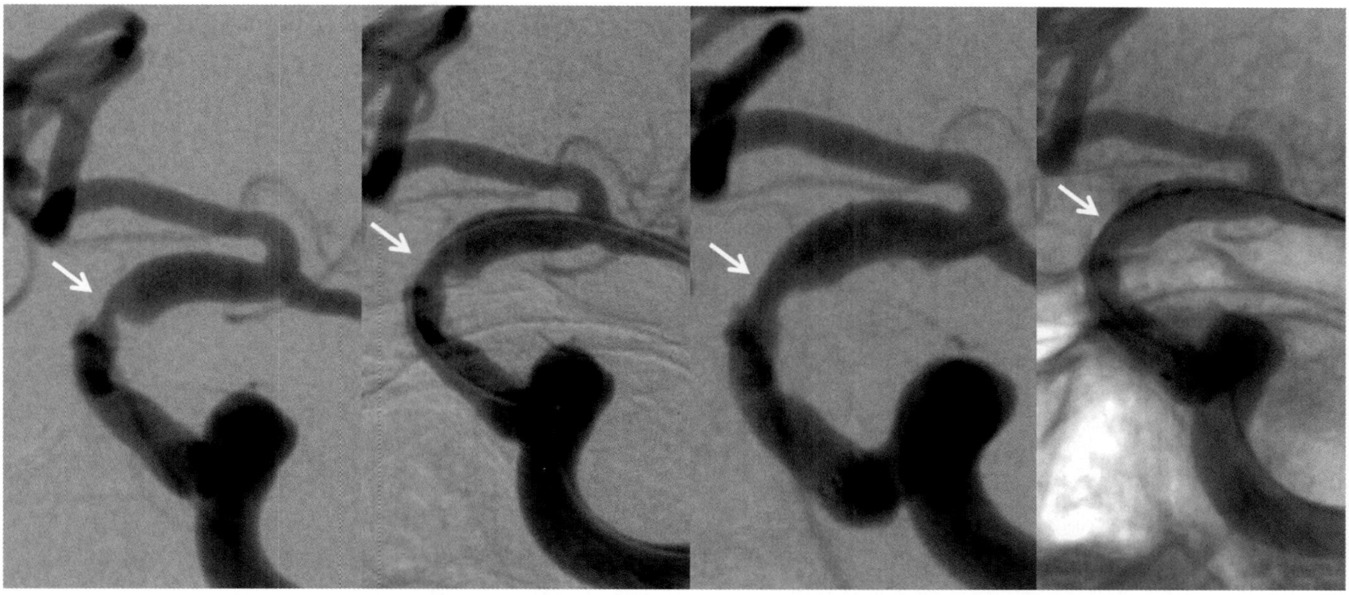

Fig. 12.4 Minimal additional luminal gain provided by stent placement. **(A)** Subtracted angiogram in the PA projection shows a high-grade stenosis of the supraclinoid segment of the left internal carotid artery, (*arrow*). **(B)** After angioplasty, there has been some improvement in the luminal diameter with ~40% residual stenosis (*arrow*). Subtracted **(C)** and native **(D)** images from post-Wingspan (Boston Scientific, Natick, MA) placement angiography demonstrate that although the stent may consolidate the effects of the angioplasty and prevent acute luminal loss from vascular recoil, it provides only minimal additional luminal gain beyond the effects of the initial post–percutaneous transluminal angioplasty result. This case example demonstrates that most of the luminal gain results from the angioplasty. Correspondingly, a suboptimal angioplasty is typically not salvaged by placement of a Wingspan. If a suboptimal angioplasty result is observed, it is technically easier to perform lesion redilation before stent placement.

After angioplasty is performed, the balloon should be retracted just proximal to the lesion and a gentle angiographic injection should be performed to exclude any procedural complications and to assess the angioplasty result. Although addition of the Wingspan will consolidate the gains of angioplasty, the additional luminal gain provided by the addition of the stent is minimal (**Fig. 12.4**). For this reason, the operator should strive for the best possible luminal gain after angioplasty. If a suboptimal result (>50% stenosis) is documented after the initial angioplasty, the existing balloon should be exchanged for a second balloon of equal diameter (or one size greater diameter) and the lesion redilated. A new balloon should be used for this procedure because after one inflation–deflation cycle, the balloon forms "wings" (as it is now no longer wrapped into its lowest profile configuration). Taking the balloon across the lesion in this form could create or exacerbate a dissection or lead to thromboemboli. A repeated predilation is probably safer than postdilating a suboptimally expanded stent. Once the stent is in place, it may provide an impediment to crossing with a second balloon. In addition, there are hazards to placing the Wingspan within a suboptimally dilated lesion (see below).

Stenting with Wingspan

After the balloon is removed over the exchange wire, the stent delivery system is introduced and positioned across the lesion. Once across the lesion, the system should be retracted until it is noted to move with a one-to-one response. At this point, the stent can be deployed by applying gentle forward pressure to the stabilizer while withdrawing the delivery catheter. In tortuosity, this can require a significant amount of stress to be placed on the delivery system to accomplish the delivery. If a considerable amount of resistance is encountered during deployment, the Wingspan delivery system should be exchanged out for a new system and the deployment reattempted. During the attempted delivery, it is critical that the proximal stabilizer does not bend and become kinked and fixed against the wire. If this occurs, both the delivery system and microwire must be removed and the lesion retraversed if stenting is to be performed. Optimally, the stent should be deployed such that the distal end of the stent extends at least 3 mm beyond the leading edge of the lesion.

Once the stent is deployed, the delivery system can be removed over the exchange wire. It is critical to closely observe the stent markers during the removal of the delivery system, as the delivery system can become engaged within the in situ stent and actually drag it proximally during removal. The piece that typically engages is the "nose cone," which lies on the distal tip of the inner delivery catheter. This nose cone measures 1.2 mm in diameter and has an angulated proximal end that can catch on the stent tines, particularly if a suboptimal angioplasty has been performed with a small balloon (e.g., 1.5 mm diameter). Any recoil of this lesion could result in luminal loss to the extent that the nose cone will not pass though the deployed stent. This catching of the nose cone on the deployed stent can also be

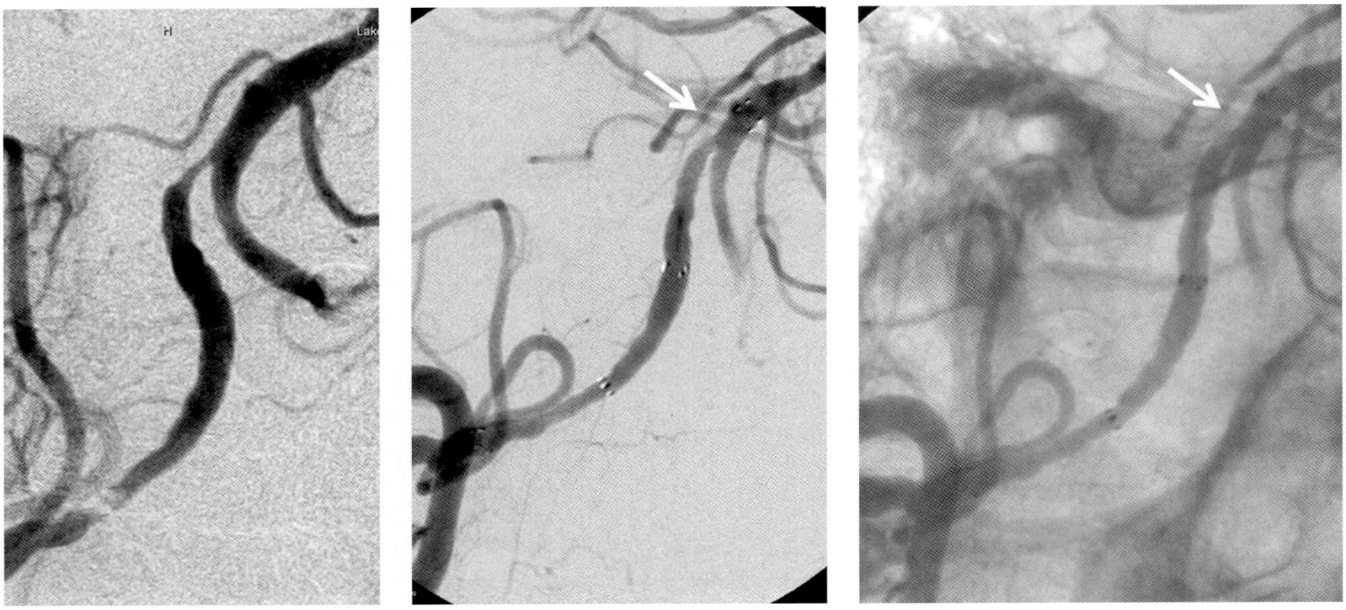

Fig. 12.5 Delivery system engaged in tortuous anatomy during attempted removal. **(A)** Subtracted image shows high-grade tandem stenoses of the right vertebral artery with occlusion of the left vertebral artery. Both lesions were treated with angioplasty and stenting. After placement of the distal Wingspan (Boston Scientific, Natick, MA), a significant amount of resistance was encountered during the removal of the delivery system. The caliber change between the basilar and vertebral arteries and the angle likely resulted in a malapposition of the Wingspan stent tines at the vertebrobasilar junction (subtracted, **B**; native, **C**). The entire system was readvanced slightly over the exchange wire. Then, the outer Wingspan delivery microcatheter was readvanced over the inner catheter to "cork" (or capture) the proximal end of the nose cone. After this was achieved, the entire delivery system was easily removed.

encountered when the device is deployed within tortuous anatomy (**Fig. 12.5**). If resistance to stent removal is encountered, several techniques can be employed:

1. The delivery system can be gently readvanced across the lesion and tried a second time.
2. The microwire can be carefully manipulated more distally within the cerebrovasculature to provide better proximal support in the region of the lesion and to slightly change the orientation of the delivery system within the deployed stent.
3. The delivery catheter can be advanced to "cork" the proximal aspect of the nose cone of the inner catheter, thereby shielding it from the stent tines.
4. The floppy exchange microwire can be exchanged for a stiffer microwire, which could change the orientation of the vessel enough to allow retraction of the delivery system.
5. Secure access in the contralateral femoral artery, and manipulate a second angioplasty balloon across the lesion, alongside the engaged delivery catheter and perform an angioplasty to further dilate the lesion and increase the luminal diameter to the extent that the delivery catheter can be removed (**Fig. 12.6**).

Final Angiography

After removal of the stent delivery system, a magnified angiographic run can then be performed in the working angle for stenting to evaluate the treated segment. In this scenario, the operator should inspect the lesion for adequate dilation. If >50% stenosis remains, the operator can consider performing a postdilation of the stent with a new angioplasty balloon. Also it is important to inspect the vessel just distal and proximal to the stent for dissection or spasm. Finally, the stented segment should be carefully inspected for local thrombotic complications. The regional perforators should be compared with the pretreatment angiogram to detect any new occlusion. In addition, the stent lumen should be inspected for filling defects indicative of intrastent thrombus formation.

At this point, a whole head branch vessel angiogram is performed in the standard PA and lateral projection to assess for distal branch vessel occlusion or distal wire perforation. The angiogram should be compared with the original branch vessel angiogram to assess for any missing branches. It is not uncommon after dilating a very high-grade stenosis that the flow in the distal branches while present demonstrates a slow transit time. In these situations, the vascular beds may have been supplied by long-standing leptomeningeal collateral flow patterns. These flow patterns may require some time to reorganize. As such, sluggish distal flow after a successful PTAS procedure may represent a normal finding related to competitive inflow from these established leptomeningeal collaterals.

If no complications are noted on the branch vessel angiogram, the operator may go back to the high-magnification working angles and the exchange microwire can be carefully removed under fluoroscopic observation. It is possible (but uncommon) for the microwire to become engaged within the stent. After removal of the microwire, we typically

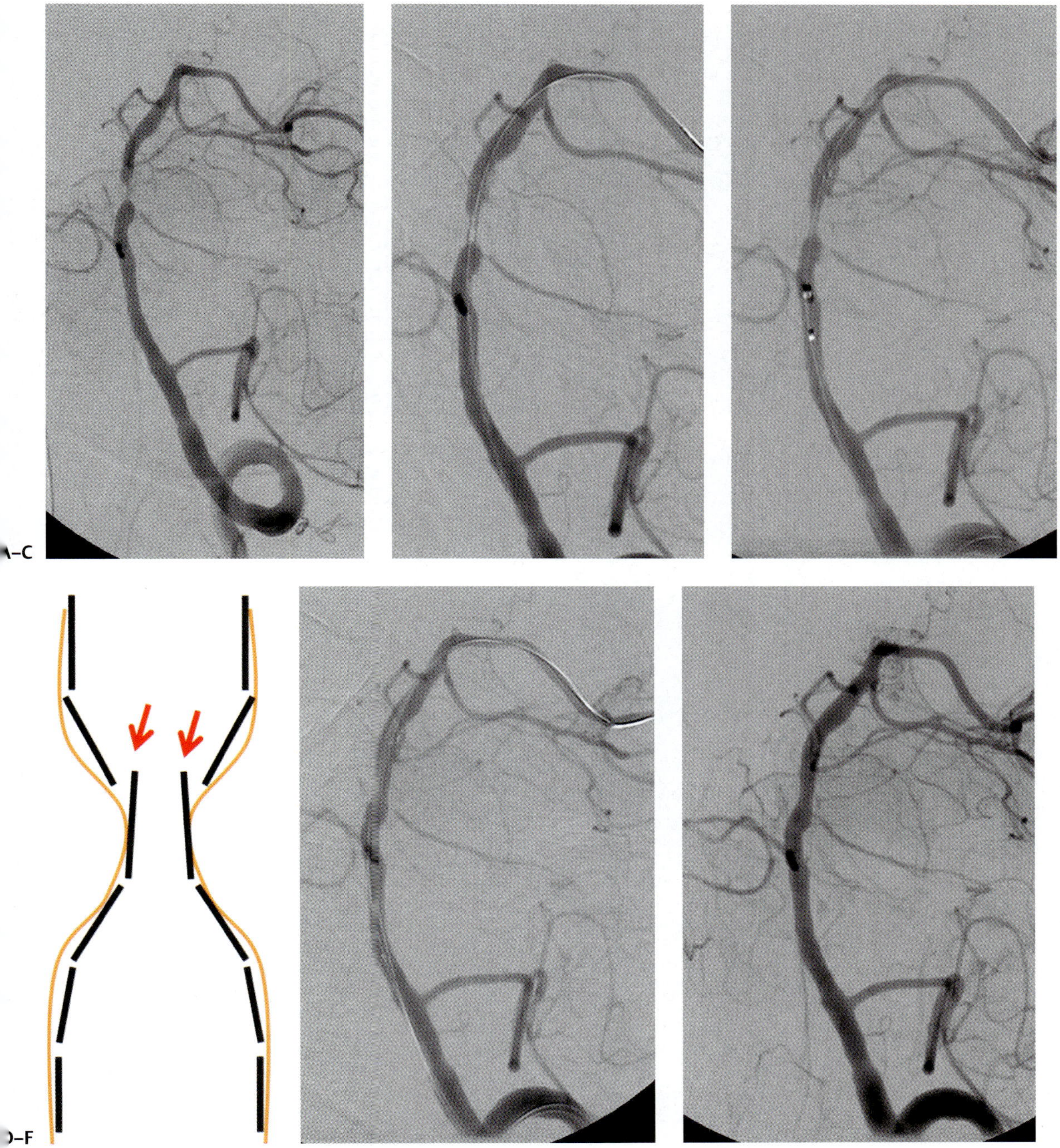

Fig. 12.6 Delivery system engaged after suboptimal angioplasty. **(A)** Subtracted image shows a very high-grade midbasilar stenosis. **(B)** Angioplasty with a 1.5-mm Gateway balloon (Boston Scientific, Natick, MA) yielded minimal luminal gain. Despite this suboptimal result, a slightly oversized 3.5 × 15-mm Wingspan stent (Boston Scientific, Natick, MA) was placed with the intention of consolidating the angioplasty result and possibly adding further to the luminal diameter. **(C)** After the deployment of the stent, however, only minimal improvement was noted. In addition, when attempts were made to retrieve the delivery system, it became engaged within the stent tines at the level of the stenosis. Attempts to advance the delivery system forward to "cork" the nose cone were also met with resistance at the stenosis. **(D)** A schematic drawing shows the putative mechanism of this engagement with the residual hourglass-shaped stenosis causing stent tines to overhang the proximal and distal (*arrows*) margins. Ultimately, the contralateral femoral artery was punctured and a second guiding catheter was placed within the left subclavian artery. Through this access, a second Gateway balloon was advanced across the stenosis and a second angioplasty was performed. **(E)** Postdilation created a luminal gain, which was sufficient to allow retrieval of the delivery system. **(F)** Completion angiography in the working projection demonstrates optimal luminal gain. The patient emerged from anesthesia at neurologic baseline.

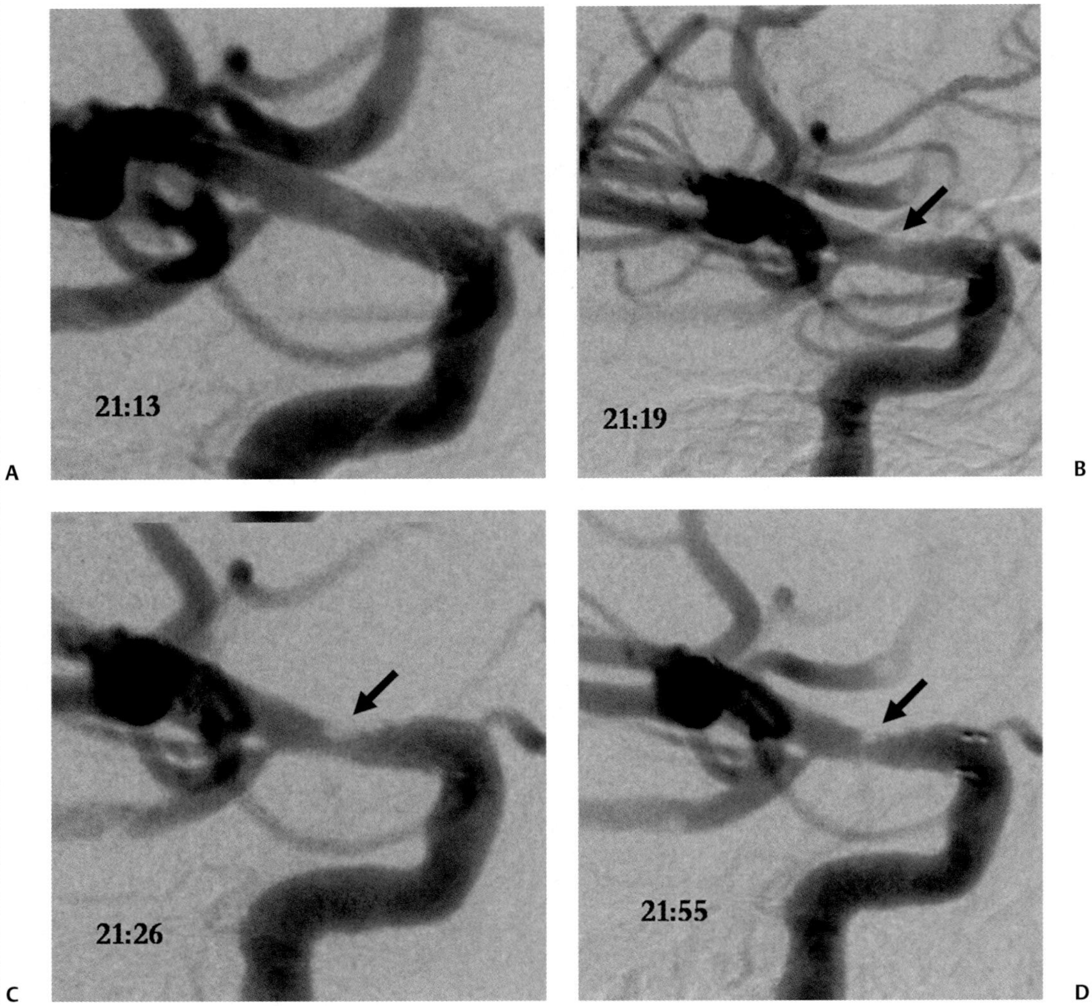

Fig. 12.7 Local thrombus formation after stenting – importance of delayed angiographic imaging. **(A)** Immediate postprocedural subtracted angiogram is made in high magnification in the working angle for angioplasty and stenting and demonstrates no significant residual stenosis. **(B)** A delayed angiogram 6 minutes later demonstrates a small amount of thrombus (*arrow*) accumulating within the midportion of the stent. **(C)** A second delayed angiogram 13 minutes poststenting demonstrates further accumulation of thrombus with enlargement of the lucent intrastent defect (*arrow*). **(D)** Twenty minutes after the intraarterial infusion of 14.5 mg of abciximab, follow-up angiogram shows the acute procedural thrombus to have almost completely resolved (*arrow*). Acute procedural thrombus is composed essentially entirely of activated platelets. As such, the thrombus mass can almost always be controlled and ultimately dissipated with the intraarterial infusion of a IIb/IIIa inhibitor. Complete thrombus dissolution is not required provided that the thrombus mass is stable over time or slowly resolving and brisk antegrade flow is maintained. Under these conditions, the thrombus mass will typically progress toward resolution with time (and without additional pharmacotherapy). Although the IIb/IIIa receptor inhibitors are often very effective in this scenario, the thrombolytic agents (e.g., tissue plasminogen activator) frequently are not, and may be more likely to elicit hemorrhagic complications.

observe the lesion angiographically for an additional 5 to 10 minutes with at least one additional angiogram performed to assess for local thrombus formation (**Fig. 12.7**).

Postdilation

In the event that the final luminal diameter after PTAS is unacceptable, the operator may consider postdilation of the residual stenosis. This is typically reserved for cases in which a residual stenosis of >50% is noted. The lesion should be assessed prior to removal of the exchange guidewire to avoid the need to renavigate a microwire across the newly deployed stent. When postdilation is to be performed, a new angioplasty balloon should be used. Reusing a previous balloon can be hazardous because the low crossing profile of a "wrapped" balloon is altered with inflation and deflation. Once inflated and deflated, the balloon will have "wings," which substantially increase the crossing profile, leading to the possibility of catching on or disrupting the stent and probably increasing the risk of procedural emboli.

Local or Distal Thrombus Treatment

Any local thrombus formation can be managed with the administration of an intraarterial IIb/IIIa receptor antagonist (e.g., abciximab). We have typically used abciximab for this purpose, administering small aliquots 2 to 5 mg intraarterially through the guiding catheter. In most cases one or two small boluses are sufficient to eradicate any procedural thrombus (which is theoretically composed entirely of platelets).

◆ Postprocedure Management

After the procedure is completed, the heparin is not reversed with protamine but rather allowed to dissipate with time. The femoral access is controlled with a closure device (e.g., StarClose, Abbott, Abbott Park, IL; Angio-Seal, St. Jude Medical, St. Paul, MN). The patient is then monitored in a neurologic intensive care unit for 24 hours. Blood pressure is tightly controlled, targeting a systolic pressure of <120 mm Hg.

References

1. Chimowitz MI, Lynn MJ, Howlett-Smith H, et al; Warfarin-Aspirin Symptomatic Intracranial Disease Trial Investigators. Comparison of warfarin and aspirin for symptomatic intracranial arterial stenosis. N Engl J Med 2005;352(13):1305–1316
2. Kasner SE, Lynn MJ, Chimowitz MI, et al; Warfarin Aspirin Symptomatic Intracranial Disease (WASID) Trial Investigators. Warfarin vs aspirin for symptomatic intracranial stenosis: subgroup analyses from WASID. Neurology 2006;67(7):1275–1278
3. Kasner SE, Chimowitz MI, Lynn MJ, et al; Warfarin Aspirin Symptomatic Intracranial Disease Trial Investigators. Predictors of ischemic stroke in the territory of a symptomatic intracranial arterial stenosis. Circulation 2006;113(4):555–563
4. Turan TN, Maidan L, Cotsonis G, et al; Warfarin-Aspirin Symptomatic Intracranial Disease Investigators. Failure of antithrombotic therapy and risk of stroke in patients with symptomatic intracranial stenosis. Stroke 2009;40(2):505–509
5. Fiorella D, Thiabolt L, Albuquerque FC, Deshmukh VR, McDougall CG, Rasmussen PA. Antiplatelet therapy in neuroendovascular therapeutics. Neurosurg Clin N Am 2005;16(3):517–540, vi
6. Lotrionte M, Biondi-Zoccai GG, Agostoni P, et al. Meta-analysis appraising high clopidogrel loading in patients undergoing percutaneous coronary intervention. Am J Cardiol 2007;100(8):1199–1206
7. Patti G, Colonna G, Pasceri V, Pepe LL, Montinaro A, Di Sciascio G. Randomized trial of high loading dose of clopidogrel for reduction of periprocedural myocardial infarction in patients undergoing coronary intervention: results from the ARMYDA-2 (Antiplatelet therapy for Reduction of Myocardial Damage during Angioplasty) study. Circulation 2005;111(16):2099–2106
8. Cuisset T, Frere C, Quilici J, et al. Benefit of a 600-mg loading dose of clopidogrel on platelet reactivity and clinical outcomes in patients with non-ST-segment elevation acute coronary syndrome undergoing coronary stenting. J Am Coll Cardiol 2006;48(7):1339–1345
9. Montalescot G, Sideris G, Meuleman C, et al; ALBION Trial Investigators. A randomized comparison of high clopidogrel loading doses in patients with non-ST-segment elevation acute coronary syndromes: the ALBION (Assessment of the Best Loading Dose of Clopidogrel to Blunt Platelet Activation, Inflammation and Ongoing Necrosis) trial. J Am Coll Cardiol 2006;48(5):931–938
10. Prabhakaran S, Wells KR, Lee VH, Flaherty CA, Lopes DK. Prevalence and risk factors for aspirin and clopidogrel resistance in cerebrovascular stenting. AJNR Am J Neuroradiol 2008;29(2):281–285
11. Nahab F, Lynn MJ, Kasner SE, et al; NIH Multicenter Wingspan Intracranial Stent Registry Study Group. Risk factors associated with major cerebrovascular complications after intracranial stenting. Neurology 2009;72(23):2014–2019
12. Wojak JC, Dunlap DC, Hargrave KR, DeAlvare LA, Culbertson HS, Connors JJ III. Intracranial angioplasty and stenting: long-term results from a single center. AJNR Am J Neuroradiol 2006;27(9):1882–1892
13. Connors JJ III, Wojak JC. Percutaneous transluminal angioplasty for intracranial atherosclerotic lesions: evolution of technique and short-term results. J Neurosurg 1999;91(3):415–423
14. Connors JJ III, Wojak JC. Intracranial angioplasty. J Invasive Cardiol 1998;10(5):298–303
15. Marks MP, Wojak JC, Al-Ali F, et al. Angioplasty for symptomatic intracranial stenosis: clinical outcome. Stroke 2006;37(4):1016–1020

Chapter 13

Extracranial Vertebral Artery Angioplasty and Stenting

Fernando Viñuela and William J. Mack

◆ Background and Indications

Stenoocclusive disease of the extracranial vertebral artery may represent a serious disorder with a high potential for death and disability if left untreated. Twice as common in men than women, vessel stenosis usually develops after the age of 60 years. Although often asymptomatic, the 5-year risk of disease progression and development of posterior fossa stroke is estimated to range between 20 and 60%, with a documented mortality rate as high as 30%.[1,2]

Vertebrobasilar ischemia often remains undiagnosed secondary to nonspecific clinical symptoms, and difficulties in noninvasive visualization of the extradural vertebral arteries. The significance of vertebral artery stenosis, therefore, may be underestimated in current clinical practice.

Presenting symptoms may include a constellation of headache, nausea, vomiting, vertigo, imbalance, cranial neuropathy, visual disturbances, and decreased level of consciousness, but an ischemic event often manifests as isolated dizziness.[3] Often, it is unclear as to whether the symptoms of vertebrobasilar territory ischemia result from thromboembolic events or from hypoperfusion. Classically, embolic events present as sudden, maximal-onset clinical events referable to high-flow vascular territories, whereas hypoperfusion states result in slower, fluctuating, often positional symptomatology due to reduced distal perfusion pressures secondary to critical or tandem stenoses. Clinical presentation coupled with results of noninvasive cerebral imaging modalities, such as magnetic resonance imaging/angiography (MRI/MRA) and computed tomography angiogram (CTA)/CT perfusion in conjunction with digital subtraction angiography delineate well the pathophysiology of vertebrobasilar ischemia (**Fig. 13.1**).

The vertebral artery arises most frequently from the posterosuperior wall of the subclavian artery. However, it can also arise from the aortic arch, the innominate artery, or the common carotid artery. The vertebral artery is divided into four anatomic segments. The first portion extends from its origin at the subclavian artery to the foramen transversarium at the level of the C6 vertebral body. The second segment travels through the foramen transversarium of the cervical vertebrae to the atlas. The third portion leaves the foramen transversarium of the atlas and extends posteriorly and horizontally on the superior surface of the posterior arch of the atlas until it reaches the dura. The fourth segment pierces the atlantooccipital membrane and the dura and enters the intracranial cavity through the foramen magnum extending to the pontomedullary junction, where it joins with the contralateral vertebral artery to form the basilar artery.

Less than 5% of vertebral arteries terminate in the posterior inferior cerebellar artery (PICA). These vessels are usually diminutive, and care must be taken to avoid vessel rupture or infarction due to forceful injections during angiography. The anterior spinal artery most often originates from the intradural vertebral artery. Muscular branches of the cervical vertebral artery anastomose with the ascending cervical, posterior deep cervical, and the external carotid artery branches, most notably the occipital and ascending pharyngeal divisions. Although a greater number of collateral vessels portends better outcome in the setting of vertebral stenoocclusive disease, it is important to be mindful of these branches when manipulating the catheter and wire during angiography.[4]

The vertebral artery ranges in diameter from 3 to 5 mm. Unilateral vertebral artery stenosis is usually well tolerated due to compensation by the contralateral vertebral artery or cerebral collateral network. This is the reason for the clinically silent nature of many vertebrobasilar disturbances. However, the risk of in situ thrombus formation and distal embolization remains a potential issue even for patients with compensated perfusion from the contralateral vertebral artery.

The most frequent cause of vertebral artery stenosis is atherosclerosis, and less commonly vasculitis, dissection, or extrinsic compression. Occlusive disease of the proximal and cervical portions of the vertebral artery represents a risk for posterior circulation ischemia. Atherosclerotic processes most frequently afflict the vertebral origin.[5] The extracranial vertebral artery is most susceptible to traumatic injury or spontaneous dissection where it is most mobile, at the entrance to the foramen transversarium at C6 and after it exits the foramen above C2. Narrowing in the third segment can result from an altered head position, most notably extension and rotation.[6]

Medical treatment for vertebral artery stenosis has historically included the use of antiplatelet agents along with systemic anticoagulation. The efficacy is uncertain.

Surgical bypass, endarterectomy, and reconstruction are technically challenging and carry a risk of thromboembolic complications, lung injury, and nerve damage, including Horner syndrome in a significant number of cases.[7,8]

In symptomatic patients with collateral channels that are poorly demonstrated angiographically, who have failed medical therapy, and for whom surgical bypass procedures present unacceptable risk, balloon-assisted stent angioplasty is reported to be of benefit. There are no clear inclusion

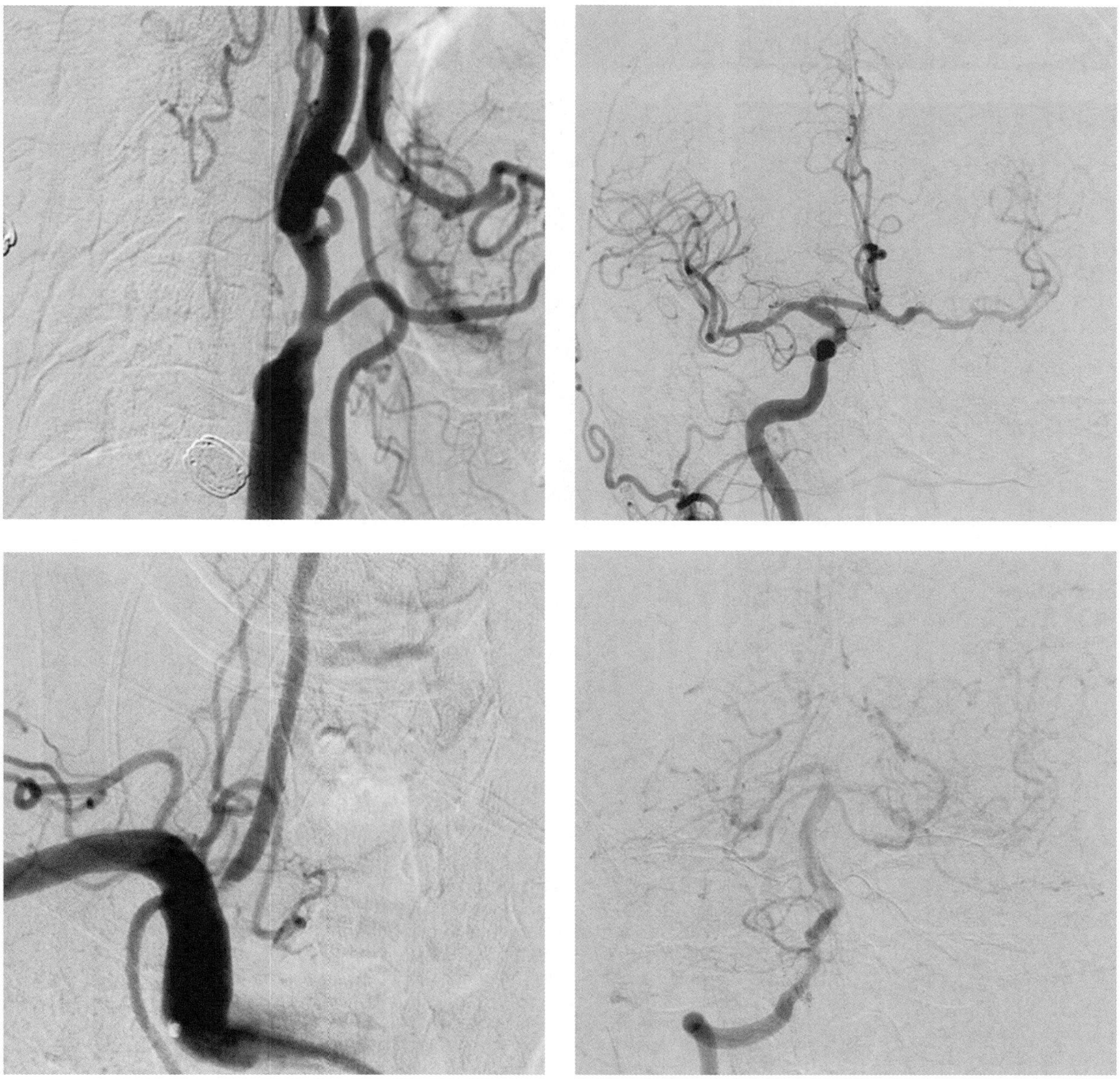

Fig. 13.1 Diagnostic cerebral angiography in a patient presenting with left hemispheric strokes. **(A)** Cervical angiogram of the left common carotid artery demonstrates complete occlusion of the internal carotid artery distal to the bifurcation. **(B)** Intracranial right common carotid artery angiogram demonstrates filling across the anterior communicating artery to opacify the left anterior and middle cerebral arteries. **(C,D)** Right subclavian angiograms demonstrate stenosis at the ostium of the right vertebral artery and filling of the left middle cerebral artery through the posterior communicating artery. Although the left posterior communicating is quite large, there is relatively little flow through this vessel due to high-grade narrowing of the bilateral vertebral arteries (not shown). *(continued)*

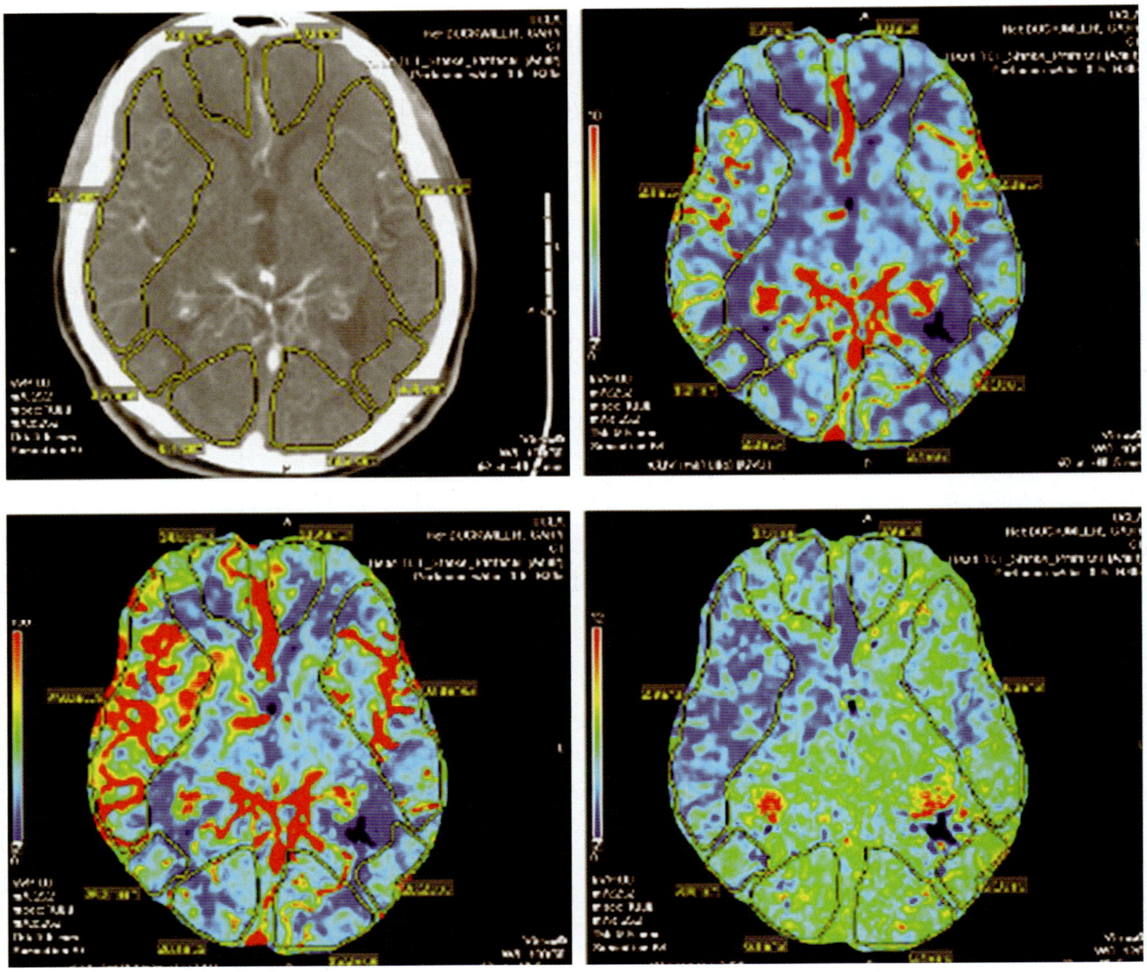

E

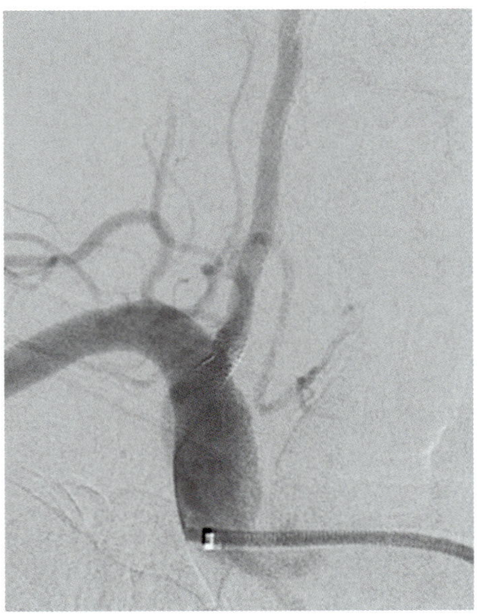

F

Fig. 13.1 *(continued)* **(E)** CT perfusion. There is an increase in mean transit time and reduction cerebral blood flow in the left middle cerebral artery (MCA) territory, suggesting ischemia. **(F)** Poststenting angiogram. Because of the high-grade bilateral vertebral origin stenoses, coupled with a chronic left internal carotid artery occlusion, which is relying on poor collateral posterior circulation flow through the left posterior communicating artery, angioplasty and stenting of the right vertebral artery origin were undertaken using a self-expanding stent. Note the proximal stent positioning within the subclavian artery to address plaque extension through the vertebral artery ostium.

criteria or guidelines used for patient selection. Most agree that vertebral artery angioplasty and stenting is indicated for patients with greater than 70% vessel stenosis and symptoms anatomically referable to the territory of the affected vertebral artery who have failed medical therapy. However, the anatomy of collateral circulation, the vascular contribution of the contralateral vertebral artery and the configuration of Willisian collaterals (most notably the posterior communicating arteries) factor into preoperative decision making in patients with less obvious symptomatology and those with less severe stenoses.

◆ Technique

Techniques specific to vertebral artery stenting procedures encompass preoperative patient selection and management, anatomic, and technical procedural considerations, and postoperative assessment and medical care. In anticipation of vertebral artery angioplasty and stenting, double antiplatelet therapy (Plavix [Bristol-Myers Squibb, New York, NY] 75 mg and aspirin 325 mg) is administered daily 3 days prior to the intervention and on the morning of the stenting procedure to decrease the risk of thromboembolic complications. In emergency cases, patients are loaded with 300 mg of Plavix and 650 mg of aspirin immediately before the procedure.

Most of our procedures are performed under monitored anesthesia care, allowing for continuous neurologic assessment during the procedure. Alternatively, general anesthesia may be utilized for uncooperative patients or those with exceedingly challenging vascular anatomy.

Arterial access is obtained via the transfemoral route, but radial artery access can be used to navigate unfavorable arch anatomy. Following arterial access a bolus of intravenous heparin is administered at 50 U/kg and redosed at 1000 U each subsequent hour (this regimen typically maintains an activated coagulation time of >250 seconds).

Detailed diagnostic cerebral angiography is undertaken; paying particular attention to the bilateral cervical vertebral arteries, their origins at the subclavian arteries, the presence and configurations of the posterior communicating arteries and anastomoses with the external carotid, ascending cervical, and posterior deep cervical arteries within the suboccipital carrefour. An anterior posterior view with a Townes angulation may be helpful to delineate the morphology of the vertebral artery ostium.

A 6 French-guide catheter or shuttle sheath is advanced over a 0.035-inch wire into the subclavian artery. These delivery systems effectively maintain position and accommodate most stents utilized in the exocranial vertebral artery system. If more stability is needed, a combination of shuttle sheath and guide catheter may be utilized. Alternatively, a 0.014- or 0.018-inch "buddy" wire can be placed in the distal subclavian to assist in stabilization of the guide catheter.

Based upon the diagnostic angiograms, a best working projection is determined. Additionally, measurements of the stenotic diameter, the length of the lesion and the diameter of the native vertebral artery distal to the stenosis are obtained (**Fig. 13.2**). Using a roadmapping technique, a microguidewire and microcatheter system are carefully advanced past the stenotic lesion. Once positioned distally, the microwire is removed and a 0.014-inch exchange length wire is position distally, often in the ipsilateral or contralateral posterior cerebral artery (**Fig. 13.3**). A significant length of wire is stabilized distal to the stenosis and visualized during the entire procedure to avoid recrossing a critical stenosis, especially following balloon angioplasty.

We customarily practice balloon predilation of tight stenoses to help ensure safe advancement of a self-expanding stent past the stenotic lesion. The balloon is measured to the length of the stenotic lesion and sized according to 80% of the native vessel diameter. Balloon inflation occurs slowly to nominal pressure to lessen the incidence of thromboembolism during the resultant vessel dissection during angioplasty. Balloon deflation must also be undertaken in a controlled, deliberate fashion. Slow inflation of balloons and deployment of stents under continuous fluoroscopy also aids in the prevention of inadvertent migration within the vessel secondary to "watermelon seeding."

Stent diameter is calibrated to 100% of the distal vertebral artery diameter and length is measured to traverse the entire lesion with a margin of several millimeters, both proximally and distally. The proximal end of the stent may require positioning within the subclavian artery to address plaque extension from vertebral artery ostium lesions (**Fig. 13.1F**). Monorail, rapid exchange, designs of both the balloon and stent systems increases ease and control of exchanges and is often preferable when limited

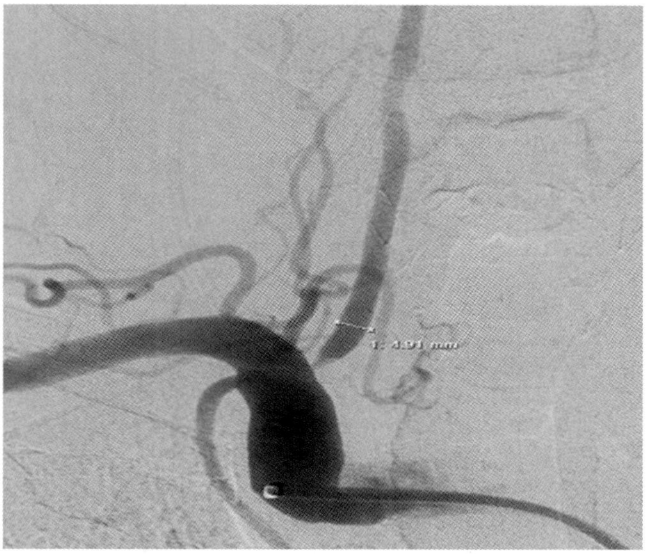

Fig. 13.2 Angiogram-demonstrating computer-generated measurement of the distal (nonstenotic) vertebral artery. Values are also obtained for the narrowed vessel diameter and the length of the stenotic segment.

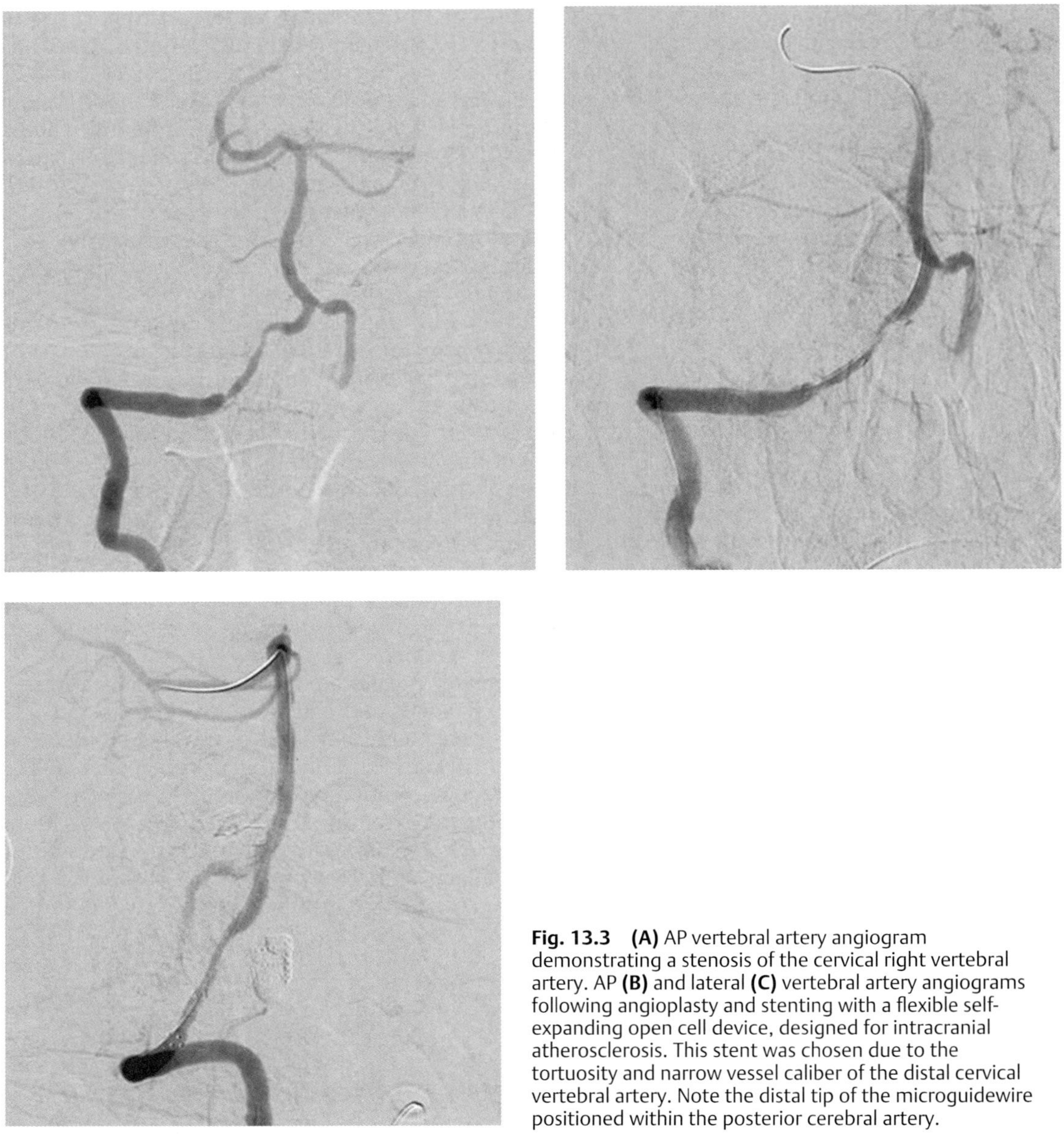

A

B

C

Fig. 13.3 **(A)** AP vertebral artery angiogram demonstrating a stenosis of the cervical right vertebral artery. AP **(B)** and lateral **(C)** vertebral artery angiograms following angioplasty and stenting with a flexible self-expanding open cell device, designed for intracranial atherosclerosis. This stent was chosen due to the tortuosity and narrow vessel caliber of the distal cervical vertebral artery. Note the distal tip of the microguidewire positioned within the posterior cerebral artery.

assistance is available. Stent selection is largely based on operator preference but is also determined by ease of access and vessel configuration. Although balloon-mounted stents (**Fig. 13.4**) combine a low profile and high radial force, self-expanding stents (**Fig. 13.1F**) are often preferable for utilization in larger diameter vessels. The strong muscularis layer of the vertebral artery origin coupled with plaque extension into the subclavian artery necessitates a stent with a high radial force.

Depending on the residual stenosis following stent deployment and distal perfusion and transit times, poststent balloon dilation may be undertaken (**Fig. 13.5**). A residual "waist" within the stented vessel segment is angioplastied by either withdrawing the balloon proximally on balloon-mounted stents or advancing a new balloon through a self-expanding stent. A balloon sized to 100% of the vertebral artery diameter distal to the stenosis is utilized. It is critical that balloon angioplasty remains within the confines of the stented arterial segment to prevent dissection of unprotected vascular intima. Oversizing the balloon diameter can perforate a vessel or extrude embolic material through the stent. Overinflation, past burst pressure, can result in vessel damage or air embolus as a result of balloon rupture. Following poststenting balloon angioplasty, it is important to fully deflate the balloon and withdraw slowly under fluoroscopy to avoid stent migration secondary to entanglement with the wings of the balloon. Postintervention cervical and intracranial angiograms are performed in the anteroposterior, lateral, and oblique projections to obtain posttreatment measurements and assess for dissections or distal embolus.

Intravenous heparin is discontinued at the conclusion of the procedure. Vessel closure is often performed with a closure device and manual pressure, as the patients have

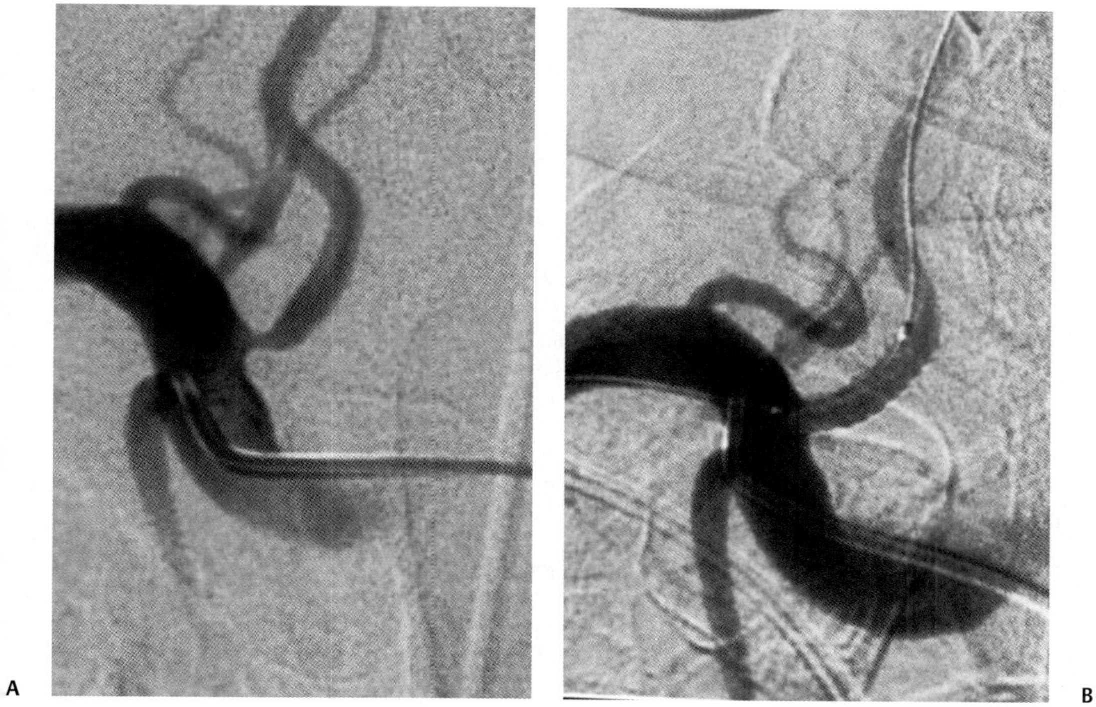

Fig. 13.4 Right subclavian artery angiograms before (A) and after (B) angioplasty and stenting with a balloon-mounted coronary stent.

received double antiplatelet therapy and intravenous anticoagulation. The patient remains in the neurologic intensive care unit or in a monitored neurologic/cardiac bed overnight and is usually discharged home the following day. Aspirin is continued indefinitely and Plavix, most commonly in our practice, for at least 3 months.

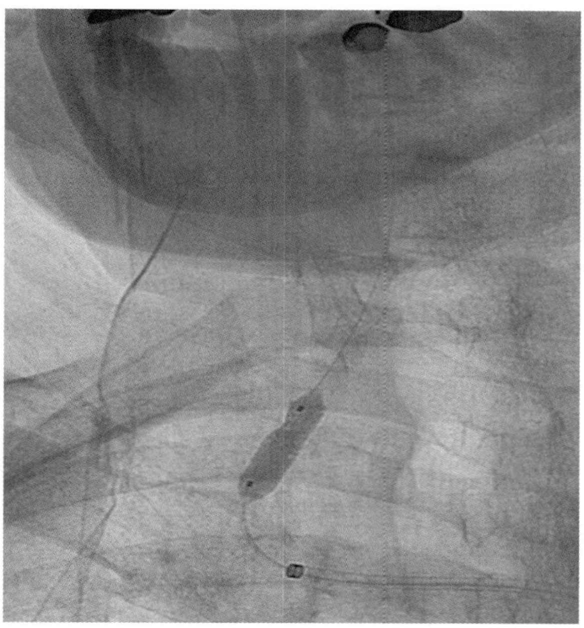

Fig. 13.5 Postangioplasty balloon dilation of a right vertebral artery origin stenosis. The inflated balloon is contained almost completely within the radiopaque markers of the stent. There is a small, retained waist in the distal region of the stented segment.

◆ Complications and Complication Avoidance

The objective of vertebral artery stenting procedures is to achieve a technically successful result with complication avoidance and resolution of the patients' clinical symptoms. Attainment of these goals hinges upon the prevention of periprocedural thromboembolic events and the deterrence of in-stent stenosis and adverse neurologic sequelae in the postoperative period.

Limitation of periprocedural thromboembolic complications is achieved through administration of double antiplatelet agents before, during, and after the intervention. Intravenous anticoagulation and meticulous assessment of catheter flushing helps prevent in situ thrombus formation. Additionally, technical modifications during the procedure, such as slow balloon inflation/ deflation and careful fluoroscopic visualization of the wire tip throughout the procedure limit the impact of mechanical vessel manipulation and crossing frequency of a stenotic lesion or dissection.

Distal embolic protection devices have become commonplace in carotid artery angioplasty and stenting. Their use is far less frequent in exocranial vertebral artery stenting procedures (**Fig. 13.6**). Because of smaller vessel caliber, the angle of the vertebral artery origin, and the tortuosity of the proximal vessel segment, we seldom find an occasion in which the benefits clearly outweigh the risks of deployment and retrieval.

Because of the frequency of vessel recoil and dissection seen with angioplasty alone, the use of stents has been heralded as a safer, more durable revascularization technique.[9–13] Complications of dissection by angioplasty can be reduced with stent deployment. Reduction of delayed thrombus

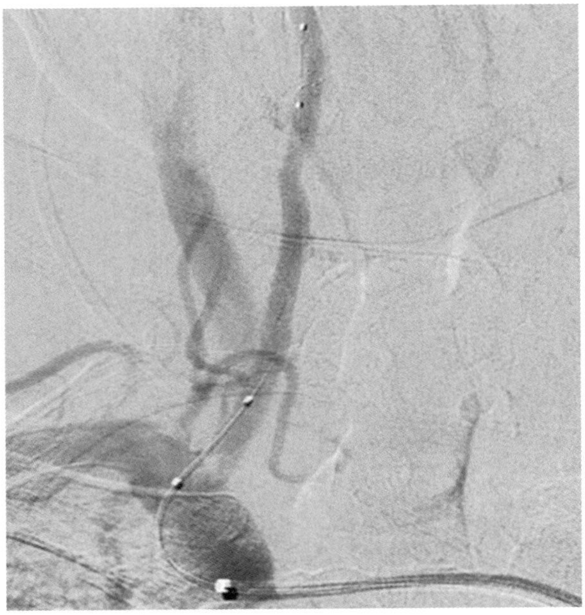

Fig. 13.6 Subclavian angiogram demonstrating a microguidewire and distal embolic protection device placed within the right vertebral artery. The device is located distally in a straight segment of the vessel wide enough to accommodate it.

formation and embolic events may be due to a protective layer of fibrous and neointimal tissue overgrowing the stent mesh and covering the atherogenic vessel wall.[14]

Straightening of a tortuous vertebral artery origin by placement of a stent, however, may accelerate a restenosis due to hemodynamic alteration and vessel wall injuries incurred during the stenting procedure.[15] Extracranial vertebral artery stenting procedures have a high rate (quoted between 10 and 43% in the largest series to date) of restenoses, but most remain asymptomatic.[16]

The Stenting of Symptomatic Atherosclerotic Lesions in the Vertebral or Intracranial Arteries (SSYLVIA) multicenter assessment of restenosis rates and their associations with clinical symptoms and specific risk factors established diabetes, greater postprocedure stenosis, smaller pretreatment vessel size and location at the vertebral ostium as independent risk factors for restenosis. The investigators noted a restenosis rate of 67% for vertebral ostium lesions and 25% for pre-PICA vertebral lesions, suggesting that ostial recoil may require a more robust stent.[16] Careful preoperative selection and diligent postoperative monitoring are therefore of paramount importance to the outcome of stenting procedures. If restenosis does occur, it most frequently occurs during the first year after the procedure. We monitor patients with noninvasive imaging in the postoperative period, but only treat if the restenosis is symptomatic. Typically, we perform initial CTA or MRA 3 months from the date of the procedure.

Initial vertebral artery stenting procedures made use of coronary balloon-mounted stents or other peripheral stents not specifically designed for intracranial use. Difficulty with navigation and tortuosity of cervicocerebral vasculature resulted in relatively high rates of procedural complications and in-stent restenosis.[7,9,13] As technology improves, the breadth of cases successfully treatable by this procedure increases significantly. Smaller, more flexible self-expanding stents have recently been approved under Food and Drug Administration (FDA) humanitarian device exemption for the indication of intracranial atherosclerosis. Small size and open cell design renders the stent flexible enough to navigate tortuous cervicocerebral vessels, while maintaining necessary radial force, thus lessening the likelihood of vessel wall injury in cases with very tortuous anatomy (**Fig. 13.3**). In-stent restenosis has decreased following cardiac angioplasty and stenting procedures with the advent of drug-eluting stents.[17] These stents may be useful in small or tortuous vertebral arteries. Investigations are currently aimed at reducing myointimal hyperplasia and resultant restenoses through the use of drug-eluting stents and technical improvements to existing device design.

References

1. Zaytsev AY, Stoyda AY, Smirnov VE, et al. Endovascular treatment of supra-aortic extracranial stenoses in patients with vertebrobasilar insufficiency symptoms. Cardiovasc Intervent Radiol 2006;29(5):731–738
2. Cartlidge NE, Whisnant JP, Elveback LR. Carotid and vertebral-basilar transient cerebral ischemic attacks: a community study, Rochester, Minnesota. Mayo Clin Proc 1977;52(2):117–120
3. Adams RD, Victor M, Ropper AH. Principles of Neurology. New York: McGraw-Hill, 1997:793–780
4. Morris P. Practical Neuroangiography. Philadelphia: Lippincott Williams & Wilkins; 2007
5. Cloud GC, Markus HS. Diagnosis and management of vertebral artery stenosis. QJM 2003;96(1):27–54
6. Wehman JC, Hanel RA, Guidot CA, Guterman LR, Hopkins LN. Atherosclerotic occlusive extracranial vertebral artery disease: indications for intervention, endovascular techniques, short-term and long-term results. J Interv Cardiol 2004;17(4):219–232
7. Imparato AM. Vertebral arterial reconstruction: a nineteen-year experience. J Vasc Surg 1985;2(4):626–634
8. Spetzler RF, Hadley MN, Martin NA, Hopkins LN, Carter LP, Budney J. Vertebrobasilar insufficiency. Part 1: Microsurgical treatment of extracranial vertebrobasilar disease. J Neurosurg 1987;66:646–661
9. Malek AM, Higashida RT, Phatouros CC, et al. Treatment of posterior circulation ischemia with extracranial percutaneous balloon angioplasty and stent placement. Stroke 1999;30(10):2073–2085
10. Albuquerque FC, Fiorella D, Han P, Spetzler RF, McDougall CG. A reappraisal of angioplasty and stenting for the treatment of vertebral origin stenosis. Neurosurgery 2003;53(3):607–614
11. Chastain HD II, Campbell MS, Iyer S, et al. Extracranial vertebral artery stent placement: in-hospital and follow-up results. J Neurosurg 1999;91(4):547–552
12. Jenkins JS, White CJ, Ramee SR, et al. Vertebral artery stenting. Catheter Cardiovasc Interv 2001;54(1):1–5
13. Ko YG, Park S, Kim JY, et al. Percutaneous interventional treatment of extracranial vertebral artery stenosis with coronary stents. Yonsei Med J 2004;45(4):629–634
14. Wakhloo AK, Tio FO, Lieber BB, Schellhammer F, Graf M, Hopkins LN. Self-expanding nitinol stents in canine vertebral arteries: hemodynamics and tissue response. AJNR Am J Neuroradiol 1995;16(5):1043–1051
15. Mukherjee D, Roffi M, Kapadia SR, et al. Percutaneous intervention for symptomatic vertebral artery stenosis using coronary stents. J Invasive Cardiol 2001;13(5):363–366
16. SSYLVIA Study Investigators. Stenting of Symptomatic Athlerosclerotic Lesions in the Vertebral or Intracranial Arteries (SSYLVIA): study results. Stroke 2004;35(6):1388–1392
17. Regar E, Serruys PW, Bode C, et al; RAVEL Study Group. Angiographic findings of the multicenter Randomized Study with the Sirolimus-Eluting Bx Velocity Balloon-Expandable Stent (RAVEL): sirolimus-eluting stents inhibit restenosis irrespective of the vessel size. Circulation 2002;106(15):1949–1956

Chapter 14

Therapeutic Internal Carotid Artery Occlusion

Brian Hoh

◆ Background

John Hunter is credited as the first to describe therapeutic proximal occlusion to treat an aneurysm. On December 12, 1785, Hunter successfully treated a patient with a popliteal aneurysm by ligating the superficial femoral artery.[1] Hunterian ligation has been a primary therapy to treat peripheral aneurysms, and has been used as a treatment for cerebral aneurysms. Advancements in microsurgical techniques and endovascular therapies have led to direct clipping or coiling as the primary treatment for cerebral aneurysms, largely supplanting Hunterian proximal occlusion; in certain cerebral aneurysms, however, therapeutic proximal occlusion still plays an important role as a treatment option. Large and giant internal carotid artery (ICA) aneurysms are the most commonly treated aneurysms by this technique. Extracranial-intracranial (EC-IC) bypass is discussed in other chapters, so this chapter will limit discussion to therapeutic ICA occlusion as a stand-alone treatment.

◆ Indications

Therapeutic ICA occlusion is most commonly employed to treat large and giant complex cerebral aneurysms of the ICA. Other indications include trauma, neoplastic invasion, and encasement of the carotid artery.

Giant cerebral aneurysms of the internal carotid artery portend a serious natural history, with a 40% risk of subarachnoid hemorrhage (SAH) over 5 years.[2] Large and giant ICA aneurysms can also cause significant cranial nerve dysfunction by mass effect. Therapeutic ICA occlusion is an effective treatment option in patients with ICA aneurysms that are not favorable for surgical clipping or endovascular coiling.[3]

Drake described using proximal "Hunterian" carotid artery occlusion to treat 160 patients with giant aneurysms of the anterior circulation, of which 90% of patients had a satisfactory outcome. Obliteration of the aneurysm by thrombosis was complete in all but four patients, and hemodynamic ischemic infarction occurred only after two of the carotid occlusions.[4]

Larson et al[5] described long-term follow-up (mean 76 months) in 58 patients that they treated for ICA aneurysms (40 intracavernous, 5 petrous carotid, 3 cervical carotid, and 10 ophthalmic segment). Patients presented with symptoms of mass effect ($n = 45$), thromboembolic transient ischemia or stroke ($n = 6$), SAH ($n = 4$), and epistaxis ($n = 3$). Carotid occlusion was performed in 55 patients (with EC-IC bypass in three patients). Postoperatively and on long-term follow-up, six patients had transient ischemia that resolved, two patients had delayed infarction, one patient had aneurysm enlargement, two patients had delayed SAH, and three patients died from treatment.

Van Rooij and Sluzewski[6] described the effects of therapeutic carotid occlusion on cranial nerve dysfunction in 31 patients they treated with cavernous ICA aneurysms. Cranial nerve dysfunction resolved in 19 patients, improved in 9 patients, and remained unchanged in 3 patients.

◆ Test Occlusion

Before performing therapeutic ICA occlusion, tolerance to carotid occlusion must be determined. If a patient cannot tolerate carotid occlusion, EC-IC bypass is indicated. The method for determining tolerance to carotid occlusion is controversial. Several different techniques have been described. These include carotid balloon test occlusion with hypotensive challenge and clinical testing,[7] carotid balloon test occlusion with single photon emission computed tomography (SPECT),[8] carotid balloon test occlusion with stable xenon-enhanced CT,[9,10] carotid balloon test occlusion with transcranial Doppler ultrasonography,[11] carotid balloon test occlusion with measuring distal ICA stump pressure,[12] and carotid balloon test occlusion with venous phase timing.[13] In our practice, we perform carotid balloon test occlusion with hypotensive challenge, clinical testing, and SPECT.

◆ Technique

Our technique of therapeutic ICA occlusion consists of a staged procedure: (1) determining tolerance to carotid occlusion by carotid balloon test occlusion with hypotensive challenge, clinical testing, and SPECT; (2) this is followed at a later date by intentional endovascular sacrifice of the ICA with coil embolization. We perform occlusion in stages to allow time to evaluate the SPECT and to counsel the patient regarding the results of the SPECT and their therapeutic options, whether therapeutic ICA occlusion as a stand-alone treatment or in conjunction with EC-IC bypass.

We determine tolerance to carotid occlusion by carotid balloon test occlusion with hypotensive challenge, clinical testing, and SPECT. This procedure requires coordination between multiple team members: the neurointerventionalist, the anesthesiologist, the neurologist, and the nuclear medicine radiologist. We have a neurologist conduct a baseline neurologic examination of the patient before the procedure. The procedure is performed with the patient awake with monitored anesthesia care. The anesthesiologist must understand the goals of the procedure and how sedatives or other medications could interfere with the clinical testing of the patient during the test occlusion. Arterial blood pressure monitoring is necessary, so a radial arterial line can be placed or the femoral arterial sheath can be transduced. The baseline mean arterial pressure should be noted. The groin is infiltrated with local anesthetic and femoral access is obtained with a micropuncture kit. We use a 6F femoral sheath if a radial arterial line has been placed, or a 7F femoral sheath if arterial blood pressure monitoring is being transduced from the femoral sheath. We perform full cerebral angiography to assess the contralateral carotid artery, the patency of the Circle of Willis, and the extent of collaterals to the carotid cerebral circulation to be tested. Intravenous systemic heparinization is administered and activated clotting times (ACTs) are checked to target a goal 250 to 300 seconds. A 6F guiding catheter connected to the usual heparinized flush system is positioned in a stable proximal location in the ICA to be tested. We perform the carotid test occlusion with a 7 × 7–mm HyperForm Occlusion Balloon System (ev3 Endovascular, Inc., Plymouth, MN) over a 0.010-inch MTI guidewire. We position the balloon at the location of the intended permanent occlusion if possible, otherwise at the petrous segment of the ICA. We inflate the balloon with a 50/50 iodixanol 320 mg/mL (GE Healthcare, Waukesha, WI) and saline solution using a Cadence 1 mL Precision injector syringe (ev3 Endovascular, Inc.) slowly until the ICA is completely occluded. We perform an ICA injection to confirm that the ICA is completely occluded by the balloon. With complete balloon occlusion of the ICA, the neurologist performs a neurologic examination. If there is a neurologic deficit, we quickly deflate the balloon, conclude the procedure, and determine that the patient did not tolerate carotid occlusion. If the patient remains neurologically baseline, we instruct the anesthesiologist to lower the mean arterial pressure to 66% of the baseline mean arterial pressure. With hypotension, the neurologist examines the patient again, and if there is a neurologic deficit, the balloon is quickly deflated, the blood pressure is normalized, and the procedure concluded. If the patient remains neurologically baseline, we continue the hypotension and balloon occlusion for 30 minutes, while the neurologist performs frequent periodic neurologic examinations. We check ICA angiograms periodically to confirm that the balloon continues to be completely occlusive. The nuclear medicine team administers intravenous 30 mCi technetium-99m bicisate (ethyl cysteinate dimmer; ECD) during hypotension and balloon occlusion. After 30 minutes of hypotension and balloon occlusion, we deflate the balloon and perform a final control ICA angiogram. The catheters and femoral sheath are removed, and either a closure device or manual compression is used to perform hemostasis at the femoral arteriotomy site. The patient is then transported to the nuclear medicine department to undergo the SPECT scan.

We review the SPECT scan with the nuclear medicine radiologist. If there is any evidence of decreased perfusion, we consider it a failure to tolerate carotid occlusion (**Fig. 14.1**). We discuss the findings with the patient and review the treatment options.

If carotid occlusion is tolerated, we proceed to the next stage, which is definitive intentional endovascular sacrifice of the ICA. We had previously performed this with detachable silicone balloons (Boston Scientific, Natick, MA), but these are no longer available, so we perform permanent ICA occlusion with coil embolization.

We perform permanent ICA occlusion with the patient awake with monitored anesthesia care. Either a radial arterial line is placed or the femoral arterial sheath can be transduced for arterial blood pressure monitoring. The groin is infiltrated with local anesthetic and femoral access is obtained with a micropuncture kit. We give intravenous heparin for a target ACT of 250 to 300 seconds. We position an 8F Merci balloon guide catheter (Concentric Medical, Mountain View, CA) in the proximal ICA or in the common carotid artery. We perform coil occlusion of the ICA with the balloon inflated to serve as proximal control to prevent thromboembolism. Whenever possible, we perform the coil occlusion at the location of the lesion, otherwise we occlude the ICA at the petrous segment. We oversize the coils and use long-length coils so that they can anchor themselves and prevent against distal coil migration. Hypertension and hypervolemia are induced during the procedure and postprocedure to support hemodynamic collateral perfusion. The patient is monitored with neurologic examinations. We conclude the procedure when there is complete occlusion of flow in the ICA (**Fig. 14.2**). Hypertension and hypervolemia are maintained for at least 24 hours postprocedure and then weaned.

◆ Complications and Complication Avoidance

The most feared complication of therapeutic ICA occlusion is hemodynamic ischemic stroke. The first and most important step in avoiding this complication is determining tolerance to carotid occlusion. This requires expertise and experience with a chosen method of carotid occlusion testing. Coordination and communication between the team members involved is critical. The anesthesiologist must understand the level of patient participation required to properly monitor the patient neurologically during the carotid balloon occlusion. The neurologist must understand the eventual goal of therapeutic carotid occlusion. The nuclear medicine radiologist must understand the perfusion findings of interest in the study.

We perform permanent carotid occlusion with the patient awake, with hypertension and hypervolemia, and if there is any change in neurologic status, we increase the level of hypertension and hypervolemia. We continue hypertension and hypervolemia for at least 24 hours postprocedure, which we believe promotes expansion of pial collateralization to the occluded carotid territory.

A cerebrovascular surgeon who can perform EC-IC bypass must be available to perform emergent cerebral revascularization, if in the postprocedure period, the patient declines and does not respond to hypertension and hypervolemia.

Thromboembolic stroke is also a complication of therapeutic carotid occlusion, which can occur while coils are being deployed in the ICA. To prevent thromboembolism, we perform our procedures with systemic heparinization and

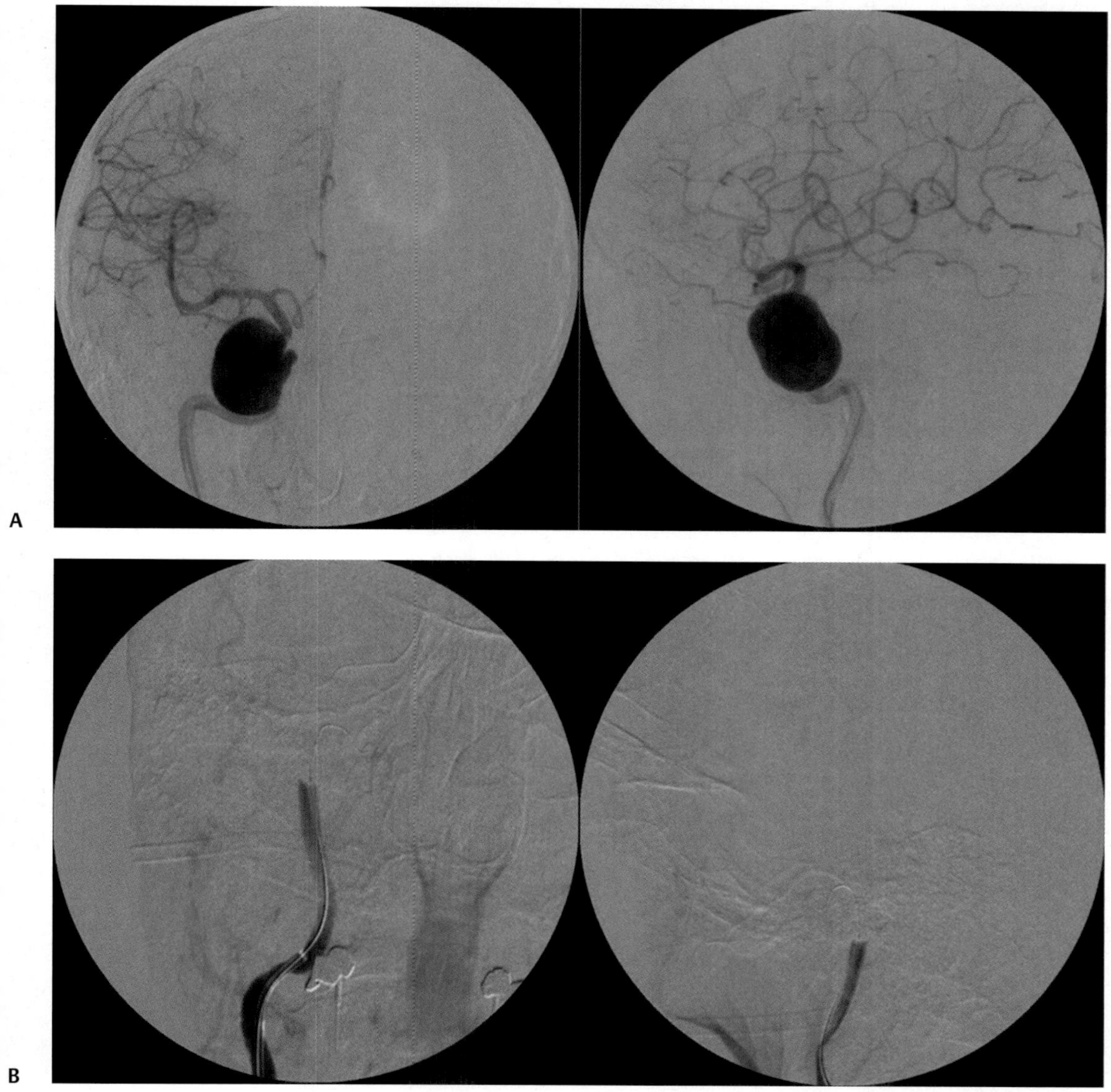

Fig. 14.1 A 54-year-old woman with new-onset right cranial nerve IV and right cranial nerve VI palsies. **(A)** AP and lateral right internal carotid artery (ICA) injection digital subtraction angiograms (DSAs) demonstrate a giant right cavernous ICA aneurysm. **(B)** AP and lateral right ICA injection DSAs during right ICA balloon test occlusion. *(continued)*

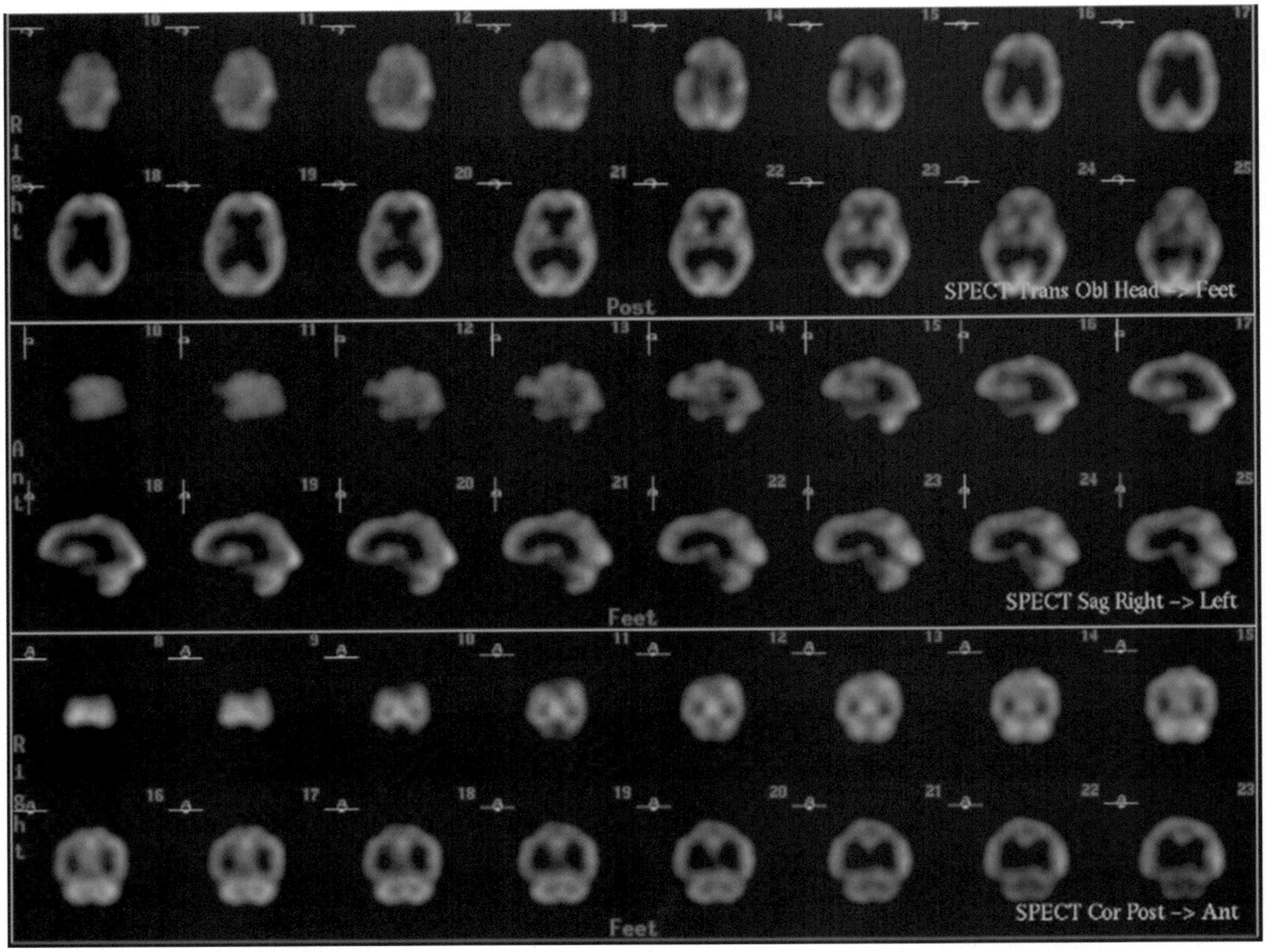

C

Fig. 14.1 *(continued)* **(C)** SPECT with 30 mCi technetium-99m bicisate (ethyl cysteinate dimmer, ECD) demonstrates decreased perfusion in the right cerebral hemisphere most pronounced in the middle cerebral artery territory.

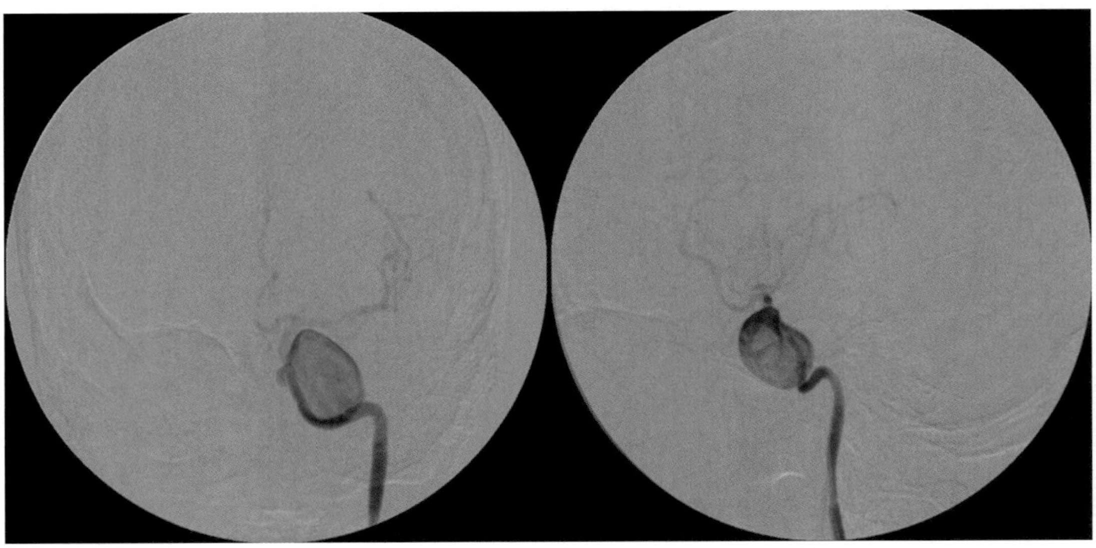

A

Fig. 14.2 A 49-year-old woman with new-onset left cranial nerve VI palsy. **(A)** AP and lateral left internal carotid artery (ICA) injection digital subtraction angiograms (DSAs) demonstrate a giant left cavernous ICA aneurysm. *(continued)*

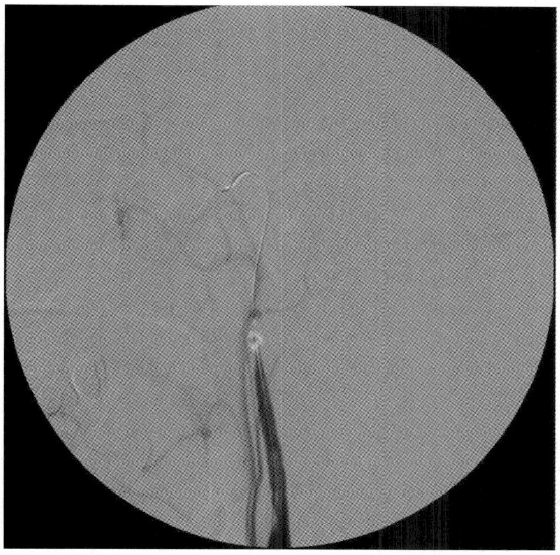

B

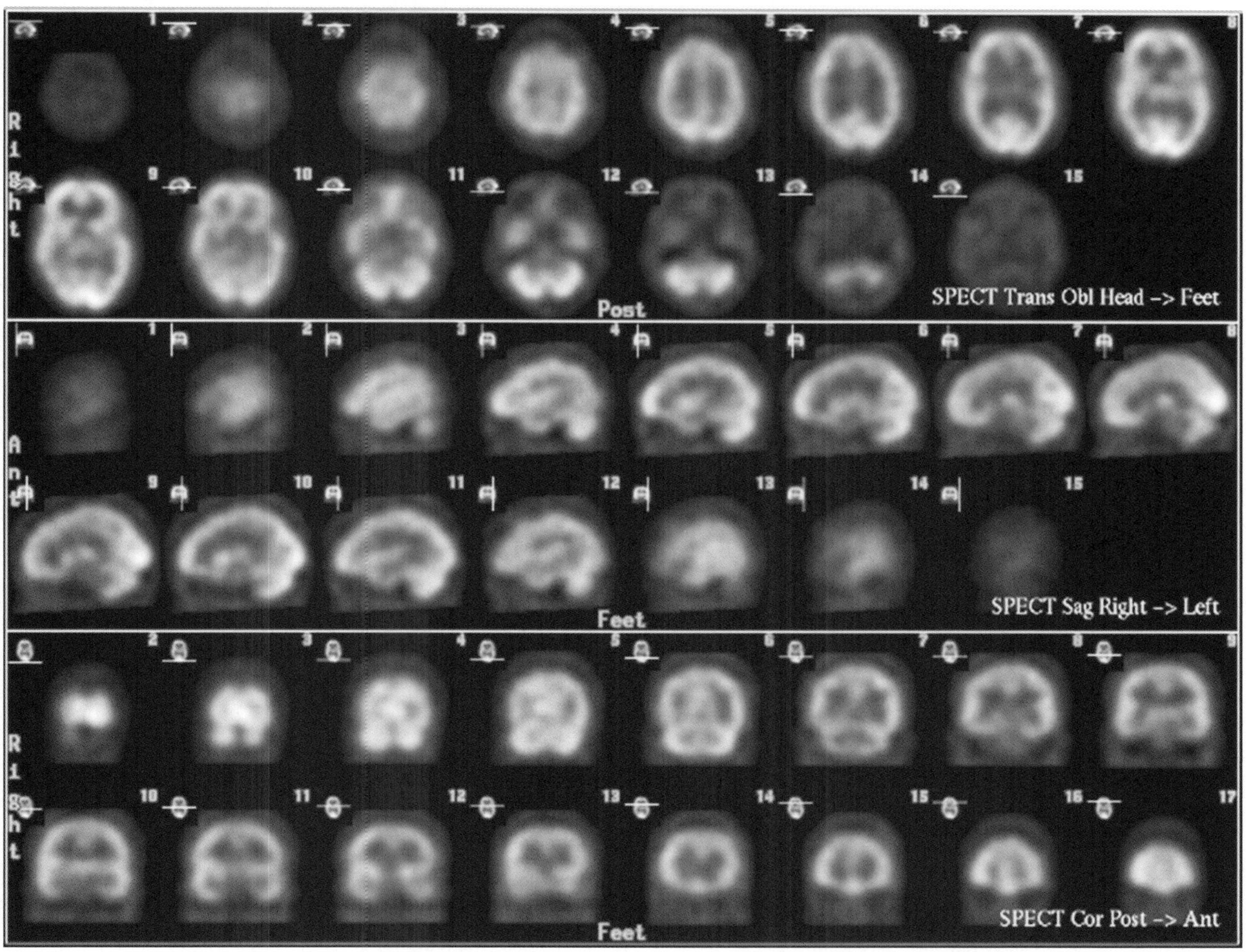

C

Fig. 14.2 *(continued)* **(B)** Lateral left ICA injection DSA during left ICA balloon test occlusion. **(C)** SPECT with 30 mCi technetium-99m bicisate (ethyl cysteinate dimmer, ECD) demonstrates symmetric perfusion in bilateral cerebral hemispheres. *(continued)*

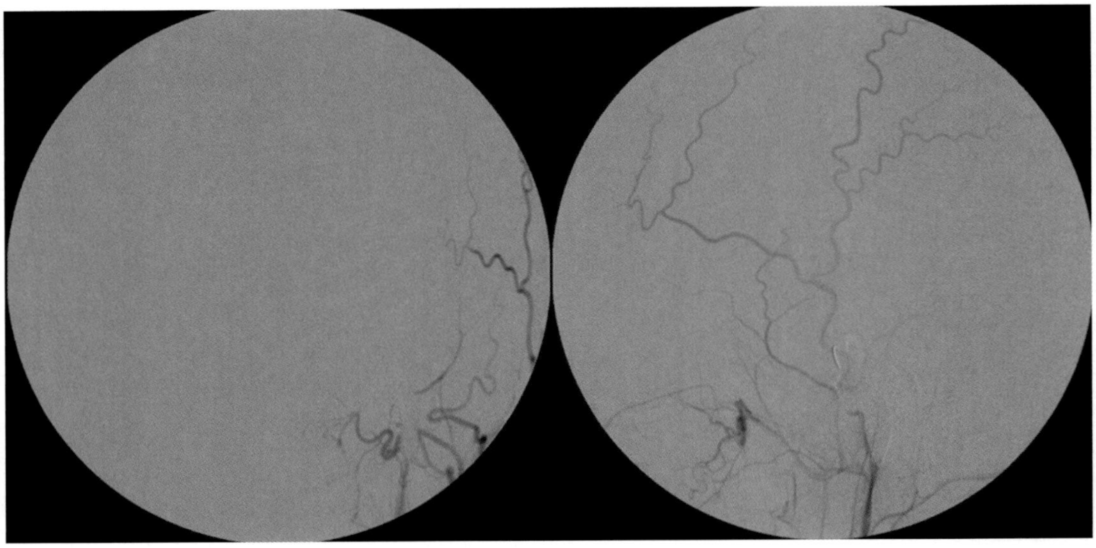

D

Fig. 14.2 *(continued)* **(D)** AP and lateral left common carotid artery injection DSAs after coil embolization demonstrates complete occlusion of the left ICA.

ACT checked to achieve a target ACT goal of 250 to 300 seconds. Additionally, we perform coil occlusion of the carotid artery using a balloon guide catheter. We inflate the balloon during the coil occlusion to serve as proximal control to reduce the risk of distal thromboembolism.

Distal coil migration can also occur. We use oversized and longer length coils to help anchor the coils to prevent their migration. Proximal control with the balloon guide catheter also serves to reduce the risk of migration of coils.

◆ Conclusions

Therapeutic ICA occlusion is a historic but still effective method for treating certain large and giant complex cerebral aneurysms of the ICA, as well as certain cases of trauma or neoplastic invasion or encasement of the carotid artery. There are several different methods of determining tolerance to carotid occlusion, and expertise and experience with a chosen method is critical. Coordination and communication between the multiple team members involved is necessary. Several key steps can be critical in avoiding complications when performing permanent occlusion of the carotid artery.

References

1. Schechter DC, Bergan JJ. Popliteal aneurysm: a celebration of the bicentennial of John Hunter's operation. Ann Vasc Surg 1986;1(1):118–126
2. Wiebers DO, Whisnant JP, Huston J III, et al; International Study of Unruptured Intracranial Aneurysms Investigators. Unruptured intracranial aneurysms: natural history, clinical outcome, and risks of surgical and endovascular treatment. Lancet 2003;362(9378):103–110
3. Hoh BL, Putman CM, Budzik RF, Carter BS, Ogilvy CS. Combined surgical and endovascular techniques of flow alteration to treat fusiform and complex wide-necked intracranial aneurysms that are unsuitable for clipping or coil embolization. J Neurosurg 2001;95(1):24–35
4. Drake CG, Peerless SJ, Ferguson GG. Hunterian proximal arterial occlusion for giant aneurysms of the carotid circulation. J Neurosurg 1994;81(5):656–665
5. Larson JJ, Tew JM Jr, Tomsick TA, van Loveren HR. Treatment of aneurysms of the internal carotid artery by intravascular balloon occlusion: long-term follow-up of 58 patients. Neurosurgery 1995;36(1):26–30
6. van Rooij WJ, Sluzewski M. Unruptured large and giant carotid artery aneurysms presenting with cranial nerve palsy: comparison of clinical recovery after selective aneurysm coiling and therapeutic carotid artery occlusion. AJNR Am J Neuroradiol 2008;29(5):997–1002
7. Standard SC, Ahuja A, Guterman LR, et al. Balloon test occlusion of the internal carotid artery with hypotensive challenge. AJNR Am J Neuroradiol 1995;16(7):1453–1458
8. Kaminogo M, Ochi M, Onizuka M, Takahata H, Shibata S. An additional monitoring of regional cerebral oxygen saturation to HMPAO SPECT study during balloon test occlusion. Stroke 1999;30(2):407–413
9. Linskey ME, Jungreis CA, Yonas H, et al. Stroke risk after abrupt internal carotid artery sacrifice: accuracy of preoperative assessment with balloon test occlusion and stable xenon-enhanced CT. AJNR Am J Neuroradiol 1994;15(5):829–843
10. Mathis JM, Barr JD, Jungreis CA, et al. Temporary balloon test occlusion of the internal carotid artery: experience in 500 cases. AJNR Am J Neuroradiol 1995;16(4):749–754
11. Sorteberg A, Bakke SJ, Boysen M, Sorteberg W. Angiographic balloon test occlusion and therapeutic sacrifice of major arteries to the brain. Neurosurgery 2008;63(4):651–660, 660–661
12. Tomura N, Omachi K, Takahashi S, et al. Comparison of technetium Tc 99m hexamethylpropyleneamine oxime single-photon emission tomograph with stump pressure during the balloon occlusion test of the internal carotid artery. AJNR Am J Neuroradiol 2005;26(8):1937–1942
13. Abud DG, Spelle L, Piotin M, Mounayer C, Vanzin JR, Moret J. Venous phase timing during balloon test occlusion as a criterion for permanent internal carotid artery sacrifice. AJNR Am J Neuroradiol 2005;26(10):2602–2609

Chapter 15

Acute Stroke Revascularization

Sabareesh K. Natarajan, Adnan H. Siddiqui, Erik F. Hauck, L. Nelson Hopkins, and Elad I. Levy

◆ Background

Until recently, the only medical therapy approved by the Food and Drug Administration (FDA) for acute stroke treatment was intravenous (IV) recombinant tissue plasminogen activator (tPA) administered within 3 hours of symptom onset for patients eligible for thrombolysis[1,2] (**Table 15.1**). The new American Heart Association/American Stroke Association (AHA/ASA) guidelines[1] recommend evaluating patients for IV tPA 3 to 4.5 hours after stroke symptom onset using the same eligibility criteria as the 0- to 3-hour time window along with any one of the additional exclusion criteria shown in **Table 15.1** (based on data from the European Cooperative Acute Stroke Study [ECASS] III[2]).

◆ Patients Who Are Not Candidates for Intravenous Thrombolysis or in Whom It Fails

Patients who do not meet the eligibility criteria for intravenous thrombolytic (IVT) therapy, who fail to improve neurologically after thrombolytic therapy, or who improve and then worsen (patients with reocclusion) are candidates for endovascular revascularization therapies. At our center, 94 patients with a mean presentation National Institutes of Health Stroke Scale (NIHSS) score of 14.7 were treated by endovascular interventions within 3 hours of stroke symptom onset.[3] In all these patients, tPA IVT was contraindicated or had failed. Partial to complete recanalization (Thrombolysis in Myocardial Infarction [TIMI] score of 2 or 3) was achieved in 62 of 89 (70%) patients presenting with significant occlusion (TIMI 0 or 1). Postprocedure symptomatic intracranial hemorrhage (SICH) occurred in five patients (5.3%), which was purely subarachnoid hemorrhage in three of these patients. The total mortality rate, including procedural mortality, progression of disease, or other comorbidities, was 26.6%. Overall, 36.7% of patients had a modified Rankin scale score (mRS) of ≤2 at discharge. Mean NIHSS at discharge was 6.5, representing an overall 8-point improvement in NIHSS score.

◆ Endovascular Therapy Leads to Higher Recanalization Rates and Improved Outcomes

In the Mechanical Embolus Removal in Cerebral Ischemia (MERCI),[4] Multi MERCI,[5] and the combined analysis of Interventional Management of Stroke (IMS) I and II Studies,[6] functional outcome (measured by mRS score of ≤2 at 3 months) was significantly better and the 3-month mortality was significantly lower in patients who had TIMI 2 or 3 recanalization than in patients in whom vessels failed to recanalize after endovascular therapy. Rha and Saver[7] reviewed 53 studies including 2,066 patients and found that good functional outcomes (mRS score ≤2) at 3 months were more frequent in patients with vessel recanalization than without vessel recanalization. The 3-month mortality rate was reduced in patients whose vessels were recanalized. Higher rates of recanalization were achieved with endovascular methods, particularly mechanical therapies, and consequently, were associated with better outcomes.

◆ Multimodal Computed Tomographic Imaging to Assess the Ischemic Penumbra (The Therapeutic Target)

The obvious advantages of computed tomography (CT) over other penumbral imaging techniques are its ubiquitous

Table 15.1 Eligibility Criteria for Intravenous Thrombolysis after Stroke Symptom Onset

For Patients Presenting within the 3-Hour Time Window before Beginning Treatment
Diagnosis of ischemic stroke causing measurable neurologic deficit
Neurologic signs not clearing spontaneously
Neurologic signs not minor and isolated
Caution should be exercised in treating a patient with major deficits
Stroke symptoms should not be suggestive of SAH
No head trauma or stroke in the previous 3 months
No myocardial infarction in the previous 3 months
No gastrointestinal or urinary tract hemorrhage in the previous 21 days
No major surgery in the previous 14 days
No arterial puncture at a noncompressible site in the previous 7 days
No previous ICH
Blood pressure not elevated (systolic $<$185 mm Hg; diastolic $<$110 mm Hg)
No evidence of active bleeding or acute trauma (fracture)
Not taking an oral anticoagulant or, if anticoagulant being taken, international normalized ratio $\leq$1
If receiving heparin in previous 48 hours, activated partial thromboplastin time must be within normal range
Platelet count $\geq$100,000 mm^3
Blood glucose concentration $\geq$50 mg/dL (2.7 mmol/L)
No seizure with postictal residual neurologic impairment
No multilobar infarction seen on NCCT scan (hypodensity $>$1/3 cerebral hemisphere)
Patient or family members understand the potential risks and benefits from treatment
Additional Eligibility Criteria for Patients Presenting between 3 and 4.5 Hours after Onset
$\leq$80 years
If taking oral anticoagulants, international normalized ratio $<$1.7
Baseline NIHSS score $\leq$25
No history of both stroke and diabetes

Abbreviations: ICH, intracranial hemorrhage; NCCT, noncontrast computed tomographic scan; NIHSS, National Institutes of Health Stroke Scale; SAH, subarachnoid hemorrhage

Source: del Zoppo GJ, Saver JL, Jauch EC, Adams HP, Jr. Expansion of the time window for treatment of acute ischemic stroke with intravenous tissue plasminogen activator. A Science Advisory from the American Heart Association/American Stroke Association. Stroke 2009; 40:2945–2948; and Adams HP, Jr., del Zoppo G, Alberts MJ, et al. Guidelines for the early management of adults with ischemic stroke: a guideline from the American Heart Association/American Stroke Association Stroke Council, Clinical Cardiology Council, Cardiovascular Radiology and Intervention Council, and the Atherosclerotic Peripheral Vascular Disease and Quality of Care Outcomes in Research Interdisciplinary Working Groups: the American Academy of Neurology affirms the value of this guideline as an educational tool for neurologists. Stroke 2007;38:1655–1711.

availability, speed of imaging, cost-effectiveness, and accessibility in the emergency department. We use a combined multimodal CT stroke protocol consisting of noncontrast CT (NCCT), CT perfusion (CTP), and CT angiography (CTA) to select patients for endovascular thrombolysis. Other groups[8–10] have similarly noted benefits of combined CTA and CTP imaging in rapid assessment of acute stroke. CTP imaging is helpful in evaluating the ischemic core [very low cerebral blood flow (CBF; $>$70% reduction), very low cerebral blood volume (CBV; $<$2 mL/100 g),[11] and extremely prolonged transit time].[12–14] In our experience, patients with large ischemic cores and even small ischemic cores in the basal ganglia region have a high risk for SICH and poor outcome. We try to avoid endovascular thrombolysis in these patients; and, if compelled to intervene due to the presence of a large penumbra, avoid pharmacologic thrombolysis and glycoprotein (GP) IIb/IIIa antagonists. The disadvantages of CTP are radiation exposure, incomplete validation, and qualitative differences in postprocessing software.

◆ Patient Selection and Complication Avoidance

Better patient selection decreases complications, including SICH. The three major criteria for selection of a patient for endovascular thrombolysis are (1) contraindication for IV tPA or neurologic condition that did not improve or worsened after initial improvement with IV tPA; (2) time window from stroke symptom onset (as discussed above); and (3) ischemic penumbra – the therapeutic target (as discussed above). On the basis of these concepts and our experience, mechanical revascularization therapy is the first choice at our center for patients who present after 3 hours of stroke symptom onset and patients with wake-up strokes (in whom the time of stroke symptom onset is unknown) after evaluating and confirming the presence of large vessel occlusion. Intraarterial pharmacologic thrombolysis is used only if the site of occlusion is distal and not reachable for mechanical therapy or as an adjunct to treat distal embolization should it occur after mechanical therapy.

Although IV tPA between 3 and 4.5 hours after stroke symptom onset has been endorsed by the recent AHA/ASA guidelines,[1] we believe that all patients with acute ischemic stroke should be evaluated for intraarterial therapies. At our center, patients who present up to 4.5 hours after stroke symptom onset with a large vessel occlusion and have no risks of SICH by clinical, radiologic, and physiologic data are candidates for bridging therapy (IVT and intraarterial thrombolysis [IAT]). Bridging therapy allows a full IV tPA dose to be initiated; and if there is no significant improvement at 30 minutes, the patient is prepared for intraarterial therapy. For those patients who are at higher risk of SICH on the basis of CTP criteria, irrespective of the time window of presentation, mechanical thrombolysis can be considered; and we defer using pharmacologic thrombolysis in these patients to the attending stroke neurologist.

Our center's current protocol for selection of treatment strategies and posttreatment management after revascularization of acute ischemic stroke patients is shown in **Table 15.2**. It is important to remember that CTP is only one of the risk-assessment tools for decision-making in these

Table 15.2 Protocol for Stroke Revascularization at the Authors' Center

All patients with a clinical diagnosis of acute ischemic stroke undergo multimodal CT stroke imaging that includes cranial NCCT, CTA from the aortic arch through the cranial vertex, and CTP whole-brain studies.
After hemorrhagic stroke is ruled out, patients with large vessel occlusion (cervical ICA, petrous ICA, intracranial ICA, MCA-M1, MCA-M2, A1, intracranial VA, BA, PCA-P1, PCA-P2) and/or with contraindications for IVT are assessed for endovascular revascularization.
Patients who have a high risk for SICH – (1) ischemic core in the basal ganglia region, and/or (2) large cortical or subcortical ischemic core on CTP (>50% of at-risk territory) – are identified.
Patients who have known stroke symptom onset, are within 4.5 hours of stroke onset, and are not at high risk for SICH are evaluated for IVT.
Patients with large vessel occlusion, at low risk for SICH, and within the 4.5-hour time window have bridging therapy (IVT + endovascular revascularization).
Patients who do not improve at least 4 points on the NIHSS after IVT or improve and then deteriorate after IVT are again evaluated for endovascular revascularization after a repeat cranial NCCT to exclude ICH.
Patients who are candidates for endovascular revascularization are carefully selected for angiography after weighing the benefit of reperfusion with the risk of SICH based on multimodal CT stroke imaging findings.
All patients who are selected for intervention on the basis of angiographic results receive sufficient heparin to maintain the activated coagulation time between 250 and 320 seconds for the duration of the procedure. Patients who are not taking aspirin or clopidogrel (or ticlopidine) are treated with aspirin (325 mg; enteric-coated, if necessary) immediately before the procedure.
Mechanical revascularization therapies – wire manipulation, Merci device (Concentric Medical, Mountain View, CA), Penumbra device (Penumbra Inc., Alameda, CA) – are the primary options for endovascular recanalization.
IAT with t-PA is used for occlusions that are not reachable with current devices or as an adjunct after mechanical revascularization for distal emboli (only in patients with low risk of SICH).
Wingspan (Boston Scientific, Natick, MA) or Enterprise (Codman Neurovascular, Raynham, MA) stent placement is used as a bailout for patients in whom vessels cannot be recanalized with current FDA-approved modalities and who have an occlusion at a site that can be stented under Humanitarian Device Exemption and FDA-approved trials. Patients considered for stent placement are given a loading dose of either clopidogrel (600 mg) or ticlopidine (1 g) and aspirin 650 mg.
GP IIb/IIIa inhibitors are used only if intraluminal thrombus formation is seen after endovascular recanalization.
Patients receiving stents are placed on dual antiplatelet therapy for 3 months and aspirin for life. All other patients with acute ischemic stroke are maintained on aspirin for life.
Patients are observed in the intensive care unit for 12–24 hours after treatment, and a blood pressure of ~150/90 mm Hg is maintained to avoid reperfusion injury.
All patients have standardized rehabilitation and disposition methods determined by the same stroke neurology team.
All patients are placed on a standardized risk modification regimen that includes control of hypertension, diabetes mellitus, and hyperlipidemia; an exercise program; smoking cessation; and treatment for obesity.

Abbreviations: AHA/ASA, American Heart Association/American Stroke Association; BA, basilar artery; CT, computed tomography; CTA, computed tomographic angiography; CTP, computed tomographic perfusion; FDA, Food and Drug Administration; GP, glycoprotein; IA, intraarterial, IAT, intraarterial thrombolysis; ICA, internal carotid artery; IV, intravenous; IVT, intravenous thrombolysis; MCA, middle cerebral artery; mRS, modified Rankin Scale; NCCT, noncontrast CT scan; NIHSS, National Institutes of Health Stroke Scale; PCA, posterior cerebral artery; SICH, symptomatic intracranial hemorrhage; tPA, tissue plasminogen activator; VA, vertebral artery patients. The final decision to revascularize and the choice of thrombolytic modality are made after integrating the CTP findings with the clinical presentation and patient factors and a discussion that involves the neurointerventionist and the stroke neurologist.

◆ Technique

Mechanical Thrombolysis or Embolectomy

Mechanical recanalization systems can be divided into two major groups, proximal or distal devices, according to where they apply force on the thrombus. Proximal devices apply force to the proximal base of the thrombus. This group includes various aspiration catheters. Distal devices approach the thrombus proximally, but then are advanced by the guidewire and microcatheter across the thrombus to be unsheathed distally, where force is applied to the distal base of the thrombus. This group includes snare-, basket-, and coil-like devices. In an animal model,[15] proximal devices were faster in application and associated with a low complication rate. The distal devices were more successful at removing thrombotic material, but their method of application and attendant thrombus compaction increased the risk of thromboembolic events and vasospasm.[16,17] Advantages and disadvantages of mechanical revascularization strategies overall are summarized in **Table 15.3**.[18] The current FDA-approved embolectomy devices are the Penumbra (proximal device; Penumbra Inc., Alameda, CA) and the Merci retriever (distal device; Concentric Medical Inc., Mountain View, CA).

Table 15.3 Advantages and Disadvantages of Mechanical Revascularization

Advantages
Devices used for mechanical thrombolysis or embolectomy lessen and may even preclude the use of pharmacologic thrombolytics, thus reducing the incidence of SICH.
These devices may extend the treatment window beyond 6–8 hours from onset.
Mechanical fragmentation of the clot increases the surface area of clot available for endogenous and exogenous fibrinolysis.
Recanalization time may be faster.
Devices used for mechanical thrombolysis may be effective for thrombi or other material resistant to thrombolytics that occlude the vessel.
Mechanical thrombolysis has emerged as the key option for patients who have a contraindication for pharmacologic thrombolysis, such as recent surgery or abnormal hemostasis,[18] or have a late presentation.[4,5,20]
Disadvantages
Technical difficulty of navigating mechanical devices through the tortuous intracranial vasculature
Excessive trauma to the vasculature
Distal embolization from fragmented thrombus

Abbreviations: SICH, symptomatic intracranial hemorrhage

Microguidewire Manipulation and Snare

The most common method for mechanical thrombus disruption is probing the thrombus with a microguidewire. This technique appears to be useful in facilitating pharmacologic thrombolysis.[19]

Merci Device

The Merci retrieval system is a shaped wire constructed of nitinol. The flexible corkscrew-like tip can easily be delivered through a microcatheter into the vessel distal to the occlusion site. When deployed, this device returns to its preformed coiled shape to ensnare the thrombus. The thrombus is bypassed and the retriever deployed from inside the catheter distal to the thrombus. The corkscrew-like tip is pulled back slowly to ensnare the clot as a corkscrew would ensnare a cork. The retriever is then retracted into the guide catheter under proximal flow arrest. Different versions of this device are available (**Fig. 15.1**): in the first-generation devices (X5 and X6), the nitinol wire was shaped in helical-tapering coil loops. The second-generation devices (L4, L5, and L6) differ from the X devices by the inclusion of a system of arcading filaments attached to a nontapering helical nitinol coil, which has a 90-degree angle in relation to the proximal wire component. The third-generation devices (V series) have variable pitch loops under a linear configuration with attached filaments. The retriever device is deployed through a 2.4F microcatheter (14X or 18L, Concentric Medical). The recent addition of a 4.3F distal access catheter has provided additional coaxial support to the system, resulting in improved deliverability with the potential for simultaneous thromboaspiration as well. Merci devices are available in various diameters from 1.5 to 3 mm, depending on the caliber of the occluded vessel. An illustrative case of Merci retrieval is provided in **Fig. 15.2**.

Merci devices are regularly used in combination with proximal balloon occlusion in the internal carotid artery (ICA), in addition to aspiration from the guiding catheter, to reduce the risk of distal thromboembolism. In general, an 8F to 9F sheath and balloon catheter of similar size are used. After placement of the balloon catheter in the ICA, a microcatheter, in combination with a microwire, is navigated to the occlusion site. This catheter is then advanced beyond the thrombus. An injection of contrast material distal to the thrombus is recommended to estimate the length of the occlusion and illustrate the anatomy of the distal vessel. The device is then introduced into the microcatheter and unsheathed behind the thrombus. The balloon at the tip of the guiding catheter is inflated. During slow retraction of the device and mobilization of the thrombus, aspiration is applied at the guiding catheter. The device and thrombus are retrieved into the guiding catheter, and the balloon is deflated. In clinical practice, the entire procedure often has to be repeated multiple times to recanalize the vessel.

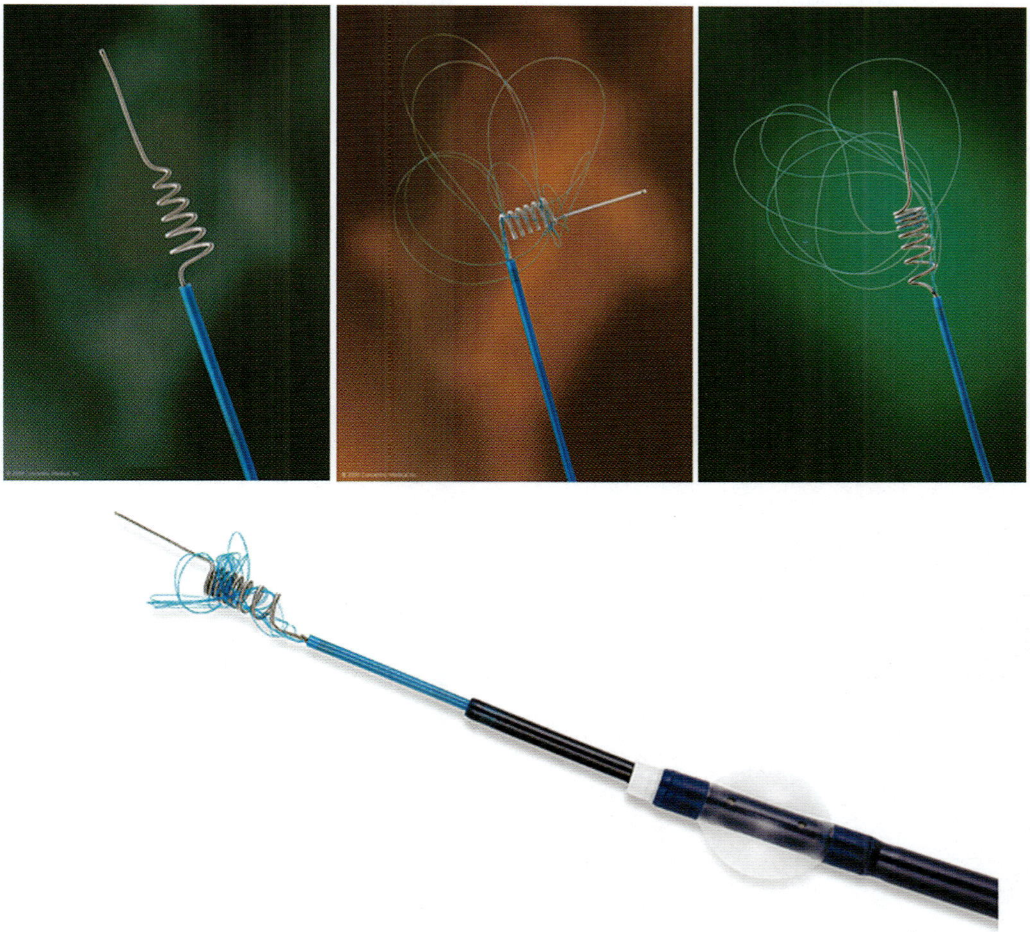

Fig. 15.1 Types of Merci devices. **(A)** Type X. **(B)** Type L. **(C)** Type V. **(D)** Catheter system. (Courtesy of Concentric Medical, Mountain View, CA).

Furthermore, the application of the balloon catheter might be limited in cases of high-grade ICA stenosis.

The Merci device often requires three or four passes before flow is restored. This process delays the time to recanalization in these patients. The aforementioned new distal access catheter available for use with the Merci device allows placement of smaller triple coaxial guide catheter near the lesion of interest for repeated quick access to the lesion and to transmit the traction force better in a straighter angle at a shorter distance.

FDA approval of the Merci device in 2004 was based on a review of data obtained in the multicenter Merci Trial that involved 141 patients (mean age 60 years; mean NIHSS score 20) ineligible for standard thrombolytic therapy.[4,20] The Multi-MERCI Trial[5] was a prospective, multicenter, single-arm registry that included 164 patients (mean age 68 years; mean NIHSS score 19) treated with different Merci retrieval systems (X5, X6, and L5). Patients with persistent large vessel occlusion after IVT (with tPA) were also included in the study, and adjunctive IAT (using tPA) was allowed. Use of the Merci device has also increased recanalization rates with intracranial ICA occlusion.[21] Two ongoing prospective randomized trials are using the device, the MR and Recanalization of Stroke Clots Using Embolectomy Trial (MR Rescue) and the IMS III Trial.[22]

Penumbra Device

From a procedural point of view, the technique with a proximal device, such as the Penumbra, is comparable to that for IAT. Access is usually gained with a 6F to 8F sheath. After placement of the guiding catheter, the device is navigated to the proximal surface of the clot. This approach omits repetitive crossing of the occlusion site. The Penumbra catheter is used in parallel with the Penumbra separator and an aspiration source to aspirate clot from the occluded vessel. The Penumbra separator is deployed from the Penumbra catheter. The Penumbra separator is advanced and retracted through the Penumbra catheter at the proximal margin of the primary occlusion. The main purpose of the Penumbra separator is to clear the Penumbra catheter, and thus keep the suction on the clot open and not to dislodge the clot itself. Direct thrombus extraction can also be attempted with the ring retriever that is part of the Penumbra system while a balloon-guided catheter is used to temporarily arrest flow. Both the microcatheter (**Fig. 15.3**) and separator are available in various sizes

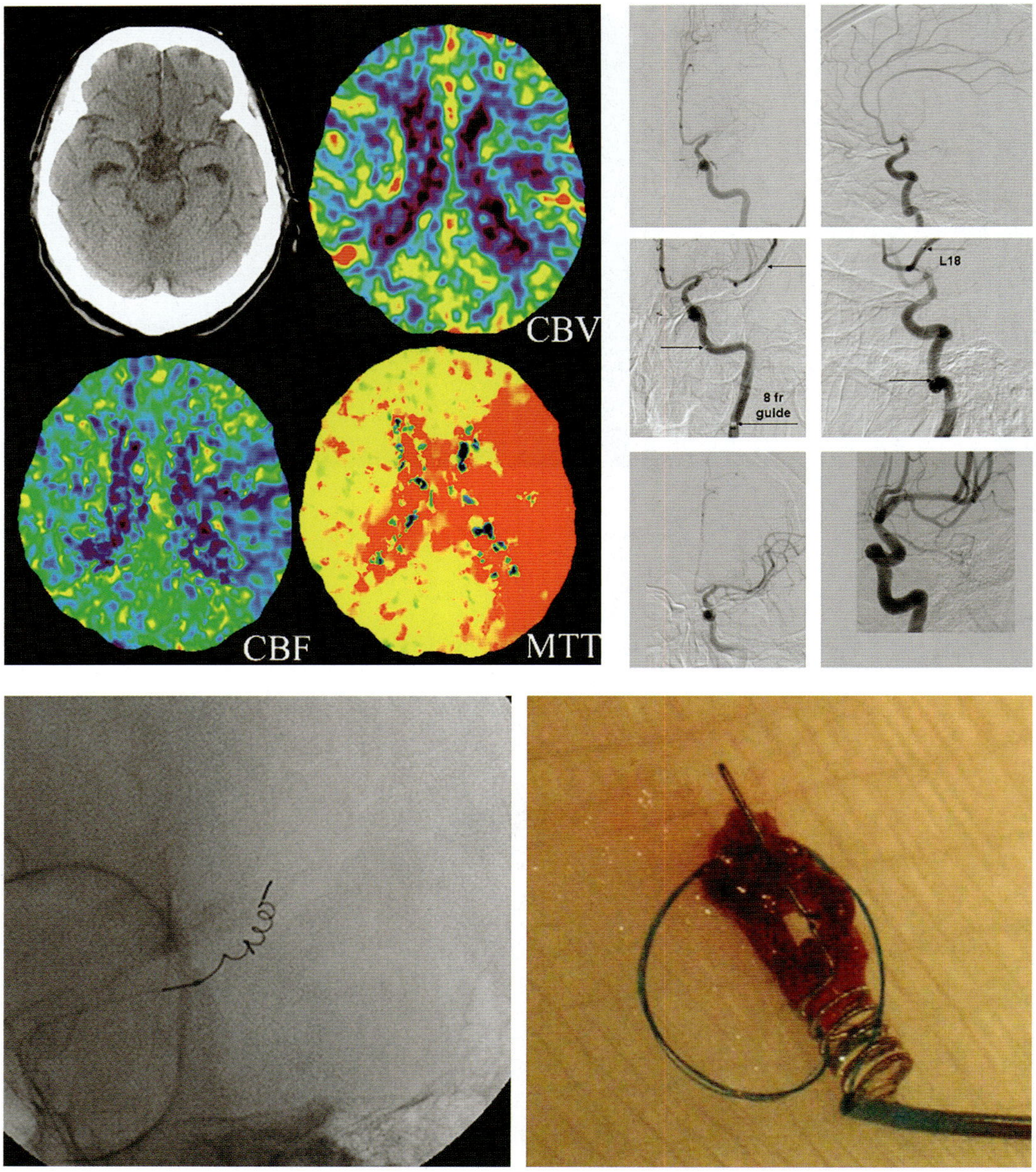

A B C D

Fig. 15.2 A 77-year-old man presented with acute aphasia and hemiparesis. His NIH Stroke Scale Score (NIHSS) was 19. Time of stroke symptom onset was <3 hours. His past medical history was significant for atrial fibrillation, coronary artery disease, aortic stenosis, prostate cancer, colon cancer, dyslipidemia, anxiety, and chronic pain. His sodium warfarin was discontinued 7 days earlier because of a serious gastrointestinal hemorrhage. Cranial noncontrast CT scan (**A,** *top row, left*) showed no acute hypodensities or hyperdensities. Intravenous tissue plasminogen activator was contraindicated because of the patient's recent hemorrhage. CT perfusion images (*remaining images in* **A**) demonstrating left-sided hypoperfusion within the middle cerebral artery (MCA) territory with mostly "preserved" cerebral blood volume, an indicator of possibly good outcome if the MCA can be recanalized. The patient was taken to the angiography suite for an attempt at clot retrieval with the Merci device (Concentric Medical, Mountain View, CA). **(B)** Preprocedure (*upper row*), intraprocedure (*middle row*), and postprocedure (*lower row*) angiograms. Femoral artery access was obtained with an 8F sheath. An initial diagnostic angiogram confirmed the left M1 occlusion (**B,** *upper row*). An 8F Concentric balloon guide catheter (Concentric Medical) was then positioned over a VTK catheter (Cook, Bloomington, IN) and 0.038-inch exchange wire (Terumo, Tokyo, Japan) in the left internal carotid artery (ICA). From here, the L 18 Merci delivery catheter (Concentric Medical), placed within the distal access catheter (Concentric Medical), was advanced across the lesion and positioned distally within an M2 division of the MCA. A dual injection demonstrates the extent of the lesion (**B,** *middle row, right column*). The V 2.5 Merci retriever device was then deployed distal to the lesion, and the clot was engaged. **(C)** At this point, the ICA was occluded with the balloon catheter and flow reversal was begun by suction-aspiration through the guide. **(D)** During flow reversal, the clot was dislodged and retrieved. Follow-up angiographic runs demonstrated TIMI 3 (thrombolysis in myocardial infarction score) flow (**B,** *bottom row*). The patient recovered from his symptoms while on the angiography table. By the following day, he was completely asymptomatic (NIHSS 0).

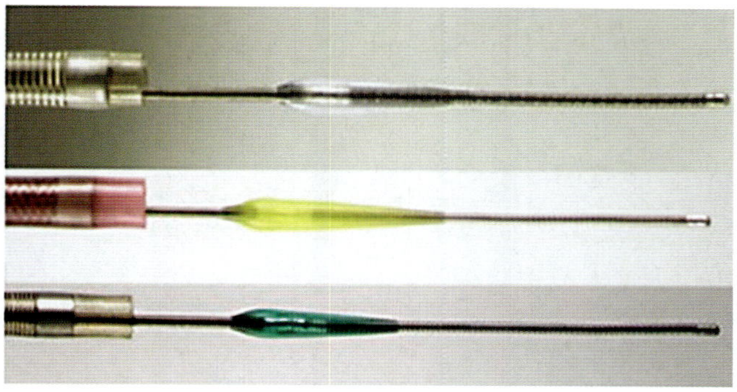

Fig. 15.3 Penumbra device. From bottom to top, the sizes are 026, 032, and 041. (Courtesy of Penumbra Inc., Alameda, CA)

and diameters to adjust the device to different anatomic settings. The Penumbra system also comes with a triple coaxial smaller guide that can be placed distally called the Neuron catheter. This catheter serves the same purposes as the distal access catheter that comes with the Merci device. The use of the Penumbra system in a patient with acute ischemic stroke is illustrated in **Fig. 15.4**.

A prospective, single-arm, independently monitored trial was performed to assess the efficiency and safety of the Penumbra system.[23] In a prospective multicenter single-arm trial of 125 patients with acute stroke who underwent revascularization with the Penumbra device, TIMI 2 or 3 recanalization was achieved in 81.6% patients with an SICH rate of 11.2% and only 25% of patients achieved mRS ≤ 2.[24] On the average, 40 minutes

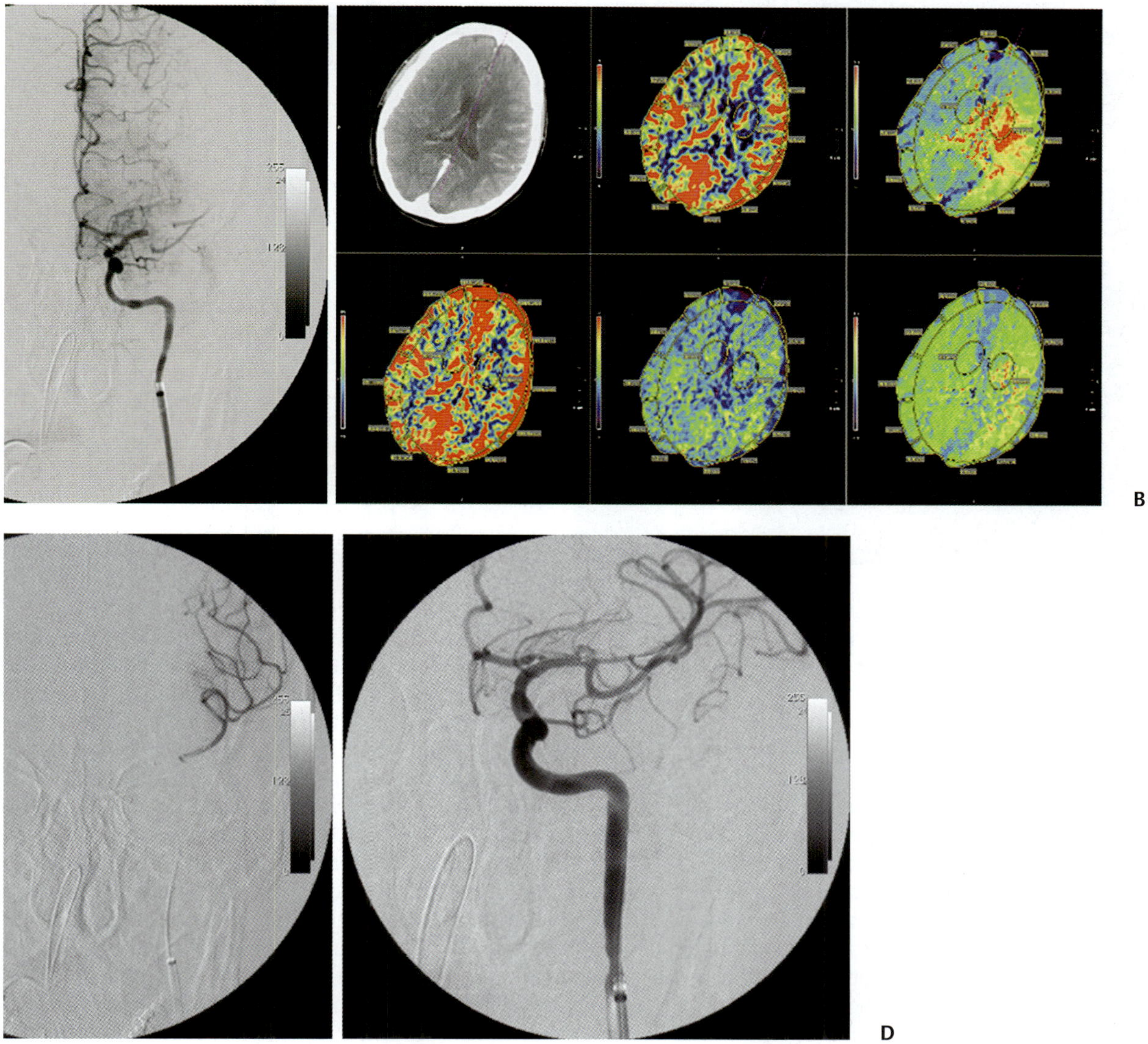

Fig. 15.4 **(A)** Selective angiogram of the left internal carotid artery (ICA) showing occlusion of the middle cerebral artery (MCA) bifurcation. **(B)** CT perfusion (CTP) images showing minimal core (decreased cerebral blood volume) and penumbra (increased cerebral blood flow, mean transit time, and time to peak) in the left MCA territory. **(C)** Selective microrun of the M2 vessel after the lesion has been crossed with a microcatheter. **(D)** Selective angiogram of the left ICA with the Penumbra device (Penumbra Inc., Alameda, CA) in the superior branch of the MCA showing good flow through that branch. *(continued)*

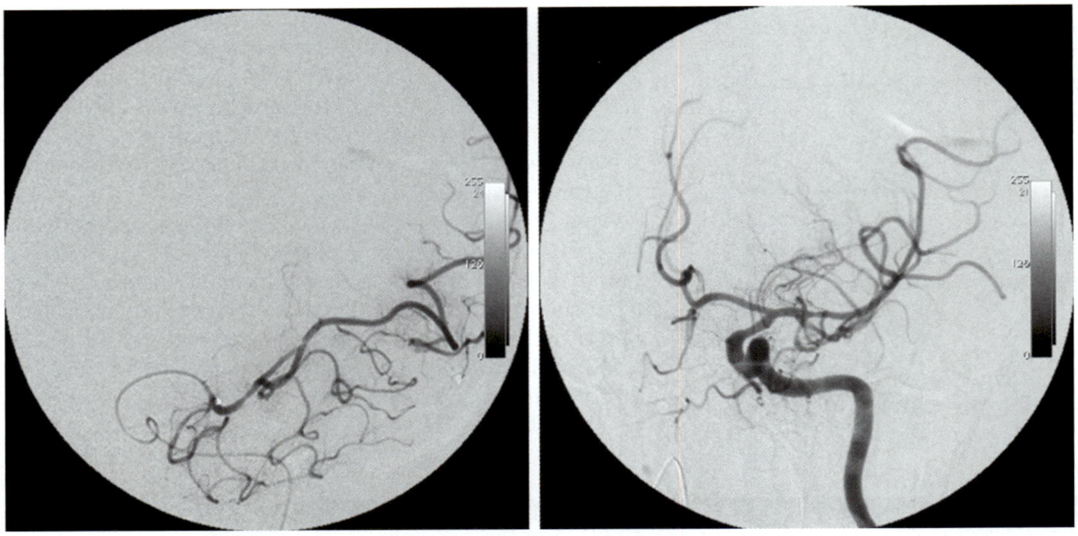

E F

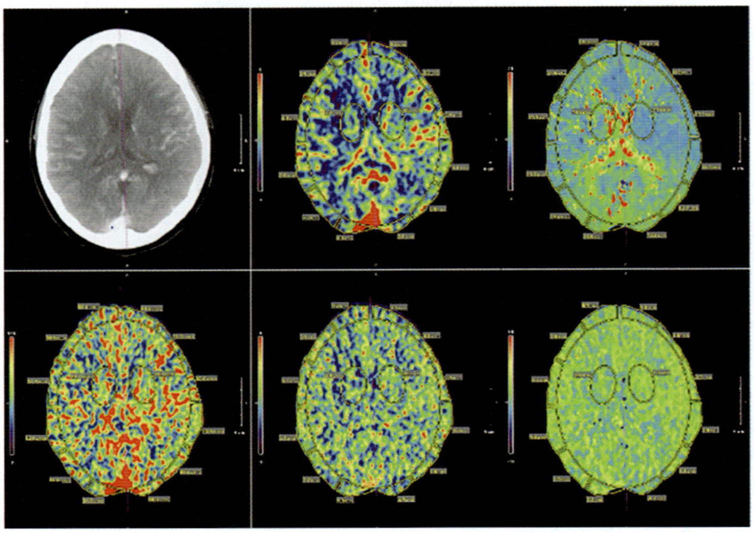

G

Fig. 15.4 *(continued)* **(E)** Selective angiogram of the inferior MCA branch with the Penumbra device in situ showing good flow. **(F)** Final angiogram showing TIMI 3 (thrombolysis in myocardial infarction score) recanalization of the MCA bifurcation. **(G)** CTP images after recanalization showing corrected cerebral blood flow, mean transit time, and time-to-peak maps. (From Natarajan SK, Siddiqui AH, Hopkins LN, Levy EI. Endovascular thrombolysis: pharmacologic and mechanical. In Bendok BR, Batjer HH, Naidech AM, Walker MT, eds. Hemorrhagic and Ischemic Stroke: Surgical, Interventional, Imaging, and Medical Approaches. New York: Thieme; in press.)

elapsed from the time the Penumbra device was deployed near the clot until complete flow restoration was achieved.

Stent-Assisted Thrombolysis

Self-expanding stents (SESs) designed specifically for the cerebrovasculature are available. These stents can be delivered to target areas of intracranial stenosis with a success rate of >95% with an increased safety profile because they are deployed at significantly lower pressures than balloon-mounted coronary stents.[25] Advantages and disadvantages of stent-assisted revascularization for acute ischemic stroke are summarized in **Table 15.4**. With the stent-for-stroke technique, vessel recanalization is instantaneous, and the chance of early reocclusion after treatment is decreased. Reocclusion after IVT (34%) and pharmacologic IAT (17%) has been shown and is associated with poor outcome.[26]

The stent length should cover at least 2 mm of normal vessel on either side of the lesion. The optimal diameter of the stent chosen for insertion should match the size of the normal vessel diameter. If the vessel tapers, the stent should be sized appropriately to match the portion of the vessel with the larger diameter. Standard femoral or radial artery access is obtained, and a 6F (or larger) guide catheter is placed in the target vessel proximal to the occlusion. To minimize the release of distal emboli, the occlusion is crossed in a fashion similar to that used for the Merci clot retriever. First, a .014-inch steerable wire is softly advanced through the clot. A low-profile catheter is then advanced over the wire distal to the occlusion. Following microangiographic confirmation that the microcatheter is distal to the occlusion, an exchange wire is brought through the microcatheter and anchored distal to the occlusion. The microcatheter is removed, and the stent delivery catheter delivered over the exchange wire. To minimize the release of debris, the stent is deployed first distal to the occlusion (thus trapping any debris that may be later released between the stent and the vessel wall), then through the occlusion, and finally just proximal to the occlusion (**Fig. 15.5**). Stent-assisted revascularization in a patient with acute ischemic stroke is illustrated in **Fig. 15.6**.

Table 15.4 Advantages and Disadvantages of Stent-Assisted Revascularization

Advantages	
	Immediate restoration of flow in the occluded vessel
	High recanalization rates
	Decreased chances of early reocclusion after treatment
	Recanalization time may be faster.
	Stents with radial expansive force like the Wingspan (Boston Scientific, Natick, MA) can be used in atherothrombotic lesions with proven safety.
Disadvantages	
	A great proportion of strokes are caused by emboli in a normal intracranial vessel and, in such cases, only embolectomy and not a permanent scaffold may be needed.
	Stent navigability and deployment is possible only in the proximal vessels around the circle of Willis and not in the distal intracranial vasculature.
	Patients need to be on dual antiplatelet therapy for 3 months after stent placement; this may potentially increase the ICH rate and complicate additional invasive procedures sometimes required by the recovering stroke patient.

Abbreviations: ICH, intracranial hemorrhage

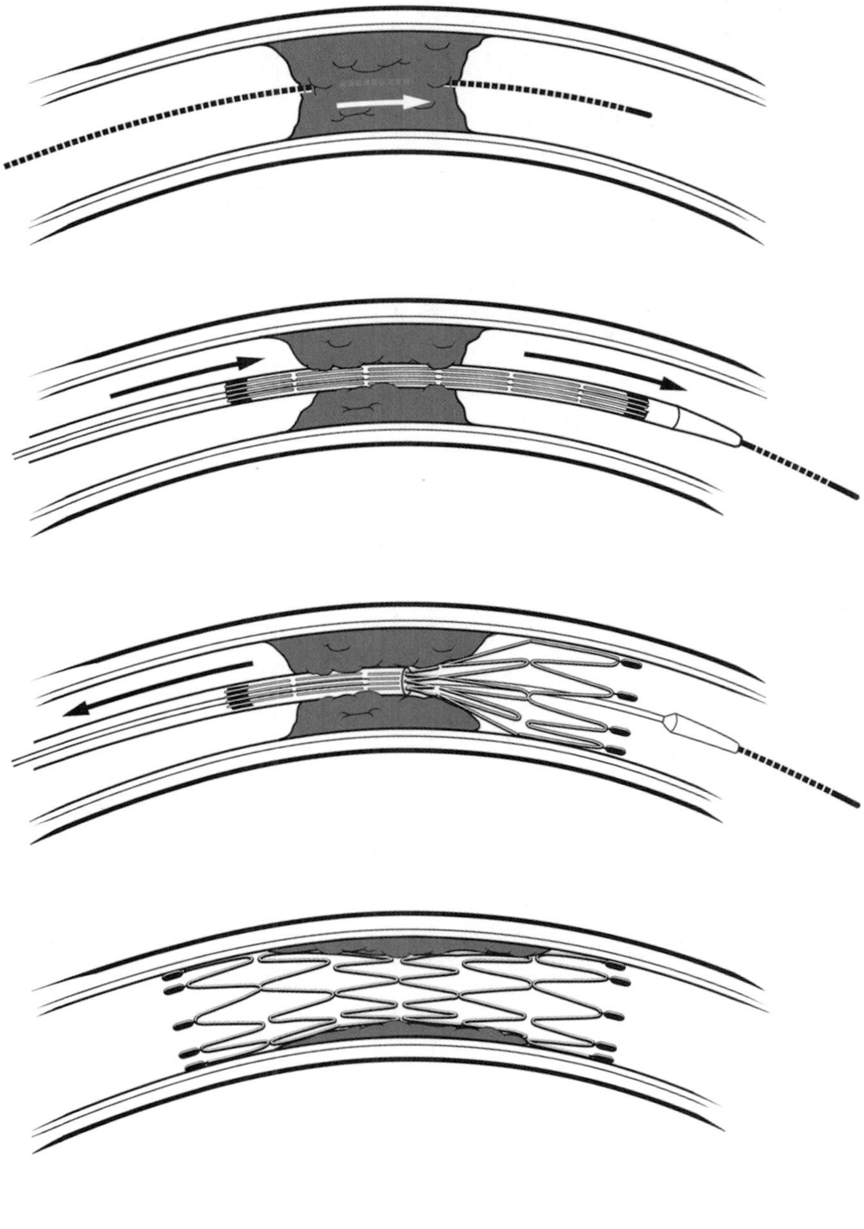

Fig. 15.5 Wingspan stent (Boston Scientific, Natick, MA) for recanalization. *Top to bottom*: occlusive clot crossed with a microwire; placement of stent across the occlusion; deployment of stent, thus trapping the occlusion; and recanalization. (From Levy EI, Mehta R, Gupta R, et al. Self-expanding stents for recanalization of acute cerebrovascular occlusions. AJNR Am J Neuroradiol 2007; 28:816–822. Reprinted with permission.)

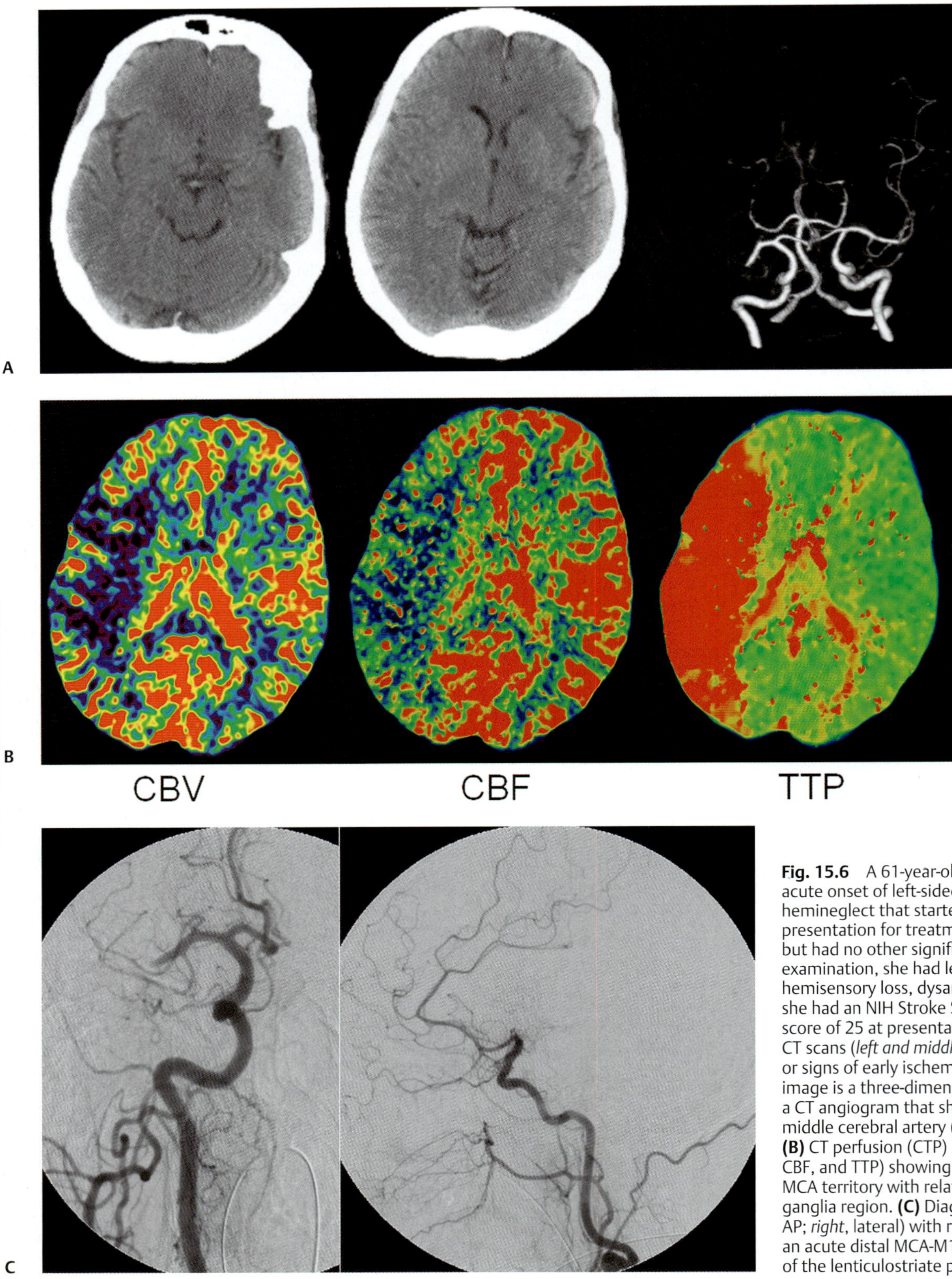

Fig. 15.6 A 61-year-old woman had acute onset of left-sided weakness and left hemineglect that started 7 hours before presentation for treatment. She was a smoker, but had no other significant comorbidities. On examination, she had left-sided hemiplegia, hemisensory loss, dysarthria, and aphasia; she had an NIH Stroke Scale Score (NIHSS) score of 25 at presentation. **(A)** Noncontrast CT scans (*left and middle images*) show no bleed or signs of early ischemic changes; the right image is a three-dimensional reconstruction of a CT angiogram that shows acute right distal middle cerebral artery (MCA)-M1 occlusion. **(B)** CT perfusion (CTP) images (*left to right:* CBV, CBF, and TTP) showing a large CBV lesion in the MCA territory with relative sparing of the basal ganglia region. **(C)** Diagnostic angiograms (*left*, AP; *right*, lateral) with right ICA injection show an acute distal MCA-M1 occlusion with sparing of the lenticulostriate perforators. *(continued)*

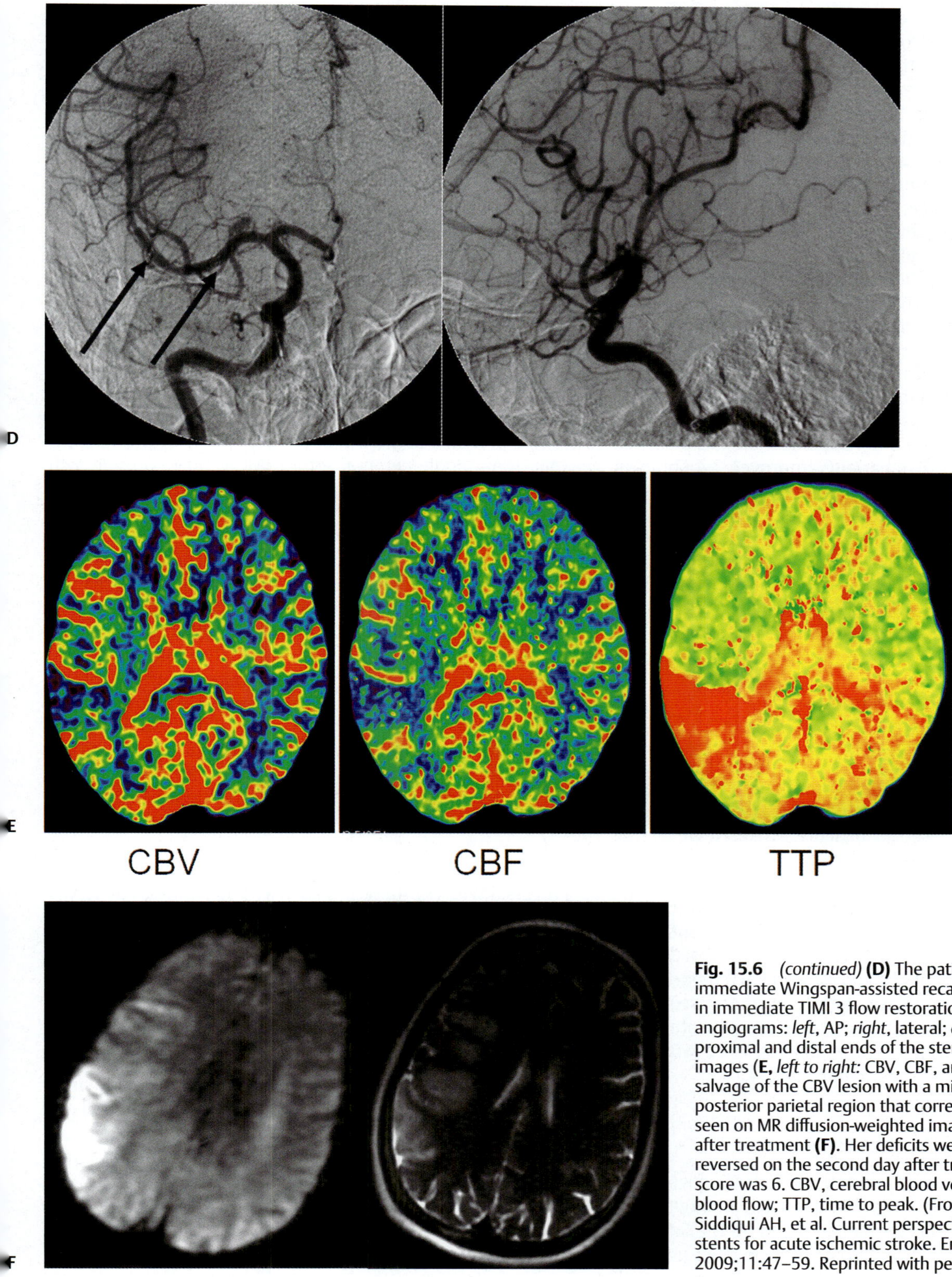

Fig. 15.6 *(continued)* **(D)** The patient underwent immediate Wingspan-assisted recanalization that resulted in immediate TIMI 3 flow restoration (immediate poststent angiograms: *left*, AP; *right*, lateral; *arrows* show the proximal and distal ends of the stent). Posttreatment CTP images (**E,** *left to right:* CBV, CBF, and TTP) show complete salvage of the CBV lesion with a minimal infarct core in the posterior parietal region that corresponds to the lesion seen on MR diffusion-weighted images on the first day after treatment **(F)**. Her deficits were almost completely reversed on the second day after treatment; her NIHSS score was 6. CBV, cerebral blood volume; CBF, cerebral blood flow; TTP, time to peak. (From Levy EI, Natarajan SK, Siddiqui AH, et al. Current perspective on self-expanding stents for acute ischemic stroke. Endovascular Today 2009;11:47–59. Reprinted with permission.)

Several retrospective case series reported successful use of SESs for acute stroke treatment, with higher rates of recanalization than other recanalization modalities.[27–29] On the basis of this preliminary data, we received FDA approval for a pilot study, Stent-Assisted Recanalization in Acute Ischemic Stroke (SARIS),[30] to evaluate the Wingspan stent (Boston Scientific, Natick, MA) for revascularization in patients who did not improve after IVT or had a contraindication for IVT. Average presenting NIHSS score was 14. Seventeen patients presented with a TIMI score of 0 and 3 patients with a TIMI score of 1. Intracranial SESs were placed in 19 of 20 enrolled patients. One patient experienced recanalization of the occluded vessel with positioning of the Wingspan stent delivery system prior to stent deployment. In two patients, the tortuous vessel did not allow tracking of the Wingspan stent. The more navigable Enterprise stent (Codman Neurovascular, Raynham, MA) was used in both these cases. Twelve patients had other adjunctive therapies. TIMI 2 or 3 recanalization was achieved in 100% of patients; 65% of patients improved >4 points in NIHSS score after treatment. One patient (5%) had SICH, and two had asymptomatic ICH. At the time of the 1-month follow-up evaluation, 12 of 20 (60%) patients had an mRS ≤2 and 9 (45%) had an mRS ≤1. Mortality at 1 month was 25%. None of these patients died due to stent placement-related causes; all deaths were due to the severity of the initial stroke and associated comorbidities.

Stent Platform-Based Therapies

Temporary Endovascular Bypass

The need for an aggressive antithrombotic regimen after stent implantation remains one of the major limitations to the use of stents in the setting of acute stroke. However, the advent of closed-cell stents has allowed resheathing/removal of the stent after recanalization is achieved, obviating the need for dual antiplatelet therapy, which could potentially increase the risk of hemorrhagic conversion of the infarct. In addition, this technique should eliminate the risk of delayed in-stent stenosis. Kelly et al[31] and Hauck et al[32] reported the use of the Enterprise stent as a temporary endovascular bypass in acute stroke. In both cases, the Enterprise stent was partially deployed for some time and retrieved with successful recanalization of the occluded vessel.

Stent Platform-based Thrombectomy Device

The Solitaire FR Revascularization Device (ev3 Endovascular, Inc., Plymouth, MN) is a recoverable self-expanding thrombectomy device that was developed based on the Solitaire/Solo stent (ev3 Endovascular, Inc.).[33] The advantage of this device is that it is a fully recoverable SES-platform–based device that can be used as both a temporary endovascular bypass and a thrombectomy device. The device restores flow immediately and avoids the placement of a permanent stent, and thus, the necessary antithrombotic therapy and risk of in-stent stenosis. Moreover, it can be electrolytically detached like a coil in case a permanent stent is necessary, such as in the setting of an atherothrombotic lesion. We evaluated the safety and efficacy of this device in a canine intracranial stroke model with soft and firm clots.[33a] The device could be easily deployed and recovered; it restored TIMI 2 or 3 flow immediately in all cases. Minimal residual clot in two of four instances required a second pass for complete clot retrieval. Minimal vasospasm was observed in two of four cases.

Extracranial Carotid Revascularization

Acute strokes related to isolated proximal (extracranial) ICA occlusions typically have a better prognosis, given the compensatory collateral flow at the level of the external carotid artery–ICA anastomosis (e.g., ophthalmic artery) and/or circle of Willis. However, patients with an incomplete circle of Willis or with tandem occlusions of the intracranial ICA–middle cerebral artery (MCA) often present with severe strokes and are potential candidates for urgent revascularization. Stent placement in the proximal cervical vessels may also be required to gain access to the intracranial thrombus with other mechanical devices or catheters. Furthermore, brisk antegrade flow is essential for the maintenance of distal vascular patency, as is particularly evident in patients with severe proximal stenoses who commonly develop rethrombosis after vessel recanalization. Recent case series have shown success and good outcome after endovascular treatment of acute ischemic stroke due to proximal extracranial ICA occlusions.[34–38] The distal intracranial lesions seen after stenting of extracranial lesions may be due to emboli caused by reopening of the occluded ICA. This could be prevented or at least minimized by using a balloon guide catheter, such as the Concentric guide (Concentric Medical), or a sheath, such as the Gore flow-reversal device (W.L. Gore & Associates, Flagstaff, AZ), for temporary flow arrest or flow reversal with aspiration, especially when antegrade flow is first restored. The operator needs to ensure that the inner diameter of the balloon guide catheter is large enough to accommodate the chosen stent system.

Endovascular Pharmacologic Thrombolysis

To perform IAT, a microcatheter is placed proximal to or directly into the thrombus. A long 6F or 7F sheath is placed into the femoral artery, and a 6F or 7F guiding catheter is advanced into the ICA or vertebral artery of the affected side. A microcatheter is then navigated to the occlusion site over a microwire. An illustrative case of IAT in a patient with acute ischemic stroke is provided in **Fig. 15.7**. Theoretical advantages and disadvantages of IAT are presented in **Table 15.5**.

The safety and efficiency of IAT for treatment of acute ischemic stroke were evaluated in the first Prolyse in Acute Cerebral Thromboembolism Trial (PROACT I).[39] The results of this trial suggested an enhanced recanalization with prourokinase and a positive trend toward better neurologic outcome and survival rate. PROACT II[40] was a large-scale, multicenter, randomized (2:1), phase III trial and demonstrated the beneficial effect of IAT on recanalization rates and clinical outcomes of patients with M1 and M2 occlusions. A metaanalysis of PROACT I and II data showed an odds ratio (OR) of better outcome with treatment of 2.49 ($p = 0.022$), which was greater than the OR (2.13) in the original PROACT II analysis.[41] These studies established superiority of IAT within 6 hours over antithrombotic therapy for MCA M1 and M2 occlusions. The superiority of IAT over IVT has not been demonstrated by randomized clinical studies. The FDA did not approve prourokinase, and it is currently not available for clinical use. Current AHA/ASA guidelines[1,42] recommend the use of IAT with tPA within 6 hours from symptom onset for selected patients who have major stroke due to MCA occlusion and who are not eligible for IVT. Therefore, at present, this approach should not preclude IV administration of tPA in all other eligible patients. There is no level 1 data of the efficacy of IAT for distal ICA or posterior circulation occlusion.

Special Situations Where Endovascular Revascularization Is Increasingly Used

Wake-Up Strokes

Approximately 16 to 28% of ischemic stroke patients awaken with their deficits.[43,44] In wake-up strokes, the onset of symptoms is defined as the "time last seen well." Because this is the time the patient went to sleep, these patients are usually placed outside the window for thrombolysis or are ineligible for entry into reperfusion clinical trials. Barreto et al[45] reported that patients with wake-up stroke have better outcomes when they are treated. Adams et al,[46] in their post hoc analysis of wake-up stroke in the Abciximab in Emergency Stroke Treatment Trial-II, reported poorer outcomes after treatment. In our series, Natarajan et al[47] reported on 30 patients with stroke onset >8 hours and wake-up stroke (mean presentation NIHSS, 13) who were selected for treatment on the basis of CTP imaging results. A combination of endovascular revascularization strategies resulted in TIMI 2 or 3 recanalization in 67% of patients, with an SICH rate of 10%. At 3 months, 20% of patients improved to an mRS score of <2, and the mortality was 33.3%. Janjua et al[48] used clinical diffusion-mismatch criteria (patients with NIHSS >8 with limited abnormality on diffusion-weighted imaging) to evaluate the benefit of endovascular interventions in 11 patients with large vessel occlusion presenting >8 hours after stroke symptom onset. At 1 week after treatment, 72% of the patients overall and 100% of patients having successful revascularization had decreases of >4 points on the NIHSS.

Posterior Circulation Stroke

Posterior circulation stroke differs from anterior circulation stroke in several aspects. The evolution of clinical symptoms is often gradual, making precise assessment of the onset of symptoms and of the time window for treatment difficult.

A

B

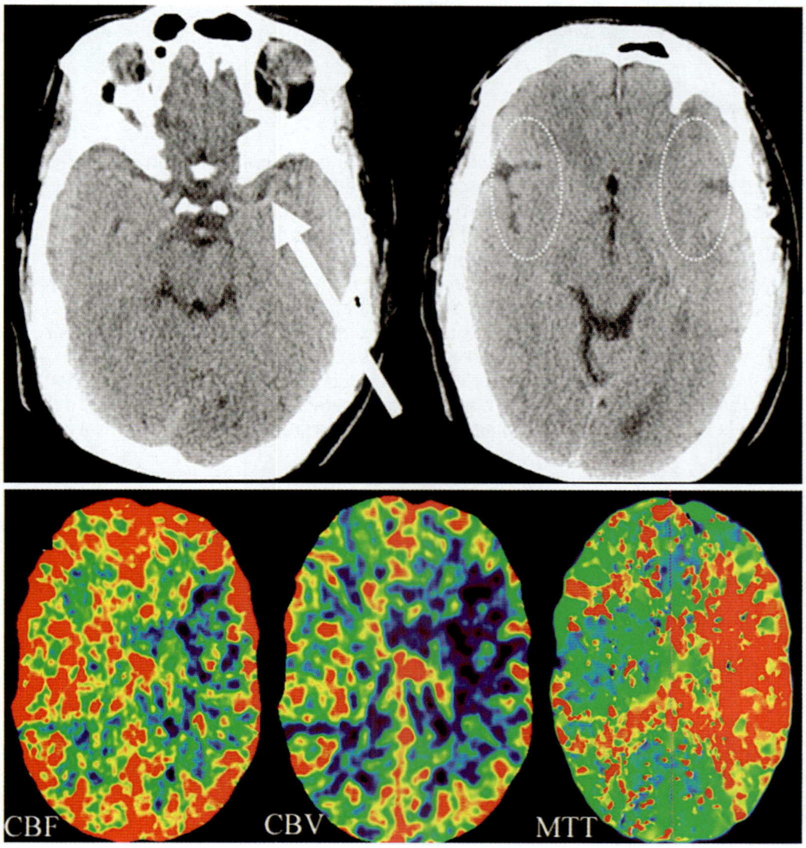

Fig. 15.7 This 46-year-old man presented with right-sided weakness, lethargy, and slurred speech 5 hours after onset. His NIH Stroke Scale Score (NIHSS) was 16 at presentation. **(A)** Cranial noncontrast CT scans showed no evidence of intracranial hemorrhage, but some left-sided edema (*arrow* shows middle cerebral artery occlusion and the ovals show edema in comparison to the other side). **(B)** CT perfusion images showed decreased cerebral blood flow in the left hemisphere with markedly decreased cerebral blood volume (CBV). As the patient was young and within 5 hours of stroke onset, we decided to attempt revascularization, despite the decreased CBV, which, based on our observations, was suggestive of irreversible cerebral infarction with little chance of recovery. The patient was taken to the angiography suite for revascularization. *(continued)*

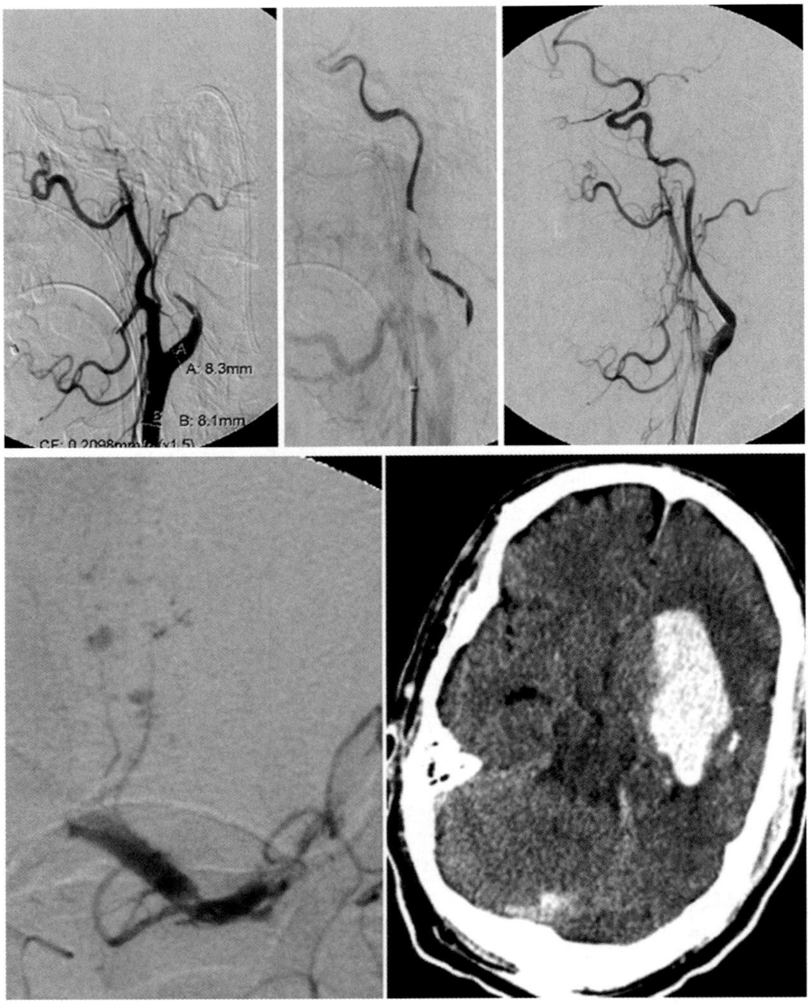

C D E

Fig. 15.7 *(continued)* **(C)** Diagnostic angiography showed a left carotid dissection with left M1 occlusion. After carotid revascularization with the Wallstent (Boston Scientific, Natick, MA), revascularization of the MCA was attempted with a temporary endovascular bypass. The bypass failed. Even though flow was established immediately, the bypass thrombosed within minutes. At this time, 7 hours had passed since the time of symptom onset. We decided to proceed with tPA IAT at this point. After injection of the first 2 units of reteplase, no recanalization was achieved. Two additional units were infused. **(D)** Follow-up angiography now demonstrated contrast extravasation in the area of the lenticulostriate arteries. The patchy extravasation mimicked a blossoming bouquet of flowers ("bouquet sign"), which was warning enough to not further proceed with additional revascularization attempts. **(E)** Postprocedure CT scan revealed hemorrhagic conversion in the infarct core region. The patient remained clinically stable and is now undergoing a course of rehabilitation therapy and is slowly recovering from his infarct. The take-home message from this case is to be conservative with intraarterial tPA administration more than 6 hours after symptom onset and to look for signs that may predict a higher risk of hemorrhage, such as contrast extravasation in the area of the lenticulostriate arteries. Further, this case confirms the theory that decreased CBV at baseline is a negative predictor with respect to the achievement of successful revascularization with clinical improvement.

Table 15.5 Advantages and Disadvantages of Pharmacologic Intraarterial Thrombolysis

Advantages
Angiographic evaluation reveals the precise occlusion site, the extent of collaterals, and assesses the grade of recanalization during treatment.
An effective concentrated dose of thrombolytic agent is delivered directly to the thrombus, thus reducing the systemic side effects.
The approach facilitates combination with mechanical recanalization techniques.
Disadvantages
Time-consuming procedure that delays the initiation of treatment, compared with intravenous thrombolysis
Manipulation of cervical and cranial vessels with the risk of periintervenional complications
Demands highly specialized centers with high human and financial resources

Atherothrombosis (unstable plaque with thrombus) is more common. The risk of reocclusion after recanalization is therefore higher.[49–52] The natural history shows a poor outcome with a high mortality rate of 70 to 80%, unless recanalization is achieved.[49,53] A metaanalysis of IAT in basilar artery occlusion[54] showed a recanalization rate of 64%, with a mortality rate of 87% in patients in whom recanalization was not achieved, with a significant ($p < 0.001$) reduction in mortality to 37% in patients in whom recanalization was achieved. A metaanalysis of either IVT or IAT for basilar artery occlusion[55] showed that the likelihood of good outcome was 2% without recanalization. Recanalization was achieved more frequently with IAT (65% vs 53%, $p = 0.05$), but the outcomes after IAT and IVT were similar. Levy et al[56] performed a metaanalysis for predictors of outcome after IAT for vertebrobasilar artery occlusion and found that failure to recanalize was associated with a higher mortality rate (relative risk 2.34; 95% confidence interval 1.48–3.71). Studies have suggested extending the time window for treatment beyond or up to 24 hours postictus.[51,57,58]

Distal Internal Carotid Artery Occlusion

Small retrospective case series[59,60] show the safety and efficacy of IAT with acceptable recanalization rates and outcomes in patients with distal ICA occlusion. The ability to recanalize distal ICA occlusions is low because of a larger clot burden in these cases. These occlusions are associated with poor outcome because the regions supplied by perforators arising from the A1 and M1 are ischemic. These perforators are essentially end arteries, and the regions they supply do not have collateral blood supply.

IVT and IAT Bridging Therapy

At many centers, accessible occlusions in the anterior circulation are treated with IAT, either in patients in whom reperfusion did not occur after IVT or even as a first line of treatment. In the IMS II trial,[61] combination IV and intraarterial therapy resulted in a better outcome than placebo treatment in the National Institutes of Neurological Disorders and Stroke (NINDS) trial;[62] further, if secondary outcome measures (mRS score, NIHSS score, and Barthel Index) were considered, a statistically better outcome was seen with combination therapy in IMS II than with IV treatment in NINDS. Recanalization was achieved only after rescue intraarterial therapy in most patients in the NINDS trial. A bridging strategy between IVT and IAT has the advantage of not delaying IV therapy, while identifying nonresponders with persisting large artery occlusion.

The bridging therapy approach is being tested in IMS III, with initial IV tPA followed by artery reopening by thrombolysis or clot retrieval if vessel occlusion is demonstrated.[22] Patients are randomized to receive IV tPA followed by IAT or standard-dose (0.9 mg/kg) IV rtPA alone in a 2:1 ratio. Patients in the IVT–IAT group receive a lower dose of IV tPA (0.6 mg/kg, 60 mg maximum) for 40 minutes followed by immediate angiography. If a treatable thrombus is not visualized, no intraarterial therapy is administered. If an appropriate thrombus is identified, the neurointerventionist may select either the EKOS microcatheter (EKOS Corp., Bothell, WA) or the Merci retriever to infuse intraarterial tPA, according to user preference. The trial investigators are currently exploring incorporation of the Penumbra system as another mechanical option. A maximum dose of 22 mg of tPA may be administered intraarterially. Intraarterial treatment must begin within 5 hours and must be completed within 7 hours of stroke onset. The primary outcome measure is the rate of good clinical outcomes (mRS score ≤ 2) at 90 days. The primary safety measure is mortality at 3 months and SICH within the 24 hours of randomization. Trial enrollment began in July of 2006. The planned sample size is 900 patients. A summary of the trials using combination IVT and IAT (IMS I[63] and IMS II[64]) is included in **Table 15.6**.[65]

IAT versus IVT

The outcome and morbidity of patients treated with IVT and IAT were compared at two different stroke treatment centers.[66] Patients were selected based on the presence of a hyperdense MCA sign on CT imaging, indicating an M1 occlusion. Fifty-five patients were treated with IAT using urokinase (UK); 59 patients underwent IVT with tPA. Although the time to treatment was significantly ($p = 0.0001$) longer in the IAT group (mean 244 minutes) than in the IVT group (mean 156 minutes), the study revealed a more frequent favorable outcome for patients treated with intraarterial UK (53%) compared with patients treated with IVT (23%; $p = 0.001$). In addition, the mortality rate was reduced in the IAT group compared with the IVT group (4.7% vs 23%; $p = 0.001$).

◆ Discussion

Results for the important published interventional stroke trials are summarized in **Table 15.6** (a summary of NINDS[62] and ECASS III[67] data has been included for comparison in the same table). On the basis of all studies noted in this table, improved outcome rates fluctuate from 25 to 45%. Thus, despite better recanalization rates, outcomes improved marginally. These data beg the question as to what is the relationship between recanalization and good outcomes. We hypothesize that it depends on what is being revascularized. Revascularization of an ischemic or completely infarcted core will likely cause breakthrough hemorrhage and this risk will likely increase with an increasing delay in treatment, and the risk will further increase in those situations in which thrombolytic therapies are utilized. This results in an increase in SICH rates that is concurrent with increasing revascularization rates, as noted above. Therefore, as the success of the revascularization strategy improves, more ICH occurs because of breakthrough bleeding in ischemic cores. Simply increasing recanalization rates does not proportionally improve outcomes. Part of the reason the final outcomes are relatively fixed is that all the aforementioned studies relied on simple cranial NCCT imaging. Consequently, as recanalization rates increase, good clinical outcomes rise and then fall because of the poor patient

Table 15.6 Summary of Important Published Interventional Stroke Trials (Data from IV tPA trials NINDS and ECASS III Included for Comparison)

Study	No. of Patients	Type of Study	Treatment	Time Window from Symptom Onset (h)	Mean Presentation NIHSS	Recanalization Rate (%)	SICH Rate (%)	mRS ≤2 or ≤1* at 3 Months (%)	Mortality at 3 Months (%)	Main Results
NINDS[62]	333 (168 vs 165)	RCT	IV tPA (0.9 mg/kg) vs placebo	0–3	14 vs 15	NR	6.4 vs 0.6	39 vs 26*	21 vs 24	1. No difference between groups at 24 h (trend in favor of treatment) 2. Significant improvement in functional status at 90 d in treated group ($p = 0.30$) 3. Significant difference in SICH rates ($p < 0.001$)
ECASS III[67]	821 (418 vs 403)	RCT	IV tPA (0.9 mg/kg) vs placebo	3–4.5	10.7 vs 11.6	NR	2.4% vs 0.2%	52.4 vs 45.2*	7.7 vs 8.4	1. Significant improvement in functional status at 3 months ($p = 0.04$) 2. Significant difference in SICH rates ($p = 0.008$) 3. No difference in mortality ($p = 0.68$)
PROACT I[39]	40 (26 vs 14)	RCT	IA r-prourokinase (6 mg) + IV heparin (high or low dose) vs IV heparin (high or low dose)	0–6	17 vs 19	57.7 vs 14.3	15.4 vs 7.1	30.8 vs 21.4*	26.9 vs 42.9	1. Significant higher recanalization efficacy with IAT ($p = 0.17$) 2. No significant difference in SICH ($p = 0.64$)

PROACT II[40]	180 (121 vs 59)	RCT	IA r-prourokinase (9 mg) + IV heparin (low dose) vs IV heparin (low dose)	0–6	17 vs 17	66 vs 18	10 vs 2	40 vs 25	25 vs 27	1. Significant better outcome at 3 months ($p = 0.04$) and significant higher recanalization rate ($p < 0.001$) in the treatment group 2. Difference in SICH not significant ($p = 0.06$)
IMS I[63]	80 (IAT-62)	Prospective	IV tPA (0.6 mg/kg) + IA tPA (4 mg in clot+9 mg/h) (if clot identified by angiography after IVT) + low-dose IV heparin	0–3	18	56	6.30	43, 30*	16%	Results compared with NINDS tPA and placebo arms 1. Significant better 3-month outcomes when compared with NINDS placebo OR >2 2. Difference in mortality or SICH not significant
IMS II[61]	81 (IAT-55)	Prospective	IV tPA (0.6 mg/kg) + IA tPA (22 mg over 2 h using EKOS or normal catheter) (if clot identified by angiography after IVT) + low-dose IV heparin	0–3	19	58	9.90	46	16	Results compared with NINDS tPA and placebo arms 1. Significant better 3-month outcomes when compared with NINDS placebo OR >2.7

(continued)

Table 15.6 Summary of Important Published Interventional Stroke Trials (Data from IV tPA trials NINDS and ECASS III Included for Comparison) *(continued)*

Study	No. of Patients	Type of Study	Treatment	Time Window from Symptom Onset (h)	Mean Presentation NIHSS	Recanalization Rate (%)	SICH Rate (%)	mRS ≤2 or ≤1* at 3 Months (%)	Mortality at 3 Months (%)	Main Results
										2. Better outcomes in the recanalized cohort when compared with nonrecanalized ($p = 0.046$) 3. Difference in mortality or SICH not significant
MERCI[4,20]	141	Prospective	IA Merci (I generation) + IAT, no IVT	0–8	20	60.3 (48 device alone)	7.80	36	34	Better functional outcome at 3 months in recanalized patients when compared with nonrecanalized patients ($p = 0.01$)
Multi MERCI[5]	164	Prospective	IA Merci (I & II generation) + IAT + IVT allowed	0–8	19	68 (55 device alone)	9.80	36	26	Higher rates of recanalization with 2nd-generation devices
Penumbra[65]	125	Prospective	IA Penumbra + IAT	0–8	17	81.6 (device alone)	11.20	25	32.80	Higher rates of recanalization when compared with previous mechanical revascularization therapies

Abbreviations: ECASS, European Cooperative Acute Stroke Study; h, hours; IA, intraarterial; IAT, intraarterial thrombolysis; IMS, Interventional Management of Stroke; IV, intravenous; IVT, intravenous thrombolysis; MERCI, Mechanical Embolus Removal in Cerebral Ischemia; mRS, modified Rankin scale; NINDS, National Institute of Neurological Disorders and Stroke; NR, not reported; PROACT, Prolyse in Acute Cerebral Thromboembolism; OR, odds ratio; RCT, randomized controlled trial; tPA, recombinant tissue plasminogen activator; SICH, symptomatic intracranial hemorrhage.
Note: Results are presented for treatment group versus control group for RCTs.

selection – a factor in all these studies. We strongly believe that revascularization of large cores of ischemic and infarcted brain does not improve outcomes and ultimately leads to worse outcomes secondary to ICH. It is also evident that the vast majority of patients who present with acute ischemic stroke will have some area of established core infarct and a variable degree of penumbra. The precise risk-benefit ratio for intervention in the varied ratios of core versus penumbra is not known. Similarly, this ratio of infarcted core versus salvageable penumbra will change based on individual collateral supply and time from occlusion. Our experience has led us to believe that the relative benefit of revascularization recedes when the core exceeds 50% of at-risk territory. Further, select areas such as the basal ganglia, which are defined by perforator segments (end arteries) on the anterior cerebral artery and MCA, also seem to form a high-risk SICH area when they form part of the infarct core.

◆ Conclusions

- Neurologic outcome after stroke intervention depends on the volume of the ischemic core or infarcted brain, the time window to recanalization, the ability to have sustained flow restoration, and the morbidity of SICH associated with the treatment.
- Current treatment options for acute ischemic stroke are aiming at an early and sustained restoration of flow to the penumbra, increasing the time window for treatment, and decreasing the rates of SICH.
- Endovascular interventions, especially mechanical thrombolysis, are more efficient than IV or intraarterial pharmacologic thrombolysis in opening up the vessels without the increased risk of SICH associated with the use of pharmacologic thrombolysis.
- Although recanalization rates have increased with endovascular therapies, SICH rates also have increased whereas outcomes have improved only marginally.
- Better standards and protocols for physiologic imaging with good reproducibility, improvements in mechanical revascularization strategies, and newer thrombolytics allow selection of patients who may benefit from endovascular revascularization even up to 24 to 36 hours after stroke symptom onset.

Better patient selection and the addition of neuroprotective strategies may improve outcomes in the future.

References

1. del Zoppo GJ, Saver JL, Jauch EC, Adams HP, Jr. Expansion of the time window for treatment of acute ischemic stroke with intravenous tissue plasminogen activator. A Science Advisory from the American Heart Association/American Stroke Association. Stroke 2009;40:2945–2948
2. Hacke W, Kaste M, Bluhmki E, et al; ECASS Investigators. Thrombolysis with alteplase 3 to 4.5 hours after acute ischemic stroke. N Engl J Med 2008;359(13):1317–1329
3. Mathews MS, Sharma J, Snyder KV, et al. Safety, effectiveness, and practicality of endovascular therapy within the first 3 hours of acute ischemic stroke onset. Neurosurgery 2009;65(5):860–865
4. Smith WS, Sung G, Starkman S, et al; MERCI Trial Investigators. Safety and efficacy of mechanical embolectomy in acute ischemic stroke: results of the MERCI trial. Stroke 2005;36(7):1432–1438
5. Smith WS, Sung G, Saver J, et al; Multi MERCI Investigators. Mechanical thrombectomy for acute ischemic stroke: final results of the Multi MERCI trial. Stroke 2008;39(4):1205–1212
6. Tomsick T, Broderick J, Carrozella J, et al; Interventional Management of Stroke II Investigators. Revascularization results in the Interventional Management of Stroke II trial. AJNR Am J Neuroradiol 2008;29(3):582–587
7. Rha JH, Saver JL. The impact of recanalization on ischemic stroke outcome: a meta-analysis. Stroke 2007;38(3):967–973
8. Esteban JM, Cervera V. Perfusion CT and angio CT in the assessment of acute stroke. Neuroradiology 2004;46(9):705–715
9. Kloska SP, Nabavi DG, Gaus C, et al. Acute stroke assessment with CT: do we need multimodal evaluation? Radiology 2004;233(1):79–86
10. Maruya J, Yamamoto K, Ozawa T, et al. Simultaneous multi-section perfusion CT and CT angiography for the assessment of acute ischemic stroke. Acta Neurochir (Wien) 2005;147(4):383–391
11. Tan JC, Dillon WP, Liu S, Adler F, Smith WS, Wintermark M. Systematic comparison of perfusion-CT and CT-angiography in acute stroke patients. Ann Neurol 2007;61(6):533–543
12. Hellier KD, Hampton JL, Guadagno JV, et al. Perfusion CT helps decision making for thrombolysis when there is no clear time of onset. J Neurol Neurosurg Psychiatry 2006;77(3):417–419
13. Parsons MW, Pepper EM, Chan V, et al. Perfusion computed tomography: prediction of final infarct extent and stroke outcome. Ann Neurol 2005;58(5):672–679
14. Wintermark M, Meuli R, Browaeys P, et al. Comparison of CT perfusion and angiography and MRI in selecting stroke patients for acute treatment. Neurology 2007;68(9):694–697
15. Gralla J, Schroth G, Remonda L, et al. A dedicated animal model for mechanical thrombectomy in acute stroke. AJNR Am J Neuroradiol 2006;27(6):1357–1361
16. Gralla J, Burkhardt M, Schroth G, et al. Occlusion length is a crucial determinant of efficiency and complication rate in thrombectomy for acute ischemic stroke. AJNR Am J Neuroradiol 2008;29(2):247–252
17. Gralla J, Schroth G, Remonda L, Nedeltchev K, Slotboom J, Brekenfeld C. Mechanical thrombectomy for acute ischemic stroke: thrombus-device interaction, efficiency, and complications in vivo. Stroke 2006;37(12):3019–3024
18. Nogueira RG, Smith WS; MERCI and Multi MERCI Writing Committee. Safety and efficacy of endovascular thrombectomy in patients with abnormal hemostasis: pooled analysis of the MERCI and multi MERCI trials. Stroke 2009;40(2):516–522
19. Barnwell SL, Clark WM, Nguyen TT, O'Neill OR, Wynn ML, Coull BM. Safety and efficacy of delayed intraarterial urokinase therapy with mechanical clot disruption for thromboembolic stroke. AJNR Am J Neuroradiol 1994;15(10):1817–1822
20. Gobin YP, Starkman S, Duckwiler GR, et al. MERCI 1: a phase 1 study of Mechanical Embolus Removal in Cerebral Ischemia. Stroke 2004;35(12):2848–2854
21. Flint AC, Duckwiler GR, Budzik RF, Liebeskind DS, Smith WS; MERCI and Multi MERCI Writing Committee. Mechanical thrombectomy of intracranial internal carotid occlusion: pooled results of the MERCI and Multi MERCI Part I trials. Stroke 2007;38(4):1274–1280
22. Khatri P, Hill MD, Palesch YY, et al; Interventional Management of Stroke III Investigators. Methodology of the Interventional Management of Stroke III Trial. Int J Stroke 2008;3(2):130–137
23. Bose A, Henkes H, Alfke K, et al; Penumbra Phase 1 Stroke Trial Investigators. The Penumbra System: a mechanical device for the treatment of acute stroke due to thromboembolism. AJNR Am J Neuroradiol 2008;29(7):1409–1413
24. Penumbra Pivotal Stroke Trial Investigators. The penumbra pivotal stroke trial: safety and effectiveness of a new generation of mechanical devices for clot removal in intracranial large vessel occlusive disease. Stroke 2009;40(8):2761–2768
25. Henkes H, Miloslavski E, Lowens S, Reinartz J, Liebig T, Kühne D. Treatment of intracranial atherosclerotic stenoses with balloon dilatation and self-expanding stent deployment (WingSpan). Neuroradiology 2005;47(3):222–228

26. Qureshi AI, Siddiqui AM, Kim SH, et al. Reocclusion of recanalized arteries during intra-arterial thrombolysis for acute ischemic stroke. AJNR Am J Neuroradiol 2004;25(2):322–328
27. Levy EI, Mehta R, Gupta R, et al. Self-expanding stents for recanalization of acute cerebrovascular occlusions. AJNR Am J Neuroradiol 2007;28(5):816–822
28. Zaidat OO, Wolfe T, Hussain SI, et al. Interventional acute ischemic stroke therapy with intracranial self-expanding stent. Stroke 2008;39(8):2392–2395
29. Brekenfeld C, Schroth G, Mattle HP, et al. Stent placement in acute cerebral artery occlusion: use of a self-expandable intracranial stent for acute stroke treatment. Stroke 2009;40(3):847–852
30. Levy EI, Siddiqui AH, Crumlish A, et al. First Food and Drug Administration-approved prospective trial of primary intracranial stenting for acute stroke: SARIS (stent-assisted recanalization in acute ischemic stroke). Stroke 2009;40(11):3552–3556
31. Kelly ME, Furlan AJ, Fiorella D. Recanalization of an acute middle cerebral artery occlusion using a self-expanding, reconstrainable, intracranial microstent as a temporary endovascular bypass. Stroke 2008;39(6):1770–1773
32. Hauck EF, Mocco J, Snyder KV, Levy EI. Temporary endovascular bypass: a novel treatment for acute stroke. AJNR Am J Neuroradiol 2009;30:1532–1533
33. Yavuz K, Geyik S, Pamuk AG, Koc O, Saatci I, Cekirge HS. Immediate and midterm follow-up results of using an electrodetachable, fully retrievable SOLO stent system in the endovascular coil occlusion of wide-necked cerebral aneurysms. J Neurosurg 2007;107(1):49–55
33a. Natarajan SK, Siddiqui AH, Hopkins LN, Levy EI. Retrievable, detachable stent-platform–based clot-retrieval device (Solitaire™ FR) for acute stroke revascularization: first demonstration of feasibility in a canine stroke model. Vasc Dis Manag 2010;7:E120–E125
34. Jovin TG, Gupta R, Uchino K, et al. Emergent stenting of extracranial internal carotid artery occlusion in acute stroke has a high revascularization rate. Stroke 2005;36(11):2426–2430
35. Nikas D, Reimers B, Elisabetta M, et al. Percutaneous interventions in patients with acute ischemic stroke related to obstructive atherosclerotic disease or dissection of the extracranial carotid artery. J Endovasc Ther 2007;14(3):279–288
36. Dabitz R, Triebe S, Leppmeier U, Ochs G, Vorwerk D. Percutaneous recanalization of acute internal carotid artery occlusions in patients with severe stroke. Cardiovasc Intervent Radiol 2007;30(1):34–41
37. Lavallée PC, Mazighi M, Saint-Maurice JP, et al. Stent-assisted endovascular thrombolysis versus intravenous thrombolysis in internal carotid artery dissection with tandem internal carotid and middle cerebral artery occlusion. Stroke 2007;38(8):2270–2274
38. Miyamoto N, Naito I, Takatama S, Shimizu T, Iwai T, Shimaguchi H. Urgent stenting for patients with acute stroke due to atherosclerotic occlusive lesions of the cervical internal carotid artery. Neurol Med Chir (Tokyo) 2008;48(2):49–55, discussion 55–56
39. del Zoppo GJ, Higashida RT, Furlan AJ, Pessin MS, Rowley HA, Gent M. PROACT: a phase II randomized trial of recombinant pro-urokinase by direct arterial delivery in acute middle cerebral artery stroke. PROACT Investigators. Prolyse in Acute Cerebral Thromboembolism. Stroke 1998;29(1):4–11
40. Furlan A, Higashida R, Wechsler L, et al. Intra-arterial prourokinase for acute ischemic stroke. The PROACT II study: a randomized controlled trial. Prolyse in Acute Cerebral Thromboembolism. JAMA 1999;282(21):2003–2011
41. Wechsler LR, Roberts R, Furlan AJ, et al; PROACT II Investigators. Factors influencing outcome and treatment effect in PROACT II. Stroke 2003;34(5):1224–1229
42. Adams HP Jr, del Zoppo G, Alberts MJ, et al; American Heart Association; American Stroke Association Stroke Council; Clinical Cardiology Council; Cardiovascular Radiology and Intervention Council; Atherosclerotic Peripheral Vascular Disease and Quality of Care Outcomes in Research Interdisciplinary Working Groups. Guidelines for the early management of adults with ischemic stroke: a guideline from the American Heart Association/American Stroke Association Stroke Council, Clinical Cardiology Council, Cardiovascular Radiology and Intervention Council, and the Atherosclerotic Peripheral Vascular Disease and Quality of Care Outcomes in Research Interdisciplinary Working Groups: the American Academy of Neurology affirms the value of this guideline as an educational tool for neurologists. Stroke 2007;38(5):1655–1711
43. Fink JN, Kumar S, Horkan C, et al. The stroke patient who woke up: clinical and radiological features, including diffusion and perfusion MRI. Stroke 2002;33(4):988–993
44. Serena J, Dávalos A, Segura T, Mostacero E, Castillo J. Stroke on awakening: looking for a more rational management. Cerebrovasc Dis 2003;16(2):128–133
45. Barreto AD, Martin-Schild S, Hallevi H, et al. Thrombolytic therapy for patients who wake-up with stroke. Stroke 2009;40(3):827–832
46. Adams HP Jr, Leira EC, Torner JC, et al; AbESTT-II Investigators. Treating patients with 'wake-up' stroke: the experience of the AbESTT-II trial. Stroke 2008;39(12):3277–3282
47. Natarajan SK, Snyder KV, Siddiqui AH, Ionita CC, Hopkins LN, Levy EI. Safety and effectiveness of endovascular therapy after 8 hours of acute ischemic stroke onset and wake-up strokes. Stroke 2009;40(10):3269–3274
48. Janjua N, El-Gengaihy A, Pile-Spellman J, Qureshi AI. Late endovascular revascularization in acute ischemic stroke based on clinical-diffusion mismatch. AJNR Am J Neuroradiol 2009;30(5):1024–1027
49. Zeumer H, Freitag HJ, Grzyska U, Neunzig HP. Local intraarterial fibrinolysis in acute vertebrobasilar occlusion. Technical developments and recent results. Neuroradiology 1989;31(4):336–340
50. Hacke W, Zeumer H, Ferbert A, Brückmann H, del Zoppo GJ. Intra-arterial thrombolytic therapy improves outcome in patients with acute vertebrobasilar occlusive disease. Stroke 1988;19(10):1216–1222
51. Becker KJ, Monsein LH, Ulatowski J, Mirski M, Williams M, Hanley DF. Intraarterial thrombolysis in vertebrobasilar occlusion. AJNR Am J Neuroradiol 1996;17(2):255–262
52. Jahan R. Hyperacute therapy of acute ischemic stroke: intraarterial thrombolysis and mechanical revascularization strategies. Tech Vasc Interv Radiol 2005;8(2):87–91
53. Archer CR, Horenstein S. Basilar artery occlusion: clinical and radiological correlation. Stroke 1977;8(3):383–390
54. Smith WS. Intra-arterial thrombolytic therapy for acute basilar occlusion: pro. Stroke 2007; 38(2, Suppl)701–703
55. Lindsberg PJ, Mattle HP. Therapy of basilar artery occlusion: a systematic analysis comparing intra-arterial and intravenous thrombolysis. Stroke 2006;37(3):922–928
56. Levy EI, Firlik AD, Wisniewski S, et al. Factors affecting survival rates for acute vertebrobasilar artery occlusions treated with intra-arterial thrombolytic therapy: a meta-analytical approach. Neurosurgery 1999;45(3):539–545, discussion 545–548
57. Zeumer H, Hacke W, Ringelstein EB. Local intraarterial thrombolysis in vertebrobasilar thromboembolic disease. AJNR Am J Neuroradiol 1983;4(3):401–404
58. Zeumer H, Freitag HJ, Zanella F, Thie A, Arning C. Local intra-arterial fibrinolytic therapy in patients with stroke: urokinase versus recombinant tissue plasminogen activator (r-TPA). Neuroradiology 1993;35(2):159–162
59. Arnold M, Nedeltchev K, Mattle HP, et al. Intra-arterial thrombolysis in 24 consecutive patients with internal carotid artery T occlusions. J Neurol Neurosurg Psychiatry 2003;74(6):739–742
60. Jansen O, von Kummer R, Forsting M, Hacke W, Sartor K. Thrombolytic therapy in acute occlusion of the intracranial internal carotid artery bifurcation. AJNR Am J Neuroradiol 1995;16(10):1977–1986
61. Investigators IMS; IMS II Trial Investigators. The Interventional Management of Stroke (IMS) II Study. Stroke 2007;38(7):2127–2135
62. National Institute of Neurological Disorders and Stroke rt-PA Stroke Study Group. Tissue plasminogen activator for acute ischemic stroke. N Engl J Med 1995;333:1581–1587
63. Investigators IMS; IMS Study Investigators. Combined intravenous and intra-arterial recanalization for acute ischemic stroke: the Interventional Management of Stroke Study. Stroke 2004;35(4):904–911
64. IMS II Trial Investigators. The Interventional Management of Stroke (IMS) II Study. Stroke 2007;38(7):2127–2135
65. Penumbra Pivotal Stroke Trial Investigators. The penumbra pivotal stroke trial: safety and effectiveness of a new generation of mechanical devices for clot removal in intracranial large vessel occlusive disease. Stroke 2009;40(8):2761–2768
66. Mattle HP, Arnold M, Georgiadis D, et al. Comparison of intraarterial and intravenous thrombolysis for ischemic stroke with hyperdense middle cerebral artery sign. Stroke 2008;39(2):379–383
67. Hacke W, Kaste M, Bluhmki E, et al; ECASS Investigators. Thrombolysis with alteplase 3 to 4.5 hours after acute ischemic stroke. N Engl J Med 2008;359(13):1317–1329

Chapter 16

Venous Sinus Thrombosis Recanalization Techniques

Gregory J. Velat and J Mocco

◆ Background

Cerebral venous sinus thrombosis (CVST) is a relatively rare disease that accounts for less than 1% of all strokes.[1] The exact incidence of CVST is unknown, but ranges from 0.03% to as high as 9% on autopsy series.[2–5] Various factors are believed to contribute to CVST. Hypercoagulable states, infection of cranial sinuses and otitis, as well as the use of oral contraceptives have all been implicated as causative factors. Interestingly, as high as 40% of cases are thought to be idiopathic.[6] CVST is more common in young women, particularly during puerperium. [7,8]

Headache is the most common presentation and is estimated to occur in up to 80% of cases.[8] Other symptoms related to elevated intracranial pressure are common including nausea with or without emesis and visual disturbances. Focal neurologic deficits or seizures may occur in conjunction with venous hypertension or related cerebral infarction or hemorrhage.[9]

◆ Indications

The natural course of CVST is variable, and treatment guidelines are not well established. The goal of therapy is to recanalize the affected venous sinus(es) to improve clinical signs and symptoms. Patients with elevated intracranial pressure secondary to venous hypertension should be treated aggressively with mannitol, hyperventilation, and/or cerebrospinal fluid diversion in accordance with their neurologic status. Seizures should be controlled with anticonvulsants. Systemic and/or direct thrombolysis should be initiated once the patient has been stabilized from a respiratory and hemodynamic standpoint. Rapid deterioration in a patient's neurologic status requires emergent intervention.

◆ Techniques

Systemic Thrombolysis

Multiple publications have described the successful treatment of CVST with resolution of neurologic symptoms using heparin. Two small randomized controlled trials have evaluated the effects of systemic heparinization in the treatment of CVST.[10,11] One study found an eightfold increased likelihood of patients with CVST having improved neurologic function at 3 days, 8 days, and 3 months after systemic anticoagulation with heparin compared with controls.[11] A retrospective analysis of a subgroup of patients with CVST in this study showed that systemic heparinization in the setting of intracranial hemorrhage was safe. The second study, however, failed to demonstrate improved outcomes in patients who received low-molecular-weight heparin relative to controls.[10] Neither study demonstrated improved overall survival with heparin therapy. The International Study on Cerebral Vein and Dural Sinus Thrombosis (ISCVT) was a multinational prospective observational study that enrolled 624 adult patients diagnosed with CVST.[12] Although the choice of therapy was not regimented, 520 (83%) of the patients were anticoagulated acutely with either intravenous (IV) heparin (64%) or low-molecular-weight heparin (35%). At a median follow-up of 16 months, 57% of patients were asymptomatic and ~32% of patients had mild or moderate impairments. Patient factors predictive of worse outcome on multivariate analysis included coma at the time of presentation, thrombosis of deep cerebral veins, cancer, and central nervous system infection. Systemic thrombolysis using urokinase and recombinant tissue plasminogen activator (rtPA) has been performed in animals[13] and human case reports exist.[14] Although evidence suggests that these agents may effect sinus recanalization, the increased anecdotal risk of hemorrhagic complications makes them less attractive options.

The goal of systemic heparin therapy is to maintain the activated partial thromboplastin time at 2 to 2.5 times normal. Once the patient's neurologic condition has stabilized, Coumadin therapy is initiated with an INR goal between 2 to 3 for 6 months. Prolonged anticoagulation (>6 months) is recommended for patients with hereditary thrombophilias or recurrent CVST.[15]

Direct Thrombolysis

Direct thrombolysis is reserved for patients who derive no clinical benefit from systemic anticoagulation or for patients with rapidly deteriorating neurologic status. Various techniques for direct thrombolysis have been described in multiple case series (**Table 16.1**). The earliest published reports involved prolonged local infusions of urokinase into the superior sagittal sinus through direct sinus cannulation following either midline craniotomy[16] or percutaneous transcranial puncture.[17] Advances in endovascular technology have nearly obviated the need for direct sinus cannulation. Since its initial description by Tsai and colleagues,[18] transfemoral venous puncture has become the preferred method of accessing the intracranial venous sinuses. Sinus recanalization, as confirmed by serial intracranial venography, is typically achieved through prolonged infusions of urokinase (no longer commercially available in the United States) or rtPA. Patients typically remain on systemic anticoagulation for 6 months following direct thrombolysis.

Direct chemical thrombolysis may be augmented by various mechanical thrombolytic techniques. Balloon catheter thrombectomy,[19–21] rheolytic therapy using the AngioJet catheter system (Possis Medical, Minneapolis, MN),[22–26] and snare devices[27] have been used successfully to achieve sinus recanalization in combination with various systemic or direct thrombolytic therapies. Only one prospective study of direct thrombolysis for CVST has been published to date.[21] It used a combination of mechanical and chemical

Table 16.1 Direct Thrombolysis for Treatment of Cerebral Venous Sinus Thrombosis (CVST)

Author, Year	*N*	Agent	Dosage	Results
Scott et al, 1988[16]	1	Urokinase	240,000 U/h × 3 h; 60,000 U/h × 8 h	Significant neurologic improvement to mild dysphasia at 4 weeks
Higashida et al, 1989[27]	1	Urokinase	1,000 U/h × 2 h	Normal development at 3 years of age
Barnwell et al, 1991[31]	3	Urokinase	58,000 U/h × 4–10 d	2 patients showed clinical improvement 1 patient with partial resolution of CVST failed to improve clinically
Tsai et al, 1992[18]	5	Urokinase	200,000–600,000 U	Neurologic recovery in all patients
Smith et al, 1994[29]	7	Urokinase	20,000–150,000 U/h × 163 h (range 88–244 h)	Neurologic improvement[6] Surgery for dural arteriovenous fistula[1]
Horowitz et al, 1995[32]	12	Urokinase	50,000–500,000 U bolus 73,600 U/h for 50 h	Good to excellent outcomes[10] Functional sinus patency achieved[11]
Barnwell et al, 1995[33]	6	Urokinase	100,000 U bolus 40,000–80,000 U/h for up to 48 h	Completely recovery[3] Blindness[1] Death[2]
Kim & Suh, 1997[28]	9	rtPA	10 mg bolus over 10 min, 50 mg over 3 h, 5 mg continuous infusion for maximum daily dose of 100 mg	Complete sinus recanalization in all patients between 8 and 43 h
Rael et al, 1997[34]	1	Urokinase	250,000 U bolus × 2, 80,000 U/h for 165 h	Normal neurologic function at 30 d
Phillips et al, 1999[35]	6	Urokinase	200,000–1,000,000 U	Neurologic improvement in all patients
Frey et al, 1999[30]	12	rtPA	Mean rtPA dose = 46 mg (23–128 mg) Mean infusion time = 29 h (13–77 hour)	Flow restored[9] Worsening intracranial hemorrhage[2]
Yamini, 2001[36]	1	rtPA	25 mg bolus, 1 mg/min infusion for 19 h	Complete neurologic recovery
Wasay et al, 2001[37]	20	Urokinase	250,000 U bolus, 80,000 U/h for 16–18 h	Excellent neurologic function[16] Mild[3] and moderate[1] neurologic deficits
Ming et al, 2002[38]	5	Urokinase	200,000 U/15 min	Excellent clinical improvement in all patients
Stam et al, 2008[21]	20	Urokinase	120,000–600,000 U bolus, 100,000 U/h × 24 h	Neurologic recovery,[12] permanent neurologic disability,[2] death[6]
Sujith et al, 2008[39]	3	Urokinase	3,000,000–3,600,000 U over 24–48 h	Neurologic improvement in all patients

Abbreviations: rtPA, recombinant tissue plasminogen activator thrombolytic techniques on 20 patients, 12 of which were comatose prior to treatment. Fifteen patients underwent chemical thrombolysis with direct urokinase infusion into the superior sagittal and straight sinuses combined with thrombosuction via a rheolytic catheter and thrombectomy using a Fogarty catheter. Nine patients fully recovered, but six patients died of complications related to CVST.

Procedural Description

Systemic anticoagulation is the first-line therapy for CVST. For patients with worsening neurologic status despite systemic thrombolysis, however, direct thrombolysis with or without mechanical thrombolysis should be performed emergently. Joint transfemoral arterial (5F) and venous (6F) access should be attained. We recommend performing a four-vessel diagnostic cerebral arteriogram to estimate the extent of sinus involvement prior to beginning direct thrombolysis. A 6F Envoy catheter (Codman Neurovascular, Raynham, MA) is then advanced over a 0.035-inch guidewire up to the distal cervical internal jugular vein. A Prowler 14 microcatheter (Codman Neurovascular) is then advanced over a Synchro-2 microwire (Boston Scientific, Natick, MA) to the proximal portion of the thrombosed venous sinus. Using a gentle rapid rotating motion, the microwire is then advanced through the thrombus to avoid vessel wall perforation. The selection of microcatheter and microwire may be altered if difficulty is encountered while attempting to navigate through the thrombus. With the microcatheter positioned proximal to the thrombosed sinus, direct thrombolysis may be initiated. We recommend using a continuous rtPA infusion at 2 mg/h until the sinus is recanalized. In cases of multiple thrombosed sinuses, two microcatheters may be used. Once the microcatheter(s) and access sheath(s) have been secured, the patient is transported to the intensive care unit for frequent neurologic checks while the thrombolytic agent is being infused. Intracranial venography is then performed every 12 hours until sinus patency is achieved. Patients are then placed on systemic anticoagulation for 6 months with follow-up magnetic resonance venography to confirm sustained sinus patency.

Case Illustration

A 45-year-old woman presented with worsening headaches and right-sided hemiparesis. Initial noncontrast head computed tomography (CT) showed a hypodense region in the left thalamus that corresponded to restricted diffusion of the left caudate, thalamus, and basal ganglia on diffusion-weighted magnetic resonance imaging (MRI) (**Fig. 16.1**). Initial MR venography revealed thrombin in the superior sagittal sinus. Neurologically, the patient was awake and alert with a dense right-sided hemiparesis and brisk localization in the left upper extremity. She remained dysphasic. The patient was placed initially on systemic heparin therapy, but she became unarousable and was flexing only on the left side. She underwent rapid-sequence intubation and received mannitol for presumed elevated intracranial pressure.

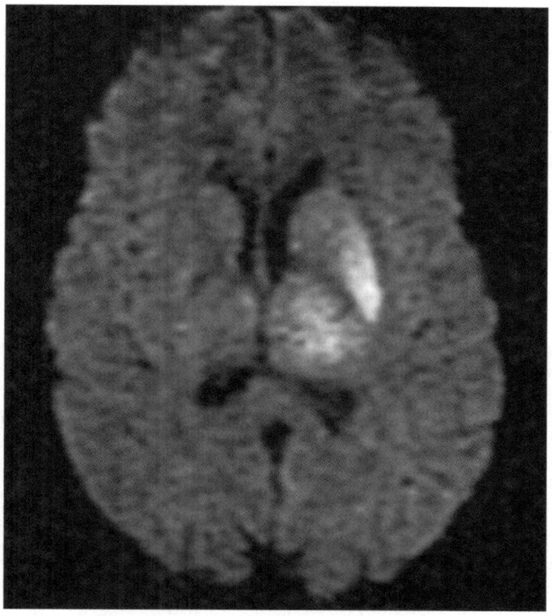

Fig. 16.1 Diffusion-weighted MRI shows acute infarction of the left caudate, thalamus, and basal ganglia.

Repeat head CT scan revealed progression of thrombus, now involving the posterior superior sagittal sinus and torcula. The patient was taken emergently to the angiography suite for planned endovascular intervention. Transfemoral access was attained bilaterally using a 5F sheath placed into the left femoral artery and a 6F sheath placed into the right femoral vein. A diagnostic arteriogram was performed, confirming significant thrombus in the posterior superior sagittal sinus, torcula, and left transverse sinus. The 6F guide catheter was parked in the distal right internal jugular vein. Next, a Prowler 14 microcatheter and Synchro-2 microwire were advanced through the right transverse sinus and torcula into the posterior superior sagittal sinus. Significant thrombus was encountered as the microwire and microcatheter were successfully advanced to the proximal portion of the thrombus using gentle mechanical thrombolysis (**Fig. 16.2A**). Because of the significant amount of clot, a second Prowler 14 microcatheter and Synchro-2 microwire were introduced in the proximal right transverse sinus (**Fig. 16.2B**). rtPA was then infused through the microcatheters directly into the superior sagittal and proximal right transverse sinuses at 2 mg/h. The sheaths were sutured in place, and the patient was transported back to the intensive care unit for frequent neurologic checks. The patient's neurologic examination improved to localizing in the left upper extremity several hours after the intervention. A venogram was performed at 12 hours, which revealed partial recanalization of the posterior superior sagittal and left transverse sinuses (**Fig. 16.2C**). A significant amount of thrombus was still seen at the torcula. The direct rtPA infusion was continued for an additional 12 hours (48 mg total of rtPA). The repeat venograms at 24 hours revealed complete recanalization of the affected sinuses (**Fig. 16.2D**).

At this time, the two microcatheters were removed. The patient was started on therapeutic systemic heparin therapy and was converted over to Coumadin. Her neurologic status improved to opening her eyes spontaneously with brisk localization in the left upper extremity and stable right-sided hemiparesis. She was eventually extubated and discharged to rehabilitation. At 6-month follow-up, the patient had regained significant strength on her right side as well as some speech function. MRV revealed complete recanalization of the superior sagittal and bilateral transverse sinuses (**Fig. 16.2E**).

◆ Complications and Complication Avoidance

The major risk of thrombolysis to treat CVST is intracranial hemorrhage. Relative contraindications to systemic

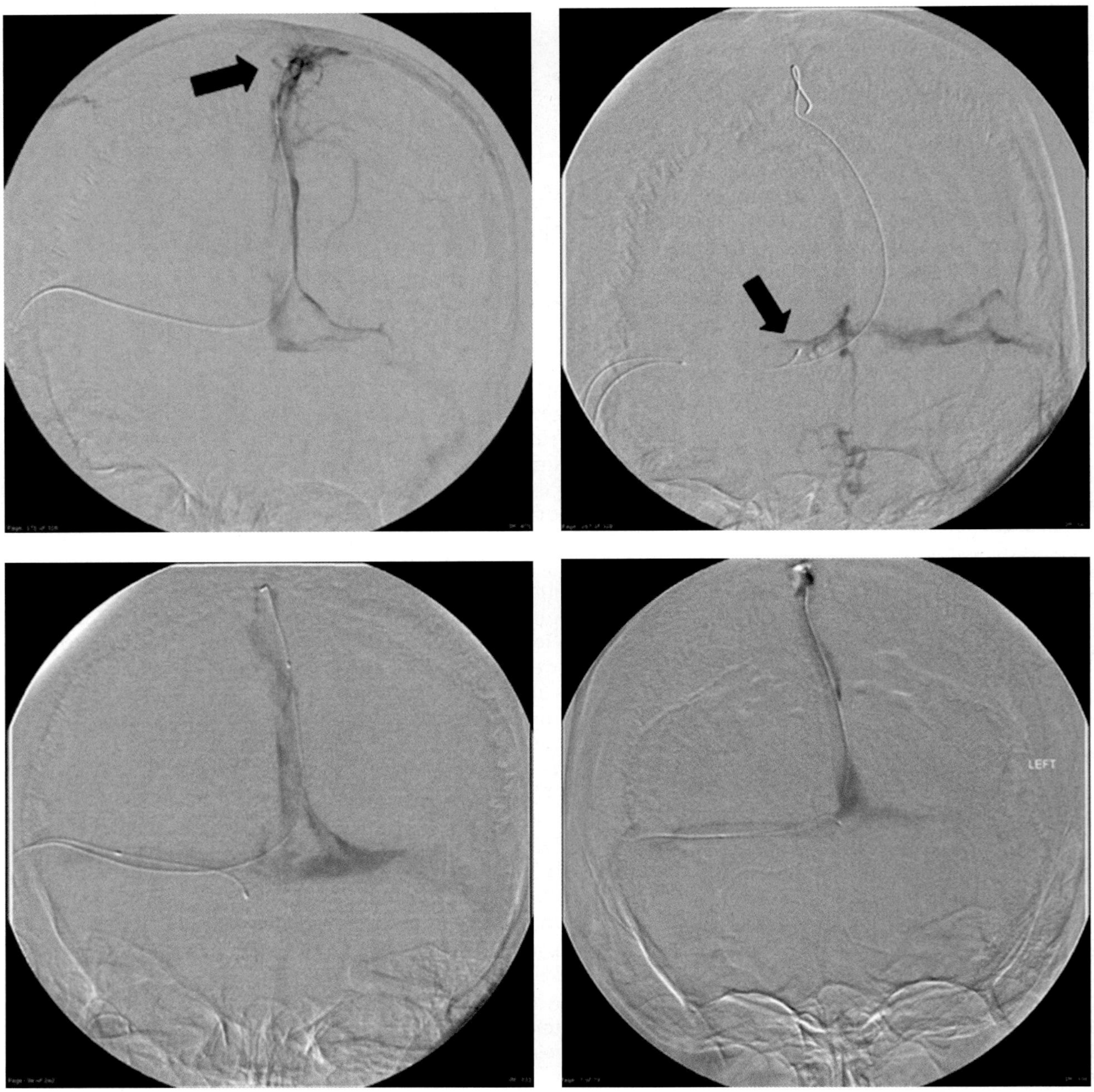

Fig. 16.2 **(A)** Venogram reveals significant thrombus involving the posterior superior sagittal sinus. The microcatheter was advanced through the right transverse sinus and torcula, and its tip (*arrow*) lies proximal to the thrombus in the superior sagittal sinus. **(B)** Venogram shows placement of the second microcatheter into the proximal right transverse sinus (*arrow*). **(C)** Venogram made 12 hours after rtPA infusion reveals significant recanalization of the posterosuperior and left transverse sinuses. **(D)** Venogram made 24 hours after rtPA infusion shows improved venous outflow through the posterosuperior sagittal and left transverse sinuses. *(continued)*

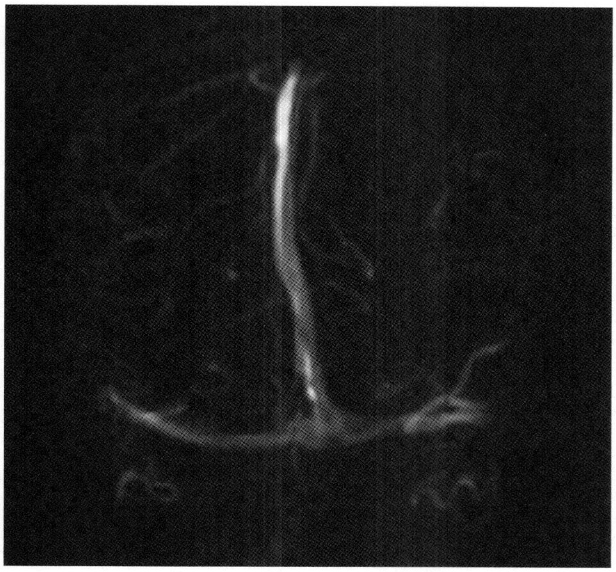

E

Fig. 16.2 *(continued)* **(E)** MR venogram from 6 months after intervention shows complete resolution of thrombus in the superior sagittal and transverse sinuses.

thrombolytic therapy include intracranial hemorrhage, recent major surgery, trauma, and active gastrointestinal bleeding. Endovascular interventions may be complicated by retroperitoneal hemorrhage,[28] pseudoaneurysm formation,[23] infection at the percutaneous femoral puncture site,[29] and progression of intracranial hemorrhage.[24,30] Mechanical thrombolysis may be complicated by injury to the sinus endothelium that may result in rethrombosis or dislodgement and spread of microemboli into the pulmonary system.[26] Rheolytic therapy–associated anemia has also been observed.[15] Endovascular approaches may be limited by patient anatomic factors and catheter properties. In cases of extreme vessel tortuosity, transjugular venous access may be required. More robust microcatheters and microwires may be used cautiously to navigate through thick thrombus. Transcranial sinus cannulation may be reserved for cases in which transfemoral or transjugular access is not attainable.

References

1. Masuhr F, Mehraein S, Einhäupl K. Cerebral venous and sinus thrombosis. J Neurol 2004;251(1):11–23
2. Barnett HJM, Hyland HH. Noninfective intracranial venous thrombosis. Brain 1953;76(1):36–49
3. Ehler H, Courville CB. Thrombosis of cerebral veins in infancy and childhood: review of literature and report of five cases. J Pediatr 1936;8:600–623
4. Erez N, Babuna C, Uner A. Low incidence of thromboembolic disease: an evaluation of obstetric and gynecologic patients in Istanbul. Obstet Gynecol 1966;27(6):833–837
5. Towbin A. The syndrome of latent cerebral venous thrombosis: its frequency and relation to age and congestive heart failure. Stroke 1973;4(3):419–430
6. Diaz JM, Schiffman JS, Urban ES, Maccario M. Superior sagittal sinus thrombosis and pulmonary embolism: a syndrome rediscovered. Acta Neurol Scand 1992;86(4):390–396
7. Ameri A, Bousser MG. Cerebral venous thrombosis. Neurol Clin 1992; 10(1):87–111
8. Bousser MG, Chiras J, Bories J, Castaigne P. Cerebral venous thrombosis: a review of 38 cases. Stroke 1985;16(2):199–213
9. Paciaroni M, Palmerini F, Bogousslavsky J. Clinical presentations of cerebral vein and sinus thrombosis. Front Neurol Neurosci 2008;23: 77–88
10. de Bruijn SF, Stam J. Randomized, placebo-controlled trial of anticoagulant treatment with low-molecular-weight heparin for cerebral sinus thrombosis. Stroke 1999;30(3):484–488
11. Einhäupl KM, Villringer A, Meister W, et al. Heparin treatment in sinus venous thrombosis. Lancet 1991;338(8767):597–600
12. Ferro JM, Canhão P, Stam J, Bousser MG, Barinagarrementeria F; ISCVT Investigators. Prognosis of cerebral vein and dural sinus thrombosis: results of the International Study on Cerebral Vein and Dural Sinus Thrombosis (ISCVT). Stroke 2004;35(3):664–670
13. Alexander LF, Yamamoto Y, Ayoubi S, al-Mefty O, Smith RR. Efficacy of tissue plasminogen activator in the lysis of thrombosis of the cerebral venous sinus. Neurosurgery 1990;26(4):559–564
14. Di Rocco C, Iannelli A, Leone G, Moschini M, Valori VM. Heparin-urokinase treatment in aseptic dural sinus thrombosis. Arch Neurol 1981;38(7):431–435
15. Einhäupl K, Bousser MG, de Bruijn SF, et al. EFNS guideline on the treatment of cerebral venous and sinus thrombosis. Eur J Neurol 2006;13(6):553–559
16. Scott JA, Pascuzzi RM, Hall PV, Becker GJ. Treatment of dural sinus thrombosis with local urokinase infusion: case report. J Neurosurg 1988;68(2):284–287
17. Higashida RT, Helmer E, Halbach VV, Hieshima GB. Direct thrombolytic therapy for superior sagittal sinus thrombosis. AJNR Am J Neuroradiol 1989; **10**(5, Suppl)S4–S6
18. Tsai FY, Higashida RT, Matovich V, Alfieri K. Acute thrombosis of the intracranial dural sinus: direct thrombolytic treatment. AJNR Am J Neuroradiol 1992;13(4):1137–1141
19. Chaloupka JC, Mangla S, Huddle DC. Use of mechanical thrombolysis via microballoon percutaneous transluminal angioplasty for the treatment of acute dural sinus thrombosis: case presentation and technical report. Neurosurgery 1999;45(3):650–656
20. Soleau SW, Schmidt R, Stevens S, Osborn A, MacDonald JD. Extensive experience with dural sinus thrombosis. Neurosurgery 2003; 52(3):534–544
21. Stam J, Majoie CB, van Delden OM, van Lienden KP, Reekers JA. Endovascular thrombectomy and thrombolysis for severe cerebral sinus thrombosis: a prospective study. Stroke 2008;39(5):1487–1490
22. Agner C, Deshaies EM, Bernardini GL, Popp AJ, Boulos AS. Coronary Angiojet catheterization for the management of dural venous sinus thrombosis. Technical note. J Neurosurg 2005;103(2):368–371
23. Baker MD, Opatowsky MJ, Wilson JA, Glazier SS, Morris PP. Rheolytic catheter and thrombolysis of dural venous sinus thrombosis: a case series. Neurosurgery 2001;48(3):487–493, discussion 493–494
24. Chow K, Gobin YP, Saver J, Kidwell C, Dong P, Viñuela F. Endovascular treatment of dural sinus thrombosis with rheolytic thrombectomy and intra-arterial thrombolysis. Stroke 2000;31(6):1420–1425
25. Curtin KR, Shaibani A, Resnick SA, Russell EJ, Simuni T. Rheolytic catheter thrombectomy, balloon angioplasty, and direct recombinant tissue plasminogen activator thrombolysis of dural sinus thrombosis with preexisting hemorrhagic infarctions. AJNR Am J Neuroradiol 2004;25(10):1807–1811
26. Zhang A, Collinson RL, Hurst RW, Weigele JB. Rheolytic thrombectomy for cerebral sinus thrombosis. Neurocrit Care 2008;9(1):17–26
27. Newman CB, Pakbaz RS, Nguyen AD, Kerber CW. Endovascular treatment of extensive cerebral sinus thrombosis. J Neurosurg 2009;110(3): 442–445
28. Kim SY, Suh JH. Direct endovascular thrombolytic therapy for dural sinus thrombosis: infusion of alteplase. AJNR Am J Neuroradiol 1997; 18(4):639–645
29. Smith TP, Higashida RT, Barnwell SL, et al. Treatment of dural sinus thrombosis by urokinase infusion. AJNR Am J Neuroradiol 1994;15(5): 801–807
30. Frey JL, Muro GJ, McDougall CG, Dean BL, Jahnke HK. Cerebral venous thrombosis: combined intrathrombus rtPA and intravenous heparin. Stroke 1999;30(3):489–494
31. Barnwell SL, Higashida RT, Halbach VV, Dowd CF, Hieshima GB. Direct endovascular thrombolytic therapy for dural sinus thrombosis. Neurosurgery 1991;28(1):135–142

32. Horowitz M, Purdy P, Unwin H, et al. Treatment of dural sinus thrombosis using selective catheterization and urokinase. Ann Neurol 1995;38(1):58–67
33. Barnwell SL, Nesbit GM, Clark WM. Local thrombolytic therapy for cerebrovascular disease: current Oregon Health Sciences University experience (July 1991 through April 1995). J Vasc Interv Radiol 1995; 6(6 Pt 2, Suppl)78S–82S
34. Rael JR, Orrison WW Jr, Baldwin N, Sell J. Direct thrombolysis of superior sagittal sinus thrombosis with coexisting intracranial hemorrhage. AJNR Am J Neuroradiol 1997;18(7):1238–1242
35. Philips MF, Bagley LJ, Sinson GP, et al. Endovascular thrombolysis for symptomatic cerebral venous thrombosis. J Neurosurg 1999;90(1):65–71
36. Yamini B, Loch Macdonald R, Rosenblum J. Treatment of deep cerebral venous thrombosis by local infusion of tissue plasminogen activator. Surg Neurol 2001;55(6):340–346
37. Wasay M, Bakshi R, Kojan S, Bobustuc G, Dubey N, Unwin DH. Nonrandomized comparison of local urokinase thrombolysis versus systemic heparin anticoagulation for superior sagittal sinus thrombosis. Stroke 2001;32(10):2310–2317
38. Ming S, Qi Z, Wang L, Zhu K. Deep cerebral venous thrombosis in adults. Chin Med J (Engl) 2002;115(3):395–397
39. Sujith OK, Krishnan R, Asraf V, Rahman A, Girija AS. Local thrombolysis in patients with dural venous thrombosis unresponsive to heparin. J Stroke Cerebrovasc Dis 2008;17(2):95–100

IV

Neuro-Critical Care

Chapter 17

Stabilization of Patients with Acute Ischemic Stroke

Tariq Janjua

"The brain cells are dying faster than you are thinking."

Early management of acute ischemic stroke (AIS) is best conducted in an environment that is conducive to prevention, early recognition, and preemptive management of complications. The early phase of AIS requires management of both neurologic and nonneurologic factors. Central nervous system issues can be divided into protection of the newly restored perfusion as well as prevention or treatment of the complications secondary to the original ischemic insult. The highest mortality from AIS is present during the first weeks after the stroke; in the Northern Manhattan Stroke Study (NOMASS), the early mortality rate from AIS approached 75%.[1] Impaired consciousness on admission, vertebrobasilar involvement, and early transtentorial herniation are the most significant predictors of higher mortality.[2] Increasing age has also been identified as an independent factor for increasing medical complication and mortality rates (**Table 17.1**).[3]

The Glasgow Coma Score (GCS) and NIH Stroke Scale Score (NIHSS) are major predictors for instability during the early phase of management. With every point increase in NIHSS score, one can expect a 24% reduction in the ultimate outcome quality.[4] It has become clear with experience that when the NIHSS score approaches and exceeds 16, the risk for complications is high, the ultimate neurologic outcome is predictably worse, and the patient will benefit from admission to the neurocritical care unit. Expert neurocritical care skills are beneficial to preempt and reverse cerebral edema and medical complications in this setting.

Early Stabilization of Acute Ischemic Stroke

Multiple factors can affect the immediate stabilization of patients with AIS. Premorbid conditions such as hypertension, diabetes mellitus, unstable coronary artery disease, chronic obstructive pulmonary disease (COPD), renal failure and congestive heart failure must be appreciated and addressed. In addition, the affected vascular territory can have a significant impact on complication and mortality rates, with complete middle cerebral artery infarctions carrying a high risk of malignant cerebral edema and intracranial hypertension. Posterior circulation stroke may be complicated by airway compromise due to lower cranial nerve involvement or direct insult to or compression of brainstem respiratory centers.

Preintervention Stabilization

Prior to interventional attempts to restore cerebral perfusion, several measures must be taken to stabilize airway, breathing, and circulation.

Airway and Oxygenation

Although early recanalization of a major arterial occlusion takes precedence over most other interventions, patients with airway compromise require immediate establishment of an adequate airway, often via endotracheal intubation. It is important to perform a quick and complete neurologic examination before intubation as sedation or paralysis will confound the ability to properly document the neurologic condition. Prior to intubation, patients should be preoxygenated, and preferably two suction catheters should be prepared. Most patients have eaten within the previous 6 to 8 hours, thus rapid sequence induction with lidocaine is the most appropriate approach. We prefer to avoid the use of a paralytic agent, which may impair our ability to monitor the patient's neurologic exam. Etomidate is our drug of choice for sedation (0.3 μg/kg), followed by low-dose propofol or dexmedetomidine infusion. Endotracheal tube placement should be confirmed objectively with a chest radiograph. If

Table 17.1 Factors Associated with Increased Morality with Acute Ischemic Stroke

Impaired consciousness on presentation
Posterior circulation acute ischemic stroke
Cerebral herniation syndrome
Advancing age
Acute cerebral edema
Respiratory failure requiring intubation and mechanical ventilation
Acute myocardial infarction
NIH Stroke Scale Score ≥16

the patient is hypotensive, end tidal CO_2 may give a false indication of low exhaled CO_2, which may also result from massive pulmonary embolism.

One can start with 100% FiO_2 either with a nonrebreather mask or with mechanical ventilation. Oxygen saturation is kept close to 100%, and FiO_2 is titrated down based on the saturation. Blood gases may be checked to confirm PaO_2 is consistent with saturation.

Circulation: Cerebral Perfusion Pressure and Blood Pressure

Cerebral perfusion pressure (CPP) depends on mean arterial pressure (MAP). MAP is kept within the area under the curve (AUC) by carefully controlling the blood pressure itself. We use nicardipine or clevidipine and avoid reducing the systolic blood pressure (BP) and MAP below 25% of baseline. If the CPP drops below the AUC, phenylephrine, 25% albumin, or hypertonic saline can be used. In the tPA stroke survey, pretreatment BP was one of the main factors associated with an increased fatality rate and was also related directly to the risk of hemorrhagic conversion.[5] In our experience, the placement of an arterial line for real-time monitoring is helpful in the early management of uncontrolled BP.

In the International Stroke Trial (IST), abnormal systolic BP and MAP were directly related to poor outcome at 6 months. The early mortality rate was increased by 3.8% for every 10 mm Hg above 150 mm Hg and by 17.9% for every 10 mm Hg below 150 mm Hg.[6] **Figure 17.1** provides a representative standardized order set as used by our neurovascular service for BP control in the setting of AIS.

A. Systolic Blood Pressure (SBP)
Keep SBP ≥ ________ mmHg and ≤ _________ mmHg
Nicardipine gtt 5 – 15 mg for SBP ≥ _________
Clevidipine 2-21 mg/hour for SBP ≥ _________
Labetalol 10 – 20 mg IV every 4 – 6 hourly for SBP ≥ ________
Phenylephrine gtt 25ug – 400ug per min for SBP ≤ _________

B. Mean Arterial Blood Pressure (MAP)
Keep MAP ≥ _________ mmHg and ≤ _________ mmHg
Nicardipine gtt 5 – 15 mg for MAP ≥ _________
Clevidipine 2-21 mg/hour for SBP ≥ _________
Labetalol 10 – 20 mg IV every 4 – 6 hourly for MAP ≥ ________
Phenylephrine gtt 25ug – 400 ug per min for MAP ≤ _________

Fig. 17.1 Proposed protocol for blood pressure control in neurocritical care.

Postintervention Stabilization

Following intervention to attempt reperfusion of the involved territory, we continue the above protocols. In addition, the below mentioned measures are implemented. The neurocritical care management can be very complicated with multiple variables (**Table 17.2**).

Table 17.2 Medical Factors Complicating the Neurocritical Care Management of Acute Ischemic Stroke

Pulmonary
COPD with baseline hypoxemia
Acute bronchospasm
Respiratory failure
Aspiration pneumonitis
Acute thromboembolism with paradoxical emboli
Obstructive sleep apnea syndrome
Cardiac
Atrial fibrillation with rapid ventricular response
Decompensated congestive heart failure
Aortic stenosis–severe with fixed cardiac output
Prosthetic cardiac valve with anticoagulation
Renal
Renal transplant with immunotherapy
Renal failure with fluid restriction
Metabolic
Diabetes mellitus with DKA or hyperglycemia
SIADH
Cerebral salt wasting

Abbreviations: COPD, chronic obstructive pulmonary disease; DKA, diabetes ketoacidosis; SIADH, syndrome of inappropriate antidiuretic hormone.

Glucose Management

Preexisting diabetes mellitus in AIS patients can lead to uncontrolled hyperglycemia. The mere presence of hyperglycemia is itself predictive of a worse outcome. The National Institute of Neurological Disorders and Stroke (NINDS) recombinant tPA (rtPA) trial found admission hyperglycemia to be directly associated with a less-favorable outcome including a higher incidence of intracranial hemorrhage (ICH).[7] This was true whether or not recanalization of the affected vessel could be achieved.[8–10] A serum glucose control protocol should be used for all patients with AIS. In general, it is useful to keep glucose in the low triple-digit level. Levels above 140 mg/dL should be avoided as this can be related to hemorrhagic transformation and cerebral vasospasm.

Fluids and Electrolytes

Most patients with AIS should receive maintenance intravenous (IV) fluids unless they suffer from severe cardiac or renal dysfunction. Dehydration, which can occur due to inability to swallow, should be avoided. The serum sodium levels are checked regularly and cerebral salt wasting is treated as necessary with hypertonic saline to prevent cerebral edema and seizures. Rarely, the syndrome of inappropriate antidiuretic hormone (SIADH) may occur in these patients and should be treated if encountered.

Cardiac

In the setting of AIS, nonspecific ST and T wave changes can be seen in the absence of any serious cardiac pathology. In severe stroke, cardiac enzymes may be elevated without coronary disease simply due to excess catecholamine surge. The use of a β-blocker is sometimes helpful to control tachycardia, although one must balance any reduction in heart rate with the need to maintain CPP as the cardiac index falls. We obtain a baseline electrocardiogram (ECG) on all patients with AIS, and, if needed, follow-up ECG can be performed in 24 hours. An echocardiogram, preferably with a bubble study, is considered in young stroke patients who may have paradoxical emboli. If a patient is found to have a patent foramen ovale and higher pulmonary pressure, the lower extremities are scanned for any signs of deep vein thrombosis (DVT) and pulmonary computed tomography (CT) angiography is done to check for pulmonary embolism.

Acute myocardial infarction in conjunction with AIS represents a dangerous combination of events. These patients require special attention to cardiac dysfunction given that it impacts cerebral perfusion, and some will require percutaneous coronary angioplasty, which may necessitate the use of powerful antiplatelet agents. Hemorrhagic conversion is a limiting factor in these patients. In the Framingham Study, atrial fibrillation was directly related to mortality at 30 days in AIS patients, with the mortality rates being 25% in patients with atrial fibrillation and 14% in those without.[11] The presence of a prosthetic valve in the setting of AIS can also result in difficult management issues. In our experience, we have found it reasonably safe to withhold anticoagulation for a week or longer in these patients if necessary. Serial echocardiographic studies may be useful to exclude the development of potential embolic sources related to discontinuation of the anticoagulation.

Pulmonary Concerns

Hypoxia is avoided by routinely using supplemental oxygen. If the patient's level of consciousness is depressed, hypoventilation must be avoided. In this setting, $PaCO_2$ tension and a chest radiograph to exclude aspiration should be evaluated. Patients with major arterial occlusion and brainstem insult may need intubation for both airway control and active treatment of progressive hypoxemia. Anticipation of a difficult airway must be part of this management. Ideally, the most experienced person available should deal with the airway. As a general guideline, if the GCS falls below 8, endotracheal intubation is recommended, especially in the setting of stridor or labored respiration.

In patients with AIS, the differentiation between neurogenic and nonneurogenic pulmonary edema can be complex. Knowledge of left ventricle wall thickness and motion and other echocardiographic findings are used to differentiate between systolic and diastolic dysfunction. In this setting, the use of arterial line cardiac index or placement of a pulmonary arterial catheter can offer objective measures to assess for pulmonary artery occlusive pressure. Diuretics should be administered with caution as the resulting decreased filling pressure can diminish CPP after the intervention.

Temperature

Brain temperature, which is usually 0.5 to 1°C higher than the core body temperature, can substantially affect cerebral edema. All febrile conditions may be associated with increasing infarct size and associated cerebral edema. It is known that epidural temperature is normally elevated 1°C over rectal temperature, while intraventricular temperature is 0.2 to 0.3°C higher than the rectal temperature. There is thus a temperature gradient from gray matter to the "core" of the brain.[12] From a practical perspective, temperature can be controlled with either an intravascular or a surface cooling system. Induced hypothermia may have a role in uncontrolled cerebral edema and AIS.[13] At our center, we have actively investigated the use of therapeutic hypothermia in the setting of malignant cerebral edema.

Venous Thromboembolism

The risk of venous thromboembolism (VTE) is reduced by early patient mobilization and proper prophylactic interventions. Prophylaxis with subcutaneous low-dose heparin, 5000 IU every 8 to 12 hours is recommended. Additional benefit is added with the use of a sequential compression lower extremities device when the patient is bedridden. The use of peripherally inserted central catheters is associated with close to 25% local DVT rates, and such lines should be monitored externally for any sign of edema and using Doppler studies to assess for local clot formation. Insertion should be avoided if possible on the weak or paralyzed extremity.

Case Illustrations

Extracranial Arterial Dissection

A 52-year-old white woman was transferred from the local emergency department with headache and slurred speech. A CT scan showed acute infarction in the right middle cerebral artery (MCA) distribution. Her presenting BP was 152/90, and motor power was 5/5 in all four extremities. Magnetic resonance imaging (MRI) showed an acute infarct in the right MCA distribution. The right internal carotid artery (ICA) was occluded on the MR angiogram, which was confirmed with the angiogram showing dissection of the right ICA with thrombosis in the right MCA. Heparin was started without bolus with a partial thromboplastin time and weight-based heparin protocol. Our approach was similar to Schievink et al, who proposed a treatment algorithm for the medical management of ICA dissection.[14] This patient left the hospital 7 days later on oral anticoagulation without any focal deficit (**Fig. 17.2**).

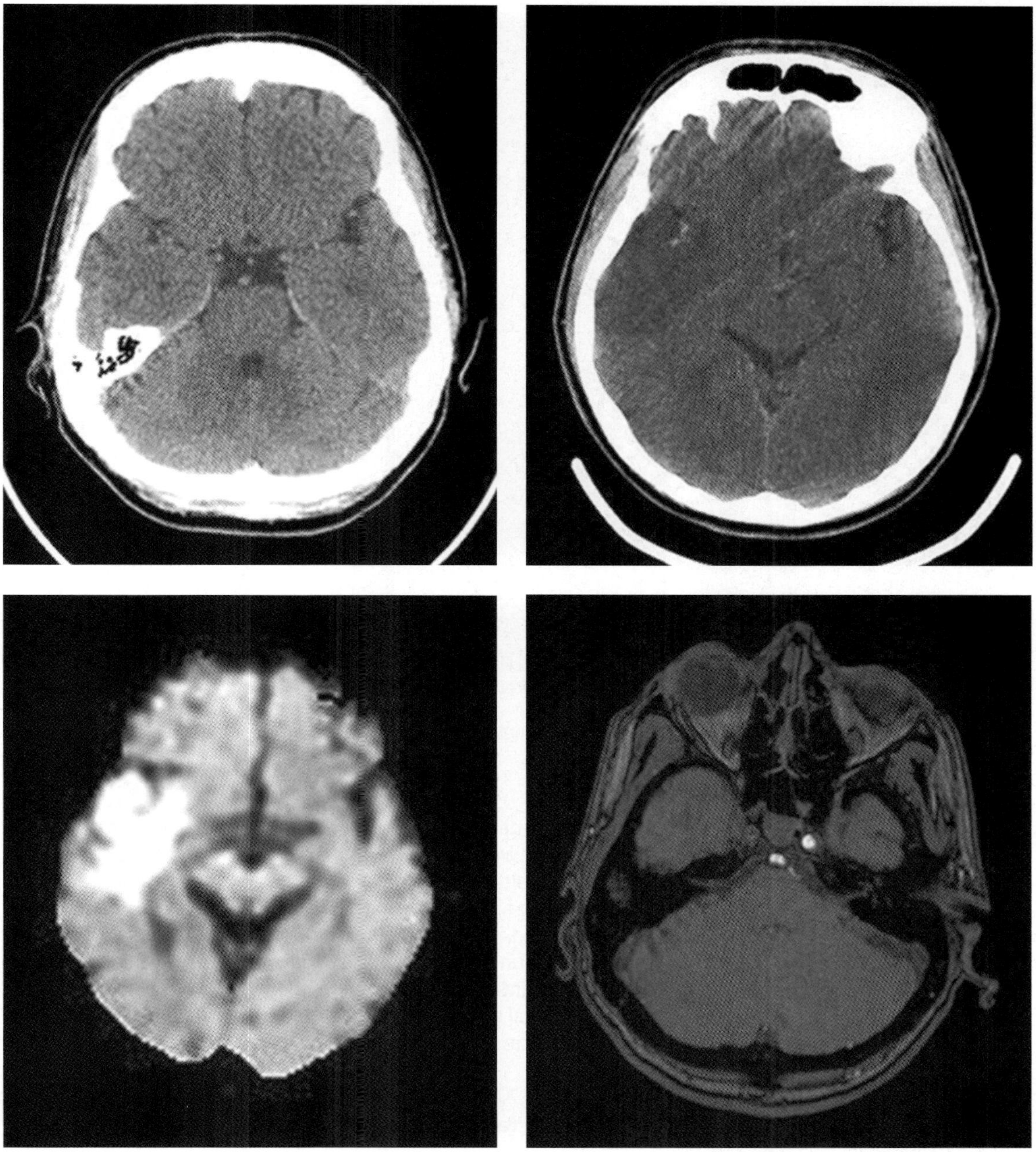

A B C D

Fig. 17.2 (A,B) CT scans showing early right middle cerebral artery territory ischemic injury. **(C)** MRI confirming the finding of the CT scan. **(D)** MR angiogram with no flow in the right internal carotid artery (ICA). *(continued)*

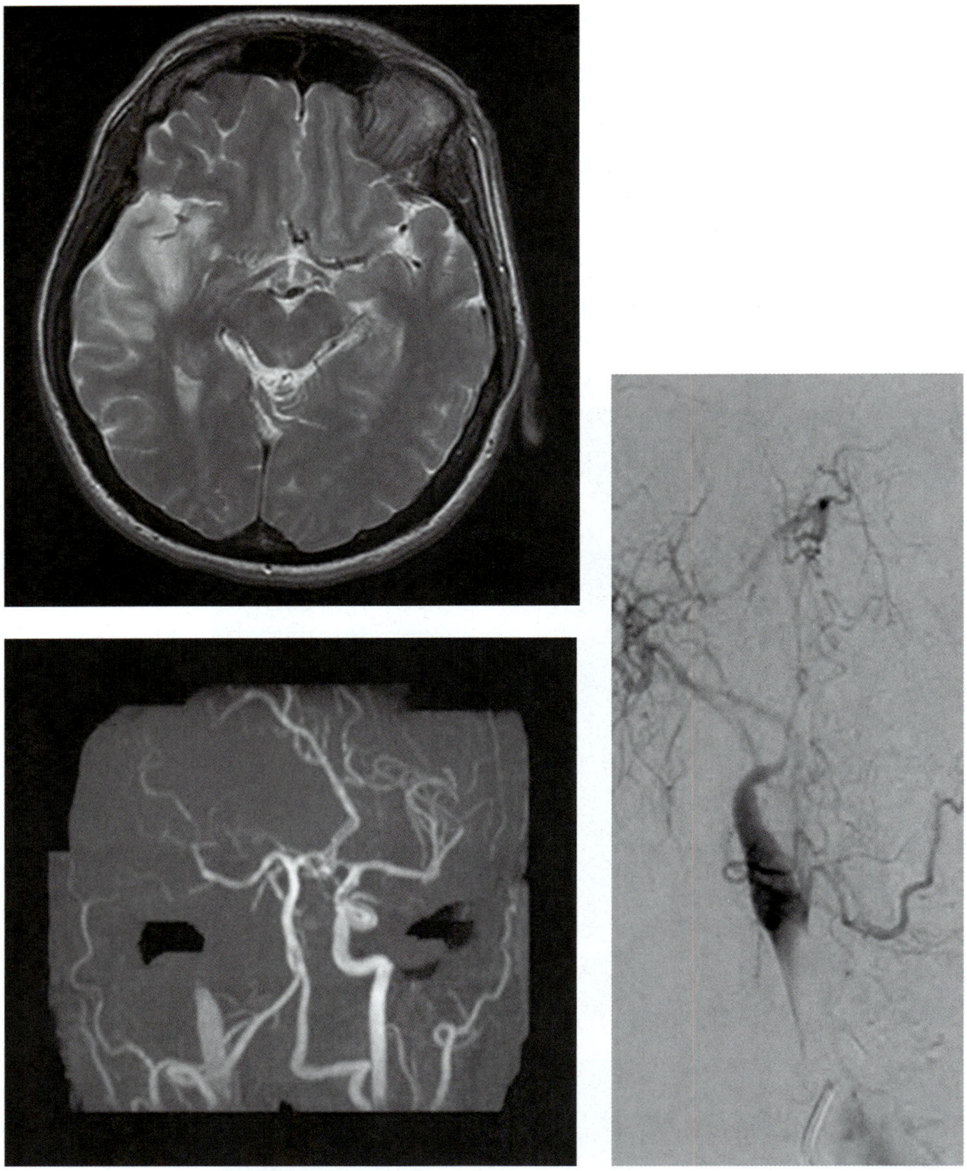

E F G

Fig. 17.2 *(continued)* **(E)** Mild cerebral edema noted on T2-weighted MRI. **(F)** MR angiogram confirming occluded right ICA. **(G)** Cerebral angiogram with limited proximal filling of the right ICA compatible with dissection.

Cerebral Vasospasm

Delayed ischemic neurologic deficit from cerebral vasospasm is a preventable condition. The mortality rate associated with vasospasm is ~15 to 20%. Cerebral autoregulation is impaired in subarachnoid hemorrhage with vasospasm. Cerebral blood flow is dependent on MAP. To lower the ICP and to increase the CPP, the following maneuvers help: central head position, elevation of the head versus lowering the head (based on the fixed blood flow physiology), reducing cerebral edema and reduction of hydrocephalus. BP is optimized by early passive increase in MAP after the cerebral aneurysm is secured. Our agent of choice for active elevation of MAP is phenylephrine. The role of calcium channel blockers is clear except when it leads to a drop in MAP, which is counterintuitive for CPP. Our approach is not to use nimodipine given that it leads to frequent drops in MAP, rather we use lower-dose continuous IV nicardipine. Volume expansion is achieved with the use of normal saline and 25% human albumin. The pulmonary artery occlusive pressure[15] can be used, or if the patient is on the ventilator, the stroke volume variation (SVV) with the arterial line in place can be used. This takes into consideration the relationship of cardiac index and cerebral blood flow. The cardiac index is kept in the range of 4.0 with the use of dobutamine.

Intracranial Arterial Stenosis

A 46-year-old woman presented with slurred speech. An MRI/MRA showed punctate areas of increased diffusion in

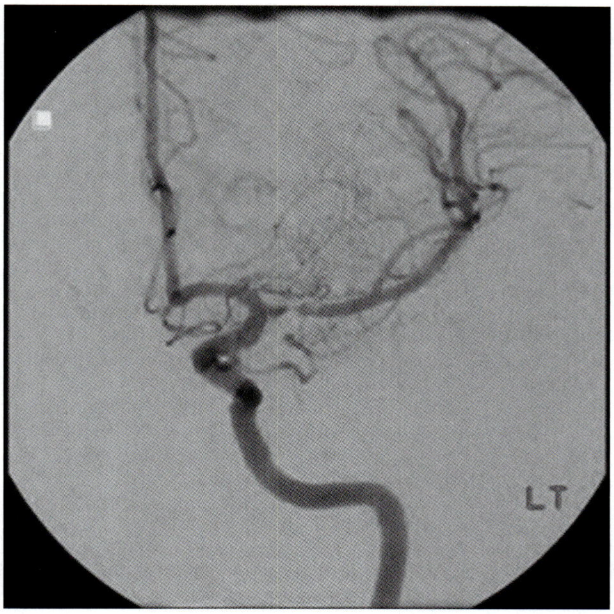

Fig. 17.3 High-grade stenosis of the left middle cerebral artery treated with left extracranial-intracranial bypass and ultimate full recovery.

the left MCA territory in a watershed distribution with poor visualization of the ipsilateral M1 segment of the MCA. The cerebral angiogram showed 90% occlusion of the left MCA M1 segment. Aggressive cerebral perfusion management is the mainstay of therapy to provide blood flow to the MCA territory and prevent severe infarction. This parallels the HHH (hypertensive, hypervolemic, hemodilution) approach used for post–subarachnoid hemorrhage cerebral vasospasm, although the use of calcium channel blockers is omitted. After stabilization, the patient underwent uneventful extracranial-intracranial bypass and left the hospital a week later (**Fig. 17.3**).

Temporal Arteritis

Temporal arteritis is a vasculopathy with middle-size arterial involvement. It should be considered in any stroke patient older than 50 years. A temporal artery biopsy is performed if the erythrocyte sedimentation rate is elevated. High-dose steroids are used even if the diagnosis is not confirmed as untreated disease may lead to acute vision loss.

Avoiding Hemorrhagic Conversion after AIS and rtPA Treatment

Uncontrolled hypertension will directly impact the incidence of ICH in rtPA patients. After rtPA infusion, patients are admitted to the neurocritical care unit, and most of these patients have arterial lines placed for BP control. Nasogastric tubes and urinary catheters are held for some time after tPA. If BP is low, it will worsen the ischemia, especially if the collateral flow is the only way of providing oxygenation to the periinfarct area. In addition to the bleeding risk, reperfusion injury can happen from glutamate and calcium influx. The lysis of clot from post-tPA period can potentially lead to distal small emboli.

For ~36 hours the major complication is hemorrhagic transformation. It may present in two ways–intracranial or systemic. The most common is systemic bleeding. In the NINDS trial[16] the incidence of systematic ICH was 6.4%; the ECASS-II trial (European Cooperative Acute Stroke Study)[17] showed an incidence of 8.8%. The amount of ischemia is one of the main contributors to hemorrhagic transformation. It is not clear if recanalization is directly attributed to this. The other factors contributing to hemorrhagic transformation are older age (usually above 75 years of age), previous head injury or surgery, inappropriate thrombolytic dose, hyperglycemia, amyloid angiopathy, and undiagnosed abnormal vasculature like an arteriovenous malformation or an aneurysm. These patients should be admitted to a neurologic intensive care unit. During close observation, the onset of ICH can be seen, with a sudden increase in BP, focal neurologic deficit, or change in level consciousness. Frequent neurologic examination is performed with GCS checks and if needed, objective measurements of the cerebral blood flow. This can be checked with near-infrared spectroscopy or transcranial Doppler. With the availability of portable CT scans, it is easy to confirm this at bedside. During management, systolic spikes are prevented. In older patients, medication such as morphine used for headache, can lead to venous pooling with a drop in cardiac output and resultant hypotension. The distinction is obvious between pre-tPA control of BP versus post-tPA. The rate of hemorrhage is higher for patients with uncontrolled BP. Once ICH is diagnosed, it should be confirmed that there are not multiple sites of bleeding. The drop in cerebral pressure from lowering the BP versus expansion of hematoma due to uncontrolled BP is the dilemma faced by most of the neurointensivists. Stopping the growth of the hematoma takes precedent over the lower flow to infarct. The sites most commonly affected by bleeding include gastrointestinal, retroperitoneal, nasal, and urinary tracts.

Some general steps for hemorrhage conversion stabilization are shown in **Table 17.3**. Surgical intervention is possible only with good fibrinogen level, adequate clotting, and a completed risk-benefit comparison. The role of neurointensivist is to support the process in a timely fashion.

Table 17.3 Steps to Prevent Hemorrhagic Transformation in Acute Ischemic Stroke

1. Stop the infusion of recombinant tissue plasminogen activator
2. Blood pressure control
3. Maintain fibrinogen level close to 350 mg/dL with cryoprecipitate
4. Surgical intervention

Future Directions

AIS management is evolving. The currently recommended time window for the use of rtPA is 4.5 hours. There are newer thrombolytics like anti-XA agents in the pipeline. The use of neuroprotective agents is being evaluated. Better and more robust multimodality monitoring technologies will change how we manage these patients. The utility of dedicated neurocritical care units will become more obvious as outcome studies become available.

References

1. Hartmann A, Rundek T, Mast H, et al. Mortality and causes of death after first ischemic stroke: the Northern Manhattan Stroke Study. Neurology 2001;57(11):2000–2005
2. van der Worp HB, Kappelle LJ. Complications of acute ischaemic stroke. Cerebrovasc Dis 1998;8(2):124–132
3. Tanne D, Gorman MJ, Bates VE, et al. Intravenous tissue plasminogen activator for acute ischemic stroke in patients aged 80 years and older: the tPA stroke survey experience. Stroke 2000;31(2):370–375
4. Adams HP Jr, Davis PH, Leira EC, et al. Baseline NIH Stroke Scale score strongly predicts outcome after stroke: a report of the Trial of Org 10172 in Acute Stroke Treatment (TOAST). Neurology 1999;53(1):126–131
5. Tanne D, Kasner SE, Demchuk AM, et al. Markers of increased risk of intracerebral hemorrhage after intravenous recombinant tissue plasminogen activator therapy for acute ischemic stroke in clinical practice: the Multicenter rt-PA Stroke Survey. Circulation 2002;105(14):1679–1685
6. Leonardi-Bee J, Bath PM, Phillips SJ, Sandercock PA; IST Collaborative Group. Blood pressure and clinical outcomes in the International Stroke Trial. Stroke 2002;33(5):1315–1320
7. Bruno A, Levine SR, Frankel MR, et al; NINDS rt-PA Stroke Study Group. Admission glucose level and clinical outcomes in the NINDS rt-PA Stroke Trial. Neurology 2002;59(5):669–674
8. Alvarez-Sabín J, Molina CA, Montaner J, et al. Effects of admission hyperglycemia on stroke outcome in reperfused tissue plasminogen activator–treated patients. Stroke 2003;34(5):1235–1241
9. Ribo M, Molina CA, Montaner J, et al. Acute hyperglycemia state is associated with lower tPA-induced recanalization rates in stroke patients. Stroke 2005;36(8):1705–1709
10. Alvarez-Sabín J, Molina CA, Ribó M, et al. Impact of admission hyperglycemia on stroke outcome after thrombolysis: risk stratification in relation to time to reperfusion. Stroke 2004;35(11):2493–2498
11. Lin HJ, Wolf PA, Kelly-Hayes M, et al. Stroke severity in atrial fibrillation: the Framingham Study. Stroke 1996;27(10):1760–1764
12. Mellergård P, Nordström CH. Epidural temperature and possible intracerebral temperature gradients in man. Br J Neurosurg 1990;4(1):31–38
13. Hemmen TM, Lyden PD. Induced hypothermia for acute stroke. Stroke 2007; 38(2, Suppl)794–799
14. Schievink WI. Spontaneous dissection of the carotid and vertebral arteries. N Engl J Med 2001;344(12):898–906
15. Mori K, Arai H, Nakajima K, Tajima A, Maeda M. Hemorheological and hemodynamic analysis of hypervolemic hemodilution therapy for cerebral vasospasm after aneurysmal subarachnoid hemorrhage. Stroke 1995;26(9):1620–1626
16. The National Institute of Neurological Disorders and Stroke rt-PA Stroke Study Group. Tissue plasminogen activator for acute ischemic stroke. N Engl J Med 1995;333(24):1581–1587
17. Hacke W, Kaste M, Fieschi C, et al; Second European-Australasian Acute Stroke Study Investigators. Randomised double-blind placebo-controlled trial of thrombolytic therapy with intravenous alteplase in acute ischaemic stroke (ECASS II). Lancet 1998;352(9136):1245–1251

Chapter 18

Perioperative Management of Patients Undergoing Revascularization

Tariq Janjua

Patients with impaired cerebral blood flow (CBF) may require either surgical or endovascular revascularization. A comprehensive team approach is required to optimize the cerebral perfusion pressure (CPP) and local metabolic needs of the brain in this setting. Familiarity with the use of multiple technologies and pharmacologic agents are important in achieving a good outcome, and maintenance of adequate CPP during this period is critically important to avoid ischemic injury. CPP is determined by multiple factors, the most important of which is the mean arterial pressure (MAP) as detailed below (**Table 18.1**). In these delicate patients, dangerous hemodynamic instability may occur at any time, including prior to and during induction, during the procedure, and in the postoperative period (**Table 18.2**).

Preoperative Preparation

Blood Pressure and Cerebral Perfusion Pressure

As mentioned, maintenance of adequate CPP is the most important factor in avoiding ischemic injury in this population. At our center, an arterial line is placed for all procedures in this patient population. Medications to optimize the systolic blood pressure (BP) and MAP are used on a routine basis to protect the CPP. In our practice, we commonly use a combination of clevidipine or nicardipine with Neo-Synephrine (Bayer Consumer Health, Morristown, NJ) to achieve an optimal MAP. If necessary, dopamine may be used for bradycardia while dobutamine is used for lower cardiac index. We monitor the cardiac index with an arterial line using a flotrac device from Edwards Life Sciences (Irvine, CA).

Airway and Oxygenation

Direct access to the airway may be limited during surgical or neurointerventional revascularization. A proper secure airway must therefore be ensured prior to the start of the procedure.

Electrolytes

Sodium, potassium, calcium, phosphorus, and magnesium are checked and corrected prior to the revascularization procedure. Sodium is kept at a high normal level to limit perioperative ictal activity and to reduce the risk of cerebral edema. The fluid of choice is generally normal saline (sodium concentration of 154 mmol/L) as compared with ringer's lactate (which has only 132 mmol/L). In addition to sodium, magnesium has been shown to play an important role in neuronal excitability.[1] Magnesium is checked and replaced, and kept at a high normal value, preferably using a standardized replacement protocol.

Cardiac

As possible given time constraints, cardiac screening is done to limit the potential perioperative risk for cardiac morbidity. Care should be used when administering a preoperative β-blocker before neurovascular procedures due to its rate-limiting effect, which can ultimately reduce the cardiac index. This may lead to a reduction in the CBF and CPP (**Table 18.3**). For carotid endarterectomy and extracranial-intracranial (EC-IC) bypass procedures, an aspirin is given to reduce the risk of postoperative stroke. Use of a β-blocker may be warranted in these procedures if there is a history of coronary artery disease.

Table 18.1 Cerebral Blood Flow Physiologic Attributes

MAP: perfusion pressure
ΔP: P1 (enter pressure) − P1 (exit pressure)
R: resistance to flow
F: flow volume
CPP = MAP − ICP

Abbreviations: MAP, mean arterial pressure; CPP, cerebral perfusion pressure; ICP, intracranial pressure.

Table 18.3 Relationship of Cardiac Index to Cerebral Perfusion Pressure

CPP α CI
CPP = MAP − ICP
Where MAP = {(CI × BSA) × SVR} + CVP
Therefore, CPP = [{(CI × BSA) × SVR} + CVP] − ICP

Abbreviations: α, directly proportional; CI, cardiac index; CPP, cerebral perfusion pressure; MAP, mean arterial pressure; ICP, intracranial pressure; BSA, body surface area; SVR, systemic volume resistance.

Special Situations

Pregnancy is a challenge during revascularization. If an endovascular procedure is contemplated, the patient is prepared by adequate shielding. The risk–benefit ratio of possible prolonged exposure is discussed with the patient.

Patients with a history of possible significant intravenous (IV) dye reactions are prepared using a steroid protocol. The tubing for the IV and the pressure monitoring is kept at a greater length than usual. The oxygen sensor is placed on the lower limb on the side of the femoral access to check for early blood flow compromise. It is preferable to use one port for medication infusion for better access, and staff can label this port with color-coded tape prior to the procedure.

Intraoperative Anesthetic Considerations

Anesthetics Effect

Different agents are used to induce and maintain the anesthesia depth in patients who will undergo a cerebral revascularization procedure. The limitation of blood flow and potential for postprocedural hyperperfusion of the brain should always be considered. Thiopental loading may reduce postcardiopulmonary bypass neurologic deficits. This agent can be used effectively during the acute resuscitation of malignant intracranial pressure, reducing the metabolic activity of the brain. Most routinely used volatile anesthetics will similarly reduce the metabolic activity of the brain, and propofol can reduce the cerebral metabolic rate of oxygen ($CMRO_2$) by 50%, which helps combat the reduced blood flow during these procedures.[2] Etomidate will suppress the electroencephalographic (EEG) results but will not cause the myocardial depression that may be seen with other previously mentioned agents. In theory, etomidate, thiopental, and ketamine can all reduce nitric oxide levels in acute ischemic stroke (AIS), which could reduce blood flow to the penumbra area.[3] In addition, etomidate is a potent suppressant of corticosteroid synthesis in the adrenal gland, which may become important in a hypotensive bypass patient.[4]

Table 18.2 Perioperative Hypertension

Presurgery and induction
Intraoperative
Recovery phase
24–48-hour postoperative period

Volatile agents for anesthesia are vasoactive with direct effect on the cerebral tone. Hypocarbia and reduction in the cerebral metabolic rate (CMR) with vasodilatation must be monitored. For most agents, when the minimal alveolar concentration (MAC) exceeds 0.6, the direct vasodilating effect becomes more pronounced. Isoflurane decreases $CMRO_2$ and has a minimal effect on the CBF at levels below 0.6 MAC. Shunting from the abnormal hemisphere to the normal hemisphere can increase potential intraoperative ischemia and is a concern at higher MAC levels. Desflurane may have a similar effect on the CBF, except the sympathetic stimulation with higher BP and CPP may be beneficial after revascularization. Sevoflurane is the least vasoactive and is most frequently used in the pediatric population. It can lead to emergence agitation, which is controlled with low-dose propofol or dexmedetomidine.[5]

The adjuvant use of opioids leads to improved intraoperative BP control and more rapid emergence from the effects of anesthesia. Opioid pain control and antitussive effects are complementary, and agents commonly used during cranial procedures are sufentanil, remifentanil, and fentanyl.

CEA requires smooth induction with a goal of minimal BP changes. Hypocapnia is avoided to prevent cerebral vasoconstriction. This is due to the steal phenomenon after hypocapnia where shunting happens from the abnormal side to the normal side. Hyperventilation may have a role to reduce the blood flow only when hyperperfusion is suspected after the procedure, although no study has shown benefit in prevention of hyperperfusion from this approach. In EC-IC bypass for moyamoya disease, it is prudent to maintain strict normocapnia to avoid vasoconstriction as well as regional steal.[6]

Bradycardia and hypotension due to carotid sinus manipulation in CEA can be reduced with local anesthetic to the carotid sinus. The same effect can be seen during the inflation of a balloon or deployment of a stent during carotid angioplasty. Atropine or glycopyrrolate is used for this, and the patient can be prepared with an external pacer in case these medications do not work. The use of local anesthetic technique for CEA has some advantages, including the ease of direct neurologic examinations, less hemodynamic instability, and reduced intraoperative shunt use. The General Anesthesia versus Local Anesthesia for Carotid Surgery (GALA) trial did not show a definite difference in outcomes between general and local anesthesia for carotid surgery. The anesthetist and surgeon, in consultation with the patient, should decide which anesthetic technique to use.[7] If a cervical plexus block is used for the regional anesthesia, possible complications, include recurrent laryngeal and glossopharyngeal nerve injury leading to hoarseness and dysphagia, respectively. Other less common complications are subarachnoid injection of local anesthesia leading to seizures, blockage of phrenic nerve with prolonged ventilator time, and Horner syndrome from sympathetic block.

For neurointerventional radiology (NIR), the sedation protocols are variable.[8] Agents like midazolam and fentanyl with low-dose propofol are used. Propofol can be replaced with dexmedetomidine or remifentanil. The airway is kept under direct watch if the patient is not intubated.

Cerebral Perfusion Pressure

The ideal CPP depends on multiple factors. During a craniotomy, when the blood flow is limited, the CPP should be kept on the high side. Long-standing hypertension suggests a higher CPP requirement, with the goal being 70 mm Hg or higher. Hypotension is avoided to minimize the time below CPP 60 mm Hg. Elevation of MAP is achieved as necessary with an α-agonist like phenylephrine and the addition of 25% albumin.

On a simple level, it should be remembered that ICP can be affected by patient positioning. With the prone position, abdominal pressure is increased, venous drainage is reduced, and the head may be below the level of the heart. Venous outflow reduction can also result from hyperrotation or hyperflexion of the neck. This surgical positioning is complicated with application of positive end expiratory pressure (PEEP) during positive pressure ventilation. AutoPEEP in patients with COPD will exacerbate this relationship. The total PEEP (intrinsic and extrinsic) during controlled mechanical ventilation for the neurovascular procedure is a better estimation of venous return than individual values.

$$PEEP_t = PEEPe + PEEPi$$

During CEA, the cross-clamping time is kept to a minimum. The need for a shunt can be determined with intraoperative use of EEG and transcranial Doppler.[9]

Blood Flow Monitoring

The manipulation of arterial CO_2 is a means for altering both the CBF and the cerebral blood volume (CBV). Hypocapnia will reduce flow and volume and thus ICP. But this should only be used if the benefit outweighs the risks involved with potentially limiting flow. If applied, hyperventilation should be terminated when the intended goal has been achieved or is no longer needed. The higher pH associated with hypocapnia may have an impact on lowering the seizure threshold. The blood–brain barrier (BBB) permeability is increased with ammonia, which may impact patients with liver impairment.

Different modalities may be used for CBF monitoring.[9] These include transcranial Doppler, NIRS, surface Doppler on the bypass track, and an EEG with signal averaging. The volume needs and responsiveness for lower BP or CPP can be measured with stroke volume variation (SVV), which is checked with the formula shown below and which can be easily calculated by looking at the compressed arterial line waveform.[10]

$$SVV = \frac{SV_{max} - SV_{min}}{SV_{mean}}$$

Where: SV_{max} is maximal stroke volume, SV_{min} is minimal stroke volume, and SV_{mean} is the mean of the given stroke volume maximum and minimum.

Coagulation

Venous air embolism (VAE) is a preventable complication of revascularization craniotomy. The factors leading to VAE include the height gradient between the heart and the site of surgery and the venous system's being open to the atmosphere. This is most problematic when operating in the posterior fossa in a sitting position, which should never be necessary for surgical revascularization including when performing posterior inferior cerebellar artery revascularization.

During surgery, a decrease in $ETCO_2$ is concerning for air embolism. Clinical examination will show signs of bronchoconstriction with hypoxemia. Rarely airlock can happen where air can block the right ventricular outflow with cardiac arrest. The presence of a patent foramen ovale can lead to right to left sudden shunt with paradoxical air embolism and stroke. If VAE is suspected, the surgical field is covered with saline followed by repositioning to make the heart higher than the head by tilting the bed down. Aspiration of air is performed with a multilumen central catheter with the tip positioned 2 cm below the superior vena cava–right atrium junction or a single-lumen catheter 3 cm above this junction. Meanwhile, the jugular veins are compressed temporarily with no PEEP on the ventilator.

There are clinical indications for anticoagulation in certain revascularization procedures. Systemic heparinization is generally performed before the cross-clamping for CEA. Long saphenous vein grafts for EC-IC bypass may require intraoperative low-dose heparin to keep the graft open. The activated clotting time (ACT) is checked during and after endovascular procedures, and heparin is given to target ACT to at least two times normal or above 250 seconds. This may be reversed at the end with protamine at the discretion of the surgeon. Antiplatelet agents are used for the purpose of management of smaller clots that may have formed during the procedure due to platelet aggregation. 2B/3A inhibitors, and agents such as bivalirudin may be used to treat acute intraluminal thrombus formation as well.[11]

Hypothermia

The jury is still out on the role of intraoperative hypothermia in cerebral revascularization. Experimental and some clinical studies have shown some evidence that mild to moderate hypothermia reduces the $CMRO_2$ and ultimately the size of ischemia.[12] During revascularization surgery, the control of temperature is important, and a perioperative increase in temperature will increase the $CMRO_2$. We have generally opted for mild hypothermia perioperatively during revascularization procedures but have not employed more aggressive cooling measures in the absence of significant ischemic injury.

Postoperative Monitoring

All postanesthesia care units should have strict monitoring guidelines for systolic BP, oxygen saturation, MAP, and neurologic examination. Obviously, the airway should be secure before the patient leaves the operating room or endovascular catheterization laboratory. Close monitoring every 5 to 10 minutes is done with a one-to-one staffing model if the level of consciousness is not fully compatible with airway protection.

Sedation and Liberation from the Airway

Postoperative mechanical ventilation is continued for a certain period if there is an oxygenation abnormality, if the airway is not patent, if the BP is very high or low, or if there is raised ICP or brainstem injury. If hypothermia is present, the patient may shiver, which can increase CO_2 production. This becomes a management issue when the spontaneous ventilation cannot maintain the demand, as in patients with chronic obstructive pulmonary disease. We have found dexmedetomidine to be a useful agent in maintaining the sedation for emergence and extubation. The aim is to avoid hypertension, tachycardia, and excessive coughing to prevent anastomotic dehiscence and bleeding.

Blood Pressure Control

Normovolemia is the goal after all revascularization. We prefer colloids in the setting of hypovolemic hypotension, and our agent of choice is 25% albumin, administered as either 50 or 100 mL every 6 to 8 hours. Hematocrit is kept above 30% or hemoglobin at 10 g/dL to improve both the oxygen-carrying capacity and also BP. Any coagulopathy is corrected if it is not iatrogenically induced on an intentional basis.

Electrolytes

Sodium is kept close to the higher end of normal range with 0.9% saline during and after the procedure. The magnesium levels are checked and kept at high-normal levels. This will keep the seizure threshold at a high level and reduce the risk of regional edema. The glucose needs at the regional level are different after revascularization due to newly improved blood flow. We target normoglycemia with the goal in the 100 to 140 range. Although hyperglycemia may increase ischemic injury, hypoglycemia may be equally dangerous, and normoglycemia should be the ultimate goal.

Seizure Prevention

CBF is improved after revascularization, which is an improved condition. But in the setting of a chronic ischemic condition, autoregulation is impaired, and the brain cannot produce normal physiologic vasoconstriction due to chronic low blood flow at baseline. This dysautoregulation may lead to a lowering of the seizure threshold. We have generally used prophylaxis in the perioperative period to decrease the risk of a seizure. Intraoperatively, the effect of anesthetics helps suppress any seizure activity, but in the recovery phase, phenytoin remains the best studied agent followed by carbamazepine, valproic acid, and levetiracetam. One newer agent for partial seizure, lacosamide, has shown promise in decreasing seizure risk in the setting of acute focal brain conditions. Both phenytoin and valproic acid are inducers of liver enzymes, which later can cause hyponatremia, another possible cause of seizures. The use of halothane should be restricted in these patients due to synergistic hepatic toxicity. If neuromuscular blocking agents are used, the paralytic effect is prolonged and caution is required due to the synergistic effects with these antiepileptics.[13]

Discharge Criteria

After revascularization, the patients are best cared for in an environment in which a close watch can be kept on the patency of the newly provided blood flow to brain. Because of complex postoperative care and monitoring requirements, neurocritical care units must stay on the cutting edge to meet those goals. The assurance of a proper airway, hemodynamic stability, and neurologic functional improvement requires frequent reassessment by neurologically trained nurses to prepare them for discharge.

References

1. Mack WJ, Kellner CP, Sahlein DH, et al. Intraoperative magnesium infusion during carotid endarterectomy: a double-blind placebo-controlled trial. J Neurosurg 2009;110(5):961–967
2. Strebel S, Lam AM, Matta B, Mayberg TS, Aaslid R, Newell DW. Dynamic and static cerebral autoregulation during isoflurane, desflurane, and propofol anesthesia. Anesthesiology 1995;83(1):66–76
3. Galley HF, Webster NR. Brain nitric oxide synthase activity is decreased by intravenous anesthetics. Anesth Analg 1996;83(3):591–594
4. Absalom A, Pledger D, Kong A. Adrenocortical function in critically ill patients 24 h after a single dose of etomidate. Anaesthesia 1999; 54(9):861–867
5. Strebel S, Lam AM, Matta B, Mayberg TS, Aaslid R, Newell DW. Dynamic and static cerebral autoregulation during isoflurane, desflurane, and propofol anesthesia. Anesthesiology 1995;83(1):66–76

6. Oshima H, Katayama Y, Hirayama T. Intracerebral steal phenomenon associated with global hyperemia in moyamoya disease during revascularization surgery. J Neurosurg 2000;92(5):949–954
7. Lewis SC, Warlow CP, Bodenham AR, et al; GALA Trial Collaborative Group. General anaesthesia versus local anaesthesia for carotid surgery (GALA): a multicentre, randomised controlled trial. Lancet 2008;372(9656):2132–2142
8. See JJ, Manninen PH. Anesthesia for neuroradiology. Curr Opin Anaesthesiol 2005;18(4):437–441
9. Rowed DW, Houlden DA, Burkholder LM, Taylor AB. Comparison of monitoring techniques for intraoperative cerebral ischemia. Can J Neurol Sci 2004;31(3):347–356
10. Berkenstadt H, Margalit N, Hadani M, et al. Stroke volume variation as a predictor of fluid responsiveness in patients undergoing brain surgery. Anesth Analg 2001;92(4):984–989
11. Memon MZ, Georgiadis AL, Vazquez G, et al. Safety and efficacy of anticoagulation with bivalirudin in neuro-endovascular procedures. Stroke 2009;40:13
12. Choi R, Andres RH, Steinberg GK, Guzman R. Intraoperative hypothermia during vascular neurosurgical procedures. Neurosurg Focus 2009;26(5):E24
13. Wright PM, McCarthy G, Szenohradszky J, Sharma ML, Caldwell JE. Influence of chronic phenytoin administration on the pharmacokinetics and pharmacodynamics of vecuronium. Anesthesiology 2004;100(3):626–633

Chapter 19

Postprocedure Complications and Complication Avoidance

Edward M. Manno and Tariq Janjua

Postoperative observation and management of postprocedural complications is a crucial role for neurocritical care. Although most neurosurgical textbooks emphasize surgical technique, little is often written addressing postprocedural complications. Treatment remains largely anecdotal based on variably sized cohorts. In this chapter we attempt to synthesize the available knowledge on the complication rates and management of the most common neurovascular procedures.

Carotid Endarterectomy

Carotid endarterectomy (CEA) for primary and secondary prevention of stroke is one of the most common surgical procedures performed in the United States.[1] Epidemiologic studies have demonstrated that the long-term benefit of surgery can be negated by excessive postoperative morbidity.[2,3] Meticulous surgical techniques and careful patient selection has been emphasized; however, despite this there still remains significant information on CEA complications.

Complications

Cranial Nerve Deficits

The most common complication post-CEA is the development of a cranial nerve deficit. Individual cranial nerve deficits occur in 6 to 17% of procedures.[4] The most common nerves involved include the facial, recurrent and superior laryngeal, hypoglossal, marginal mandibular, and the glossopharyngeal. The North American Symptomatic Carotid Endarterectomy Trial (NASCET) reported a 7.6% incidence of cranial nerve deficits.[2] The wide variation in reported deficits, however, probably represents the degree of scrutiny involved when looking for a deficit. When laryngoscopy is included, complication rates approach 16%.[5]

Fortunately, most cranial nerve deficits are temporary and resolve in 3 to 6 months. Most are not considered serious complications and are due to traction and compression injuries and not transection of the nerves. One potentially serious complication can occur if bilateral recurrent laryngeal or hypoglossal nerves are damaged during bilateral procedures. This can seriously impair respiration and airway control leading to a chronic severe cough and aspiration.[4,5] Laryngoscopic examination of these nerves prior to staged bilateral operations should be performed to ensure the integrity and function of the involved muscles and nerves.[5]

Neck Hematomas

Wound hematomas have ben estimated to occur in ~5.5% of procedures. Most are small and nonsignificant representing oozing from the surgical site, which can be aggravated by antiplatelet agents and heparinization. Rupture of the arterial suture site is rare and is usually fatal. Bleeding requiring reoperation has been reported to occur in 0.7 to 2.5% of cases.[6] Reoperation for examination should be considered for any obvious hematoma. More urgent evacuation is needed for rapidly expanding hematomas that can compromise airways. Emergent bedside evacuation is recommended in this clinical situation even prior to endotracheal intubation.[1] **Figure 19.1** shows an example of right neck hematoma next to the CEA site. This patient required an emergent tracheostomy and control of bleeding.

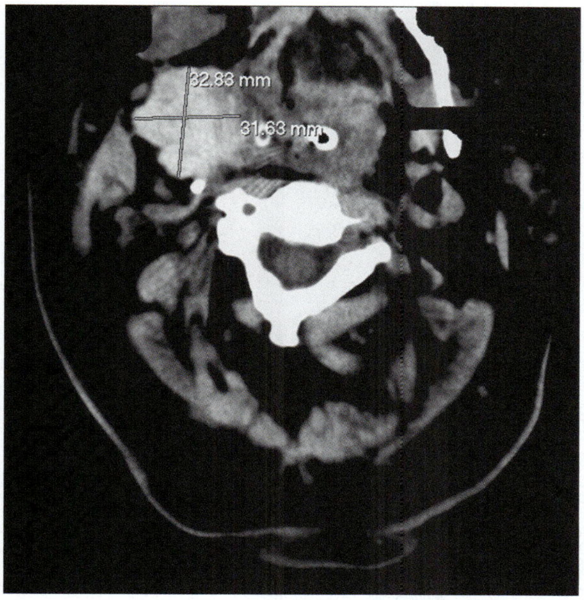

Fig. 19.1 Right neck hematoma after an elective right carotid endarterectomy.

Ischemic Stroke

Operative stroke is the measure by which CEA is evaluated. Several clinical series evaluating operative stroke during CEA were performed in the 1970s and 1980s. Most were from academic institutions using cerebral monitoring and shunting techniques. The reported stroke rates ranged between 1.6 to 6.5%.[1] In general stroke rates need to be ≤3% in asymptomatic patients and ≤6% for symptomatic patients for long-term benefit from the procedure.[7] Questions have been raised whether low-volume centers can meet these criteria.[8] Stroke rates are reported higher with contralateral carotid occlusion, ulcerated plaques, and patients with previous strokes.[1,4]

Continuous transcranial Doppler ultrasound has revealed that 30% of CEAs will have evidence for distal emboli during the procedure. Most are considered gaseous emboli and are of little significance; however, the appearance and timing of these emboli have provided clues as to when distal thrombotic emboli may occur.[9] Operative strokes are believed to occur during prepping of the site, dissection and manipulation of the carotid, and during cross clamping. Cerebral monitoring, arterial shunts, and other protective devices have all been developed to decrease the incidence of operative strokes.[9]

About half of all strokes occur postoperatively. The mechanism is presumably secondary to emboli from an acute carotid occlusion or microembolization from the denuded endothelium of the surgical site. Cerebral hypoperfusion can occur but is believed to occur less frequently than distal emboli.[9]

Antiplatelet agents are used almost universally by surgeons before, during, and after the procedure. Heparin is similarly used during surgery, but there are variations in practice as to whether anticoagulation is continued, discontinued, or reversed after surgery.[1,9,10]

The decision to consider reexploration of the site can be quite difficult because many postoperative deficits may be transient and a reoperation could potentially worsen the situation. An urgent reoperation is encouraged when a patient awakens with a severe neurologic deficit.[9]

Myocardial Infarction

Carotid artery disease is a marker for coronary artery disease. Myocardial infarctions are common post CEA occurring in 2 to 3% of patients and accounting for 40 to 50% of all late deaths.[9] Patients should have postoperative electrocardiographic (ECG) monitoring and be followed closely for signs of myocardial ischemia. A low threshold should be given to send cardiac biomarkers for suspected cardiac ischemia.

Postoperative Hyperperfusion

As our understanding of cerebral autoregulation has improved, the occurrence of postoperative hyperperfusion has become rare. Nevertheless, it remains part of the differential diagnosis of new neurologic change in the postoperative period. **Figure 19.2** shows an example of a left frontal intracranial hemorrhage that developed after an internal carotid artery stenting procedure. The repeat angiogram clearly shows hyperperfusion of the left anterior cerebral artery. This complication can be avoided by carefully controlling the blood pressure after revascularization. Anticoagulants and antiplatelet therapies are closely monitored as these can play a role in hemorrhagic conversion of the hyperperfusion areas of the brain.

Postoperative Management

Postoperative management of patients undergoing a CEA poses some specific challenges. Hemodynamic instability is common and includes persistent hypertension, bradycardia and hypotension, and normal perfusion pressure breakthrough. Careful blood pressure, fluid and electrolyte management is necessary to avoid large fluctuations in hemodynamics.

Postoperative patients are typically followed in a postanesthesia care unit for 2 to 3 hours after CEA. A slow emergence from anesthesia may be beneficial in moderating blood pressure changes postoperatively.[11] Analgesia may need to be limited to facilitate a neurologic exam. Patients may arrive in the intensive care unit (ICU) intubated. Care should be taken to inspect the surgical site for bleeding or swelling. Any deviation of the airway should prompt a return to the operating room. A neurologic assessment should focus on focal deficits and/or subtle cranial nerve deficits. A 12-lead ECG should be performed along with a thorough cardiac assessment. Most patients are admitted to the ICU overnight. Swallowing and orthostasis should be evaluated prior to dismissal from the ICU.[11,12]

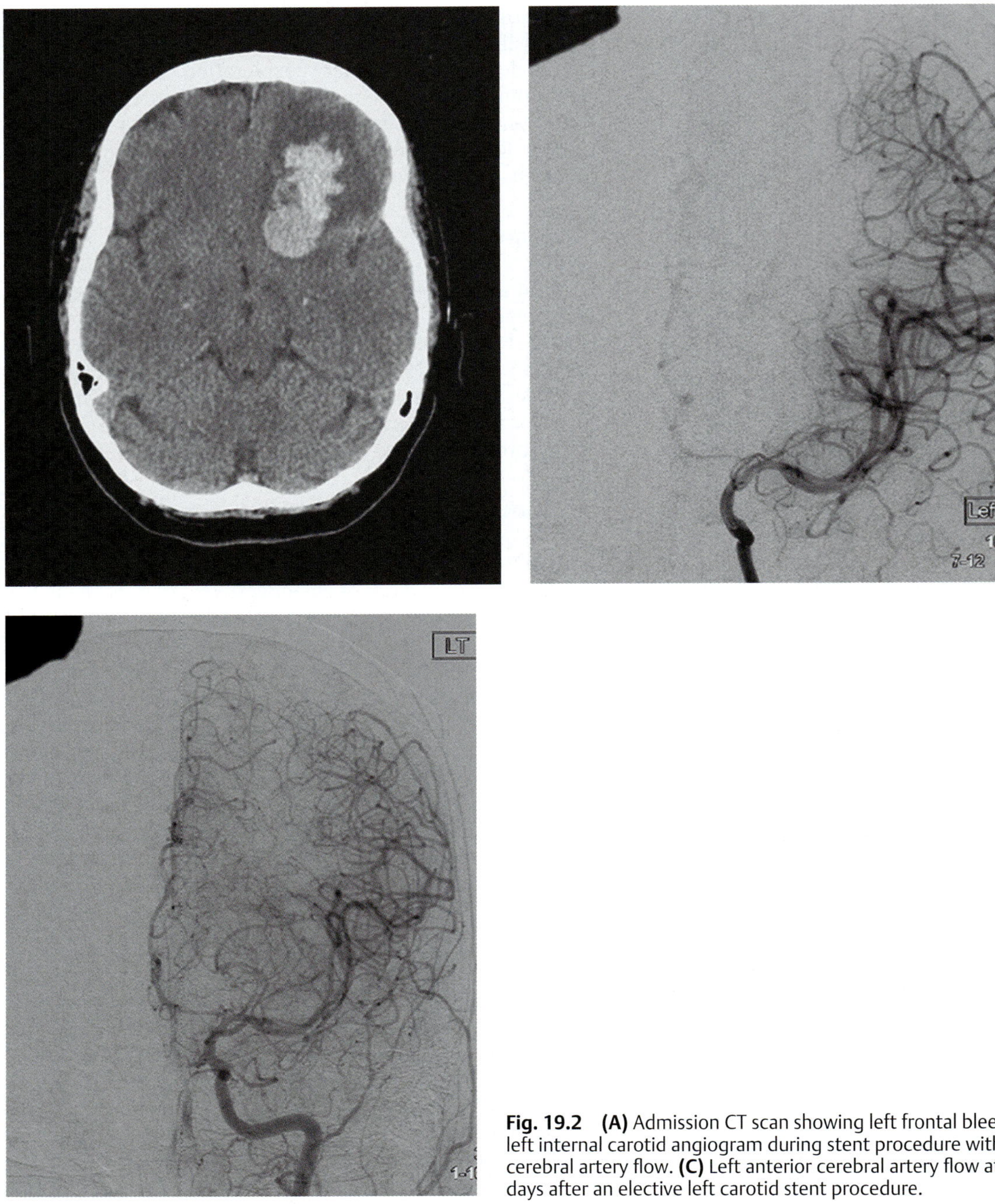

A B C

Fig. 19.2 **(A)** Admission CT scan showing left frontal bleeding. **(B)** Baseline left internal carotid angiogram during stent procedure with limited left anterior cerebral artery flow. **(C)** Left anterior cerebral artery flow at the time of admission 5 days after an elective left carotid stent procedure.

Postoperative hypertension is common, occurring in 50 to 60% of patients. Persistent hypertension is associated with worse outcomes and correlates with severe preoperative hypertension.[13] As a result, some experts recommend delaying elective surgery until preoperative hypertension is controlled.[1] Hypertension and hypotension are prevalent after carotid reconstruction and severe blood pressure fluctuations can occur after bilateral CEA.[14]

Hypertension is postulated to be mediated through damage to the sinus nerve of Hering. Under these circumstances damage to this nerve may be misinterpreted through the normal neurologic reflex arc mediated at the brainstem as a sustained reduction in blood pressure. Thus, compensatory reflex mechanisms designed to induce hypertension are initiated. Postoperative bradycardia and hypotension can also occur when the sinus nerve function is preserved. Under these circumstances carotid sinus transmural pressure is increased post CEA. This is interpreted as sustained hypertension, which initiates mechanisms to lower blood pressure.[1]

This hypothesis has been supported by several reports of successful treatment of postoperative hypertension with local anesthesia to the sinus nerve.[1,15,16] Towne, however, could not reproduce these findings with transection of the nerve.[17] Wade et al suggested that the effect of the sinus nerve decreased significantly with age and was severely attenuated in the elderly, a group commonly treated with CEA.[18] Finally, Ransen et al noted that hypovolemia was the major contributing factor to postoperative hypotension. Similarly, bradycardia was a problem only in the setting of hypovolemia. In most instances this can be easily corrected.[19]

The treatment of post-CEA hypertension is somewhat controversial. Some authors have argued that transient postoperative hypertension should not be aggressively treated to avoid significant drops in blood pressure, which could potentially be harmful. Postoperative hypertension is argued to be in reaction to and not the cause of neurologic deficits in many instances.[20]

It is generally agreed, however, that severe hypertension should be treated and that significant fluctuations in blood pressure should be avoided. The most feared consequence of uncontrolled hypertension is normal perfusion pressure breakthrough with subsequent intracerebral hemorrhage. Cerebral autoregulation is believed to be downregulated in the ipsilateral hemisphere in severe carotid stenosis due to a persistent decrease in perfusion pressure. Once the stenosis is removed the downregulated hemisphere is subjected to relative high-perfusion pressures even in the setting of normal blood pressure. Sundt et al demonstrated a significant increase in cerebral blood flow ipsilateral to a CEA in the setting of normal blood pressure.[21] Even with large increases in blood flow intracerebral hemorrhage occurs in <1% of CEAs.[1] Risk factors include a severe preoperative stenosis, preoperative hypertension, and sustained postoperative systolic pressures >180 mm Hg.[14]

Modest blood pressure management post CEA is probably prudent. Systolic blood pressure should be maintained within 20% of preoperative levels.[1,11,12] Preoperative antihypertensive medications should be continued. Nitroprusside or nicardipine drips can be initiated if needed. Esmolol drips may be preferable if bradycardia is not present. Hypotension is best treated with volume replacement. In rare instances vasopressor support with phenylephrine or norepinephrine may be required. Atropine or glycopyrrolate should be available at the bedside for postoperative bradycardia.

Carotid Angioplasty and Stenting

Carotid angioplasty and stent placement have similar complications as CEA. The most common complication reported is procedural and postprocedural embolic stroke. Several large multicenter trials have provided direct comparisons of CEA to placement of carotid stents for both symptomatic and asymptomatic carotid stenosis. The SPACE (Stent-Supported Percutaneous Angioplasty of the Carotid Artery versus Endarterectomy) and EVA-3S (Endarterectomy versus Angioplasty in Patients with Severe Symptomatic Carotid Stenosis) trials both failed to confirm noninferiority of carotid stenting to CEA.[22,23] In EVA-3S, a 2.5 increased relative risk of stroke and 30-day mortality in the carotid stent group prompted early discontinuation of the study.[23] Patients >80 years and those with hemispheric symptoms appear to be a subgroup of patients at higher risk for stroke.[23] Two-year restenosis rates were also reported higher with carotid stenting.[24]

Despite these findings carotid stenting may prove to be beneficial in patients with recurrent stenosis, history of neck radiation, or severe medical comorbidities.[25,26] Decreased medical complications with carotid stents were reported in both large trials.[22,23]

Several preliminary studies have reported a decreased incidence of stroke using a variety of procedural cerebral protective devices.[27] Multicenter trials now require these devices. In addition, 3-day pretreatment with aspirin (100–300 mg) and clopidogrel (75 mg) is often required.[28]

Bradycardia and hypotension can occur after carotid angioplasty and/or stenting. One retrospective analysis of over 400 patients reported bradycardia (<50 beats/min) and/or hypotension (systolic blood pressure less than 80 mm Hg) in 7% of carotid stents.[29] Vasopressors were required in 2% of patients.[29] Prophylactic placement and use of transcutaneous temporary cardiac pacing during carotid angioplasty and stenting has been reported.[30]

Therapeutic Occlusion of the Internal Carotid Artery

Therapeutic occlusion of the internal carotid artery can be used as treatment for cerebral aneurysms and pseudoaneurysms or for carotid blowout syndromes. Emergent occlusion of the internal carotid artery without prior evaluation with test balloon occlusion results in stroke and death rates as high as 26% and 12%, respectively.[31] Clinical testing with balloon occlusion decreases the stroke rate to <5%.[32] Adjunctive testing with cerebral blood flow measures is often used, but has not been demonstrated to decrease the procedural complication rate. Despite this, extracranial-intracranial (EC-IC) bypass is often employed prior to carotid sacrifice if ipsilateral cerebral hypoperfusion is documented with test balloon occlusion.[33]

The most common complication after sacrifice of the carotid artery is ischemic stroke. It is speculated that the etiology is embolic because prior testing usually will define patients at risk for cerebral hypoperfusion. There is some suggestion that surgical sacrifice of the vessel has higher stroke rates than balloon occlusion possibly because of greater manipulation of the vessel or the inability to use adequate anticoagulation.[34] The balloon itself can also fail and serve as a nidus for embolization.[35]

Other complications with carotid occlusion can occur. Cerebral aneurysms can become painful and cause cranial nerve deficits as they thrombose, subsequently compressing local structures.[36] Formation of new aneurysms can also occur after carotid occlusion. The presumed mechanism is through increased blood flow through the contralateral carotid artery. Anterior communicating artery aneurysms most commonly develop. Subsequently, the risk of subarachnoid hemorrhage is greatly increased.[37]

Cerebral Revascularization

Cerebral revascularization techniques continue to be used for the treatment of cerebral aneurysms, moyamoya disease, cranial base tumors, and for sacrifice of the carotid or vertebral arteries.[38–40] Saphenous vein and radial artery grafts are most commonly used. Radial artery grafts are easier to perform and may have improved longer-term patency. They however cannot be used in situations where higher flow volumes are required.[38–40] The major complication of arterial vasospasm has been overcome by expanding the vessel prior to implantation with a pressure distention technique. Saphenous vein grafts are more commonly used but are technically more challenging to place. They are used when high flow volumes are required. Focal turbulence however can lead to kinking and graft occlusion.[38–40]

Complications of bypass procedures include intraoperative and postoperative graft occlusion. Intraoperative angiography is recommended if Doppler or direct evaluation of the graft does not demonstrate good flow. Postoperative occlusion is rare if intraoperative flow is adequate. Sekhar reported a cerebral infarction rate of 16% postprocedure; however, most patients made excellent recoveries.[39] Epidural hematomas can develop in this setting.

Postoperative management may include subcutaneous heparin 5000 units every 8 hours and/or aspirin 325 mg daily. To prevent possible hyperperfusion syndromes, maintenance of systolic blood pressures below 120 mm Hg in normotensive and 140 mm Hg in hypertensive patients has been recommended for 1 week. Replacement bypasses can have blood pressure limits liberalized after 2–3 days.[40]

Indirect methods for revascularization have been developed for the pediatric population with moyamoya disease. These include encephalomyosynangiosis, encephaloduroarteriosynangiosis, encephalomyosynangiosis, encephaloduroarteriomyosynangiosis, and various combinations of these procedures. All have reported varying degrees of success, although one report suggested that encephalogaleosynangiosis was superior to encephaloduroarteriosynangiosis alone.[41] Possible complications of these procedures include focal seizures, wound infections, and chronic subdural hematomas. Ischemic symptoms in moyamoya can be aggravated by hyperventilation and hypotension and should be meticulously avoided both intraoperatively and postoperatively.[42] Direct methods of revascularization in the pediatric population have proved technically challenging but have been shown to be feasible.[43]

Intracranial Angioplasty and Stenting

The Warfarin-Aspirin Symptomatic Intracranial Disease (WASID) and GESICA studies have both reported 2-year stroke rates at 13 to 14% despite medical treatment for symptomatic intracranial stenosis.[44,45] Most of these events also appear to occur within the first month of symptoms[45] arguing for aggressive early interventional treatment. Multiple reports have suggested feasibility of both angioplasty and stenting of the intracranial arteries.[46] The GESICA study also reported a higher neurologic event rate in patients with hemodynamically significant stenosis.[45] Unfortunately, the periprocedural complication rate was 14% and 2-year subsequent stroke rates were only decreased to 7% making interventions difficult to routinely recommend.[45] Drug eluting stents may provide some additional benefit to routine stenting procedures.[47]

A retrospective review of vertebrobasilar stenting procedures reported a neurologic complication rate of 5.5% for the vertebral artery and 17.3% for the basilar artery. Mortality rates were listed as 0.3% and 3.2%, respectively.[48] The Carotid and Vertebral Artery Transluminal Angioplasty Study (CAVATAS) failed to show a benefit to endovascular treatment of vertebral artery stenosis, however, the numbers were quite limited. In addition, most patients had carotid artery territory stroke or myocardial infarctions in the follow-up period rather than a stroke in the involved vertebral artery.[49] Restenosis rates were high in the CAVATAS trial[50] and angioplasty of the vertebral origin has fallen into disfavor due to a high restenosis rate.[51] Hyperfusion as a complication after cerebral artery stenting has been reported.[52]

Venous Sinus Recanalization

Thrombolysis both with and without mechanical clot manipulation has been used to treat deteriorating patients with cerebral venous sinus thrombosis. A review of the literature reports over 100 patients in case series or reports treated with thrombolysis after failure of adequate anticoagulation.[53] Mechanical disruption or angioplasty of the dural sinus was reported in 12.2% of the cases. Most patients were young females treated within 72 hours. Urokinase was the preferred thrombolytic agent. Bleeding complications were reported in 14% of patients. Recanalization rates were ~56.5%. Good recoveries were reported in 70% of patients with most deaths attributed to previous intracerebral hemorrhages or cerebral herniation.[53] One prospective study of 20 patients reported good outcomes in 12 patients. Five patients in this series had increased cerebral hemorrhage after thrombolysis.[54]

Arterial Thrombectomy and Embolectomy

Mechanical endovascular embolectomy devices have been developed in an attempt to increase the therapeutic time window for the treatment of ischemic stroke.[55] The phase 1 study for the MERCI (Mechanical Embolus Removal in Cerebral Ischemia) retrieval device reported a large vessel recanalization rate of 45%, which increased to 64% when additional intraarterial tissue plasminogen activator was administered.[55] Newer generation devices have also been studied. The multi-MERCI trial reported successful large vessel recanalization in 69.5% of patients. This percentage increased to 69.5% with adjunctive thrombolytic therapy.[56] Symptomatic intracerebral hemorrhages occurred in 9.8% of patients and procedural complications were reported in 5.5% of patients. There was a tendency for improved clinical outcomes in patients that were successfully recanalized.[56] A new penumbra system has reported even more promising results of successful recanalization of the large basal cerebral arteries.[57]

Future Direction

Interventional procedures have become a growing part of the strategies involved in the treatment of cerebrovascular disease. As devices and techniques improve, it is hoped that complications will decrease. However, this hope may be tempered by the extension of these techniques to even sicker patients. Subsequently, the postprocedural management of these patients will become more complex and more important. Controlled studies will be needed to provide the necessary information to provide adequate information to treat this growing population.

References

1. Hertzer NR. Early complications of carotid endarterectomy: incidence, diagnosis, and management. In: Moore WS, ed. Surgery for Cerebrovascular Disease. New York: Churchill Livingstone; 1987:625–649
2. North American Symptomatic Carotid Endarterectomy Trial Collaborators. Beneficial effect of carotid endarterectomy in symptomatic patients with high-grade carotid stenosis. N Engl J Med 1991;325(7):445–453
3. European Carotid Surgery Trialists' Collaborative Group. MRC European Carotid Surgery Trial: interim results for symptomatic patients with severe (70-99%) or with mild (0-29%) carotid stenosis. European Carotid Surgery Trialists' Collaborative Group. Lancet 1991;337(8752): 1235–1243
4. Zabramski JM, Green KA, Marciano FF, Spetzler RF. Carotid endarterectomy. In: Carter LP, Spetzler RF, eds. Neurovascular Surgery. New York: McGraw-Hill: 1995:325–357
5. Hertzer NR, Feldman BJ, Beven EG, Tucker HM. A prospective study of the incidence of injury to the cranial nerves during carotid endarterectomy. Surg Gynecol Obstet 1980;151(6):781–784
6. Kunkel JM, Gomez ER, Spebar MJ, Delgado RJ, Jarstfer BS, Collins GJ. Wound hematomas after carotid endarterectomy. Am J Surg 1984;148 (6):844–847
7. Moore WS, Barnett HJM, Beebe HG, et al. Guidelines for carotid endarterectomy. A multidisciplinary consensus statement from the ad hoc Committee, American Heart Association. Stroke 1995;26(1):188–201
8. Easton JD, Sherman DG. Stroke and mortality rate in carotid endarterectomy: 228 consecutive operations. Stroke 1977;8(5):565–568
9. Bailes JE, Medary MB. Carotid endarterectomy. In: Winn HR, ed. Youman's Neurological Surgery. 5th ed. Philadelphia: Saunders; 2004: 1621–1644
10. Dirrenberger RA, Sundt TM Jr. Carotid endarterectomy. Temporal profile of the healing process and effects of anticoagulation therapy. J Neurosurg 1978;48(2):201–219
11. Gupta S, Matta BF. Anesthesia for carotid surgery. In: Matta BF, Menon DK, Turner JM, eds. Textbook of neuroanesthesia and critical care. New York: Cambridge University Press; 2000:209–226
12. Baker JD. Perioperative and post operative management of patients undergoing carotid endarterectomy. In: Moore WS, ed. Surgery for Cerebrovascular Disease. New York: Churchill Livingstone; 1987: 619–624
13. Lehv MS, Salzman EW, Silen W. Hypertension complicating carotid endarterectomy. Stroke 1970;1(5):307–313
14. Wong JH, Findlay JM, Suarez-Almazor ME. Hemodynamic instability after carotid endarterectomy: risk factors and associations with operative complications. Neurosurgery 1997;41(1):35–41
15. Cafferata HT, Merchant RF Jr, DePalma RG. Avoidance of postcarotid endarterectomy hypertension. Ann Surg 1982;196(4):465–472
16. Pine R, Avellone JC, Hoffman M, Plecha FR, Swayngim DM Jr, Urban J. Control of postcarotid endarterectomy hypotension with baroreceptor blockade. Am J Surg 1984;147(6):763–765
17. Towne JB, Bernhard VM. The relationship of postoperative hypertension to complications following carotid endarterectomy. Surgery 1980;88(4):575–580
18. Wade JG, Larson CP Jr, Hickey RF, Ehrenfeld WK, Severinghaus JW. Effect of carotid endarterectomy on carotid chemoreceptor and baroreceptor function in man. N Engl J Med 1970;282(15):823–829
19. Ranson JHC, Imparato AM, Clauss RH, Reed GE, Hass WK. Factors in the mortality and morbidity associated with surgical treatment of cerebrovascular insufficiency. Circulation 1969;39(5, Suppl 1)I269–I274
20. Satiani B, Vasko JS, Evans WE. Hypertension following carotid endarterectomy. Surg Neurol 1979;11(5):357–359
21. Sundt TM, Sandok BA, Whisnant JP. Carotid endarterectomy. Complications and preoperative assessment of risk. Mayo Clin Proc 1975; 50(6):301–306
22. Ringleb PA, Allenberg J, Brückmann H, et al; SPACE Collaborative Group. 30 day results from the SPACE trial of stent-protected angioplasty versus carotid endarterectomy in symptomatic patients: a randomised non-inferiority trial. Lancet 2006;368(9543):1239–1247
23. Mas JL, Chatellier G, Beyssen B, et al; EVA-3S Investigators. Endarterectomy versus stenting in patients with symptomatic severe carotid stenosis. N Engl J Med 2006;355(16):1660–1671
24. Eckstein HH, Ringleb P, Allenberg JR, et al. Results of the Stent-Protected Angioplasty versus Carotid Endarterectomy (SPACE) Study to treat symptomatic stenoses at 2 years: a multinational, prospective, randomised trial. Lancet Neurol 2008;7(10):893–902
25. Meschia JF, Brott TG, Hobson RW II. Diagnosis and invasive management of carotid atherosclerotic stenosis. Mayo Clin Proc 2007;82(7):851–858
26. Qureshi AI. Carotid angioplasty and stent placement after EVA-3S trial. Stroke 2007;38(6):1993–1996
27. Kastrup A, Gröschel K, Krapf H, Brehm BR, Dichgans J, Schulz JB. Early outcome of carotid angioplasty and stenting with and without cerebral protection devices: a systematic review of the literature. Stroke 2003;34(3):813–819
28. Mansour MA. Carotid artery stenting in the SPACE and EVA-3S trials: analysis and update. Perspect Vasc Surg Endovasc Ther 2008;20(1): 11–14
29. Mlekusch W, Schillinger M, Sabeti S, et al. Hypotension and bradycardia after elective carotid stenting: frequency and risk factors. J Endovasc Ther 2003;10(5):851–859
30. Im SH, Han MH, Kim SH, Kwon BJ. Transcutaneous temporary cardiac pacing in carotid stenting: noninvasive prevention of angioplasty-induced bradycardia and hypotension. J Endovasc Ther 2008;15(1): 110–116
31. Linskey ME, Jungreis CA, Yonas H, et al. Stroke risk after abrupt internal carotid artery sacrifice: accuracy of preoperative assessment with balloon test occlusion and stable xenon-enhanced CT. AJNR Am J Neuroradiol 1994;15(5):829–843
32. Mathis JM, Barr JD, Jungreis CA, et al. Temporary balloon test occlusion of the internal carotid artery: experience in 500 cases. AJNR Am J Neuroradiol 1995;16(4):749–754
33. Barnett DW, Barrow DL, Joseph GJ. Combined extracranial-intracranial bypass and intraoperative balloon occlusion for the treatment of intracavernous and proximal carotid artery aneurysms. Neurosurgery 1994;35(1):92–97
34. McIvor NP, Willinsky RA, TerBrugge KG, Rutka JA, Freeman JL. Validity of test occlusion studies prior to internal carotid artery sacrifice. Head Neck 1994;16(1):11–16
35. Swann KW, Heros RC, Debrun G, Nelson C. Inadvertent middle cerebral artery embolism by a detachable balloon: management by embolectomy. Case report. J Neurosurg 1986;64(2):309–312
36. Eskridge JM, Harris AB, Finch L, Alotis MA. Carotid sinus syndrome and embolization procedures. AJNR Am J Neuroradiol 1993;14(4):818–820
37. Timperman PE, Tomsick TA, Tew JM Jr, van Loveren HR. Aneurysm formation after carotid occlusion. AJNR Am J Neuroradiol 1995;16(2): 329–331
38. Sekhar LN, Duff JM, Kalavakonda C, Olding M. Cerebral revascularization using radial artery grafts for the treatment of complex intracranial aneurysms: techniques and outcomes for 17 patients. Neurosurgery 2001;49(3):646–658
39. Sekhar LN, Kalavakonda C. Cerebral revascularization for aneurysms and tumors. Neurosurgery 2002;50(2):321–331
40. Sekhar LN, Natarajan SK, Ellenbogen RG, Ghodke B. Cerebral revascularization for ischemia, aneurysms, and cranial base tumors. Neurosurgery 2008; 62(6, Suppl 3)1373–1408
41. Kim S-K, Wang K-C, Kim I-O, Lee DS, Cho B-K. Combined encephaloduroarteriosynangiosis and bifrontal encephalogaleo(periosteal) synangiosis in pediatric moyamoya disease. Neurosurgery 2002;50(1): 88–96
42. Garg BP, Bruno A, Biller J. Moyamoya disease and cerebral ischemia. In: Batjer HH, ed. Cerebrovascular Disease. Philadelphia: Lippincott-Raven; 1997:489–499

43. Golby AJ, Marks MP, Thompson RC, Steinberg GK. Direct and combined revascularization in pediatric moyamoya disease. Neurosurgery 1999;45(1):50–58
44. Chimowitz MI, Lynn MJ, Howlett-Smith H, et al; Warfarin-Aspirin Symptomatic Intracranial Disease Trial Investigators. Comparison of warfarin and aspirin for symptomatic intracranial arterial stenosis. N Engl J Med 2005;352(13):1305–1316
45. Mazighi M, Tanasescu R, Ducrocq X, et al. Prospective study of symptomatic atherothrombotic intracranial stenoses: the GESICA study. Neurology 2006;66(8):1187–1191
46. Ecker RD, Levy EI, Sauvageau E, Hanel RA, Hopkins LN. Current concepts in the management of intracranial atherosclerotic disease. Neurosurgery 2006; 59(5, Suppl 3)S210–S218
47. Gupta R, Al-Ali F, Thomas AJ, et al. Safety, feasibility, and short-term follow-up of drug-eluting stent placement in the intracranial and extracranial circulation. Stroke 2006;37(10):2562–2566
48. Eberhardt O, Naegele T, Raygrotzki S, Weller M, Ernemann U. Stenting of vertebrobasilar arteries in symptomatic atherosclerotic disease and acute occlusion: case series and review of the literature. J Vasc Surg 2006;43(6):1145–1154
49. Coward LJ, McCabe DJH, Ederle J, Featherstone RL, Clifton A, Brown MM; CAVATAS Investigators. Long-term outcome after angioplasty and stenting for symptomatic vertebral artery stenosis compared with medical treatment in the Carotid and Vertebral Artery Transluminal Angioplasty Study (CAVATAS): a randomized trial. Stroke 2007;38(5):1526–1530
50. McCabe DJH, Pereira AC, Clifton A, Bland JM, Brown MM; CAVATAS Investigators. Restenosis after carotid angioplasty, stenting, or endarterectomy in the Carotid and Vertebral Artery Transluminal Angioplasty Study (CAVATAS). Stroke 2005;36(2):281–286
51. Crawley F, Brown MM, Clifton AG. Angioplasty and stenting in the carotid and vertebral arteries. Postgrad Med J 1998;74(867):7–10
52. Medel R, Crowley RW, Dumont AS. Hyperperfusion syndrome following endovascular cerebral revascularization. Neurosurg Focus 2009;26(3):E4
53. Hocker SE, Dafer RM, Hacein-Bey L. Successful delayed thrombolysis for cerebral venous and dural sinus thrombosis: a case report and review of the literature. J Stroke Cerebrovasc Dis 2008;17(6): 429–432
54. Stam J, Majoie CB, van Delden OM, van Lienden KP, Reekers JA. Endovascular thrombectomy and thrombolysis for severe cerebral sinus thrombosis: a prospective study. Stroke 2008;39(5):1487–1490
55. Gobin YP, Starkman S, Duckwiler GR, et al. MERCI 1: a phase 1 study of mechanical embolus removal in cerebral ischemia. Stroke 2004;35(12):2848–2854
56. Smith WS, Sung G, Saver J, et al; Multi MERCI Investigators. Mechanical thrombectomy for acute ischemic stroke: final results of the Multi MERCI trial. Stroke 2008;39(4):1205–1212
57. Bose A, Henkes H, Alfke K, et al; Penumbra Phase 1 Stroke Trial Investigators. The Penumbra System: a mechanical device for the treatment of acute stroke due to thromboembolism. AJNR Am J Neuroradiol 2008;29(7):1409–1413

V

Special Considerations

Chapter 20

Revascularization Options for Complex Aneurysms

Manuel Ferreira, Jr., Dinesh Ramanathan, and Laligam N. Sekhar

Endovascular technology continues to advance at a dramatic rate. This is reflected in the complexity of vascular lesions treated and the decreasing number of aneurysms treated surgically. Today fewer aneurysms are uncoilable, unstentable, and unclippable. The use of revascularization techniques to treat these often complex lesions has resulted in high treatment success rates.[1–5]

What characteristics make an aneurysm untreatable? Which aneurysms are candidates for a revascularization procedure?

Usually, the lesion is part of a main parent vessel. It may be defined based on its fusiform geometry, blister type, giant size, dissecting pathology, a calcified or atherosclerotic neck, a very broad or absent neck (dome to neck ratio <1.5), a branch originating from the aneurysm, and an unstable intramural thrombus. Continued pathologic blood flow dynamics can exacerbate the pathology. Balloon and stent-assisted coiling can sometimes aid in securing these types of aneurysms; if not, then revascularization is considered.[5–7]

There are two main techniques used for revascularization. The first is an in situ bypass procedure such as side-to-side anastomosis, interposition grafting, patch grafting, and direct end-to-end resuturing. The second technique is the extracranial-intracranial (EC-IC) bypass. This includes low- and high-flow bypasses. Low-flow bypasses use external carotid artery (ECA) vasculature (superficial temporal artery [STA] and occipital artery [OA]). For high-flow bypasses, our group uses the radial artery (RA) and saphenous vein (SV) for grafting.

◆ Preoperative Evaluation and Preparation

Our patients are initially evaluated with computed tomography (CT), CT angiography (CTA), magnetic resonance imaging (MRI), and a six-vessel conventional angiogram. The CT scan can give insight into whether the aneurysm or parent vessel is calcified. The CTA gives anatomic detail of how the aneurysm relates to bony and brain structures. The MRI gives the best resolution of the brain surrounding the aneurysm. The MRI can also give additional information on the presence of thrombus within the lesion. We obtain a six-vessel angiogram to evaluate candidate vessels for the revascularization. The ECA and it branches are evaluated. Specifically, the STA and the OA are assessed for caliber and course. When the aneurysm involves the internal carotid artery (ICA) our group performs a 15-minute balloon test occlusion (BTO) with concurrent clinical examination. The BTO is also sometimes used when harvesting of the vertebral artery is anticipated. This test carries a risk of intimal dissection and/or thromboemboli. To decrease the risk, we use a low-pressure balloon and patients are placed on an aspirin regimen.

For high-flow grafting, our group has had the most success with autologous grafts using the RA, and the SV as a second choice. We have limited experience using the tibial artery, when the RA and SV are not candidates. We routinely obtain ultrasound Doppler studies for mapping and sizing of the RAs. This includes an Allen test to document the patency of the palmar arch. Ultrasound studies are also used for mapping and sizing of the SVs and tibial artery if necessary.

A multidisciplinary approach to the preoperative evaluation of the patient is used at our center.[8–10] Patients who undergo a revascularization procedure to treat an aneurysm are also seen by a cardiologist and our neuroanesthesia team. A hematologic evaluation is also performed to exclude a coagulopathy. It cannot be stressed enough that the optimization of preoperative comorbidities is directly correlated with the patient's long-term outcome. Once the patient and the lesion have been thoroughly evaluated, the treatment plan should be formulated by the whole team. This includes the neurosurgeon and his or her assistants, and the anesthesia, the monitoring, and the operating room staff.

The choice of the bypass is based on the size of the vessel to be replaced. The graft should be roughly the same size or slightly larger than the vessel. The health and caliber of the donor and recipient vessels should be assessed carefully. The collateral circulation should also be weighed in on the procedure to be performed.

The patient is given aspirin (325 mg/d) starting at least 1 week before surgery. Smokers are counseled on cessation.

◆ Anesthesia and Monitoring Considerations

The patient is given perioperative antibiotics prior to the initial skin incision. An arterial blood pressure line is used for close monitoring. A central venous line is used to assess central venous pressure throughout the surgery to maintain an ideal fluid status. The patient is kept normocapnic and normotensive throughout the operation. We monitor motor evoked potentials (MEPs), sensory evoked potentials (SSEPs), and electroencephalogram (EEG) throughout the procedure. For surgery involving the posterior circulation, we also monitor brainstem function with SSEPs and brainstem auditory evoked responses (BAERs).

The goal during temporary clip occlusion is to provide protection to brain at risk. This can be accomplished by decreasing the metabolism by the brain at risk. Both cooling and burst suppression are used. Cooling is investigational at this time: a randomized study is in progress at our center. In addition, by increasing the patient's blood pressure, perfusion via collateral vascular supply can be optimized. At the time of temporary arterial occlusion, the patient is cooled (to 34°C), the systolic blood pressure is raised by 15 to 20% and EEG burst suppression is induced. Various anesthetic agents are used for burst suppression, but we tend to use propofol because it is relatively quick acting and reversible (compared with barbiturates). This reversibility also aids in a timely postoperative neurologic examination of the patient.

For RA and SV grafts, during temporary occlusion, the patient is given 2000 to 2500 U of heparin for the prevention of thrombosis. This is not reversed at the end of the case. Prophylaxis for deep vein thromboses (DVTs) is begun on postoperative day #1.

Examination and evaluation of the bypass graft and its anastomoses is performed with the use of an intraoperative micro Doppler and indocyanine green (ICG) angiography; these techniques combined have made the need for intraoperative angiography obsolete – they provide the surgeon and team valuable data on the patency and adequacy of the graft. If the integrity of the graft is at issue, it can be corrected prior to the conclusion of the operation.

◆ Surgical Technique

Extracranial–Intracranial Bypasses

Low-flow Bypasses

Superficial Temporal Artery. The STA can be harvested for interposition grafting (see below) or for STA-MCA bypasses. The STA caliber and location is ideal for anastomosis to the distal middle cerebral artery (MCA). This is extremely useful for distal MCA (M3 or M4) aneurysms. Occasionally, the need for an STA to superior cerebellar artery (SCA) graft emerges for the treatment of posterior circulation aneurysms. The preoperative angiogram should be evaluated to determine whether to use the frontal or the temporal-parietal branch of the STA. The STA is mapped to the skin with a Doppler probe. For aneurysm operations, we prefer a flap technique for dissecting the STA because this is easily combined with the craniotomy, and both branches of the STA can be extracted if necessary (**Fig. 20.1**). The artery is dissected distal to proximal. Under the microscope, the dissection is performed. One should leave closely adherent tissue to the vessel to avoid injury. Small branches can be bipolar cauterized distal to the vessel whereas larger branches can be microclipped or ligated. The vessel is left in situ until it is needed for the bypass.

The distal anastomosis is sutured using 9–0 or 10–0 nylon sutures (**Fig. 20.2**). The heels of the graft are sutured with interrupted sutures. A single suture could be placed on the contralateral wall to prevent incorrect suturing of the edges. Running sutures, between anchored ends, are used because they are quicker than interrupted sutures. Prior to the last suture, the graft is flushed with heparinized saline to clear the air and test the anastomosis. Once the distal anastomosis is complete, the temporary clips are removed from the recipient vessel.

Occipital Artery. The occipital artery can be used to treat posterior circulation aneurysms. It can be anastomosed to the anterior or posterior inferior cerebellar artery. It can also be anastomosed to the distal posterior cerebral artery (PCA; P3 or P4) or SCA. Occasionally, the vessel is long enough to

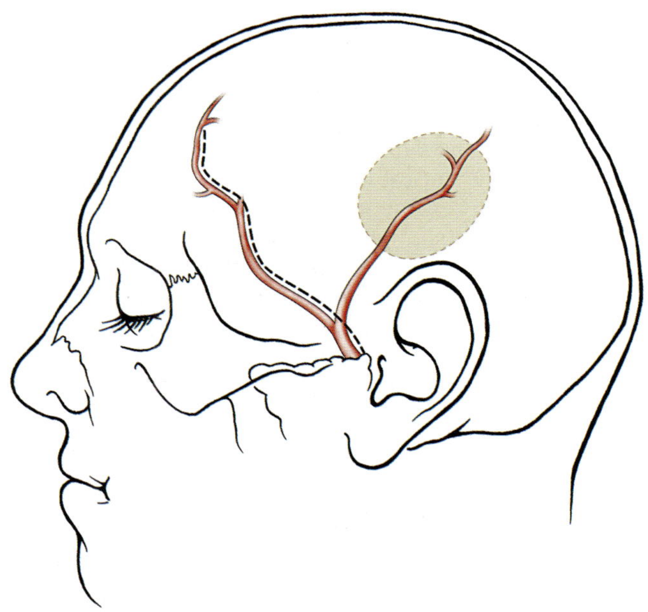

Fig. 20.1 Superficial temporal artery. Schematic showing the course of the frontal and temporal-parietal branches of the superficial temporal artery. The dashed line represents a linear incision near the vessel for a planned craniotomy at the shaded area. Alternatively, a "question mark" incision posterior to the dashed line will enable the harvesting of both vessels. (Copyright Laligam N. Sekhar.)

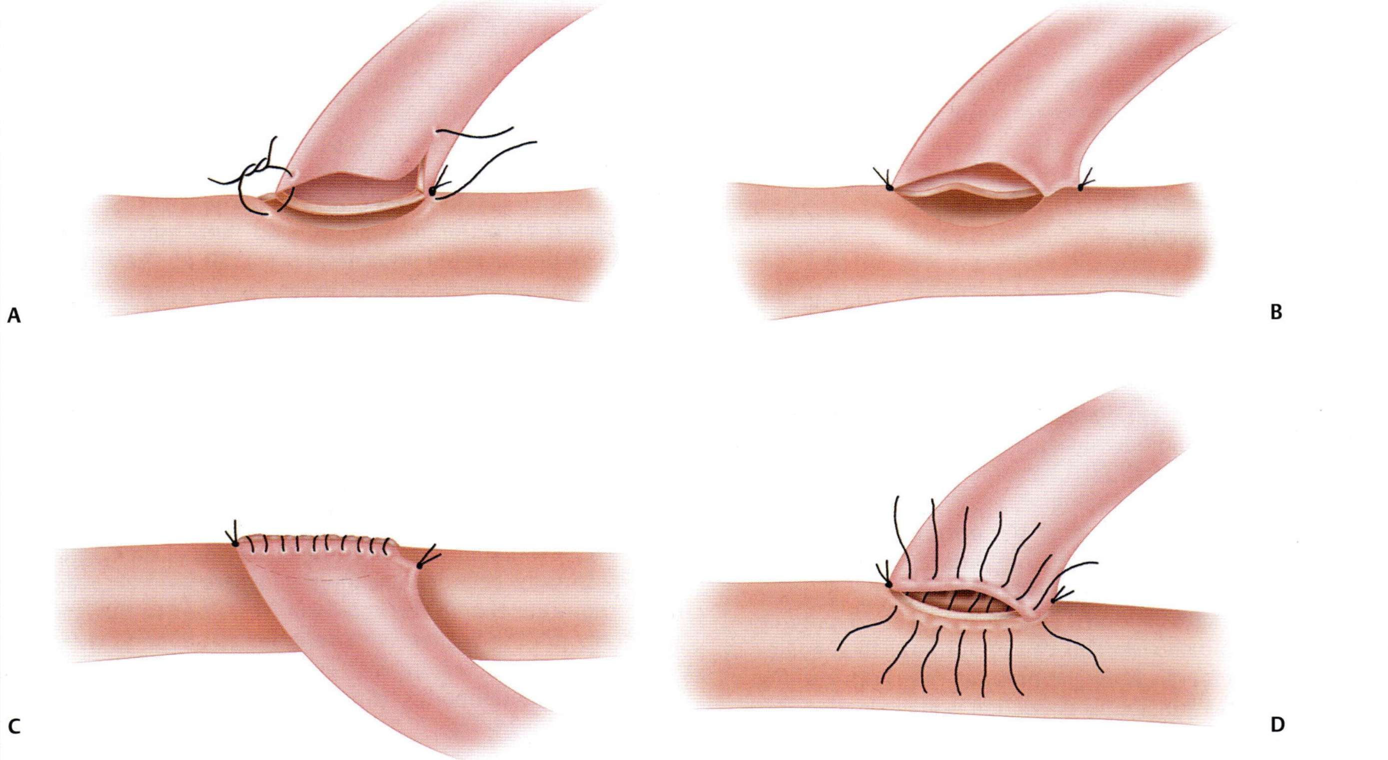

Fig. 20.2 End-to-side anastomosis. **(A)** The end of the graft has been cut in a fishmouth shape. **(B)** Anchoring interrupted sutures on each end for orienting the anastomosis is important. **(C)** The medial wall of the anastomosis has been sutured with a continuous line. **(D)** The lateral wall can be sutured with interrupted sutures or can be sutured in a running fashion. (Copyright Laligam N. Sekhar.)

use for MCA anastomoses when the STA is absent or small in caliber. This vessel should be localized with a Doppler probe and marked (**Fig. 20.3**). An inverted U-shaped incision, from the mastoid process to the midline, can be made and the flap reflected. It is found distally and traced proximally. The most difficult point of dissection is at the nuchal line, where it penetrates the muscle layers (along with the greater occipital nerve) to become more superficial. It is traced back to the digastric notch. The dissection of the OA is technically more difficult than the STA. In some patients the OA may be diseased and not exhibit good antegrade flow. In such cases, an interposition RA graft may be used instead.

High-flow Bypasses

These bypass grafts are used for the replacement of large caliber vessels (ICA, MCA, dominant vertebral artery, basilar artery). If the patient's collateral circulation is poor, anastomosis with minimal occlusion of the parent vessel is of utmost importance. This is achieved with good planning and operative technique.

Radial Artery Graft. The wall diameter is best matched to intracranial vessels, which makes this the vessel of choice in our group. The RA should be at least 0.23 cm in diameter

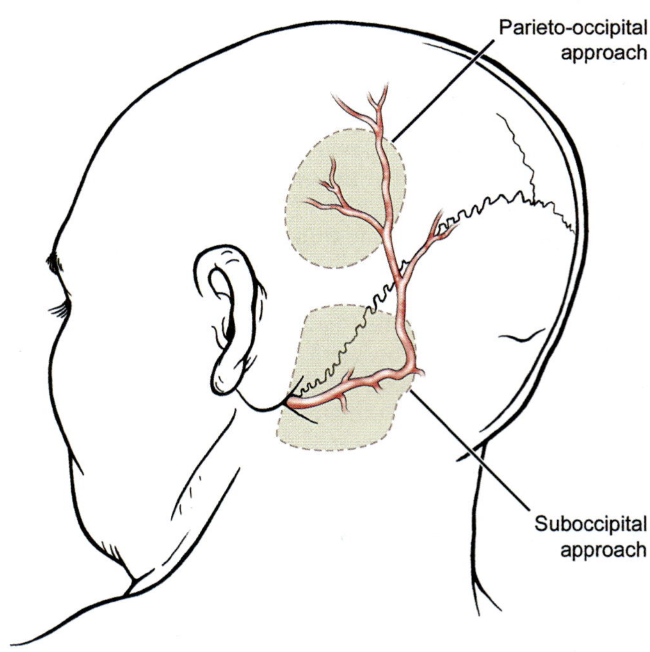

Fig. 20.3 Occipital artery. This schematic illustration depicts the course of the artery. The shaded areas show an occipital and suboccipital craniotomy and the relationship to the artery. (Copyright Laligam N. Sekhar.)

by duplex scanning. A length of ~20 cm should be available. Suturing is easier than suturing of veins. An incision is begun just over the radial pulse at the wrist. The incision is made through the dermis without harming the artery. The artery is found and bluntly dissected from the surrounding subcutaneous tissue. Closely adherent fat and soft tissue is left on the artery. Branching veins to the venous plexus surrounding the artery are bipolar cauterized and sharply cut. The venae comitantes is preserved and only denuded from the RA graft at the ends. The branch arteries are microclipped distal to the RA and cut. The artery is harvested from the wrist to the brachial artery. It is left in situ until the bypass is performed. Prior to excision, the vessel is finger occluded to confirm the absence of change in the pulse oximetry on the finger. Once the RA is harvested, the periadventitial tissue is removed 1 cm near each site of anastomosis. This is done under the microscope to prevent damaging the endothelium of the vessel.

Saphenous Vein Graft. When the RA is not available the SV is used. These veins can be extremely difficult to extract in an obese patient. The SV should be at least 0.25 cm in diameter, for a length of 20 cm by duplex scanning. Suturing is more difficult than with the RA. Prior thrombosis or venous damage can make the vessel more prone to thrombosis. The valves within the walls of the vein can also put the patient at risk for thromboembolic events. Despite these drawbacks, it has been found that the patency rates of SV grafts are good. The annual failure rate is ~1 to 1.5%.[11]

An incision is made just medial to the palpable pulse of the femoral artery (**Fig. 20.4**). This extends as far as the adductor tubercle of the thigh. We mark the course of the vein by duplex scanning, which makes it easier to dissect from distal to proximal. The upper leg and the lower thigh are preferable because the vein has a more uniform caliber. The main vein is dissected from the subcutaneous tissue with blunt dissection. Surrounding fat that is intimately associated with the vein is left attached. Branches are clamped with microclips and sharply divided. These clips should be applied away from the graft so as not to harm the graft endothelium. The vein is left in situ until just before the bypass is performed. The exact length of the vessel for the graft should be measured with a suture (from proximal to distal anastomosis) and account for the tunneling. The graft should flow in the same direction, accounting for the intraluminal valves. We do not use endoscopic harvest because this has been shown to have a higher graft failure rate in the cardiac population.[12]

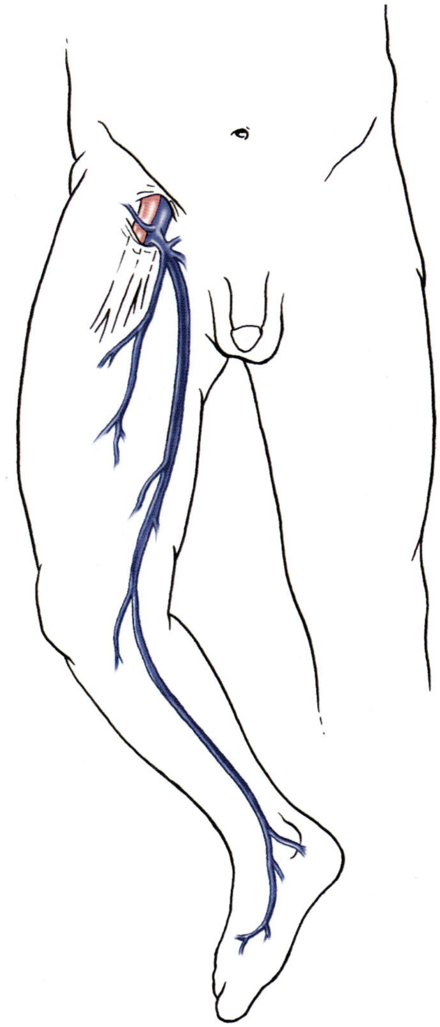

Fig. 20.4 Saphenous vein. This shows the course of the vein from the ankle to the groin, where it empties into the femoral vein. The femoral vein is located medial to the artery. The caliber of the saphenous vein decreases as the vessel runs in the distal lower extremity. (Copyright Laligam N. Sekhar.)

In Situ Bypass Procedures

Side to Side

This technique is used to reestablish flow to an adjacent vessel when obliteration of an aneurysm requires its compromise. The most common location is anterior cerebral artery (ACA; A2 to A2 or A3 to A3) or the tonsillar loop of adjacent posterior inferior cerebellar artery. In any of these examples, the technique is the same. The vessels have to be dissected from the subarachnoid space so that they come together comfortably. There should be no stretch of the vessels. A rubber dam is placed under both vessels and temporary clips applied. A 3- to 4-mm arteriotomy is made in each superomedial surface (**Fig. 20.5**). The ends are anchored with 9-0 or 10-0 nylon interrupted sutures. The posterior wall is then sutured with a running suture line. Finally, the superficial wall is sutured with a running suture.

Direct Reconstruction

When a compromised vessel cannot be mobilized for a side-to-side anastomosis or does not warrant a bypass graft, the vessel can be cut and implanted into the adjacent vessel. The cut end is fishmouthed and implanted into the recipient vessel, which

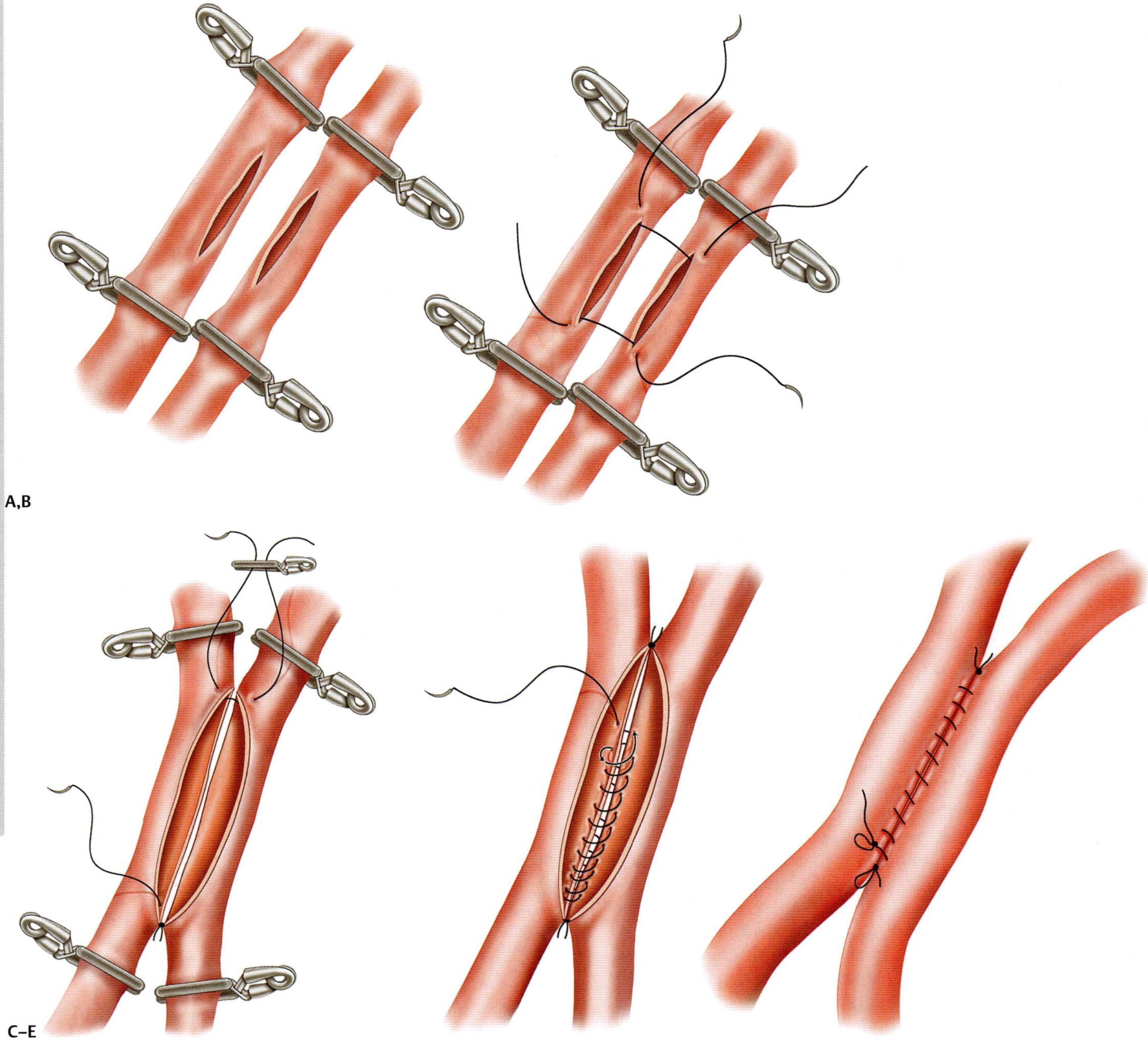

Fig. 20.5 Side-to-side anastomosis. **(A–C)** Once temporary clips are applied to both vessels, anchoring interrupted sutures are placed at each pole for orientation. **(D)** The back wall of the anastomosis is sutured first in a running fashion. **(E)** Different colored sutures demonstrate the double-running sutures from each pole of the outer wall. (Copyright Laligam N. Sekhar.)

has a fishmouth opening. End-to-end or end-to-side anastomoses can be performed (**Fig. 20.6**). A similar suturing technique (as for side-to-side anastomoses) is used.

Interposition Jump Graft

The STA, OA, RA, or SV can be used. We have also used the superior thyroid and lingual arteries when the former are not available. When the two vessels cannot be approximated to perform a tensionless anastomosis, we harvest a vessel for an interposition (**Fig. 20.7**). The suturing technique is as described above for an end-to-end anastomosis. One side should be fishmouthed. For in situ bypass procedures involving a single anastomosis, antiplatelet agents are adequate, and it is not necessary to administer heparin intravenously.

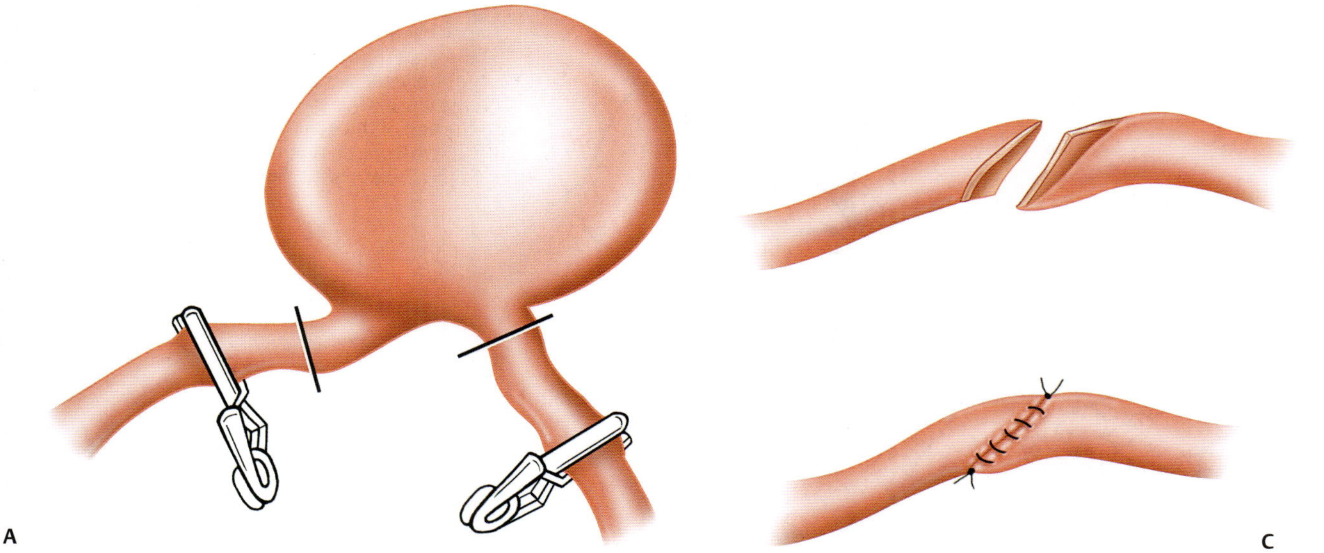

Fig. 20.6 End-to-end direct repair. **(A)** The aneurysm in this case incorporates the proximal and distal vessels. When there is sufficient length and proximal and distal ends are mobile a direct reconstruction can be done. **(B)** The cuts in the vessel ends must be complementary. **(C)** The suturing technique as described in the previous figures. (Copyright Laligam N. Sekhar.)

◆ Operative Procedure for EC-IC Bypass Revascularization

Exposure of the grafts is as previously described. We pin the patient with a radiolucent head holder in case intraoperative angiography is needed. The use of ICG angiography has made this rarely needed. While the craniotomy and exposure of the aneurysm and recipient vessel(s) is being performed, another surgeon is performing the neck dissection.

The craniotomy is tailored for the specific aneurysm and distal anastomosis. Skull base exposures are essential for basal operations because they minimize brain retraction, improve the working angles, and generally reduce the time for the bypasses.

For the carotid exposure, an oblique skin crease incision along a skin crease in the neck is used and extends to the mastoid process. Within the avascular plane just medial to the sternocleidomastoid muscle, the carotid sheath is found. Once the bifurcation is located, the common carotid artery, ICA, and ECA are isolated. The surgeon can divide the digas-

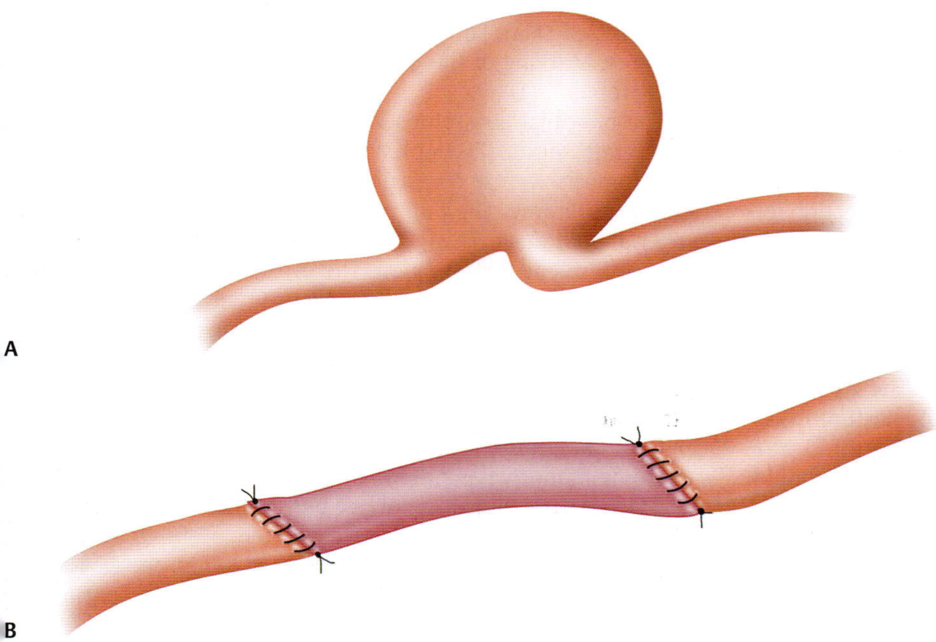

Fig. 20.7 **(A)** Interposition graft reconstruction. In the case shown, the aneurysm again incorporates the parent vessel. **(B)** When the aneurysm must be excised and the potential cut ends cannot be dissected sufficiently, a jump graft can be used. Each suture line is sutured in the manner already described. (Copyright Laligam N. Sekhar.)

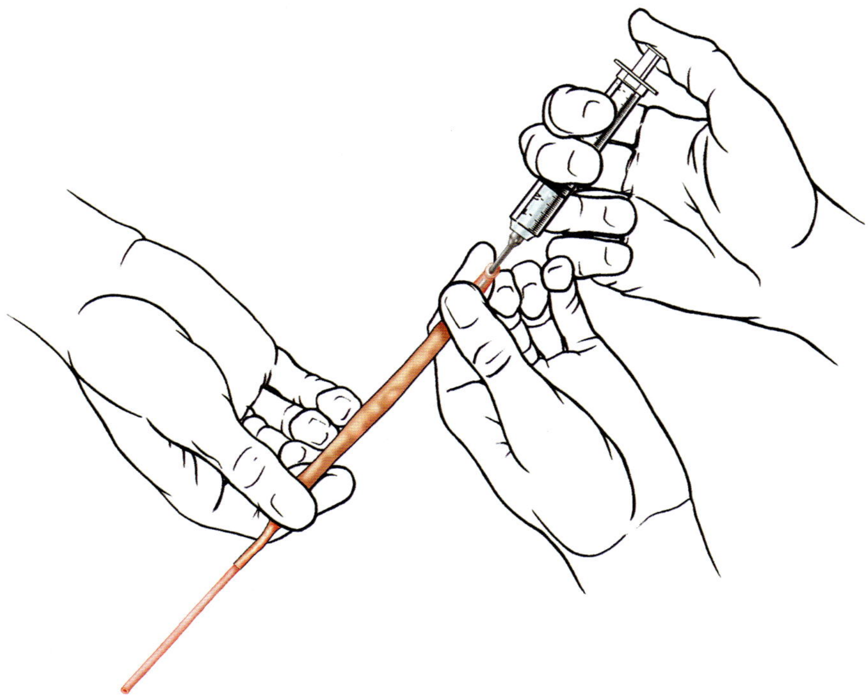

Fig. 20.8 Pressure distention technique. Heparinized saline is gently infused into one end of the graft (radial artery here, but others can be used) while the assistant gently holds pressure on the vessel. This is done sequentially marching to the end of the graft. This is performed under the microscope so that the intima is handled carefully. (Copyright Laligam N. Sekhar.)

tric muscle if needed to facilitate the graft placement. Sometimes the craniotomy and cervical incisions are connected to facilitate forming a tunnel for the graft. For SV grafts, we usually use a retroauricular tunnel, with a groove drilled in the bone. Most RA grafts are brought through a preauricular tunnel, but bony grooves may be cut at the zygoma and the temporal bone as well.

At this point, the recipient intracranial vessel is isolated. Care is taken to isolate an area void of perforators. Branch points provide additional caliber to the recipient vessel, if needed. For the MCA, either the M1 bifurcation, or a large M2 branch is usually selected. The graft is now harvested (see graft choices above). In the case of RA grafts, the artery is dilated by the pressure distension method, using heparinized saline (**Fig. 20.8**). We have found this to prevent spasm of the graft and facilitate the bypass. SV grafts are also predistended with gentle pressure of heparinized saline. Retractors should be avoided if possible. The recipient vessel is temporarily clipped (see anesthesia section for temporary clipping). Should the potentials change and reflect ischemia, the blood pressure can be increased further. We mark the artery edge with a pen to make them more visible, and to distinguish the two edges because stents are not used. The RA end is cut in an oval fashion and fishmouthed, under the operative microscope (**Fig. 20.9**). The adventitia should be removed at the edges. The distal anastomosis is sutured using 8-0 or 9-0 nylon sutures (**see Fig. 20.2**). The heels of the graft are sutured initially. A single suture should be placed on the contralateral wall to prevent the incorrect suturing of the edges. Running sutures, between anchored ends, are used because they are quicker than interrupted sutures. Prior to the last suture, the graft is forward flushed with heparinized saline to clear the air. Once the distal anastomosis is complete, the graft is occluded ~1 cm proximal to the anastomosis, and the temporary clips are removed from the recipient vessel. The distal temporary clip is removed first (before the proximal clip on the recipient artery), to check back flow into the graft. If major leaks are found, additional sutures are placed.

The graft is tunneled to the area of carotid exposure. One can use a pre- (RA graft or SV graft) or postauricular (SV graft) tunnel. When a postauricular tunnel is used, a groove is drilled in the mastoid process and suboccipital bone to accommodate the SV graft. The best way to pass the graft without torsion is to predistend it (fill it with heparinized saline) and pinch the proximal end during the passage. Marking of the graft may also be done to prevent this problem.

The proximal anastomosis is either an end-to-end or an end (graft) to side (ECA or ICA) anastomosis. For end-to-side anastomosis we use a vascular punch to create a perfectly oval arteriotomy. The punch helps to have all layers of the arterial wall flush. This is sutured in the same fashion using 7-0 Prolene or 8-0 nylon. The proximal anastomosis is flushed with heparinized saline prior to tying. In case of RA grafts, the graft is also back bled by removing the temporary clip. For SV grafts, when the proximal clips are released, a small branch may be opened distally (if necessary) to extract any air inside the graft.

Once the graft is in place, we do a Doppler study of the proximal donor vessel, the graft throughout, and the distal recipient vessel. At this point, we perform an intraoperative ICG angiogram. This has proven extremely useful in combination with Doppler to pick up any graft compromise. The surgeon should know the algorithm for troubleshooting graft complications during surgery (**Fig. 20.10**).

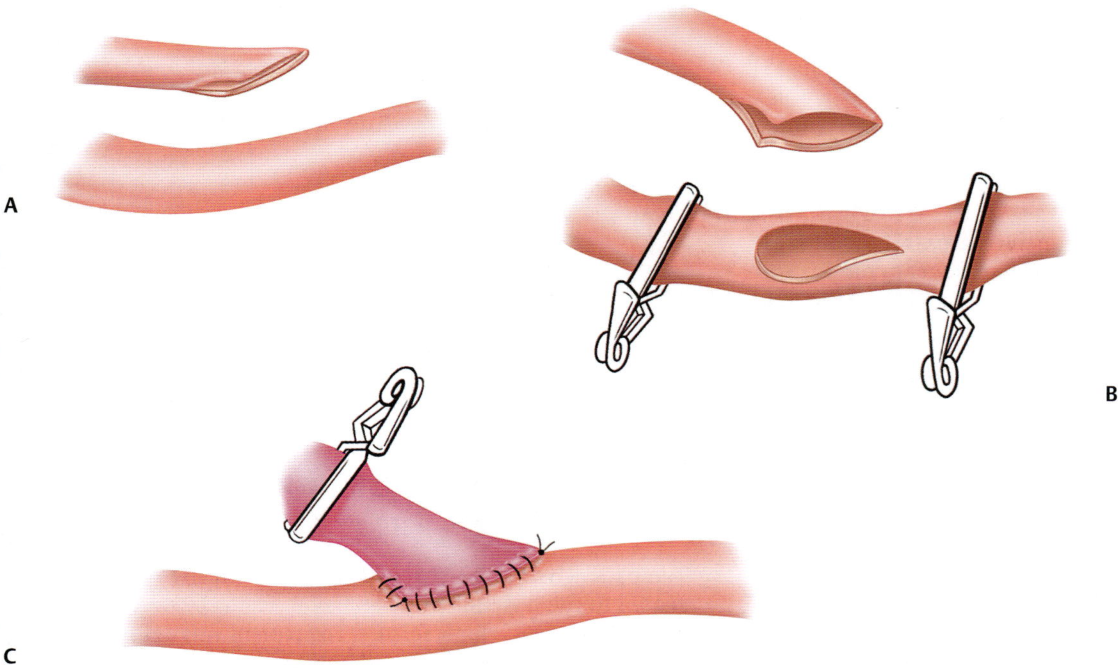

Fig. 20.9 Radial artery end-to-side anastomosis. **(A)** The end of the radial artery graft has a fishmouth cut end. **(B)** The recipient side vessel has a tear-drop cut in it to accept the radial artery graft caliber. The suturing is as described in previous figures for end-to-side anastomoses. (Copyright Laligam N. Sekhar.)

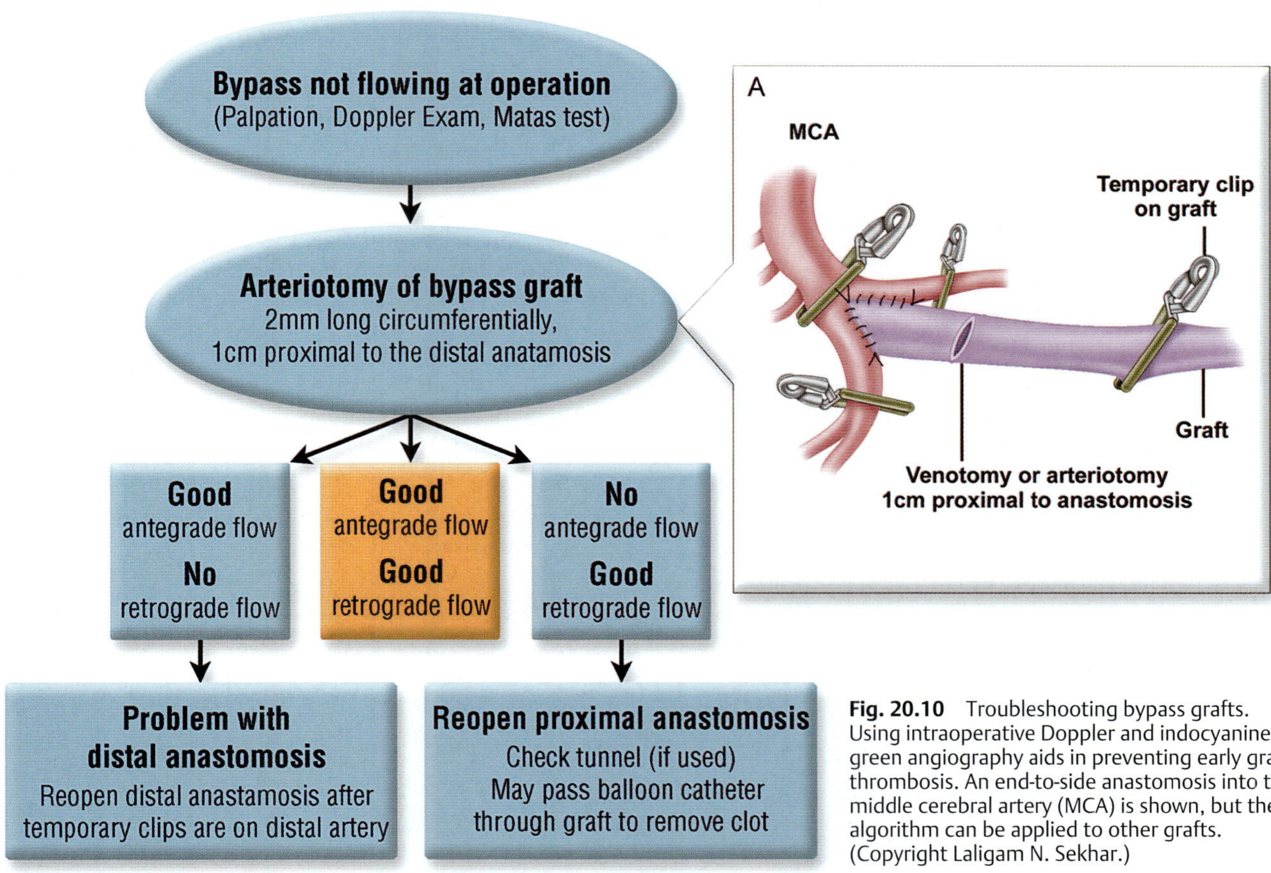

Fig. 20.10 Troubleshooting bypass grafts. Using intraoperative Doppler and indocyanine green angiography aids in preventing early graft thrombosis. An end-to-side anastomosis into the middle cerebral artery (MCA) is shown, but the algorithm can be applied to other grafts. (Copyright Laligam N. Sekhar.)

A small portion of the bone flap is removed to accommodate the graft and ensure that there is compression of the graft. The graft flow is checked again after the bone flap is replaced and the skin is closed.

◆ Postoperative Management

The patient is kept in the intensive care unit for at least 2 days. We obtain an intraarterial angiogram on postoperative day 1 for evaluation of the graft. Daily TCDs and duplex examinations are also performed until the patient is discharged. Duplex ultrasonography provides a noninvasive method for following the patency and function of high flow EC-IC bypass grafts. In fact, this could detect dysfunctional grafts, which require revision (Ferreira and Sekhar, unpublished observations). Aspirin is continued daily.

◆ Avoidance of Complications

1. Infarction: Timely technique, short temporary clip time, burst suppression, and anesthetic vigilance all reduce the incidence of stroke in these procedures.
2. Graft compromise: Technical fluency in suturing technique, proper tunneling, and adequate length of graft will prevent early compromise.
3. Epidural or subdural hematoma: The aspirin and heparin given for the success of the revascularization makes hemostasis extremely important in preventing hematomas. If subdural ooze is an issue, the heparin can be partially reversed. A subgaleal drain can be placed. Rarely, the bone flap may be left out for ~1 week.
4. Vasospasm of graft: This can occur as a result of improper manipulation. This can be avoided using the pressure distension technique mentioned earlier. If this occurs and the patient is symptomatic, endovascular angioplasty can be performed. There is a risk of thrombosis and rupture during angioplasty. The patient needs to be on dual antiplatelet therapy before this is done.
5. Wound complications: The graft harvest site and craniotomy wound can suffer from infections or hematomas. A wound revision may be needed.

◆ Case Illustrations

In the past 21 years, the senior author's experience has included 173 revascularization procedures (in 164 patients) for the management of complex cerebral aneurysm **(Table 20.1)**. The following cases illustrate the utility in these techniques for the complex aneurysms, which are refractory to the current endovascular technology. The vascular location and type of bypass performed are listed. We have also included the outcome and results for the patients who underwent cerebral revascularization procedures over this period and their outcome, using a modified Rankin Scale (mRS) (**Table 20.2**).

Table 20.1 Revascularization Procedures for Complex Cerebral Aneurysms, 1988–2009

Aneurysm	Revascularization Type					Total
	In Situ	Low Flow	High Flow			
			RAG	T	SVG	
Anterior circulation	15	18	54	2	46	135
Posterior circulation	2	13	14	0	9	38
Total	17	31	68	2	55	173

Abbreviations: RAG, radial artery graft; T, tibial arteries (anterior and posterior); SVG, saphenous vein graft.

Case #1: STA to MCA (M3) Bypass for Ruptured Fusiform Aneurysm

The patient was a 37-year-old right-handed man who presented to the hospital with the worst headache of life and a generalized tonic-clonic seizure. The patient was a Hunt-Hess 2 from a Fischer 2 subarachnoid hemorrhage. He underwent a left craniotomy for the excision of the fusiform M3 aneurysm and a STA-M3 bypass (**Fig. 20.11**). The patient made a full recovery. The aneurysm was not mycotic in nature.

Case #2: ICA to MCA (M2) Radial Artery Bypass and Proximal ICA Occlusion for a Giant Partially Thrombosed Cavernous ICA Aneurysm

The patient was a 51-year-old right-handed woman who suffered from a subacute left ophthalmoplegia. She had ptosis and restricted extraocular muscle movements in all directions. She also had no sensation in the ipsilateral V1 and V2 distribution. The patient underwent a left frontotemporal craniotomy with an orbital osteotomy. An ICA to MCA (M2) RA graft bypass and trapping of the intracavernous aneurysm was performed (**Fig. 20.12**). The initial flow of the graft was excellent. Within 20 minutes the proximal graft occluded and a patch plasty was done at the proximal anastomosis. The patient was maintained on full-dose heparin drip. The patient underwent an angioplasty of her graft on postoperative day 10 after a distal spasm and hemiparesis.

Table 20.2 Outcomes in Aneurysm Patients Undergoing Revascularization, 1988–2009

Aneurysm	mRS					Total
	0, 1	2	3	4, 5	6	
Anterior circulation	78 (61%)	35 (28%)	8 (6%)	2 (2%)	4 (3%)	127 (100%)
Posterior circulation	22 (59%)	8 (21%)	3 (9%)	0	4 (11%)	37 (100%)
Total						164

Abbreviation: mRS, modified Rankin Scale score.

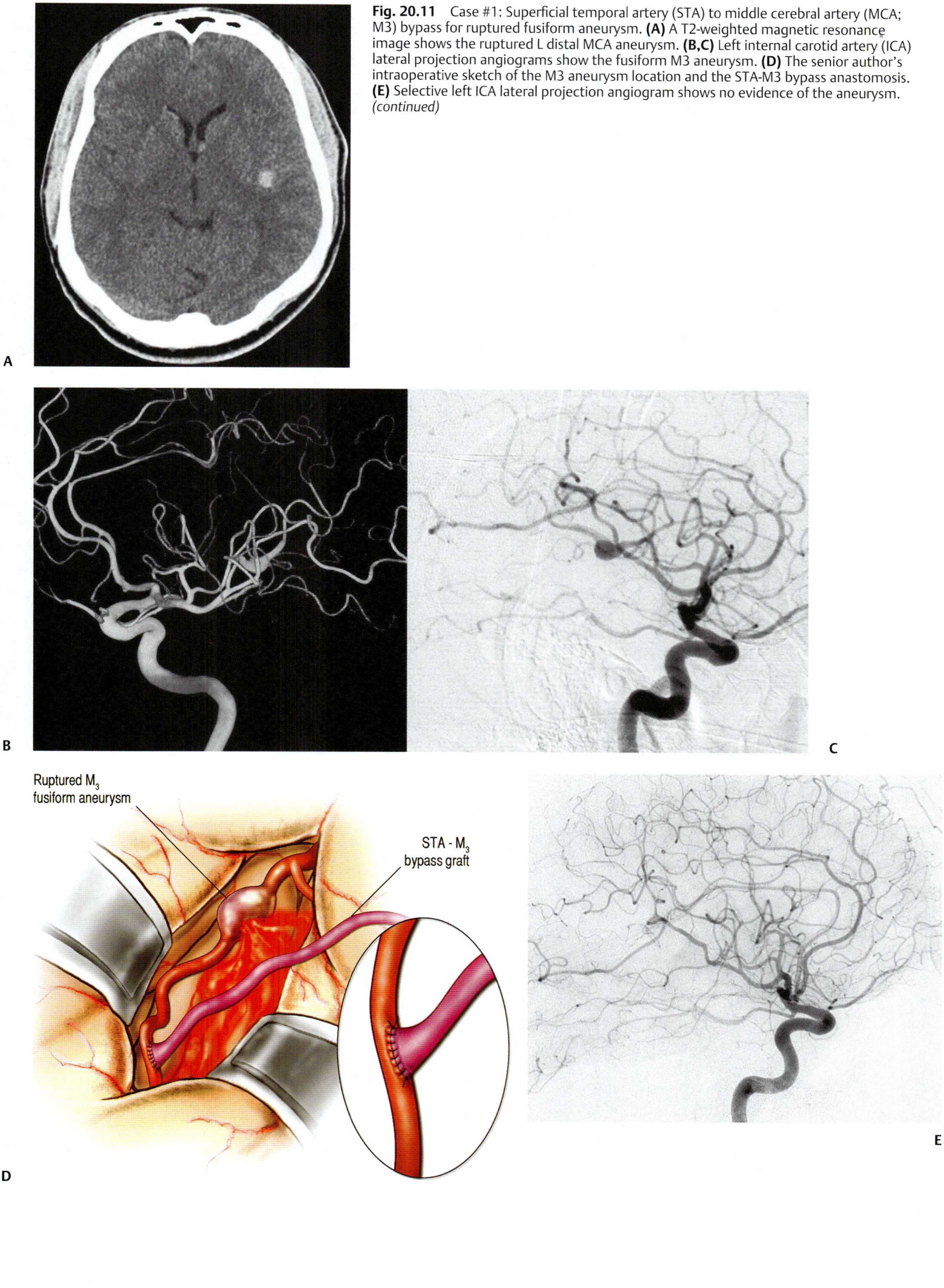

Fig. 20.11 Case #1: Superficial temporal artery (STA) to middle cerebral artery (MCA; M3) bypass for ruptured fusiform aneurysm. **(A)** A T2-weighted magnetic resonance image shows the ruptured L distal MCA aneurysm. **(B,C)** Left internal carotid artery (ICA) lateral projection angiograms show the fusiform M3 aneurysm. **(D)** The senior author's intraoperative sketch of the M3 aneurysm location and the STA-M3 bypass anastomosis. **(E)** Selective left ICA lateral projection angiogram shows no evidence of the aneurysm. *(continued)*

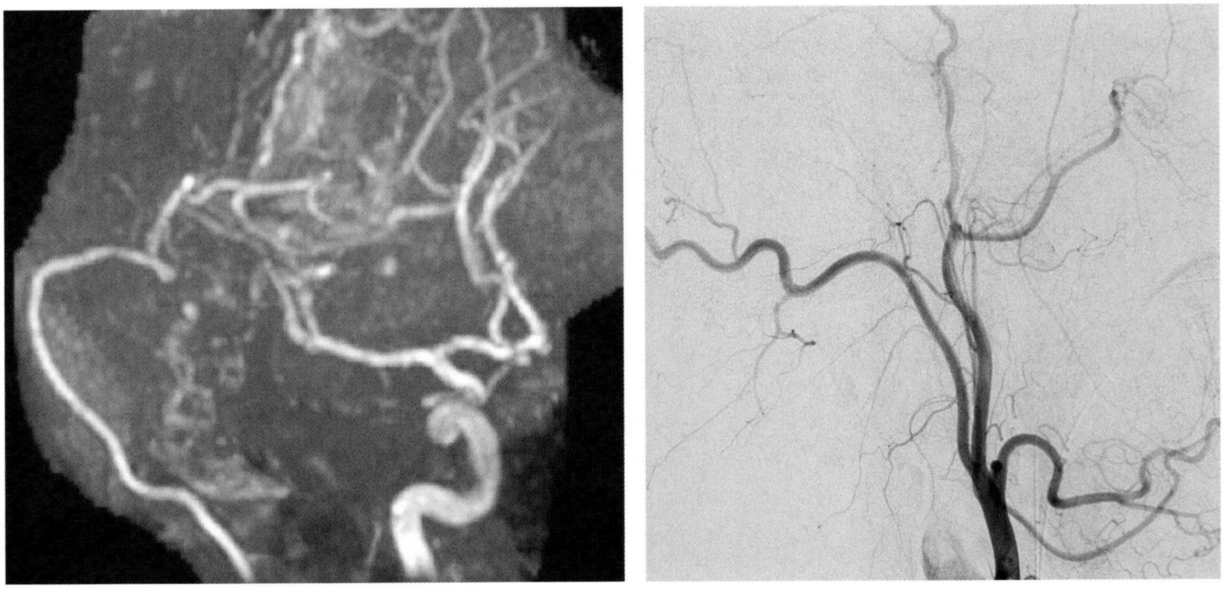

Fig. 20.11 *(continued)* **(F,G)** CT angiogram and selective left external carotid artery lateral projection angiogram show a patent STA-M3 bypass graft. (Copyright Laligam N. Sekhar.)

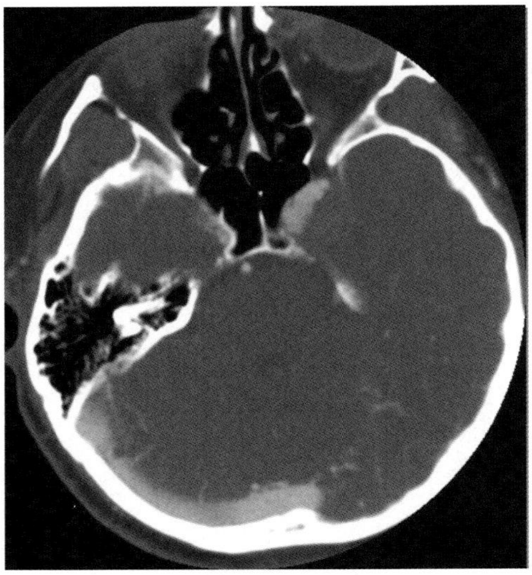

Fig. 20.12 Case #2: Internal carotid artery (ICA) to middle cerebral artery (MCA; M2) radial artery bypass and proximal ICA occlusion for a giant partially thrombosed cavernous ICA aneurysm. **(A)** CT angiogram reveals a left giant partially thrombosed cavernous ICA aneurysm. Right **(B)** and left **(C)** anteroposterior angiograms show the partially filling left cavernous segment aneurysm and the lack of significant collaterals. *(continued)*

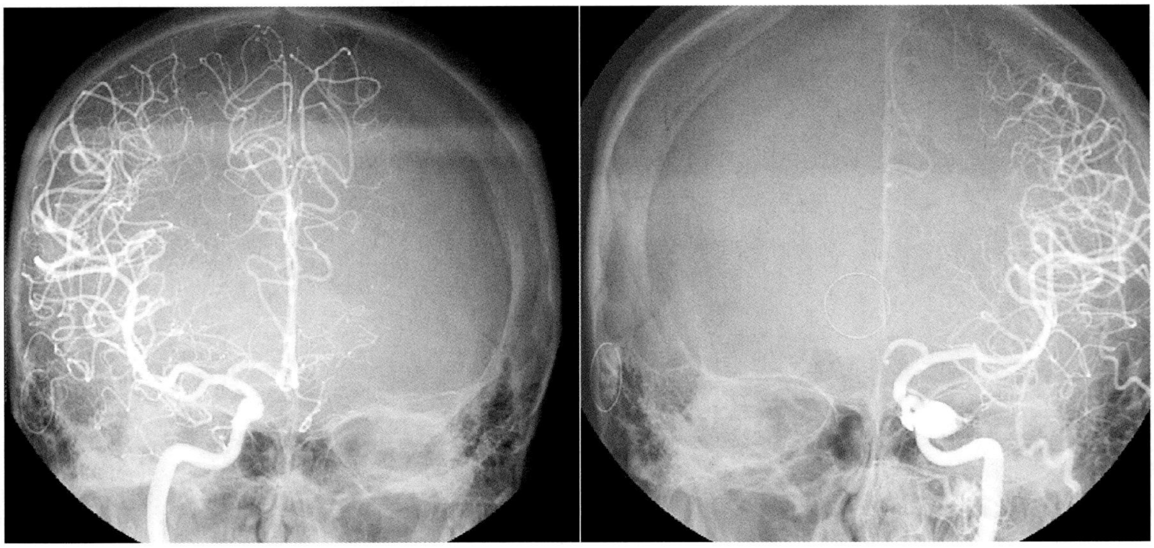

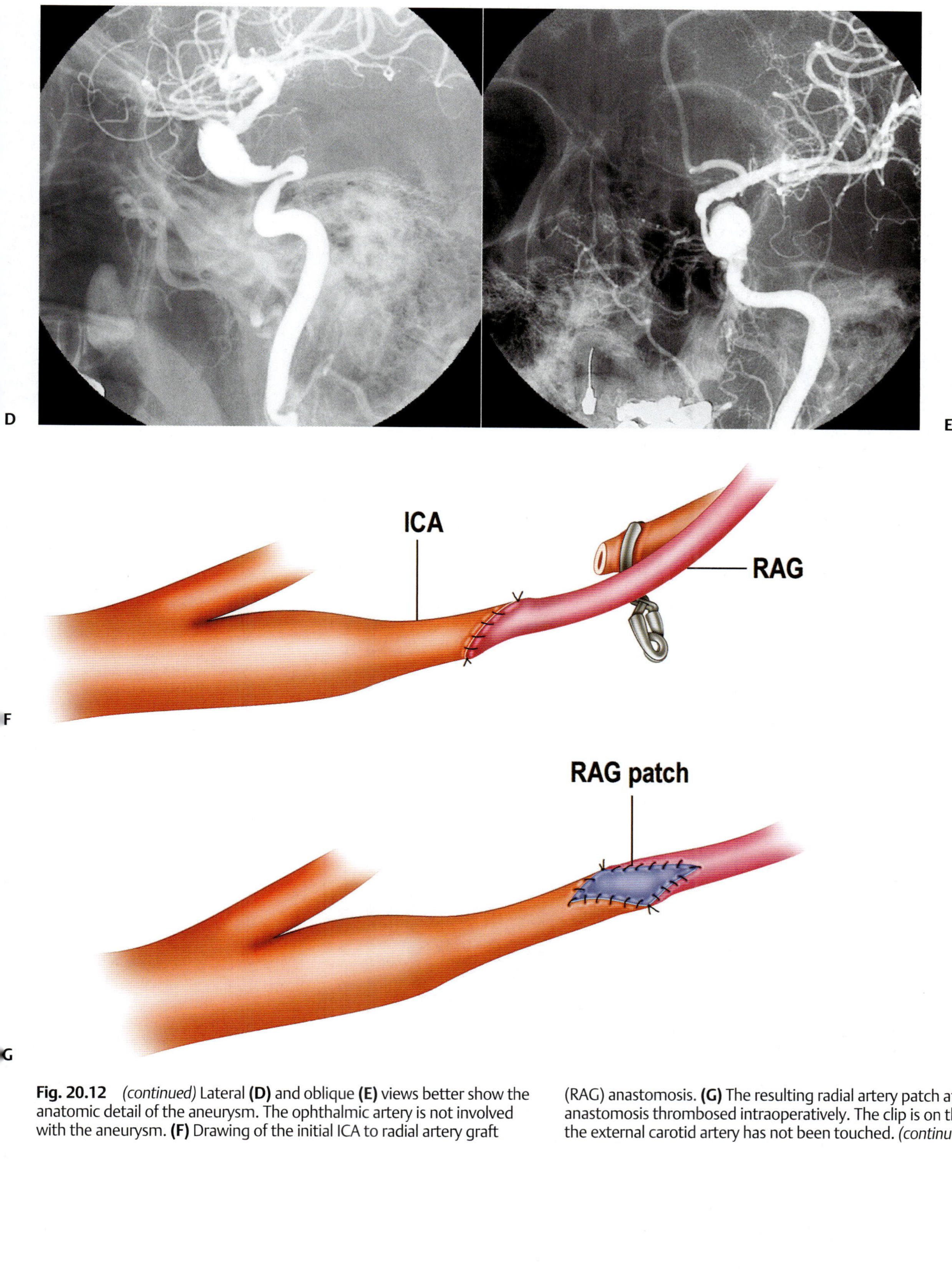

Fig. 20.12 *(continued)* Lateral **(D)** and oblique **(E)** views better show the anatomic detail of the aneurysm. The ophthalmic artery is not involved with the aneurysm. **(F)** Drawing of the initial ICA to radial artery graft (RAG) anastomosis. **(G)** The resulting radial artery patch after the proximal anastomosis thrombosed intraoperatively. The clip is on the distal ICA and the external carotid artery has not been touched. *(continued)*

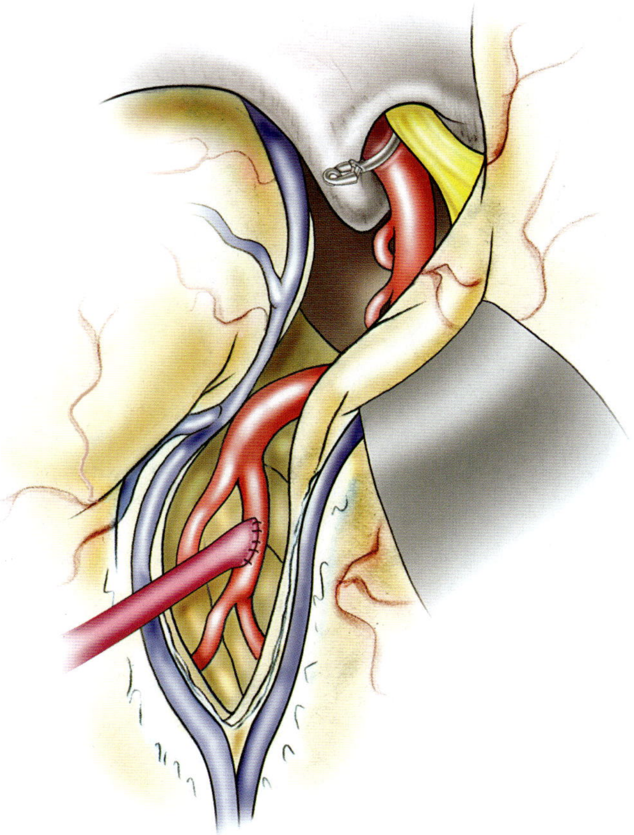

H

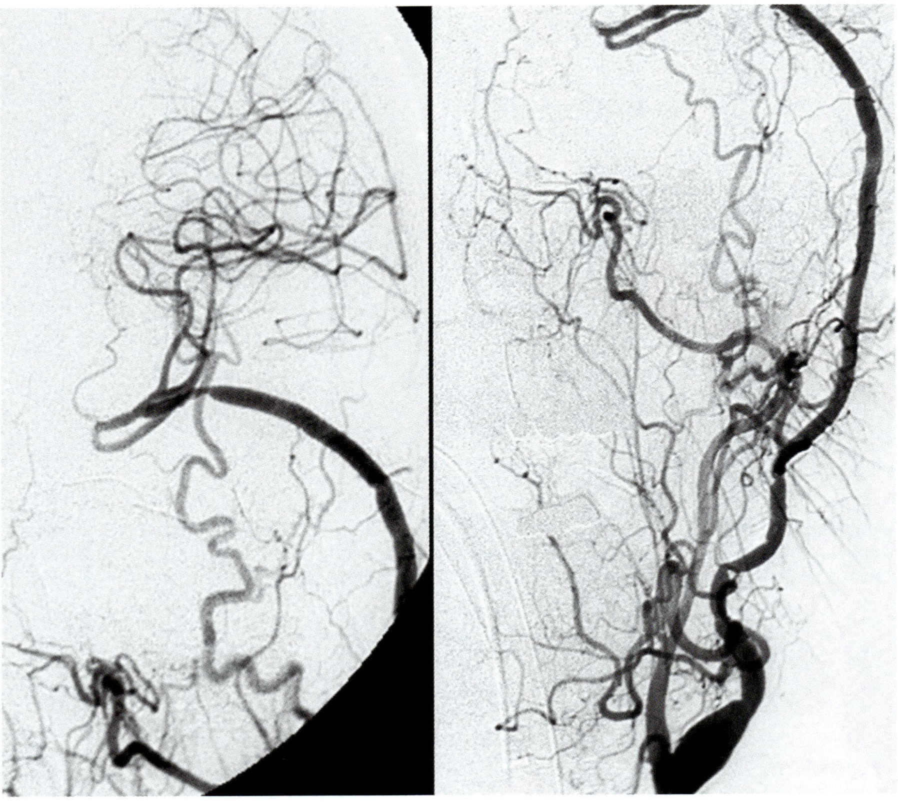

I J

Fig. 20.12 *(continued)* **(H)** The distal radial artery to M2 anastomosis. The clip is on the ICA proximal to the ophthalmic artery, which fills by retrograde flow. Postoperative distal **(I)** and proximal **(J)** anastomoses. (Copyright Laligam N. Sekhar.)

At 8-month follow-up she had near complete return of her eye movements. She had a persistent fourth nerve paralysis. Her face sensation returned to normal.

Case #3: Excision and STA to ACA (A3) Interposition Graft for Pericallosal Aneurysm Incorporating A3

The patient was a 69-year-old right-handed woman with the worst headache of life who was found to have an A2–A3 broad-necked aneurysm. The right A3 vessels were incorporated into the aneurysm. The aneurysm was excised and a STA interposition graft was used as a replacement for the parent vessel (**Fig. 20.13**). The patient made a full recovery.

Case #4: MCA (M2) to PCA (P2) RA Graft Bypass and Clipping of Giant Complex and Previously Coiled Basilar Tip Aneurysm

The patient was a 45-year-old woman who suffered a subarachnoid hemorrhage 6 years prior from a giant basilar tip aneurysm (**Fig. 20.14**). The aneurysm was initially coiled. She suffered small perforator stroke from which she recovered completely. She had persistent third nerve palsy. The aneurysm recurred due to coil compaction and she required four additional coiling procedures. An angiogram a year later revealed new coil compaction and now the right PCA origin emanated from the aneurysmal neck. She had no

A B

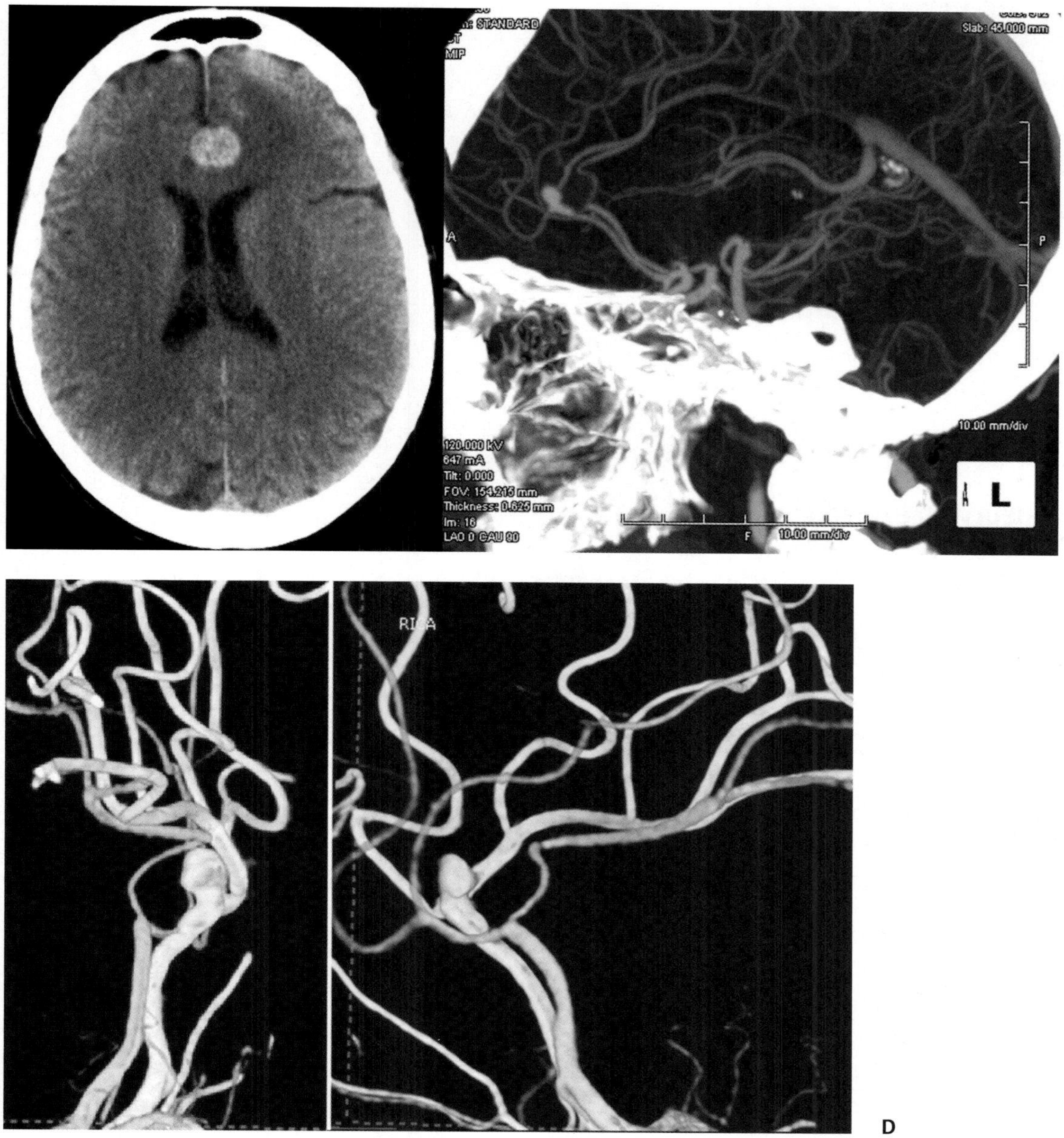

C D

Fig. 20.13 Case #3: Excision and superficial temporal artery (STA) to anterior cerebral artery (ACA; A3) interposition graft for pericallosal aneurysm incorporating A3. **(A)** CT scan reveals an interhemispheric hemorrhage. **(B)** Sagittal CT angiogram shows a broad-based pericallosal aneurysm. **(C,D)** Three-dimensional reconstruction of angiographic runs displays the broad neck anatomy and the incorporation of the A3. *(continued)*

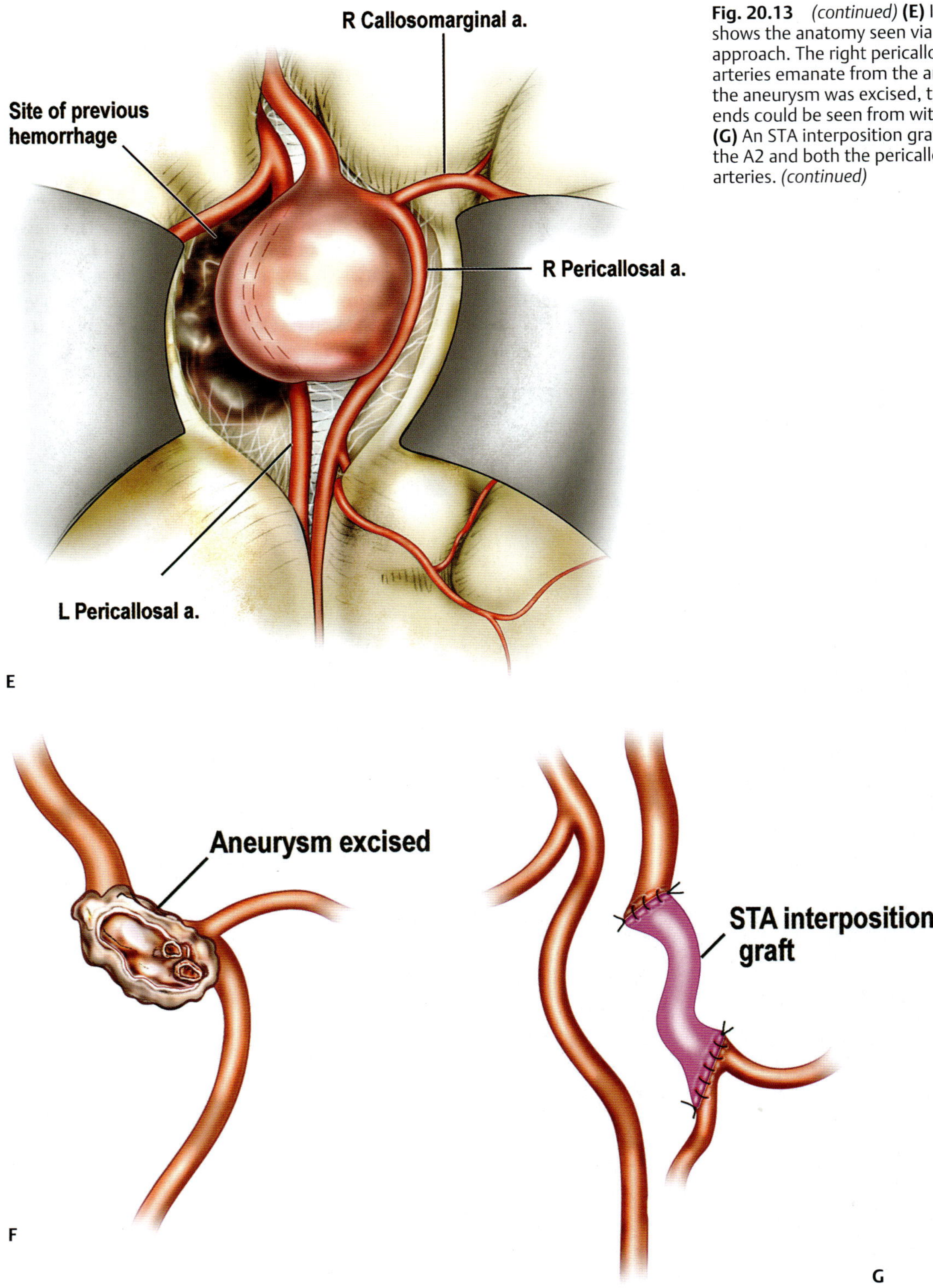

Fig. 20.13 *(continued)* **(E)** Intraoperative illustration shows the anatomy seen via an interhemispheric approach. The right pericallosal and callosomarginal arteries emanate from the aneurysmal wall. **(F)** Once the aneurysm was excised, the two proximal arterial ends could be seen from within the aneurysm dome. **(G)** An STA interposition graft was placed between the A2 and both the pericallosal and callosomarginal arteries. *(continued)*

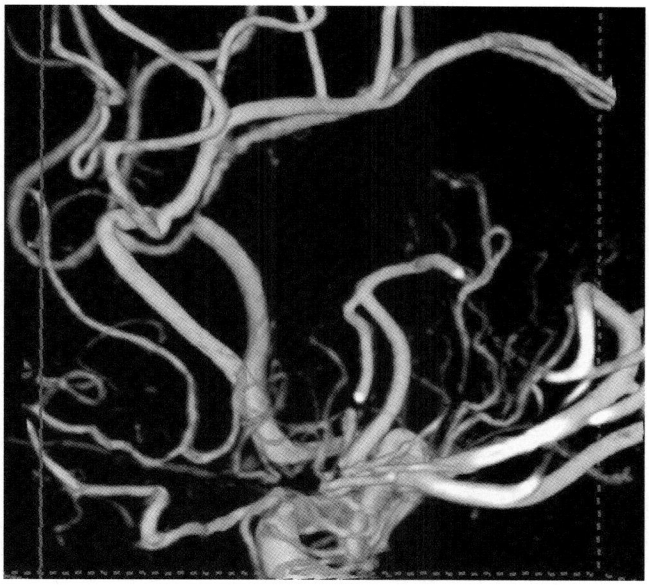

H

Fig. 20.13 *(continued)* **(H)** Postoperative angiogram reveals the absence of aneurysm and a patent graft and distal vasculature. (Copyright Laligam N. Sekhar)

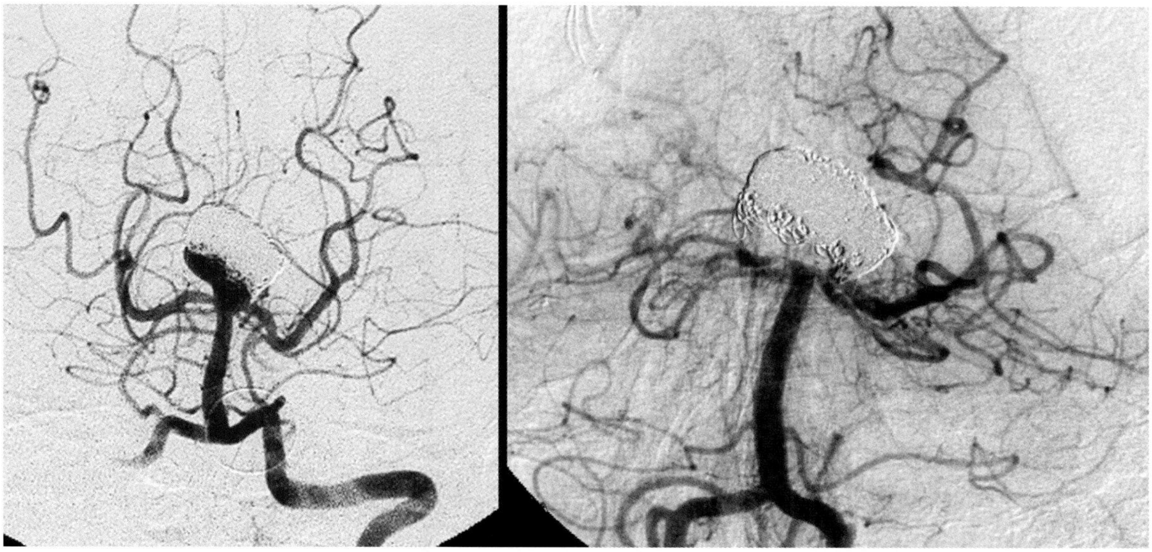

A B

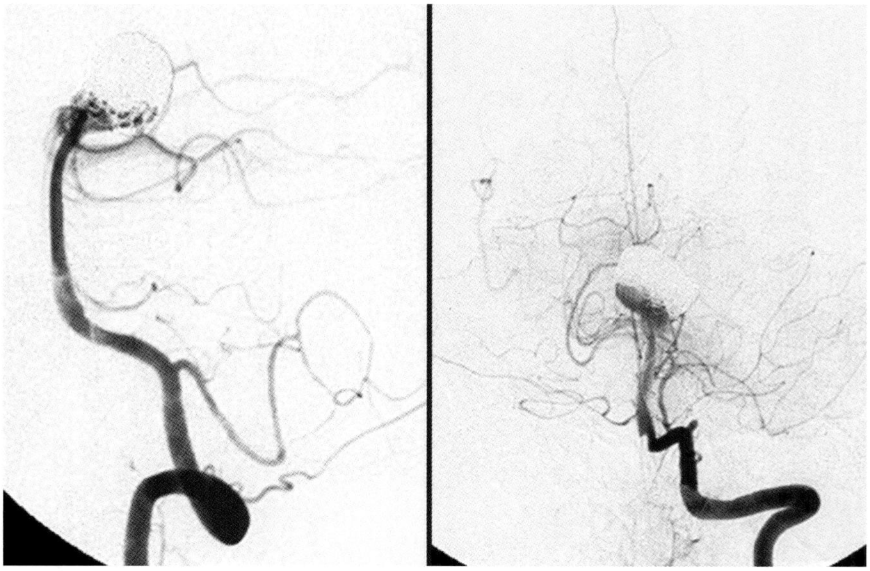

C,D

Fig. 20.14 Case #4: Middle cerebral artery (M2) to posterior cerebral artery (PCA; P2) radial artery graft bypass and clipping of giant complex and previously coiled basilar tip aneurysm. AP angiographic views, 5 years prior, showing recurrent aneurysm from coil compaction **(A)** and recoiling **(B)**. After multiple additional endovascular coilings, an angiogram revealed a recurrent aneurysm with coil compaction. **(C)** Lateral view shows the recurrent neck with the PCA emanating from it. **(D)** AP view confirms the anatomy. *(continued)*

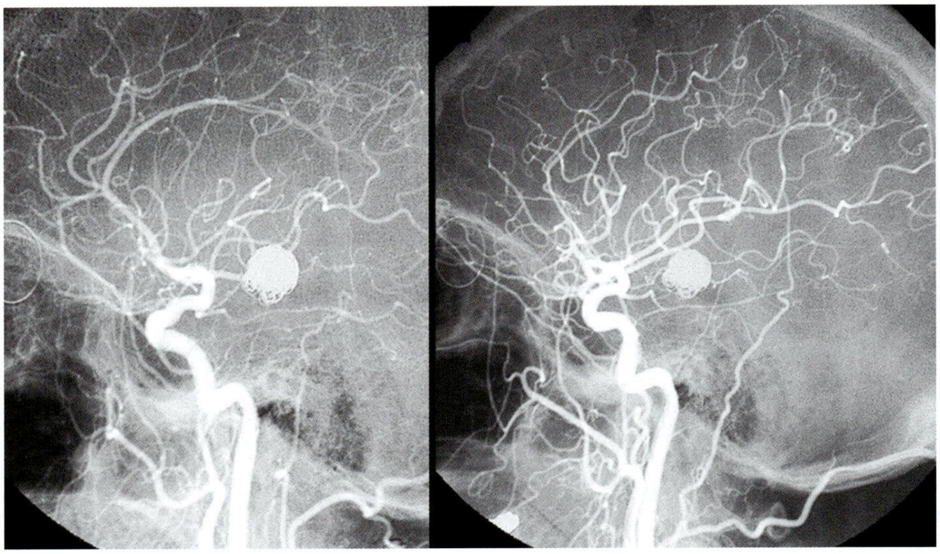

E F

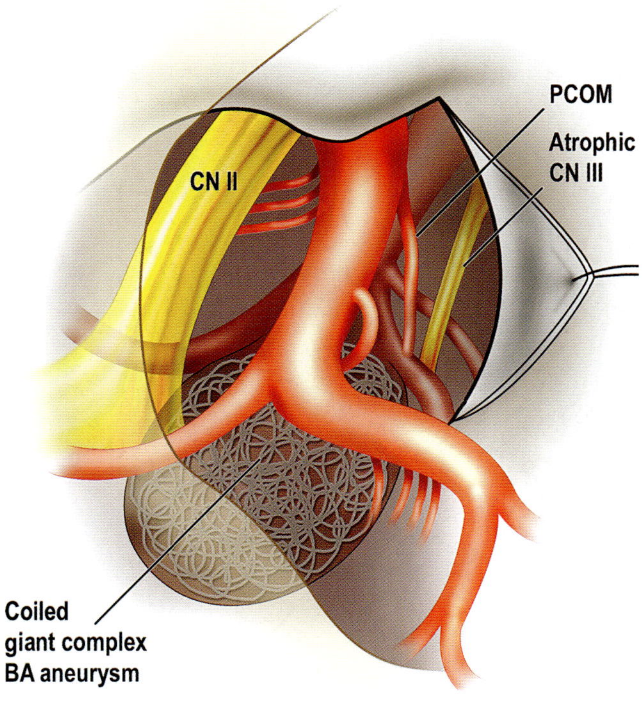

G

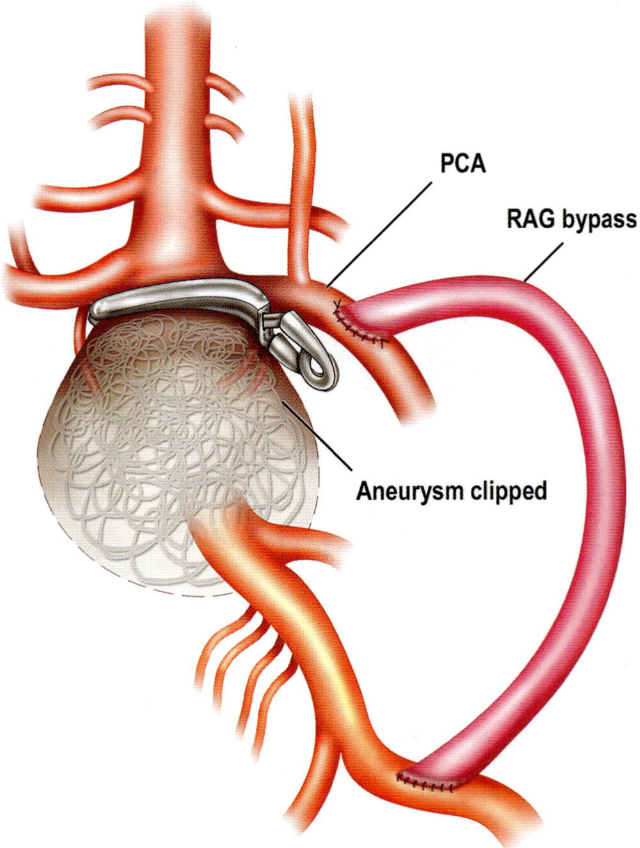

H

Fig. 20.14 *(continued)* **(E,F)** Both internal carotid artery runs reveal small posterior communicating arteries filling the PCAs. **(G)** An intraoperative cartoon shows the relevant anatomy in relation to the coil mass. **(H)** The aneurysm was clipped with a resulting stenosis of the right PCA and hence a radial artery jump graft (RAG) was placed between the M2 and P2. *(continued)*

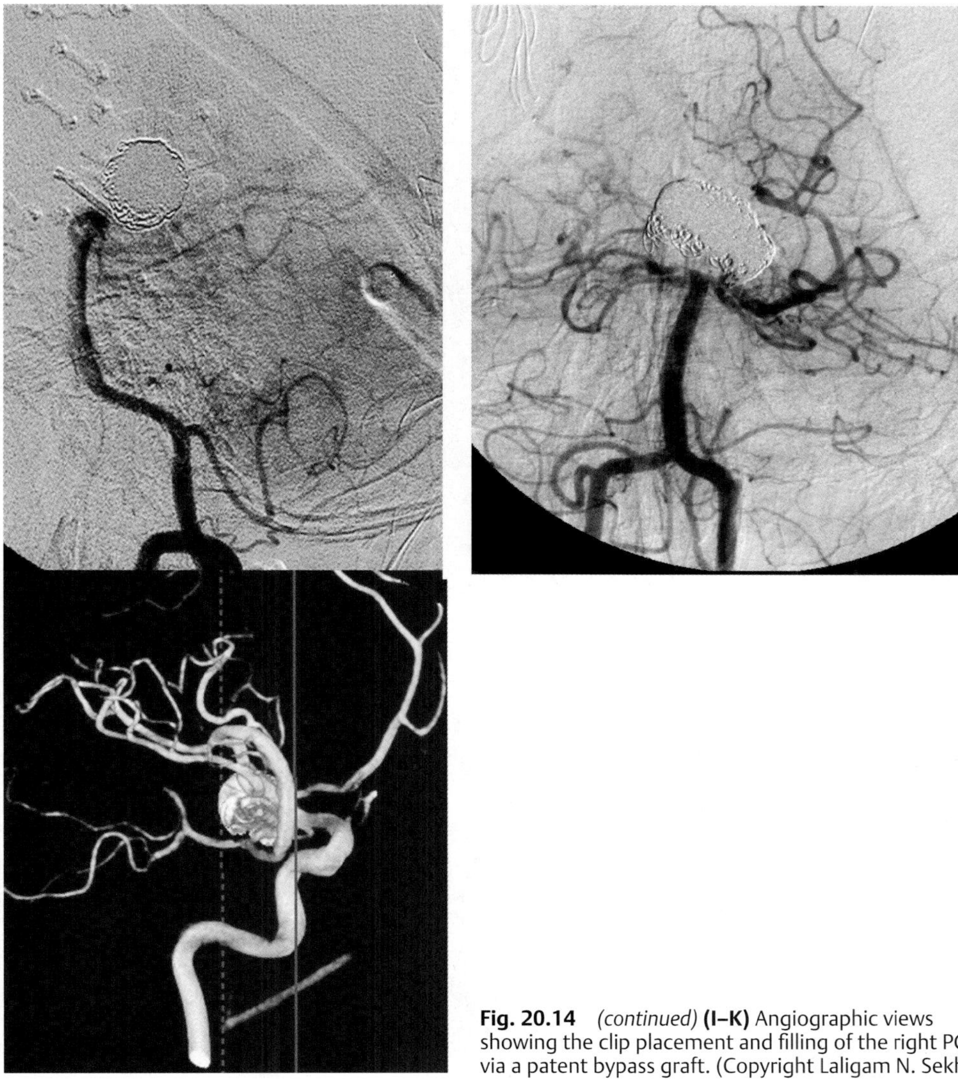

Fig. 20.14 *(continued)* **(I–K)** Angiographic views showing the clip placement and filling of the right PCA via a patent bypass graft. (Copyright Laligam N. Sekhar.)

new symptoms. A right frontal-temporal craniotomy and orbitozygomatic osteotomy was performed. An M2 to P2 RA graft bypass and clipping of the giant basilar aneurysm was successful. The patient had a transient left hemiparesis that resolved. She had had no reoccurrence at 3-year follow-up.

Case #5: Left ECA to Superior M2 RA Bypass Graft, Superior M2 Branch to Inferior M2 Side-to-Side Bypass for Giant Calcified MCA Bifurcation Aneurysm

The patient was a 68-year-old right-handed woman with a cardiac history and an incidentally found 2.5-cm giant MCA bifurcation aneurysm (**Fig. 20.15**). The MCA bifurcation emanated from the calcified neck of the aneurysm. There were also perforators emanating from the contralateral M1. The patient underwent a left frontal-temporal craniotomy with orbital osteotomy for an ECA to superior M2 RA bypass graft, superior M2 branch to inferior M2 side-to-side bypass, and clipping of the giant calcified MCA bifurcation aneurysm. The patient suffered from a transient atrial fibrillation that was controlled with medications. She returned to her preoperative baseline.

Case #6: Right Cervical ICA to Basilar Trunk Saphenous Vein Graft Bypass for Trapping of Giant Fusiform Vertebral-Basilar Aneurysm

The patient was a 15-year-old healthy girl with a growing giant fusiform vertebral-basilar aneurysm (**Fig. 20.16**). The right vertebral fed the aneurysm. The left vertebral ended in the posterior inferior cerebellar artery. The patient underwent a total petrosectomy, transpetrosal, and extreme far lateral combined approach under hypothermic circulatory arrest for the trapping and emptying of this aneurysm. The SV graft was placed from the cervical ICA, distally directly into the basilar artery and the origin of the anterior inferior cerebellar artery. At a 10-year follow-up, the patient had

(Text continued on page 222)

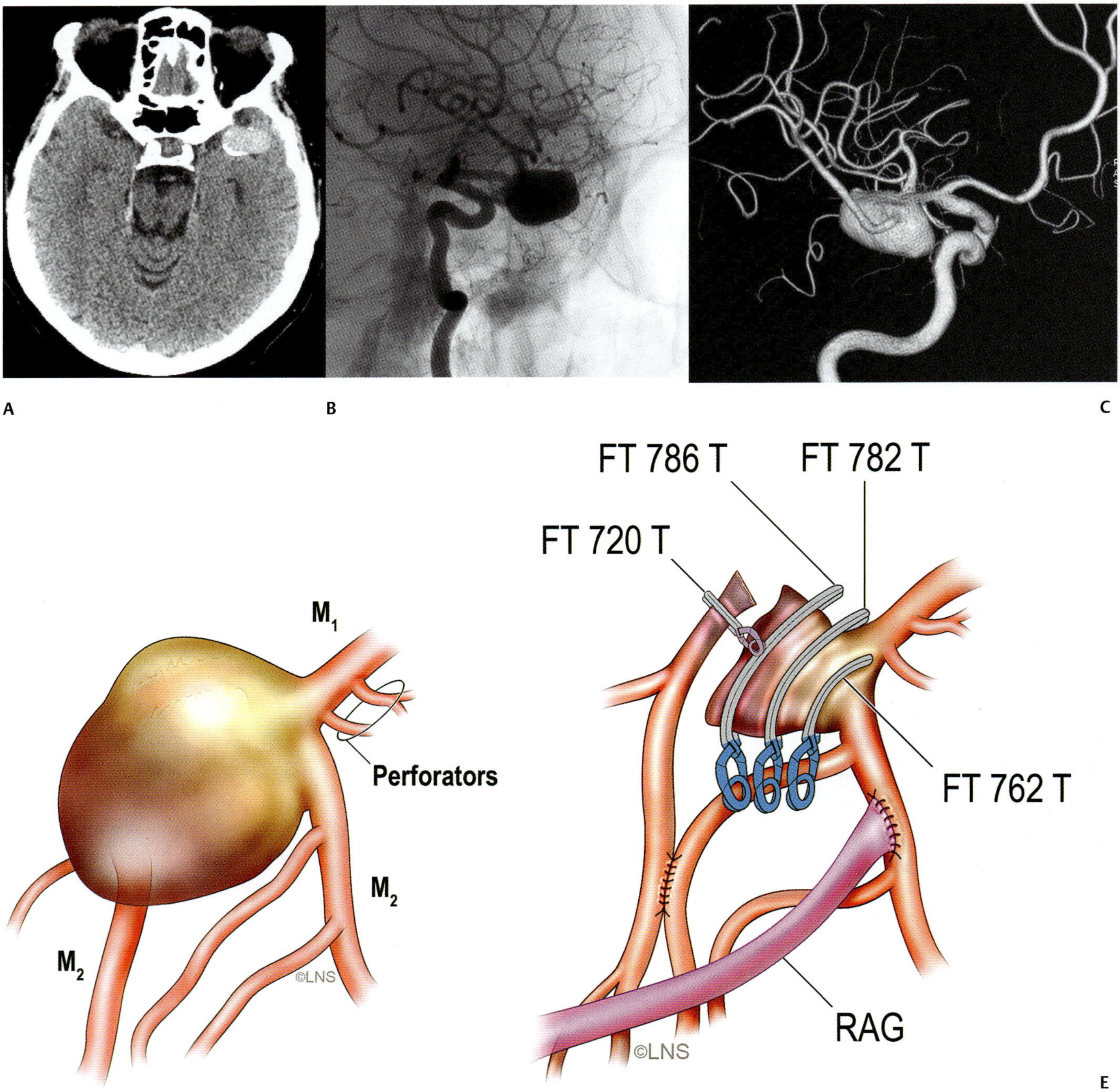

Fig. 20.15 Case #5: Left external carotid artery (ECA) to superior M2 radial artery bypass graft, superior M2 branch to inferior M2 side-to-side bypass for giant calcified middle cerebral artery bifurcation aneurysm. **(A)** CT scan reveals the calcified wall of the aneurysm. **(B)** Angiogram shows the filling of the large bifurcation aneurysm. **(C)** Three-dimensional reconstruction of the angiogram shows the bifurcation vessels emanating from the aneurysm itself. **(D)** Intraoperative drawing depicts the aneurysm and perforators. Note the atheromatous disease and calcification at the neck and branch vessels. **(E)** The aneurysm was clipped and the bifurcation vessels were reconstructed via a radial artery bypass and a side-to-side anastomosis. Postoperative angiographic views depict a patent distal anastomosis with reconstructed bifurcation *(continued)*

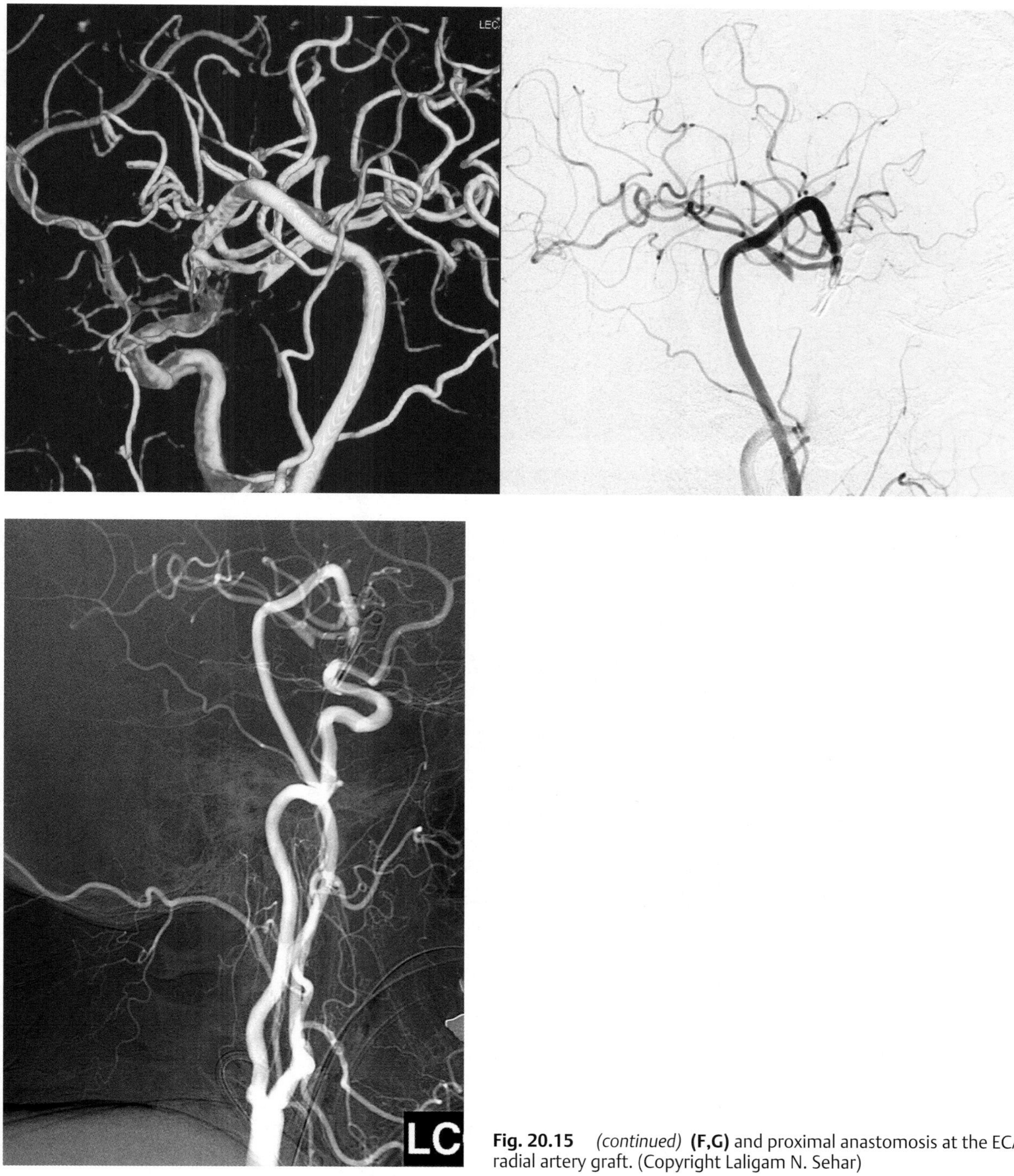

F G H

Fig. 20.15 *(continued)* **(F,G)** and proximal anastomosis at the ECA **(H)** RAG, radial artery graft. (Copyright Laligam N. Sehar)

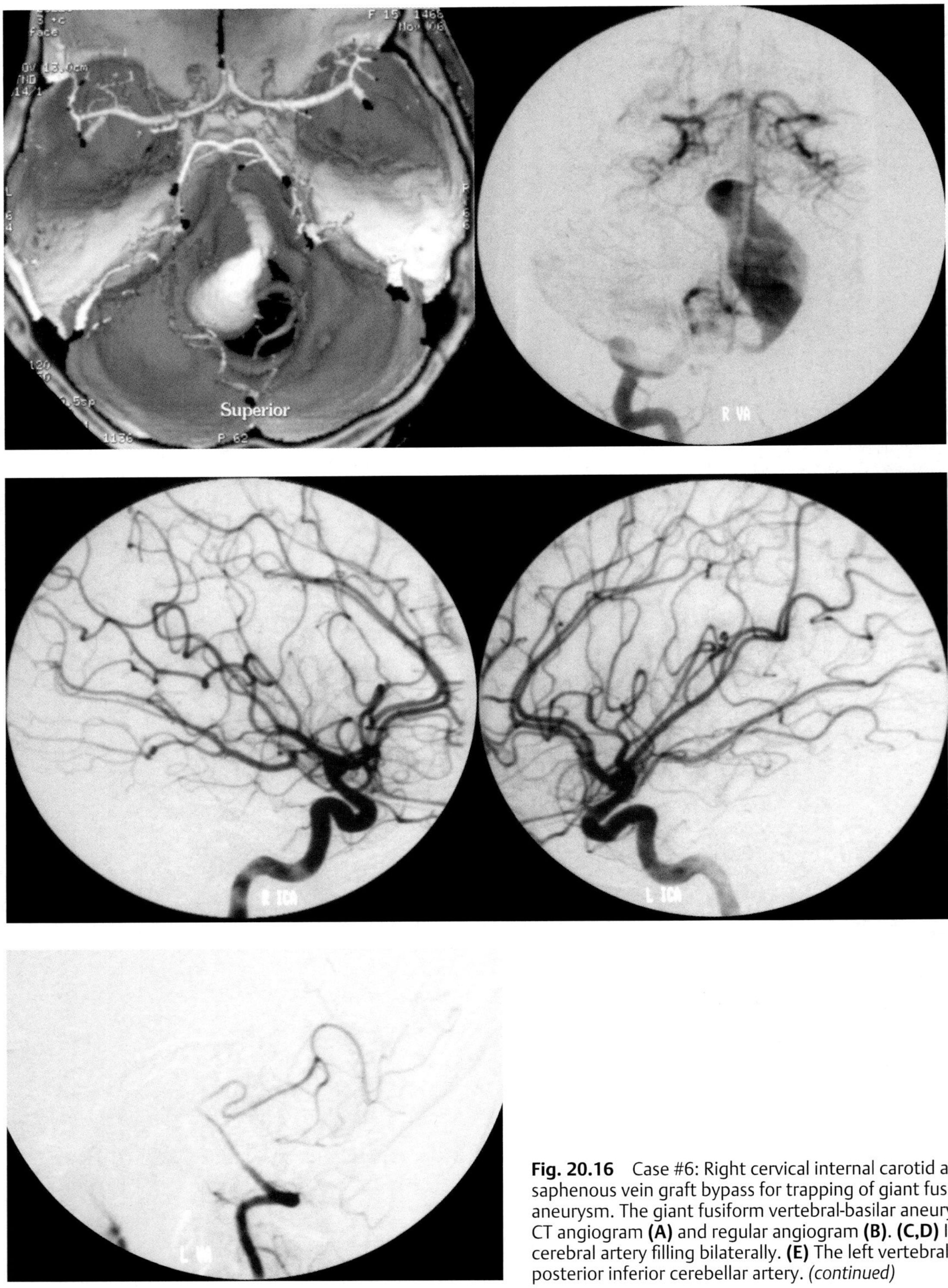

A B C D E

Fig. 20.16 Case #6: Right cervical internal carotid artery (ICA) to basilar trunk saphenous vein graft bypass for trapping of giant fusiform vertebral-basilar aneurysm. The giant fusiform vertebral-basilar aneurysm is appreciated on CT angiogram **(A)** and regular angiogram **(B)**. **(C,D)** ICA runs reveal posterior cerebral artery filling bilaterally. **(E)** The left vertebral injection ends in the posterior inferior cerebellar artery. *(continued)*

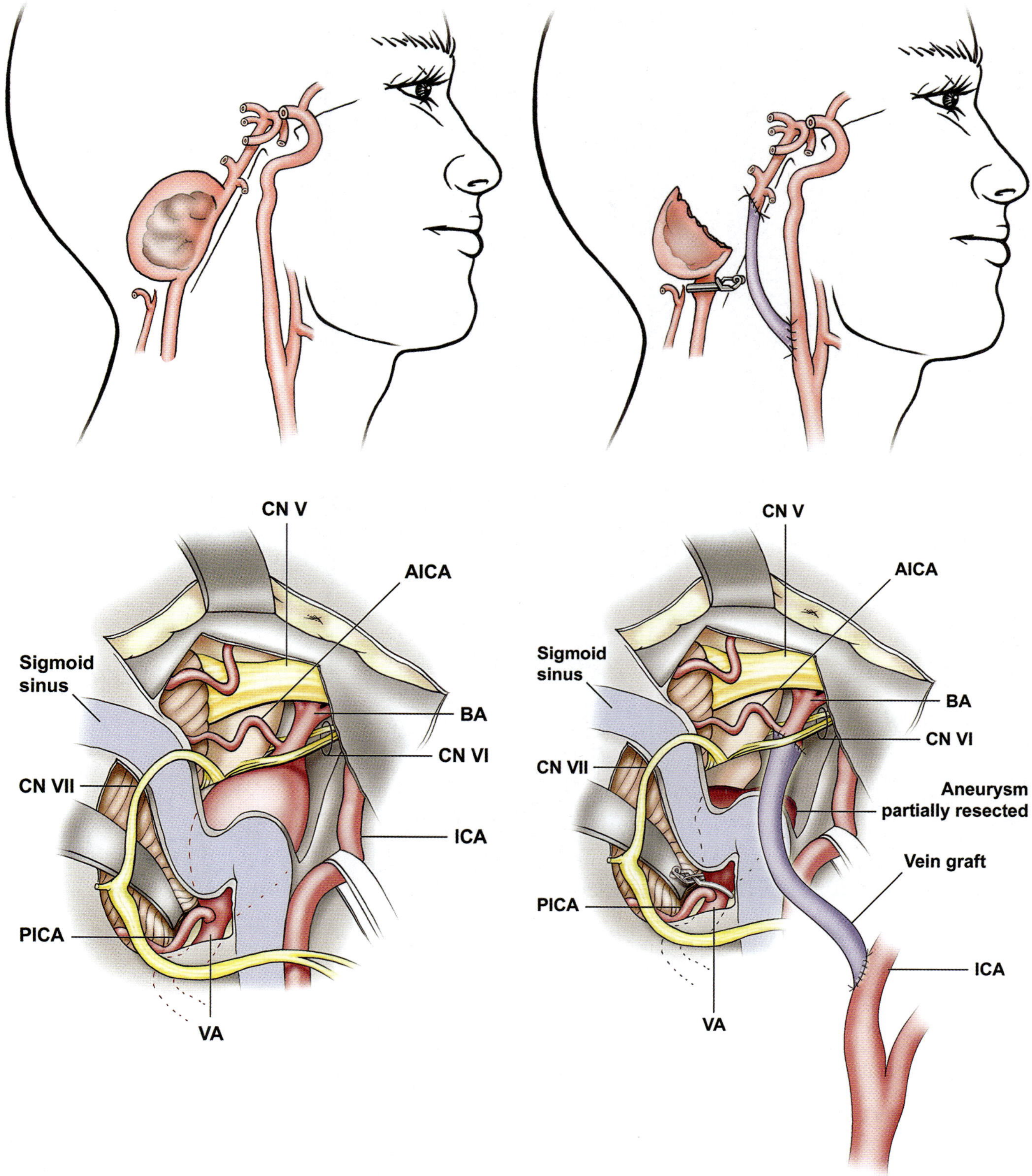

Fig. 20.16 *(continued)* **(F–I)** The preprocedure and postprocedure operative exposures. *(continued)*

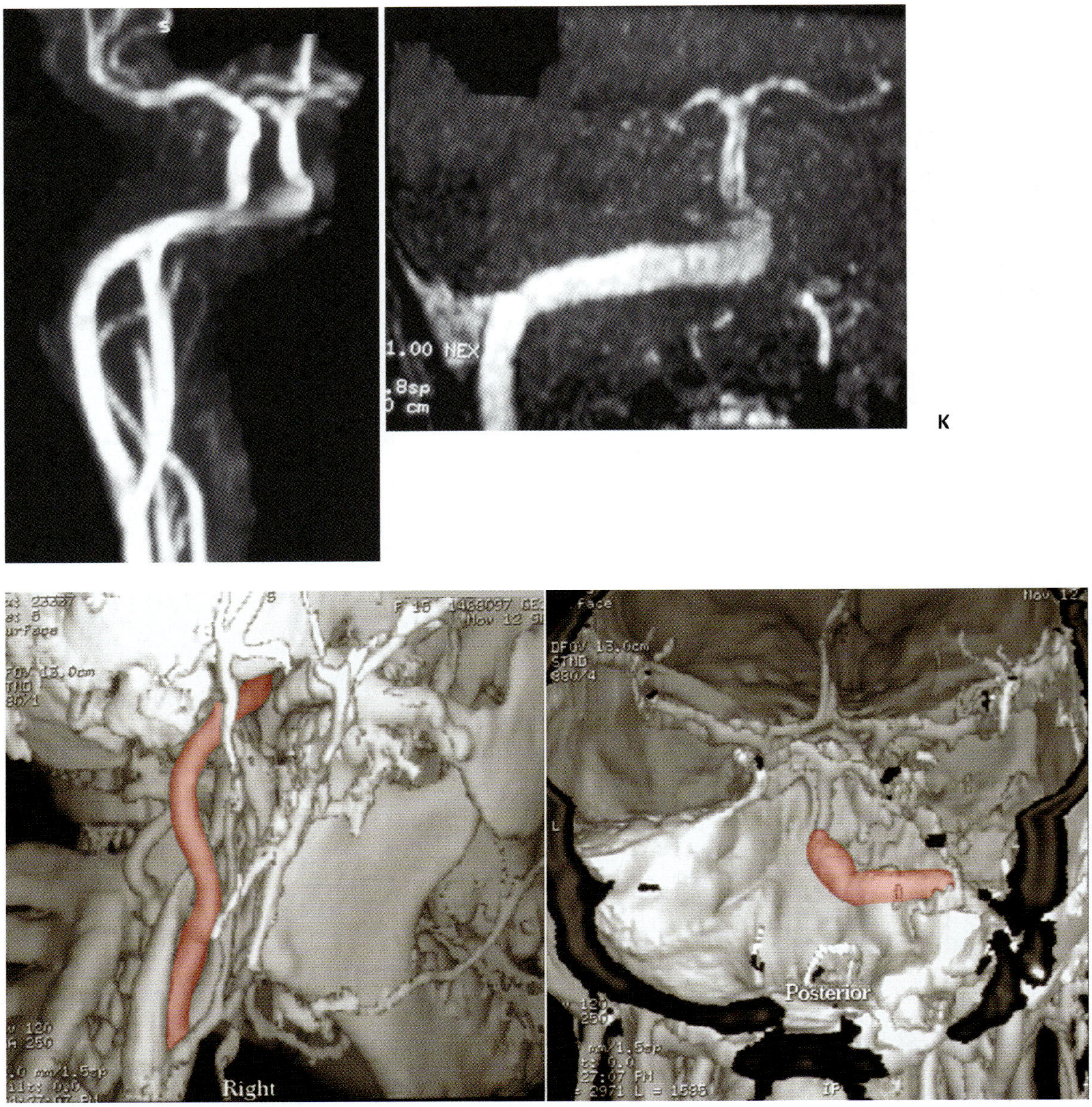

J K L M

Fig. 20.16 *(continued)* **(J,K)** Postoperative MR angiograms show a patent graft filling the posterior circulation. **(L,M)** Postoperative CT angiograms reveal the graft (*red*) in relation to the bony anatomy. CN, cranial nerve; AICA, anterior inferior cerebellar artery; PICA, posterior inferior cerebellar artery; BA, basilar artery; ICA, internal carotid artery. (Copyright Laligam N. Sekhar.)

a House-Brackman II facial paresis and no hearing on the right. She had graduated from a masters program, and was working full time. Her MRA showed a widely patent graft filling the posterior circulation.

◆ Conclusions

The overall quality of care and long-term outcome continues to improve for patients with intracranial aneurysms. The complexity of the aneurysms treated continues to increase. The field of endovascular neurosurgery has revolutionized vascular neurosurgery for the better. The coiling and stenting technology does, however, fall short in a select group of ultra-complex aneurysms. Furthermore, clip reconstruction of these aneurysms puts those patients at risk for immediate or delayed infarction as a result of poor blood flow. Revascularization techniques for the treatment of these complex aneurysms make it possible to cure those patients with minimal morbidity and mortality.

The natural history is of utmost importance when considering treatment of any aneurysm. When it is determined that the aneurysm should be treated then the risk should be weighed against the risk of the treatment. For the neurovascular center, a vascular neurosurgeon versed in revascularization techniques adds to the options for the safe treatment of these lesions.

References

1. Sekhar LN, Bucur SD, Bank WO, Wright DC. Venous and arterial bypass grafts for difficult tumors, aneurysms, and occlusive vascular lesions: evolution of surgical treatment and improved graft results. Neurosurgery 1999;44(6):1207–1223
2. Sekhar LN, Kalavakonda C. Cerebral revascularization for aneurysms and tumors. Neurosurgery 2002;50(2):321–331
3. Sekhar LN, Duff JM, Kalavakonda C, Olding M. Cerebral revascularization using radial artery grafts for the treatment of complex intracranial aneurysms: techniques and outcomes for 17 patients. Neurosurgery 2001;49(3):646–658
4. Evans JJ, Sekhar LN, Rak R, Stimac D. Bypass grafting and revascularization in the management of posterior circulation aneurysms. Neurosurgery 2004;55(5):1036–1049
5. Spetzler RF, Carter LP. Revascularization and aneurysm surgery: current status. Neurosurgery 1985;16(1):111–116
6. Sekhar LN, Stimac D, Bakir A, Rak R. Reconstruction options for complex middle cerebral artery aneurysms. Neurosurgery 2005; 56(1, Suppl):66–74
7. Sundt TM Jr, Piepgras DG, Marsh WR, Fode NC. Saphenous vein bypass grafts for giant aneurysms and intracranial occlusive disease. J Neurosurg 1986;65(4):439–450
8. Sekhar LN, Natarajan SK, Ellenbogen RG, Ghodke B. Cerebral revascularization for ischemia, aneurysms, and cranial base tumors. Neurosurgery 2008; 62(6, Suppl 3):1373–1408
9. Mohit AA, Sekhar LN, Natarajan SK, Britz GW, Ghodke B. High-flow bypass grafts in the management of complex intracranial aneurysms. Neurosurgery 2007; 60(2, Suppl 1):ONS105–ONS122
10. Sekhar LN, Natarajan SK, Britz GW, Ghodke B. Microsurgical management of anterior communicating artery aneurysms. Neurosurgery 2007; 61(5, Suppl 2):273–290
11. Regli L, Piepgras DG, Hansen KK. Late patency of long saphenous vein bypass grafts to the anterior and posterior cerebral circulation. J Neurosurg 1995;83(5):806–811
12. Markar SR, Kutty R, Edmonds L, Sadat U, Nair S. A meta-analysis of minimally invasive versus traditional open vein harvest technique for coronary artery bypass graft surgery. Interact Cardiovasc Thorac Surg 2010;10(2):266–270

Chapter 21

Evolving Technology for Open Surgical Revascularization

Tristan P. C. van Doormaal, Giuseppe Esposito, Albert van der Zwan, and Luca Regli

◆ Conventional Microanastomosis

The first vascular anastomosis was described by Eck in 1877.[1] The French physician Carrel developed and published in 1902 the first arterial end-to-side anastomosis using fine suture material and triangulation.[2] The development of neurosurgical vascular bypass techniques made a leap in the 1960s, when the merging with the development in surgical magnification led to the rapid growth of cerebral microvascular surgery.[3] Since then, to construct a microvascular anastomosis, temporary occlusion of the recipient vessel and end-to-side attachment of a donor vessel with interrupted or continuous microsutures is still the standard technique in neurosurgery and other professions using microanastomoses.

The conventional microanastomosis has several benefits. The first is the well-known reliability of the anastomosis over the long term. Enormous experimental and clinical experience has been acquired in the past 100-plus years. The second benefit is the relative flexibility of the method. The anastomosis can adapt to many different tissue conditions and localizations. Finally, the suture material is readily available and relatively inexpensive. Nevertheless, a sutured conventional microanastomosis has several disadvantages. The first disadvantage is the potential vascular wall damage caused by the penetrating needle and passage of the suture material. This can influence the local healing response and may cause an inflammatory reaction, thrombocyte aggregation, impaired endothelial function, intimal hyperplasia, and hence stenosis. Although different types of nonabsorbable suture materials, absorbable sutures, and atraumatic needles have been used to create vascular anastomoses, vascular wall damage cannot be eliminated by any of these devices.[4] The second disadvantage is the technical difficulty that is associated with conventional anastomosis creation when the depth of the anastomosis is increased and the working channel is narrow, as is often the case in vascular neurosurgery. A third disadvantage is the temporary occlusion time of the recipient artery during anastomosis attachment. This potentially results in ischemia in the flow territory of the recipient artery.[5] Moreover, the temporary clips can damage the recipient artery vessel wall. Therefore, a conventional microanastomosis is certainly not an ideal anastomosis.

◆ Ideal Microanastomosis

An ideal microanastomosis should meet several criteria. First, the attachment should not cause damage to the recipient artery. Second, it should be possible to perform the anastomosis relatively easily and quickly. For neurosurgical purposes, it is important that the anastomosis can be constructed through a narrow working channel and at increased depths without damaging or even touching surrounding intracranial structures. Third, the anastomosis should not be accompanied by typical problems like leakage in the acute phase or pseudoaneurysm formation in the chronic phase. Finally, it has to be shown that the anastomosis reendothelializes in the long term, including eventual intraluminal parts, without causing intima hyperplasia and resulting stenosis.

Several attempts have been made to invent an ideal anastomosis: sutures have been reduced or even abandoned ("sutureless") as well as temporary occlusion ("nonocclusive"). In this chapter we further describe some of the most intriguing new techniques developed to partially or fully meet the criteria of an ideal anastomosis.

◆ New Techniques

Sealants

Generally, a surgical sealant is easier and more quickly applied than a suture. Anastomosis attachment with only surgical sealant is currently impossible because the anastomotic strength is too low, resulting in leakage and pseudoaneurysm formation. However, during replacement of part of the sutures or as an adjunctive next to an anastomotic device, some sealants have been shown to be of use.[6,7] Using a sealant to replace several sutures needed to attach any type of anastomosis theoretically simplifies the procedure and reduces complications and surgery time. Furthermore, it would make an anastomosis possible on locations at which it is impossible to suture in one or more quadrants.

Four families of surgical sealants are currently available that can be used for vascular anastomosis sealing. The first group is formed by the fibrin sealants. Benefits include good applicability and nontoxicity. Several fibrin sealants are approved for intracranial use, such as Tisseel (Baxter Healthcare Corp., Deerfield, IL) and Beriplast (CSL Behring, King of Prussia, PA). Fibrin sealants have less strength than other sealant families. Moreover, the glue is very fluent at application, which can result in unintentional entering of the anastomosis or migration to other areas. However, patches coated with fibrinogen and thrombin (TachoSil; Nycomed, Zurich, Switzerland) circumvent these drawbacks and have better strength. This sealant shows less migration but with good flexibility.[8] The second category is composed of a bovine serum albumin/glutaraldehyde sealant (Bioglue, Kennesaw, GA). This sealant has good applicability and strength, but it has toxic potential. It has not been approved by the U.S. Food and Drug Administration (FDA) for intracranial use. The third group is formed by the polyethylene glycol sealants (DuraSeal, Covidien plc, Dublin, Ireland; CoSeal, Angiotech Pharmaceuticals, Vancouver, British Columbia, Canada). The benefits of these sealants include strength and nontoxicity, and they are FDA approved for intracranial use. They are difficult to apply because of low viscosity and unpractical applicators, however, and they swell within 24 to 48 hours after application. The fourth group comprises the cyanoacrylate sealants (OMNEX; Ethicon, Somerville, NJ). These sealants are strong but are histotoxic and nondeformable after polymerization, which is very fast. Hence, they are difficult to apply.

In conclusion, the optimal intracranial anastomotic sealant has not been found yet. The most promising sealant is a patch coated with fibrinogen and thrombin (TachoSil).

Clips

Another option to replace a suture is a clip. Two systems are currently on the market, and both have been used for cerebral revascularization.

The vascular closure staple (VCS) system (United States Surgical Corp., Norwalk, CT) involves titanium clips with nonpenetrating tips, housed in an automated, disposable clip applier (**Fig. 21.1**). Four different sizes of clips are available for different vessel wall thickness, from 0.9 to 3.0 mm. The clips

A 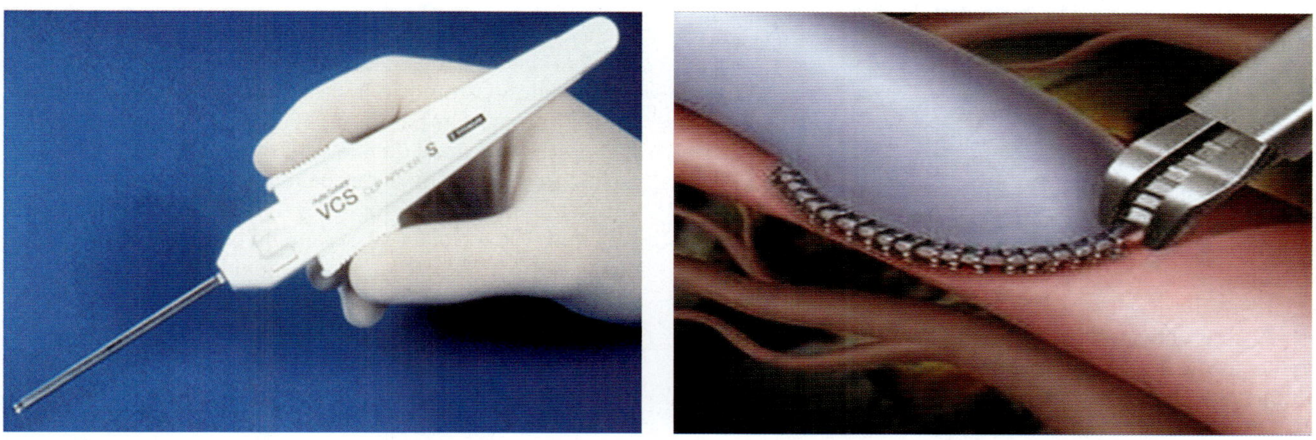 B

C 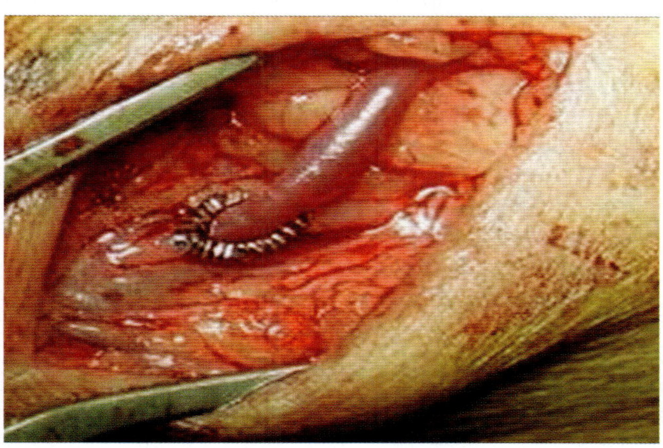

Fig. 21.1 **(A)** Vascular closure staple (VCS) applier (United States Surgical Corp., Norwalk, CT). **(B,C)** End-to-side VCS anastomosis.

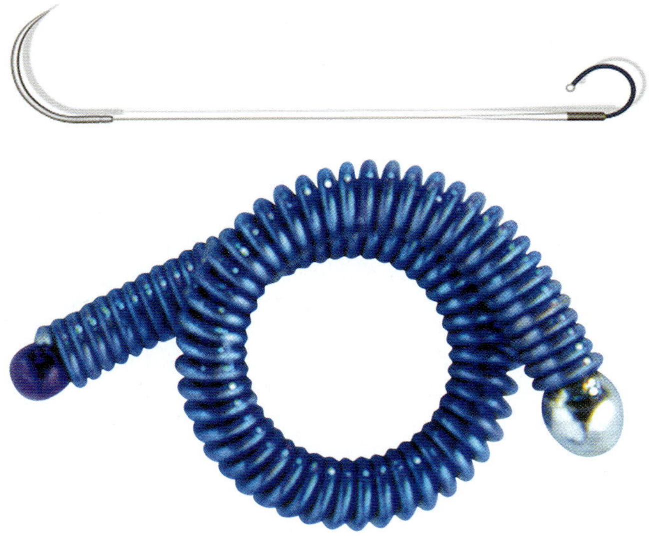

A

B

Fig. 21.2 **(A)** U-clip anastomotic device before deployment. **(B)** U-clip anastomotic device after deployment. (Courtesy of Medtronic, Inc., Minneapolis, MN.)

are applied to everted vessel edges in an interrupted fashion.[9] The main advantage of the system is that no intraluminal foreign body is present, resulting in minimal platelet aggregation and less endothelial damage than conventional suturing methods. The system does not penetrate the vessel lumen or compromise its diameter. Its main drawback is the technical challenge involved in inverting the walls of atherosclerotic vessels and joining the vessels, especially when the anastomosis is deep.[10] Microsurgical training and knowledge of clip-related pitfalls are mandatory.

The nitinol U-clip (Medtronic, Inc., Minneapolis, MN) is a self-closing vascular clip (**Fig. 21.2**). It is composed of four basic components: a self-closing clip, a release mechanism, a flexible member, and a needle. Surgical application of the U-clip is similar to conventional suture placement with the use of a standard needle driver. Once the clip is positioned, the release mechanism is activated by squeezing on the dedicated spot with the needle driver. This approximates the vessel walls by returning the U-clip to its preferred closed configuration.[11] Benefits include elimination of knot tying. Minimal anastomotic leakage and good postoperative angiographic and functional data have been reported in one patient.[12] However, the system still requires needle placement equal to a microsuture. This needle is rather big, even on the smallest available U-clip. The release mechanism requires training and can be challenging during deep anastomoses. The Spyder (Medtronic, Inc.) is a newly developed tool enabling the automatic application of six U-clips at one time. However, this device in its current form is too big for intracranial use.

Laser Welding

Another possibility to replace sutures is to weld the tissue together using a laser. The basic principle of this technique is using the thermal energy induced by the laser to create protein bonds. Neodynium YAG lasers, diode lasers, and CO_2 lasers all have been used for this purpose.[10] Advantages include reduction or suppression of bleeding, shortened operative time, and a faster and superior vascular healing process because the use of suture material is reduced. The main disadvantages are the poor anastomotic strength, especially in larger-sized vessels (therefore the laser-welded anastomosis still requires the insertion of multiple sutures) and the possibility of vascular wall heating-related damage. Advances in addressing these issues have been the use of chromophores and the addition of endogenous and exogenous material to be used as solder. In particular, the incorporation into the protein solder of a laser-absorbing chromophore makes it possible to confine the heat into the area of solder application and reduces the extent of collateral heat damage to adjacent tissues.[13,14]

Recently, a new technique was described using laser welding in combination with the topical application of indocyanine green[15] [MOLVA; minimally occlusive laser vascular anastomosis; (**Fig. 21.3**)]. This technique guarantees a minimal occlusion time of the recipient artery and increases the anastomosis strength; intraoperative thermographic analysis is used to limit the vascular wall heating-related damage. Laser welding has not yet been used on patients.

Automated End-to-Side Anastomosis: C-Port xA System

The C-port xA (Cardica, Inc., Redwood City, CA) integrates in one tool the functions necessary to enable rapid, automated end-to-side anastomosis. It was developed primarily for end-to-side coronary anastomoses (**Fig. 21.4**). A vein or arterial graft with a maximal double wall thickness of 1.4 mm is attached to the system. It can be deployed into target vessels with a minimum diameter of 1.3 mm and a wall thickness of 0.75 mm. The recipient vessel should be prepared over minimally 18 mm. The target vessel should be suitable for conventional microanastomosis and be free of arteriosclerotic disease. For deployment, the system uses a CO_2 cartridge. The system requires short temporary occlusion; average occlusion time in 10 patients was 16 ± 3.4 minutes.[9] However, the automated anastomosis time itself is 1 minute. The automated anastomosis involves the placement of 13 staples that circumferentially connect the donor and the recipient vessel end-to-side. The arteriotomy is performed at the same time by an automated knife located inside the anvil. After the anastomosis and retrieval of the device, one or more sutures are necessary to seal the small arteriotomy required to introduce the anvil into the lumen of the recipient vessel. Benefits of the system include the short temporary occlusion time. Is has been shown to be feasible on the M2 part of the middle cerebral artery on a cadaver model,[16] and good results have been reported in terms of short-term patency in 11 patients.[17,18] The disadvantages, however, are the relatively large size of the applicator and its straight shape, causing impairment of the view on the anastomosis and limiting the use of the device essentially to the M2 segments in its current design.

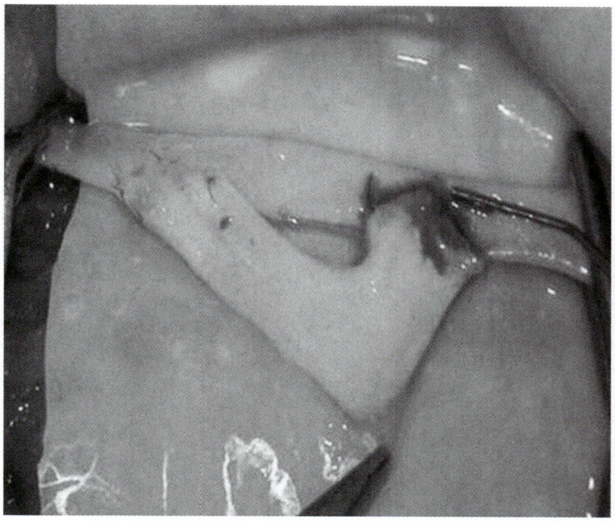
A

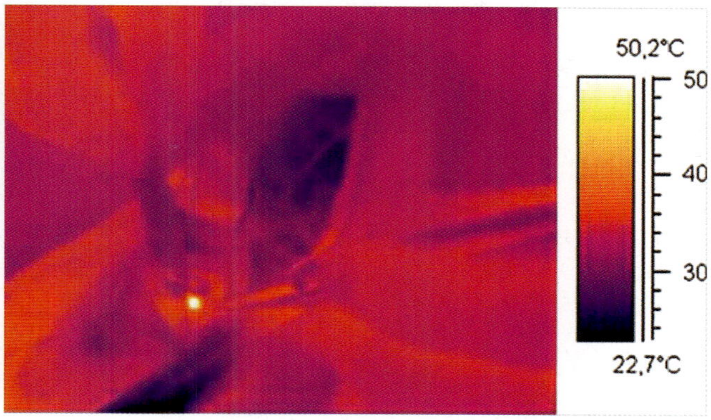

B

Fig. 21.3 **(A)** Indocyanine green application on the minimally occlusive laser vascular anastomosis (MOLVA). **(B)** Second local heating of the MOLVA by the diode laser. (From Puca A, Esposito G, Albanese A, et al. Minimally occlusive laser vascular anastomosis [MOLVA]: experimental study. Acta Neurochir [Wien] 2009;151:366. Reprinted with permission.)

As opposed to coronary anastomosis, there is not enough experience yet with cerebral revascularization to evaluate the complication rate and the long-term permeability.

Excimer Laser–Assisted Nonocclusive Anastomosis

The excimer laser–assisted nonocclusive anastomosis (ELANA) technique (**Fig. 21.5**) facilitates the construction of an end-to-side anastomosis without temporary occlusion of the recipient artery. It was primarily developed for cerebral revascularization. As a donor vessel, a vein or artery can be used with an outer circumference of minimally 2 mm and maximally 4 mm. First, a platinum ring of 2.6 or 2.8 mm is attached to the distal segment of the donor vessel using eight microsutures (**Figs. 21.5A–C**). The ring with the attached distal donor segment is subsequently stitched end-to-side to the recipient using again right microsutures (**Fig. 21.5D**). This is followed by the passing of the ELANA 2.0 laser suction catheter down the lumen of the open donor vessel. The tip of the catheter is placed against the sidewall of the recipient vessel (**Fig. 21.5E**). After 2 minutes of

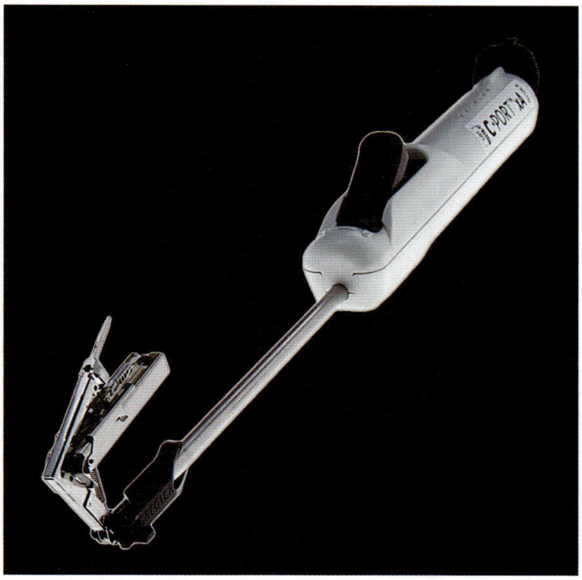

A

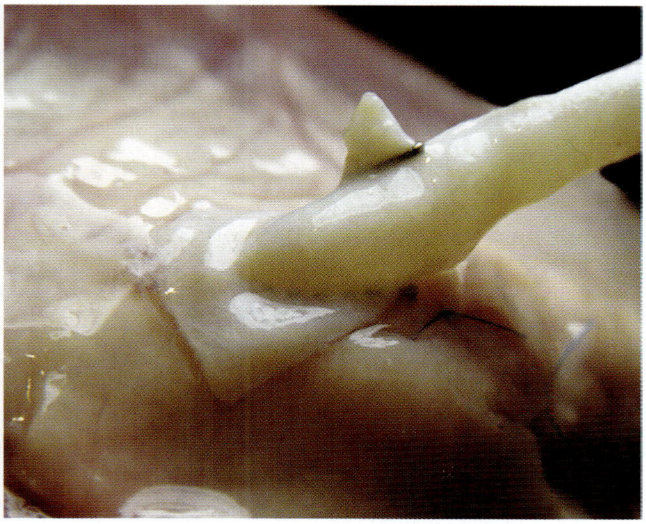
B

Fig. 21.4 **(A)** Overview of the C-Port xA applicator. **(B)** A C-Port anastomosis. (Courtesy of Cardica, Inc., Redwood City, CA.)

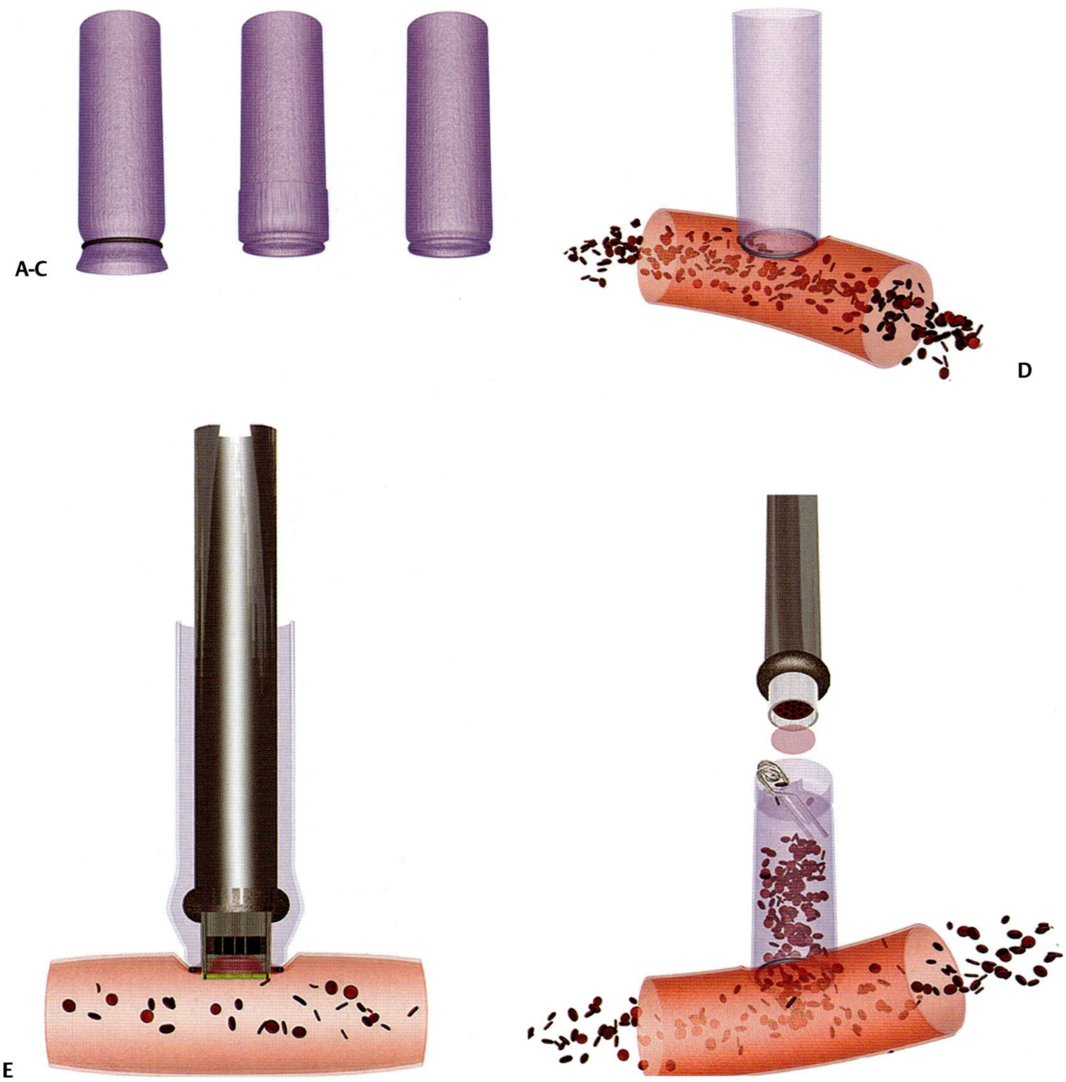

Fig. 21.5 The excimer laser–assisted nonocclusive anastomosis (ELANA) procedure. **(A–C)** The platinum ring attachment. **(D)** Attachment of the donor vessel with the ring to the recipient artery. **(E)** Insertion of the laser catheter and performance of the arteriotomy by the laser energy. **(F)** Removal of the catheter with the arteriotomy flap. A temporary clip is applied on the donor vessel to avoid retrograde flow. There is never interruption of the arterial flow in the recipient artery. (From van Doormaal TP, van der Zwan A, Verweij BH, Langer DJ, Tulleken CA. Treatment of giant and large internal carotid artery aneurysms with a high-flow replacement bypass using the excimer laser–assisted nonocclusive anastomosis technique. Neurosurgery 2008;62:1414. Reprinted with permission.)

active suctioning from the dedicated inside portion of the catheter, the laser fibers on the outside of the catheter are activated over 5 seconds. The laser broaches the recipient arterial wall and separates an arteriotomy flap from the recipient (**Fig. 21.5F**). The suction portion of the catheter maintains contact with the small arteriotomy flap, thus preventing its migration into the lumen of the recipient. Advantages of this procedure include (1) the nonocclusive character, (2) the demonstrated good functional patient outcome in a large cohort of patients (over 400 cases were performed up to mid-2009), (3) a good long-term patency rate, and (4) adequate reendothelialization.[19–22] Drawbacks of the technique are the technical challenge, which includes not only stitch placement, but also catheter insertion, and the relatively high costs of the Excimer laser system. Further developments of the ELANA technique will focus on sutureless and minimal invasive techniques.

Other Techniques

Most other developments in microanastomosis techniques are aimed at coronary end-to-side anastomoses. Several connectors have been developed to enable minimal access, reduce the technical demand, and standardize anastomosis quality. These techniques include the St. Jude connector (St. Jude Medical Inc, St. Paul, MN), the Graft Connector (Jomed International AB, Helsingborg, Sweden), the Magnetic Vascular Positioner (Ventrica, Freemont, CA), the Heartflow Anastomosis Device (Perclose Inc, Redwood City, CA), the Converge Coronary Anastomosis Coupler (Converge Medical Inc, Sunnyvale, CA), the S2 Anastomotic System (Iitech BV, Amsterdam, The Netherlands), and the Distal Anastomotic Device (Bypass Ltd, Hertzlia, Israel).[10] Theoretically, these connectors could be of use in neurosurgery. Practically, however, in their current design, none of these devices seem to meet the requirements and therefore none of them have been used yet in cerebral revascularization. The most important drawbacks of all these devices are the lack of miniaturization; limited visibility during application, resulting in suboptimal placement in areas difficult to reach; anastomosis bleeding; and intimal hyperplasia.

◆ Future

Anastomosis techniques associated with cerebral revascularization can further technically improve to meet the criteria of the ideal anastomosis: easy, fast, minimally invasive, nonocclusive, and safe. This should lead to minimal recipient artery and surrounding brain manipulation, which is traditionally associated with bypass attachment. However, the upcoming potential availability of more sutureless, nonocclusive methods that are potentially easy and safe to apply should not lead to general adaptation of cerebral revascularization in every neurosurgical clinic. Besides the creation of an anastomosis, the neurosurgeon should be trained and regularly place microsutures—not only for conventional anastomoses—but also to control leakages or other anastomosis device-related problems. To reach this goal, microsurgical training for the dedicated neurosurgeon in a readily available vascular laboratory is of vital importance. Specialized centers should be formed with close cooperation between highly trained neurosurgeons and neurointerventional specialists. The neurosurgeon in these centers should master different state of the art cerebral revascularization techniques while the neuroradiologist develops expertise in all cutting-edge endovascular techniques. Other centers in the region should refer patients and closely cooperate with the center in terms of research and resident education. This will lead to a regular performance of technically difficult cerebral revascularization procedures by the same highly trained neurosurgeons and perioperative guidance by the same specialists–anesthesiologists, neurologists, intensivists, nurses, and medical technology staff. Moreover, it will stimulate new developments in the field of cerebral revascularization that will doubtlessly lead to better functional outcome in the patients.

References

1. Hayden MG, Lee M, Guzman R, Steinberg GK. The evolution of cerebral revascularization surgery. Neurosurg Focus 2009;26(5):E17
2. Schmitt W. Our surgical heritage. Alexis Carrel (1873–1944). Zentralbl Chir 1983;108(8):495–503
3. Kriss TC, Kriss VM. History of the operating microscope: from magnifying glass to microneurosurgery. Neurosurgery 1998;42(4):899–907
4. Zeebregts CJ, Heijmen RH, van den Dungen JJ, van Schilfgaarde R. Nonsuture methods of vascular anastomosis. Br J Surg 2003;90(3):261–271
5. Lavine SD, Masri LS, Levy ML, Giannotta SL. Temporary occlusion of the middle cerebral artery in intracranial aneurysm surgery: time limitation and advantage of brain protection. J Neurosurg 1997;87(6):817–824
6. Bremmer JP, Verweij BH, Van der Zwan A, Reinert MM, Beck HJ, Tulleken CA. Sutureless nonocclusive bypass surgery in combination with an expanded polytetrafluoroethylene graft: laboratory investigation. J Neurosurg 2007;107(6):1190–1197
7. Buijsrogge MP, Scheltes JS, Heikens M, Gründeman PF, Pistecky PV, Borst C. Sutureless coronary anastomosis with an anastomotic device and tissue adhesive in off-pump porcine coronary bypass grafting. J Thorac Cardiovasc Surg 2002;123(4):788–794
8. Aziz O, Athanasiou T, Darzi A. Haemostasis using a ready-to-use collagen sponge coated with activated thrombin and fibrinogen. Surg Technol Int 2005;14:35–40
9. Kirsch WM, Cavallo C, Anton T, et al. An alternative system for cerebrovascular reconstructions: non-penetrating arcuate-legged clips. Cardiovasc Surg 2001;9(6):531–539
10. Tozzi P. Sutureless Anastomoses: Secrets for Success. Darmstadt: Steinkopff Verlag; 2007
11. Baynosa RC, Stutman R, Mahabir RC, Zamboni WA, Khiabani KT. Use of a novel penetrating, sutureless anastomotic device in arterial microvascular anastomoses. J Reconstr Microsurg 2008;24(1):39–42
12. Ferroli P, Biglioli F, Ciceri E, Addis A, Broggi G. Self-closing U-clips for intracranial microanastomoses in high-flow arterial bypass: technical case report. Neurosurgery 2007; 60(2, Suppl 1)E170
13. Bregy A, Bogni S, Bernau VJ, et al. Solder doped polycaprolactone scaffold enables reproducible laser tissue soldering. Lasers Surg Med 2008; 40(10):716–725
14. Puca A, Albanese A, Esposito G, et al. Diode laser–assisted carotid bypass surgery: an experimental study with morphological and immunohistochemical evaluations. Neurosurgery 2006;59(6):1286–1294
15. Puca A, Esposito G, Albanese A, Maira G, Rossi F, Pini R. Minimally occlusive laser vascular anastomosis (MOLVA): experimental study. Acta Neurochir (Wien) 2009;151(4):363–368
16. Bregy A, Alfieri A, Demertzis S, et al. Automated end-to-side anastomosis to the middle cerebral artery: a feasibility study. J Neurosurg 2008; 108(3):567–574
17. Hänggi D, Reinert M, Steiger HJ. C-Port Flex-A–assisted automated anastomosis for high-flow extracranial-intracranial bypass surgery in patients with symptomatic carotid artery occlusion: a feasibility study: clinical article. J Neurosurg 2009;111(1):181–187
18. Dacey RG, Zipfel GJ, Ashley WW, Chicoine MR, Reinert M. Automated, compliant, high-flow common carotid to middle cerebral artery bypass. J Neurosurg 2008;109(3):559–564
19. van Doormaal TP, van der Zwan A, Verweij BH, Han KS, Langer DJ, Tulleken CA. Treatment of giant middle cerebral artery aneurysms with a flow replacement bypass using the excimer laser–assisted nonocclusive anastomosis technique. Neurosurgery 2008;63(1):12–20
20. van Doormaal TP, van der Zwan A, Verweij BH, Langer DJ, Tulleken CA. Treatment of giant and large internal carotid artery aneurysms with a high-flow replacement bypass using the excimer laser–assisted nonocclusive anastomosis technique. Neurosurgery 2008; 62(6, Suppl 3)1411–1418
21. Klijn CJ, Kappelle LJ, van der Zwan A, van Gijn J, Tulleken CA. Excimer laser–assisted high-flow extracranial/intracranial bypass in patients with symptomatic carotid artery occlusion at high risk of recurrent cerebral ischemia: safety and long-term outcome. Stroke 2002;33(10):2451–2458
22. Brilstra EH, Rinkel GJ, Klijn CJ, et al. Excimer laser–assisted bypass in aneurysm treatment: short-term outcomes. J Neurosurg 2002;97(5): 1029–1035

Chapter 22

Evolving Technology for Endovascular Revascularization

Ziad Darkhabani, Sabareesh K. Natarajan, Erik F. Hauck, Elad I. Levy, L. Nelson Hopkins, and Adnan H. Siddiqui

During the past two decades, neuroendovascular therapy has exponentially evolved into a medical specialty of its own driven by a heterogeneous group of specialists that includes cardiologists, neurologists, radiologists, neurosurgeons, vascular surgeons, and neuroscientists in general. This evolution has been largely induced by improving materials science technology that has allowed for the development of novel devices and delivery tools that are enhanced, safe, and effective. For many indications, neuroendovascular therapy has become the standard of care, replacing or complementing traditional gold standard therapies, such as carotid endarterectomy, surgical clip ligation of intracranial aneurysms, and intravenous (IV) thrombolysis of acute stroke. Carotid stenting, coiling of intracranial aneurysms, and intraarterial (IA) thrombolysis/thrombectomy are prime examples of the ongoing endovascular evolution.[1–4] In this chapter, we focus on the newest technical developments and evolving technology of endovascular therapy with respect to intracranial revascularization for cerebral ischemia.

◆ Current Limitations of Endovascular Revascularization

Many endovascular revascularization techniques are derived from applications for treatment of peripheral or coronary vascular disease. However, unlike coronary and peripheral vessels, cerebral vessels are curved and lack structural support, being surrounded only by cerebrospinal fluid. The composition of the arterial walls is different, with intracranial arteries having loss of vasa vasorum and external elastic membranes, near absence of the adventitia, and a tunica media composed principally of smooth muscle cells.[5–8] Visualization of the intracranial vasculature has limitations. The bony cranium obscures the view. Frequently, because of vessel tortuosity, multiple angles are required to properly visualize intracranial vessels. Absolute measurements of cerebral blood flow remain a challenge. Access to the intracranial circulation can be dramatically limited because of tortuous aortic arch variations (type II or type III aortic arch). Endovascular therapy for intracranial disease, therefore, requires special devices and skills. Heterogeneity of specialists with very different training experiences substantiates this limitation. Thus, one direction of the new development is the invention, production, and application of newer catheters allowing proximal access (aortic arch, common carotid arteries) and distal access (intracranial platform catheters). In addition, modification of existing technology (i.e., coronary stents) to allow intracranial navigation (i.e., increased flexibility, softness) is another direction of the technical advancement. Further, the scientific evidence (prospective multicenter randomized controlled trials) supporting the application of endovascular procedures is still limited. A large body of evidence for neuroendovascular approaches is derived from studies that are retrospective and mostly anecdotal in nature. Because of the constant and rapid evolution/development of newer methods, evidence-based medicine lags behind. Thus, there is currently a large effort to increase level I clinical evidence to support the application of endovascular techniques as a standard of care for multiple indications, including intracranial revascularization for ischemic disease, particularly stroke. Another limit is the local availability and acceptance of endovascular technology and techniques. Frequently, institutional protocols govern the endovascular practice. Many hospitals still do not have the basic equipment (i.e., biplane angiography) to perform neuroendovascular procedures safely. The lack of these modalities is slowing the spread of endovascular evolution throughout the country as well as internationally. In summary, current endovascular therapy has some limitations, including proper visualization, technical access to the intracranial space, navigability of tools, heterogeneity of operator skills and training, scientific (data-based) validation, and local availability of the technology. But truly, only imagination is the limit for what the future holds for this field.

Intravascular Ultrasound

Intravascular ultrasound (IVUS) is a medical imaging modality that uses a specially designed catheter with a miniaturized ultrasound probe attached to the distal end of the catheter. The proximal end of the catheter is attached to computerized ultrasound equipment. IVUS allows the application of ultrasound technology to see from inside blood vessels out through the surrounding blood column, visualizing the luminal wall structure of the blood vessels. This imaging modality has become an important diagnostic and therapeutic adjunct for coronary artery angioplasty and stenting. It is used in the coronary arteries to determine the amount of atheromatous plaque built up at any particular point in the epicardium and is useful in the determination of plaque volume within the wall of the artery and/or the degree of stenosis of the artery lumen. It can be especially useful in situations in which angiographic imaging is considered unreliable, such as for the lumen of ostial lesions or where angiographic images do not visualize lumen segments adequately, such as regions with multiple overlapping arterial segments. IVUS is also used to assess the effects of treatments of stenosis, such as with hydraulic angioplasty expansion of the artery, with or without stents, and the results of medical therapy over time. It has been increasingly used in research to better understand the behavior of the atherosclerosis process in humans. We routinely use IVUS to evaluate carotid atherosclerotic disease before carotid angioplasty and stenting to establish plaque characteristics that may indicate high and low risk plaques in terms of plaque stability. Similarly, after carotid angioplasty and stenting but prior to removal of proximal or distal protection, we routinely perform IVUS to visualize any intraluminal thrombus, in particular to evaluate the cheese grating effect of the stent.[9] We have used IVUS to assist intracranial angioplasty and stent placement in a patient who underwent angioplasty and stenting for high-grade restenosis of a basilar artery atherosclerotic lesion and in another patient who underwent stenting to treat an occlusive dissection of the left internal carotid artery (ICA) that occurred during arteriovenous malformation embolization; in each case, IVUS provided important information in terms of lesion evaluation, stent selection, and stent placement.[10] Currently, however, the IVUS catheter, which measures only 1 mm in diameter, is still too stiff to be delivered reliably into the intracranial circulation, particularly into the supraclinoidal anterior circulation.

Optical Coherence Tomography

Optical coherence tomography (OCT) is a novel imaging system that is analogous to ultrasound, but imaging is performed with light instead of acoustic waves. OCT measures light reflected from turbid structures.[11–13] This technology is based on principles of low-coherence interferometry allowing the detection of back-scattered near-infrared photons from selected depths and rejection of photons being scattered from other layers. Unlike direct reflective techniques (such as angioscopy), it visualizes the depth at which back-scattering occurs. OCT provides three-dimensional information about the scattering properties of living tissue. The spatial resolution that can be reached is near-histologic (5–8 micron) scale, which makes OCT suitable for in vivo optical biopsy, allowing for the visualization of tissue cross-sectional microstructure, even without a contrast agent. Because signals from different depths are separated by the measurement approach, OCT can detect deeper events more easily than a reflection approach. Endovascular imaging using this technology has mainly been performed in coronary arteries. OCT imaging identifies the structural components of atherosclerotic plaques such as lipid-rich areas, fibrous content, calcified portions, and inflammatory plaques, and has been successfully used to identify thin-capped fibroatheromas and distinguish them from thick-capped and fibrous plaques.[14–18] OCT imaging enables visualization of stent tines postdeployment, stent-wall apposition, poststent stenosis, as well as microdissections and luminal/mural thrombus.[14–18] Feasibility studies on the use of OCT for neuroendovascular imaging in patients have been reported, although further literature in this relatively new field is scant.[11,12] Potential uses include diagnostic imaging of atherosclerotic plaques as well as of endovascular neurointerventions, such as aneurysm coiling and stenting. Similar to IVUS, development of pliable and trackable OCT delivery catheters designed for intracranial delivery hold the promise to be revolutionary during endovascular therapies for intracranial and extracranial atherosclerosis. Because of its higher resolution, OCT may provide greater data on plaque stability during extracranial atherosclerotic disease management with angioplasty and/or stenting. It could be highly valuable in the identification of true versus false lumens during endovascular management of dissections, particularly during management of intracranial dissections with stents where deployment of a device in the false lumen may have disastrous consequences. Again because of its higher resolution, this technique has the potential to deliver greater information about intracranial atherosclerotic plaques as well as thrombus morphology during revascularization of acute stroke. In cases of stent deployment, important information about stent-to-vessel wall apposition and presence of intraluminal thrombus may be obtained with OCT imaging.

Magnetic Resonance Imaging–Guided Endovascular Procedures

The safety of a percutaneous vascular intervention largely depends on accurate visualization of both the device and the surrounding anatomic structures. Fluoroscopic images provide high temporal and spatial resolution of the vascular lumen. By necessity, neuroendovascular fluoroscopic imaging is endoluminal, yielding very little information about the vascular wall and surrounding tissue. Both the patient and the examiner are exposed to radiation. Radiation exposure has immediate and long-term consequences from alopecia and skin burn to neoplasia. This is of particular importance to interventionists who spend many hours every day in an environment with an abundance of radiation. Magnetic resonance imaging (MRI) guidance has the potential to offer soft tissue contrast to visualize the vessel lumen, the vessel wall, and the surrounding structures; and this guidance can provide flow velocity data without any radiation exposure. Gadolinium-based preparations have very short intravascular retention time, and administration of the maximal approved dose of these preparations can be achieved during an interventional procedure. Wacker et al[19] were able to perform catheterization, angioplasty, and stenting in abdominal and renal vessels as small as 2 mm in pigs using MRI guidance with ultrasmall superparamagnetic iron oxide SH U 555 C as an intravascular contrast agent. Therefore, a huge potential exists for radical changes in the way interventions are performed, making them safer for both the patient and the interventional staff in the interventional suite. However, many hurdles remain before MRI guidance for neuroendovascular interventions becomes a reality. MRI hardware and sequence design have to be developed to achieve acceptable patient access and to allow real-time imaging. Further, interventional devices that allow for adequate visualization, safety, and effectiveness have to be designed for the heavy magnetic field environments.

◆ Advances in Intraarterial Pharmacology

The current direction of pharmacologic therapy for acute stroke is thrombolysis with a variety of agents resembling recombinant tissue plasminogen activator (rtPA) that can be administered IV or IA. Standard medical therapy currently approved for acute stroke by the U.S. Food and Drug Administration (FDA) and the European Union is IV alteplase (rtPA). However, IV rtPA treatment for acute stroke remains far from ideal for multiple reasons. Few patients (~3%) receive IV rtPA treatment because of the narrow window for intervention and broad ineligibility criteria.[20] Moreover, the recanalization rates from IV rtPA are of little benefit – only 10% for carotid occlusion and 30% for proximal middle cerebral artery (MCA) occlusions. The rate of clinical improvement and outcomes after IV rtPA are not satisfactory at this time (modified Rankin scale score of ≤2 in 36%).[21] All these reasons imply a need for more effective treatment strategies. IA thrombolysis alone or in combination with IV rtPA has shown promise in an acute setting in patients with thrombotic stroke.[1,22,23] The IA approach is associated with higher recanalization rates using a lower dose of thrombolytic agent and has extended the time window for treatment. Newer and experimental thrombolytic agents with different mechanisms of action are being used and explored for IA thrombolysis, including plasminogen activators, direct fibrinolytics, and fibrinogenolytic agents, as summarized in **Table 22.1**.

Table 22.1 New and Experimental Thrombolytic Agents with Potential for Application in Acute Ischemic Stroke

Plasminogen Activators	
Monteplase	Not investigated in stroke
Lanoteplase	Not investigated in stroke
Pamiteplase	Not investigated in stroke
Staphylokinase	Not investigated in stroke
Desmoteplase	Promising in some studies; from saliva of the vampire bat; more selective and potent
Fibrinolytics	
V10153	Recombinant human plasminogen activated to plasmin
Microplasmin Alfimeprase	Isolate from southern copperhead snake venom
Fibrinogenolytics	
Ancord	Isolate from Malayan pit viper venom; inactivates fibrinogen

◆ Newer Revascularization Technologies

Acute Thrombolysis Augmentation Technologies

Augmented fibrinolysis involves use of ultrasound technology. Theoretically, the ultrasonic energy changes the structure of the clot to temporarily increase its permeability while providing an acoustic pressure gradient to move a thrombolytic agent into the clot to speed its dissolution. This was first tested by using transcranial Doppler imaging while infusing IV rtPA, and initial results show some promise as reported in the Combined Lysis of Thrombus in Brain Ischemia Using Transcranial Ultrasound and Systemic tPA (CLOTBUST) Trial where 49% recanalization was achieved in middle cerebral artery (MCA) occlusions with focused transcranial Doppler during IV rtPA as compared with 30% in the cohort that received only IV rtPA.[24,25] This has been further explored by using a systemic injection of perflutren-lipid microspheres that expand when exposed to ultrasonic energy, thereby increasing the disruptive force of the ultrasonic energy.[26]

The MicroLysUS Infusion Catheter (EKOS; Bothell, WA) is a distal ultrasound transducer, which is used as a thrombolytic delivery catheter. It has been evaluated in the Interventional Management of Stroke (IMS) II trial and appeared at least as effective as a conventional microcatheter for IA rtPA delivery and thrombolysis.[23] It is being evaluated in the ongoing IMS III trial.

The OmniWave Endovascular System (OmniSonics Medical Technologies, Wilmington, MA) directs low-power ultrasonic energy down a catheter wire. This wire has been tuned to create cavitation bubbles that fracture the fibrin matrix of the thrombus without adversely damaging surrounding vessel walls. The OmniWave is currently approved for use in peripheral arterial occlusions and has not been tested in acute stroke. However, it symbolizes technologies aimed at providing adjunctive thrombus disruptive techniques to aid thrombolysis and revascularization.

Mechanical Devices for Acute Occlusion

Mechanical thrombectomy provides the distinct advantage of potentially precluding the use of adjunctive pharmacological thrombolysis. This advantage has allowed for utility of purely mechanical techniques in patients beyond the typical therapeutic windows for IV or even IA rtPA therapy after stroke symptom onset. Numerous new technologies have been developed to improve mechanical clot disruption and retrieval, and are listed below.

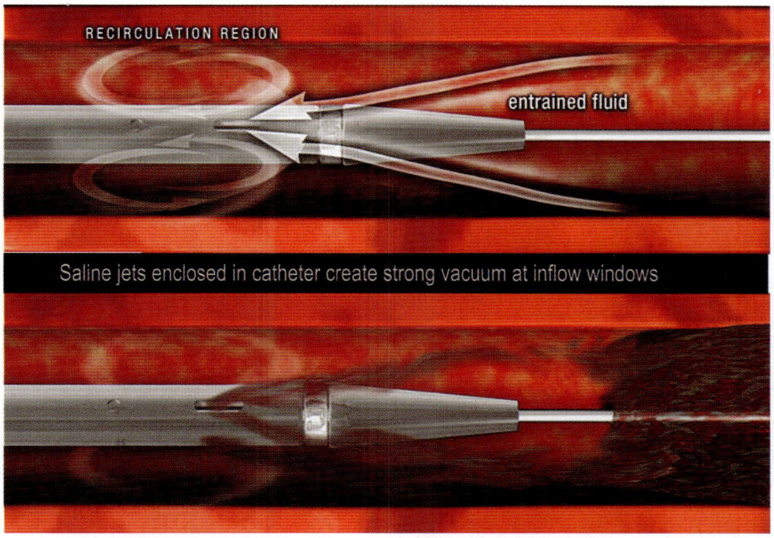

Fig. 22.1 The AngioJet system uses saline jets that are directed back into the catheter to create a low-pressure zone around the catheter tip and induce suction. (Courtesy of Possis Medical Inc., Minneapolis, MN.)

One device is the NeuroJet, which is a modification of the AngioJet device and was specifically designed for the intracranial circulation (the AngioJet is FDA-approved for peripheral and extracranial circulation use; both devices are manufactured by Possis Medical, Minneapolis MN) (**Fig. 22.1**). The device works on the principle of creating a high-pressure saline jet at the distal tip that is then immediately aspirated, creating a Venturi effect with gentle clot disruption and aspiration. There is anecdotal evidence of the utility of the AngioJet in acute stroke[27]; however, a pilot trial with the NeuroJet was aborted due to inability to navigate the tortuous intracranial circulation and proximal vessel injury.[28,29] Other devices designed primarily for the sturdier extracranial circulation that work on a similar principles include the Hydrolyzer (Cordis Endovascular, Warren, NJ), Amplatz Thrombectomy Device (Microvena, White Bear Lake, MN), and Oasis Thrombectomy Catheter (Boston Scientific, Natick, MA). The F.A.S.T. catheter (Genesis Medical Interventional, Redwood City CA), is a hybrid device that affords distal occlusion beyond the clot and local aspiration proximal to the clot. This device was developed for the peripheral circulation with intracranial models under consideration.

The Vasco 35 Catheter (Balt Extrusion, Montmorency, France) was developed for proximal thromboaspiration of clots and is approved for use in Europe. It has a distal luminal diameter of 4.2 French and aspiration is performed through a 20-mL syringe. In a comparison with another Balt device, the Catch (which is a distal basket-type retriever), the Vasco 35 was associated with a recanalization rate of only 39.4%, but, significantly, did not cause distal embolization or vessel trauma.[30]

Another variation on this theme is the Endovascular Photo Acoustic Recanalization (EPAR) system (EndoVasix, Belmont, CA; now W.L. Gore & Associates, Flagstaff, AZ) (**Fig. 22.2**). The device delivers photonic energy through a laser beam to the catheter tip, where the energy creates localized sound waves that cause the formation of microbubbles and emulsification of thrombus. There is no associated aspiration system. In a pilot study, recanalization occurred in 61.1% of patients.[31] Testing with a second laser-aided thrombus emulsification device, the LaTIS (LaTIS, Minneapolis, MN), was aborted because of difficulty navigating into the intracranial circulation.[32]

New Stent Technology for Chronic Intracranial Stenosis

Atherosclerotic stenosis of the major intracranial arteries is an important cause of ischemic stroke, especially in African Americans, Asians, and Hispanics.[33] Patients with high-grade symptomatic intracranial stenosis have a risk of stroke of ~20%, despite medical treatment with antiplatelets or anticoagulants.[34] Moreover, surgical treatment with the extracranial-intracranial bypass procedure has not been proved effective.[35] Recent series of stenting for intracranial stenosis have shown technical success rates of 83 to 100% and periprocedural stroke and death rates of 0 to 12.5%.[36–39] However, midterm results have demonstrated disappointingly high rates of restenosis.[40,41] A newer generation of stents on the market (not yet approved) for intracranial stenosis might be the future treatment for intracranial stenosis.[42]

Evolving Balloon-Expandable Stents

Stenting of intracranial stenosis was initially done with balloon-mounted (coronary) stents. These stents were not optimal for this application because their rigidity posed a limitation for access to tortuous cerebral vessels. A new generation of balloon-expandable stents, like the Pharos (Micrus Endovascular, San Jose, CA) and the Boa and Channel (Balt Extrusion, Montmorency, France), are manufactured mounted on a rapid-exchange percutaneous transluminal angioplasty catheter especially designed for intracranial endovascular applications. The Pharos stent is available in Europe and Latin America but not yet approved by the FDA. Data for the Pharos stent are available from two studies, one conducted in Europe and the other in Latin America.[43,44] Both studies concluded that Pharos stent placement for the treatment of intracranial stenosis is feasible and is associated with a high technical success rate and a low rate of restenosis.

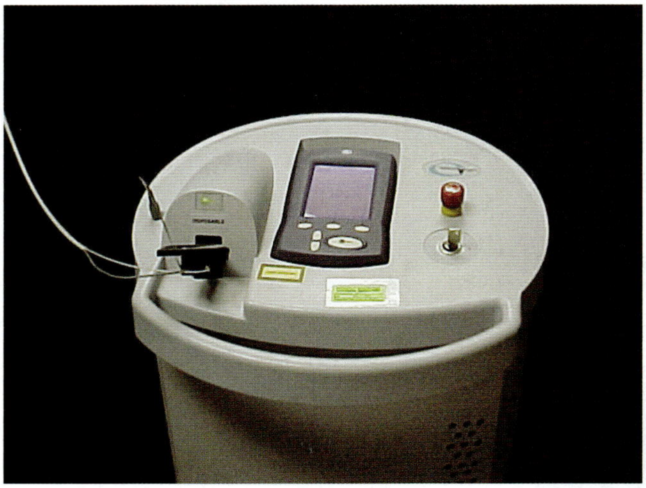

A

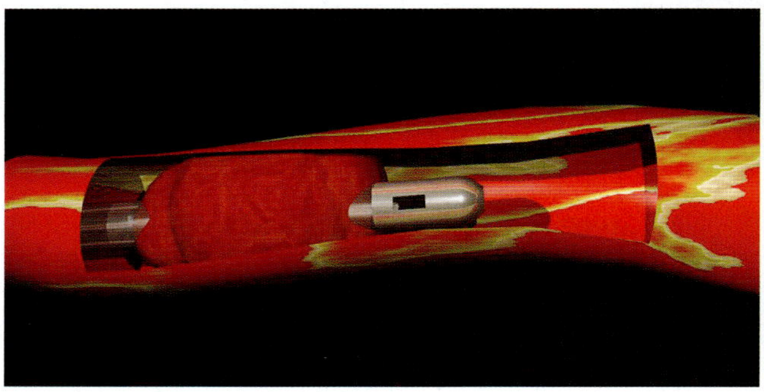

B

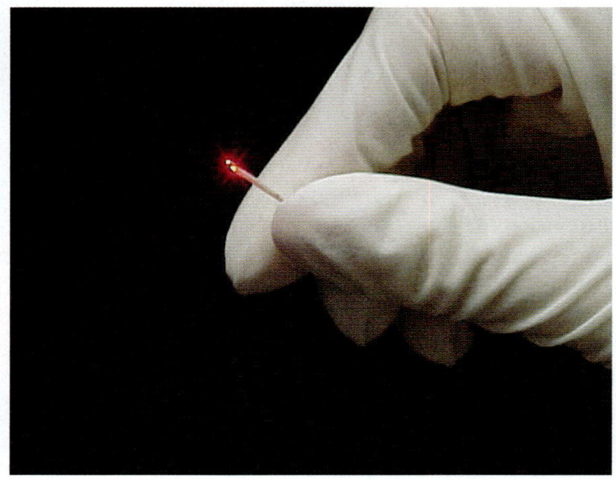

C

Fig. 22.2 Endovascular Photo Acoustic Recanalization (EPAR) system. **(A)** Laser energy source and catheter. **(B)** Image of a cerebral vessel shows the EPAR catheter tip at the treatment site, in the thrombus. **(C)** Catheter tip. (Courtesy of W.F. Gore & Associates Flagstaff AZ.)

Evolving Drug-Eluting Stents

The rate of in-stent restenosis with self-expanding bare-metal stents used for the treatment of intracranial atherosclerotic disease, such as the Wingspan stent (Boston Scientific), exceeds 30 to 40%.[40,41] In some intracranial vascular segments, specifically the supraclinoid internal carotid artery (ICA), the in-stent restenosis rate is as high as 66%. To address the issue of restenosis, the biomedical industry designed a new generation of stents providing a coating able to elute selected drugs (including sirolimus, paclitaxel, ABT578, tacrolimus, and everolimus). The drugs aim to prevent the proliferation of small muscle cells while allowing early recolonization by active endothelial cells. The drug-eluting stents (DESs) continue to attract increasing attention as potentially offering an effective means to lower the rate of restenosis,[45] and three have received approval from the FDA for coronary stenting. The first to receive approval was the sirolimus-eluting Cypher stent (Cordis, Johnson & Johnson, Warren, NJ) in 2003. Then, in 2004, a paclitaxel-eluting stent (Taxus; Boston Scientific) received approval. In 2008, the Xience V everolimus-eluting stent (Abbott Vascular, Abbott Park, IL) was approved. We have observed excellent results with the Xience stent for the treatment of vertebral artery stenosis thus far, with a reduction of in-stent restenosis by 50% from 40% (bare metal) to 20% (DES). On the horizon are DESs with different growth-arrest factors (antimitotic), like sirolimus analogues and actinomycin, or antiinflammatory (dexamethasone) or prohealing agents, such as 17β-estradiol, or an immunosuppressive medication. A new concept in DES technology is the use of plasmid DNA. The idea is to use a DES coated with a naked plasmid DNA that encodes for human vascular endothelial growth factor 2, which will result in significant reduction in restenosis. Protocols for stents releasing stem cells are in place. Newest developments include biodegradable stents, again with the goal to prevent long-term stent-related complications.[46]

◆ Global Reperfusion

Global reperfusion can be achieved using either pharmacologic approaches (hypertension, hypervolemia, hemodilution) or mechanical devices (aortic balloon occlusion). The NeuroFlo device (Co-Axia, Maple Grove, MN) is used to increase cerebral blood perfusion without increasing mean arterial pressure. The NeuroFlo device is a dual-balloon catheter uniquely designed for partial occlusion of the aorta above and below the origin of the renal arteries. The safety and efficacy of this device has been demonstrated in a clinical study.[47] The Safety and Efficacy of NeuroFlo Technology in Ischemic Stroke (SENTIS) Trial is a phase III, multicenter, randomized prospective study to evaluate cerebral perfusion augmentation with partial aortic occlusion in acute ischemic stroke compared with conventional management (control group). Follow-up evaluations were conducted at 24 hours and 90 days. Adverse events (fatal and nonfatal) were evenly distributed among the two cohorts of patients with 16 patients (34%) in each group. However, mortality was significantly lower for the treated population (6.4%) than the control population (14.9%), with more stroke progression (8.5%) and hemorrhagic transformation of the stroke area (4.3%) in the control population. Therefore, the NeuroFlo system has so far proved to be safe enough for clinical use and seems to be promising in improving survival in the acute stroke population.

◆ Flow Reversal

The rationale behind the flow-reversal technique for restoration of a completely blocked artery, such as the intracranial or even the extracranial ICA, is to perform stent-assisted revascularization during flow reversal (shunting of blood flow from intracranial to extracranial, even to a femoral vein, after passage through a filter; Gore Flow-Reversal System; W.L. Gore & Associates). At our institution, we have opened two chronic and multiple acute cases of ICA occlusion using this technique. Terada et al[48] reported a series of 15 patients in whom the flow-reversal technique was used. They used the Parodi embolic protection system (W.L. Gore and Associates) during the recanalization procedure to prevent embolic stroke by reversing the flow from the distal ICA to the common carotid artery. Recanalization of the occluded ICA was successful in 14 of 15 lesions (10 in the cervical ICA and 4 in the petrous/cavernous ICA) using the flow-reversal technique. Ischemic symptoms disappeared completely after successful recanalization, and new ischemic symptoms did not appear relative to the treated lesion. Single-photon emission computed tomographic (SPECT) findings demonstrated improvement of hemodynamic compromise in all cases. We recommend this novel technique as a modified proximal protection technique, particularly if a large clot burden is anticipated.

A more remarkable concept of flow reversal is to actually reverse the normal direction of flow (from the arterial circulation to the venous circulation) to retrogradely perfuse the capillary bed by providing arterial blood through a pump into the cerebral venous outflow. In a study conducted in baboons, catheters were deployed in the transverse sinus, and femoral arterial blood was perfused through a pump after MCA occlusion.[49] The investigators noted improved somatosensory evoked potentials and reduced infarct volumes. A device based on this concept that either unilaterally or bilaterally occludes both the ICAs and the internal jugular vein with balloon catheters is the ReviveFlow (ReviveFlow, Quincy, MA). The ReviveFlow pumps arterial blood harvested from the ICAs through a pump into the occluded internal jugular veins. This device is being evaluated in preclinical studies.

◆ Neuroprotection

This aspect of investigation into salvaging at-risk ischemic neural tissue has remained formidable and elusive. Although a plethora of pharmacologic compounds have been investigated and noted to be useful in animal studies, none have made successful transitions into completed preliminary human trials.[50,51] Such manipulation of the ischemic neuronal environment holds significant promise by extending the window of opportunity to restore flow, particularly through pharmacologic or endovascular means. A strategy that has shown some promise is global hypothermia in the setting of cardiac arrest. By lowering the oxygen consumption in the ischemic tissue, the brain is made to tolerate the effects of hypoperfusion longer than at normal body temperature. This strategy is currently being evaluated for stroke in additional clinical studies. A second strategy was borrowed from trials evaluating minocycline, a tetracycline antibiotic for neurodegenerative disease. Although no consistent benefit has been shown for amyotrophic lateral sclerosis and Parkinson disease, a preliminary study (an open-label randomized trial) in acute stroke reported significantly improved outcomes in patients at 3 months.[52] This effect seems to be mediated by the ability of minocycline to suppress activation of the microglia (the neuroinflammatory mediators), which may suppress some of the secondary pathways that augment neuronal injury following acute stroke. Neuroprotection strategies used in clinical trials and pipeline products are listed in **Table 22.2**.

Table 22.2 Strategies Used in Neuroprotection

Agents	
Albumin	Minocycline, antibiotics
Astrocyte modulator	Neutrophil adhesion molecule antagonist
Beta blocker	Nitric oxide
Calcium chelator	Opioid antagonists
CNS stimulant	Osmotic agents
Corticosteroid	Oxygenated fluorocarbon
Fibroblast growth factor	Phosphatidylcholine precurser
Flow enhancer	Potassium-channel activators
Free-radical scavengers	Prostanoid
GABA agonists	Serotonin antagonist
Ganglioside	Serotonin receptor agonist
Glycine	Serotonin reuptake inhibitor
Glutamate antagonists	Sodium channel blocker
Interleukin-1 receptor antagonist	Statin
Ion-channel modulators	Vasodilator
Iron chelator	
Magnesium	
Other Strategies	
Blood pressure related	Hypothermia
Glycemia control related	Laser system
Hemicraniectomy	Oxygen supplementation
Hemodilution	Traditional Chinese medicine
Hyperbaric oxygen	Volume expansion
Pipeline Products	
Branosyn (repinotan) (BAY x3702) DP-b99BIII-890-CL	
Cerovive (NXY-059) Branosyn (repinotan) (BAY x3702) DP-b99	
Citicoline Cerovive (NXY-059) Branosyn (repinotan) (BAY x3702)	
ONO-2506 Citicoline Cerovive (NXY-059)	
Semax ONO-2506 Citicoline	
SUN-N4057 Semax ONO-2506	
Tacrolimus SUN-N4057 Semax	
Traxoprodil (CP-101606) Tacrolimus SUN-N4057	
Traxoprodil (CP-101606) Tacrolimus	
Traxoprodil (CP-101606)	
BIII-890-CL	
DP-b99BIII-890-CL	

Abbreviations: CNS, central nervous system; GABA, gamma aminobutyric acid.

◆ Conclusion

Acute stroke remains the third most-common killer of adults and is the leading cause of adult disability. Thus far, the only FDA-approved revascularization therapy that is based on level I evidence is IV rtPA. Mechanical devices have been approved based on results from prospective, single-arm trials (level II evidence) for use in patients who do not receive or fail to improve after rtPA therapy. However, for this – the brain's greatest malady – a technologically driven revolution is under way, as noted above. The goal is revascularization of penumbral tissue. Improving emergent physiologic imaging of acute stroke patients will help identify the patients most likely to benefit and least likely to be harmed by intervention. Improving selective pharmacology will be crucial for safer thrombolysis. Many devices are on the horizon,; however, all of these approaches are uniformly plagued with the difficulties of access in typically tortuous, atherosclerotic, and noncompliant vasculature. It is expected that an ongoing evolution of material science and biomedical engineering will eventually provide viable solutions to these common problems. Which strategy will be most effective remains unknown.

References

1. Furlan A, Higashida R, Wechsler L, et al. Intra-arterial prourokinase for acute ischemic stroke. The PROACT II study: a randomized controlled trial. Prolyse in Acute Cerebral Thromboembolism. JAMA 1999;282(21):2003–2011
2. Molyneux A, Kerr R, Stratton I, et al; International Subarachnoid Aneurysm Trial (ISAT) Collaborative Group. International Subarachnoid Aneurysm Trial (ISAT) of neurosurgical clipping versus endovascular coiling in 2143 patients with ruptured intracranial aneurysms: a randomised trial. Lancet 2002;360(9342):1267–1274
3. Molyneux AJ, Kerr RS, Birks J, et al; ISAT Collaborators. Risk of recurrent subarachnoid haemorrhage, death, or dependence and standardised mortality ratios after clipping or coiling of an intracranial aneurysm in the International Subarachnoid Aneurysm Trial (ISAT): long-term follow-up. Lancet Neurol 2009;8(5):427–433
4. Zarins CK, White RA, Diethrich EB, Shackelton RJ, Siami FS; CaRESS Steering Committee and CaRESS Investigators. Carotid revascularization using endarterectomy or stenting systems (CaRESS): 4-year outcomes. J Endovasc Ther 2009;16(4):397–409
5. Glynn LE. Medial defects in the circle of Willis and their relation to aneurysm formation. J Pathol Bacteriol 1940;51:213–221
6. Lang J. Clinical Anatomy of Brain Stem Vessels. New Haven, CT: Miles Pharmaceutical; 1983
7. Stephens RB, Stilwell DL. Arteries and Veins of the Human Brain. Springfield, IL: Charles C. Thomas; 1969
8. Walmsley JG, Canham PB. Orientation of nuclei as indicators of smooth muscle cell alignment in the cerebral artery. Blood Vessels 1979;16(1):43–51
9. Wehman JC, Holmes DR Jr, Ecker RD, et al. Intravascular ultrasound identification of intraluminal embolic plaque material during carotid angioplasty with stenting. Catheter Cardiovasc Interv 2006;68(6): 853–857
10. Wehman JC, Holmes DR Jr, Hanel RA, Levy EI, Hopkins LN. Intravascular ultrasound for intracranial angioplasty and stent placement: technical case report. Neurosurgery 2006; 59(4, Suppl 2)E481–E483
11. Böhringer HJ, Lankenau E, Rohde V, Hüttmann G, Giese A. Optical coherence tomography for experimental neuroendoscopy. Minim Invasive Neurosurg 2006;49(5):269–275
12. Boppart SA. Optical coherence tomography: technology and applications for neuroimaging. Psychophysiology 2003;40(4):529–541
13. Gratton G, Fabiani M, Elbert T, Rockstroh B. Seeing right through you: applications of optical imaging to the study of the human brain. Psychophysiology 2003;40(4):487–491
14. Jang IK, Bouma BE, Kang DH, et al. Visualization of coronary atherosclerotic plaques in patients using optical coherence tomography: comparison with intravascular ultrasound. J Am Coll Cardiol 2002;39(4): 604–609
15. MacNeill BD, Lowe HC, Takano M, Fuster V, Jang IK. Intravascular modalities for detection of vulnerable plaque: current status. Arterioscler Thromb Vasc Biol 2003;23(8):1333–1342
16. Tearney GJ, Yabushita H, Houser SL, et al. Quantification of macrophage content in atherosclerotic plaques by optical coherence tomography. Circulation 2003;107(1):113–119
17. Yabushita H, Bouma BE, Houser SL, et al. Characterization of human atherosclerosis by optical coherence tomography. Circulation 2002;106(13):1640–1645
18. Yamagishi M, Terashima M, Awano K, et al. Morphology of vulnerable coronary plaque: insights from follow-up of patients examined by intravascular ultrasound before an acute coronary syndrome. J Am Coll Cardiol 2000;35(1):106–111
19. Wacker FK, Reither K, Ebert W, Wendt M, Lewin JS, Wolf KJ. MR image-guided endovascular procedures with the ultrasmall superparamagnetic iron oxide SH U 555 C as an intravascular contrast agent: study in pigs. Radiology 2003;226(2):459–464
20. Barber PA, Zhang J, Demchuk AM, Hill MD, Buchan AM. Why are stroke patients excluded from TPA therapy? An analysis of patient eligibility. Neurology 2001;56(8):1015–1020
21. Wolpert SM, Bruckmann H, Greenlee R, Wechsler L, Pessin MS, del Zoppo GJ. Neuroradiologic evaluation of patients with acute stroke treated with recombinant tissue plasminogen activator. The rt-PA Acute Stroke Study Group. AJNR Am J Neuroradiol 1993;14(1):3–13
22. Investigators IMS; IMS Study Investigators. Combined intravenous and intra-arterial recanalization for acute ischemic stroke: the Interventional Management of Stroke Study. Stroke 2004;35(4):904–911
23. IMS II Trial Investigators. The Interventional Management of Stroke (IMS) II Study. Stroke 2007;38(7):2127–2135
24. Alexandrov AV. Ultrasound identification and lysis of clots. Stroke 2004; 35(11, Suppl 1)2722–2725
25. Alexandrov AV, Molina CA, Grotta JC, et al; CLOTBUST Investigators. Ultrasound-enhanced systemic thrombolysis for acute ischemic stroke. N Engl J Med 2004;351(21):2170–2178
26. Alexandrov AV, Mikulik R, Ribo M, et al. A pilot randomized clinical safety study of sonothrombolysis augmentation with ultrasound-activated perflutren-lipid microspheres for acute ischemic stroke. Stroke 2008;39(5):1464–1469
27. Bellon RJ, Putman CM, Budzik RF, Pergolizzi RS, Reinking GF, Norbash AM. Rheolytic thrombectomy of the occluded internal carotid artery in the setting of acute ischemic stroke. AJNR Am J Neuroradiol 2001;22(3):526–530
28. Molina CA, Saver JL. Extending reperfusion therapy for acute ischemic stroke: emerging pharmacological, mechanical, and imaging strategies. Stroke 2005;36(10):2311–2320
29. Nesbit GM, Luh G, Tien R, Barnwell SL. New and future endovascular treatment strategies for acute ischemic stroke. J Vasc Interv Radiol 2004;15(1 Pt 2):S103–S110
30. Gralla J, Schroth G, Remonda L, Nedeltchev K, Slotboom J, Brekenfeld C. Mechanical thrombectomy for acute ischemic stroke: thrombus-device interaction, efficiency, and complications in vivo. Stroke 2006;37(12): 3019–3024
31. Berlis A, Lutsep H, Barnwell S, et al. Mechanical thrombolysis in acute ischemic stroke with endovascular photoacoustic recanalization. Stroke 2004;35(5):1112–1116
32. Lutsep H. Mechanical thrombolysis in acute stroke. eMedicine Neurology. Available at: http://emedicine.medscape.com/article/1163240-print. Accessed March 5, 2010
33. Benesch CG, Chimowitz MI; The WASID Investigators. Best treatment for intracranial arterial stenosis? 50 years of uncertainty. Neurology 2000;55(4):465–466
34. Chimowitz MI, Kokkinos J, Strong J, et al. The Warfarin-Aspirin Symptomatic Intracranial Disease Study. Neurology 1995;45(8):1488–1493
35. The EC/IC Bypass Study Group. Failure of extracranial-intracranial arterial bypass to reduce the risk of ischemic stroke: results of an international randomized trial. N Engl J Med 1985;313(19): 1191–1200

36. Gomez CR, Misra VK, Campbell MS, Soto RD. Elective stenting of symptomatic middle cerebral artery stenosis. AJNR Am J Neuroradiol 2000;21(5):971–973
37. Gomez CR, Misra VK, Liu MW, et al. Elective stenting of symptomatic basilar artery stenosis. Stroke 2000;31(1):95–99
38. Mori T, Kazita K, Chokyu K, Mima T, Mori K. Short-term arteriographic and clinical outcome after cerebral angioplasty and stenting for intracranial vertebrobasilar and carotid atherosclerotic occlusive disease. AJNR Am J Neuroradiol 2000;21(2):249–254
39. Rasmussen PA, Perl J II, Barr JD, et al. Stent-assisted angioplasty of intracranial vertebrobasilar atherosclerosis: an initial experience. J Neurosurg 2000;92(5):771–778
40. Albuquerque FC, Levy EI, Turk AS, et al. Angiographic patterns of Wingspan in-stent restenosis. Neurosurgery 2008;63(1):23–27
41. Turk AS, Levy EI, Albuquerque FC, et al. Influence of patient age and stenosis location on wingspan in-stent restenosis. AJNR Am J Neuroradiol 2008;29(1):23–27
42. Mocco J, Darkhabani Z, Levy EI. Pharos neurovascular intracranial stent: elective use for a symptomatic stenosis refractory to medical therapy. Catheter Cardiovasc Interv 2009;74(4):642–646
43. Freitas JM, Zenteno M, Aburto-Murrieta Y, et al. Intracranial arterial stenting for symptomatic stenoses: a Latin American experience. Surg Neurol 2007;68(4):378–386
44. Kurre W, Berkefeld J, Sitzer M, Neumann-Haefelin T, du Mesnil de Rochemont R. Treatment of symptomatic high-grade intracranial stenoses with the balloon-expandable Pharos stent: initial experience. Neuroradiology 2008;50(8):701–708
45. Steinfort B, Ng PP, Faulder K, et al. Midterm outcomes of paclitaxel-eluting stents for the treatment of intracranial posterior circulation stenoses. J Neurosurg 2007;106(2):222–225
46. Basalus MW, van Houwelingen KG, Ankone M, de Man FH, von Birgelen C. Scanning electron microscopic assessment of the biodegradable coating on expanded biolimus-eluting stents. EuroIntervention 2009; 5(4):505–510
47. Uflacker R, Schönholz C, Papamitisakis N; SENTIS trial. Interim report of the SENTIS trial: cerebral perfusion augmentation via partial aortic occlusion in acute ischemic stroke. J Cardiovasc Surg (Torino) 2008;49(6):715–721
48. Terada T, Okada H, Nanto M, et al. Endovascular recanalization of the completely occluded internal carotid artery using a flow reversal system at the subacute to chronic stage. J Neurosurg 2010;112(3):563–571
49. Frazee JG, Luo X, Luan G, et al. Retrograde transvenous neuroperfusion: a back door treatment for stroke. Stroke 1998;29(9):1912–1916
50. Donnan GA. The 2007 Feinberg lecture: a new road map for neuroprotection. Stroke 2008;39(1):242–248
51. Ginsberg MD. Neuroprotection for ischemic stroke: past, present and future. Neuropharmacology 2008;55(3):363–389
52. Lampl Y, Boaz M, Gilad R, et al. Minocycline treatment in acute stroke: an open-label, evaluator-blinded study. Neurology 2007; 69(14):1404–1410

Chapter 23

Physiologic Imaging

Jeffrey A. Bennett and Sharatchandra S. Bidari

◆ Background

The goal of physiologic imaging in cerebrovascular disease is to guide therapy toward preservation of functional brain tissue. Knowledge of the local metabolic needs of brain parenchyma is required to determine whether there is tissue at risk, realizing that certain cells in the brain have a higher adenosine triphosphate demand, such as neurons in the globus pallidus and parahippocampal gyrus, and thus are more sensitive to injury from deficient supply of oxygen and nutrients than are cells in other areas of the brain such as white matter tracts.

Anatomic imaging from magnetic resonance imaging (MRI), computed tomography (CT), and angiography is able to provide accurate characterization of arterial or venous luminal disease. CT angiography continues to rapidly improve and is making a strong bid to replace diagnostic catheter angiography. Recent developments with 320–detector row scanners even provide temporal phases on CT angiography. However, this anatomic data fails to tell the story of how well brain tissue is getting the supplies it needs. Physiologic imaging is rapidly developing to fulfill this requirement by providing measurements of cerebral hemodynamics and cerebral metabolism.

CT perfusion uses rapid intravenous (IV) bolus injection of iodinated contrast to acquire maps of cerebral blood flow, cerebral blood volume, and mean transit time, which can be used to determine tissue viability.[1] These same maps can be obtained with MRI perfusion during the IV administration of a gadolinium contrast agent.[2] These data can be compared with diffusion-weighted images to estimate ischemic core and penumbra size. A pharmacologic challenge with acetazolamide can be administered during either CT or MR perfusion to help determine cerebral blood flow reserve.[3] This can help reveal the status of collateral blood supply. Certain MR sequences, such as arterial spin labeling, are available that can provide data on brain territories supplied by individual vessels and that can help define watershed zones, which shift with various cerebrovascular injuries.[4,5] Nuclear medicine tests, especially positron emission tomography (PET), can also be used to directly measure physiologic parameters such as the regional metabolic rate of oxygen and glucose and the tissue oxygen extraction fraction (OEF).[6]

Physiologic imaging techniques will be reviewed in this chapter, with the focus on their practical use, including indications, interpretation, and potential pitfalls and artifacts. The main focus of the chapter is on CT perfusion, the tool currently being studied the most in a clinical setting.

◆ Indications

Acute stroke is the clinical context on which most research has been focused. Standard of care for acute stroke imaging remains a noncontrast head CT, as this determines whether contraindications to IV tissue plasminogen activator (tPA) exist; primarily hemorrhage, although infarct size greater than one third of the middle cerebral artery (MCA) territory also predicts increased risk of hemorrhagic transformation following IV tPA.[7] Treatments for acute stroke approved by the U.S. Food and Drug Administration (FDA) are limited to IV tPA administered within 3 hours of symptom onset and use of the Mechanical Embolus Removal in Cerebral Ischemia (MERCI) device (Concentric Medical, Mountain View, CA) within 9 hours of symptom onset. Because of the arbitrary time cutoffs, many patients presenting with acute stroke are not eligible for treatments that may salvage oligemic brain tissue. One of the main goals of physiologic imaging is to determine which patients may benefit from treatments beyond the time windows. This can be achieved by determining whether a mismatch persists between the infarcted core and surrounding ischemic penumbra. This can be determined with either CT perfusion or MR perfusion studies.[8]

A similar indication is encountered following subarachnoid hemorrhage for the determination of tissue at risk when there is vasospasm. This information can be correlated with clinical symptoms to assess the need for intraarterial intervention. If a completed infarct is seen, the study can also help the decision not to treat the vasospasm as increased risk of reperfusion hemorrhage may exist.

Clinical indications for the acetazolamide (ACZ) challenge study are to further stratify risk of infarction in patients with symptomatic or asymptomatic carotid artery stenosis or stroke risk in patients about to undergo cardiac or carotid surgery. The study may be a way to assess the effectiveness of collateral blood supply in these patients and in patients with moyamoya disease, and help determine who may benefit from extracranial-intracranial bypass surgery.

◆ Technique

MRI with diffusion-weighted images, MR perfusion, and MRA of the cervical and intracranial vessels provides essentially the same information as a CT scan of the head with CT angiography and CT perfusion. However, CT is much more accessible than MRI and is much faster, a critical concern when time is brain. Iodinated contrast is FDA-approved for CT perfusion, whereas gadolinium for MR perfusion is off-label; therefore, software companies have focused more on generating perfusion maps using CT. Also, the signal drop-out on MR perfusion based on T2* effects which is used to generate perfusion maps is not linearly related to gadolinium concentration in the brain and therefore only relative, nonquantitative maps can be produced. There is a linear relationship of tissue contrast concentration and Hounsfield unit (HU) attenuation, allowing quantitative maps with CT.

A limitation of CT perfusion is coverage. Whereas MR perfusion is of the whole brain, CT perfusion is limited by the width of the detector. This is because information is being collected from the same brain region rapidly over and over as contrast flows in and out, faster than the table can move. Therefore a 16-detector row CT scanner allows a 2-cm slab of data, which is typically reconstructed as two adjacent 10-mm-thick slices. A 64-detector row CT scanner can obtain a 4-cm slab, producing four 10-mm-thick adjacent slices. The positioning of these slices has to be chosen carefully, depending on what vascular territory is of interest. Newer 320-detector row scanners collect data over a 16-cm slab and thus can perform whole-brain CT perfusion (**Fig. 23.1**).

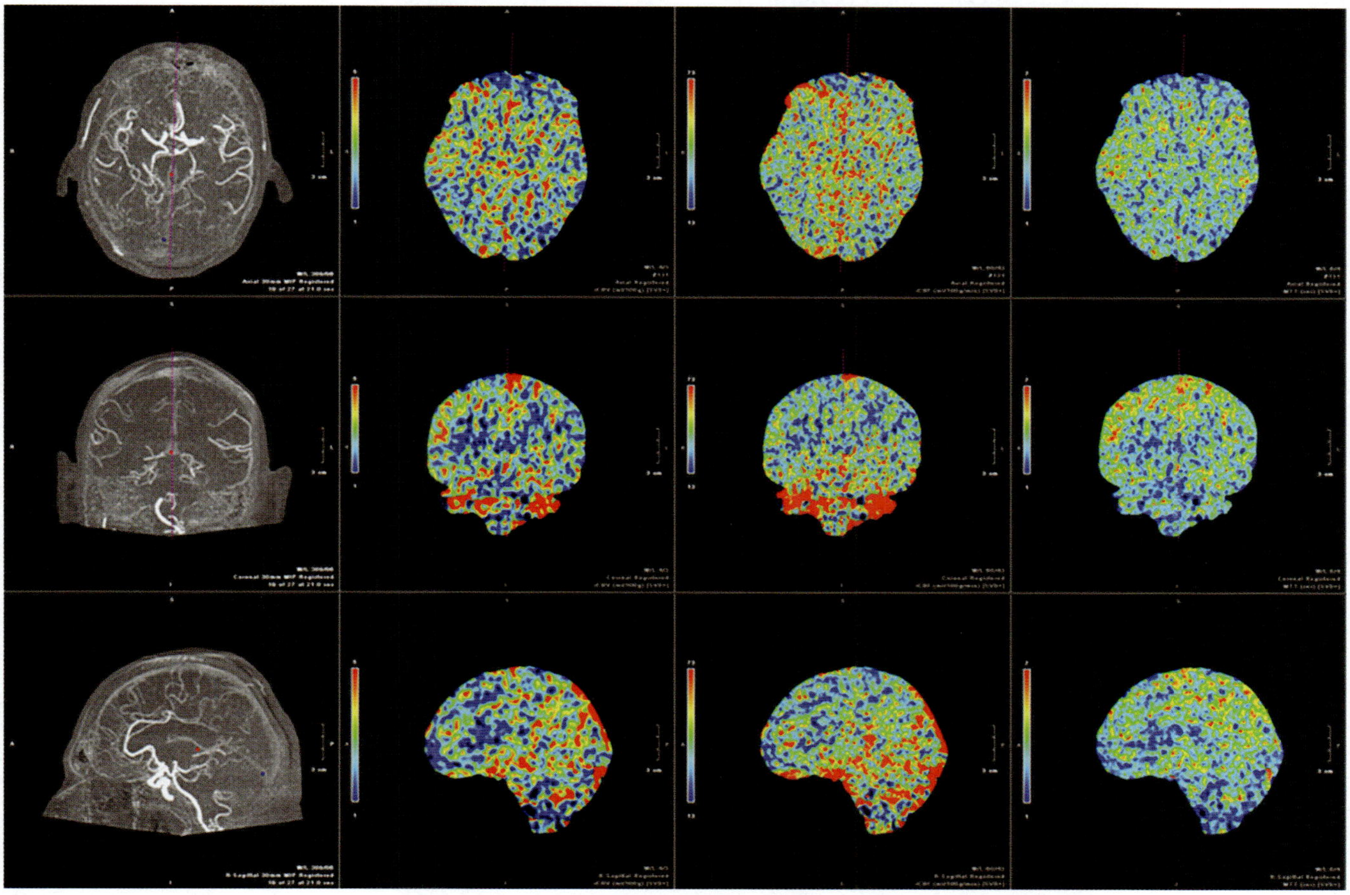

Fig. 23.1 Whole-brain CT perfusion study performed using Toshiba's Aquilon One (320-slice volume CT) shows normal mean transit time. Cerebral blood flow and cerebral blood volume color maps are shown in the axial, coronal, and sagittal planes. The images are displayed in MPR format and can be manipulated on the workstation.

CT perfusion is performed by imaging during a rapid bolus of iodinated contrast. Typically 35 to 50 mL of high-concentration contrast, 350 g/dL of iodine, is administered IV at 5 to 7 mL/s, with the faster power injector rates preferable. This is immediately followed by a 20- to 40-mL saline chaser injected at the same rate. One image per second is typically acquired for 40 seconds, followed by one image every 2 to 3 seconds for an additional 35 to 45 seconds, for a total of 75 to 90 seconds of imaging. This amount of time is necessary to collect a complete tissue concentration curve during the first pass of contrast through the capillary bed of the brain, even in patients with poor cardiac output or proximal carotid artery severe stenosis or occlusion. The optimal timing of image acquisition is still being determined, and it may be possible to increase the time between images without sacrificing data accuracy and thus decrease radiation dose.

Perfusion maps are now created by deconvolution techniques on commercially available software packages. An artery is selected, optimally one running perpendicular to the imaging plane to reduce volume averaging, as an arterial input function based on which calculations are made. A dural venous sinus is selected as a venous output function, which is necessary as a scaling factor for producing quantitative perfusion data. Maps are then constructed of mean transit time (MTT), cerebral blood flow (CBF), and cerebral blood volume (CBV). The accuracy of these maps is improved by eliminating pixels, which do not correspond with brain. This can be achieved by segmenting out pixels with HU below 0 (eliminating air and fat) and pixels with HU higher than 60 to 80 (eliminating blood, calcium, metal, etc.) Leptomeningeal blood vessels can also cause apparent falsely elevated cortical hyperperfusion. This potential pitfall can be overcome by eliminating pixels with a blood volume greater than 8 mL/min.

CT perfusion and MR perfusion have both been used to estimate cerebral vascular reserve with a pharmacologic challenge with acetazolamide, a cerebral vasodilator. Contraindications include sulfur allergy, severe kidney and liver disease, electrolyte disorders, and adrenocortical insufficiency. A baseline perfusion study is obtained. For adults, a standard dose of 1000 mg acetazolamide is then administered IV. Repeat perfusion imaging is performed 15 minutes later.

◆ Interpretation and Application

Interpretation of CT perfusion and MR perfusion studies is based on comparison of the generated maps. MTT is defined as the time taken for blood to traverse a given brain region and is measured in seconds. Cerebral blood flow is the volume of blood traversing a brain region per unit time and is measured in mL/100 g tissue per minute. Cerebral blood volume is the total amount of blood flowing through a brain region at any one time and is measured in mL/100 g tissue. **Table 23.1** provides a general guide for interpretation of CT perfusion map relations.

The core of an infarct is identified on perfusion maps as increased MTT, decreased CBF, and decreased CBV. The area of matched decreased blood volume and decreased blood flow correlates well with the ischemic core as seen on diffusion-weighted MRI (**Fig. 23.2**).[9,10] Oligemic tissue in the ischemic penumbra will also demonstrate an increased MTT and mild to moderate CBF reduction, but CBV is maintained or only minimally reduced (**Fig. 23.3**). This represents the target tissue for stroke therapy.

Physiologic imaging can be used to measure cerebrovascular reserve, or the amount of compensatory vasodilation that is present in a patient with chronic vessel stenosis. Patients who have a stenosis or occlusion of cervical or intracranial arteries undergo autoregulatory dilation of arterioles resulting in decreased vascular resistance. This can be detected on perfusion studies as a regional increase in MTT and increased CBV (**Fig. 23.4**). The CBF and OEF remain relatively unchanged until arteriolar dilation reaches its maximum. Further decreased perfusion pressure is thereafter compensated by increased oxygen extraction fraction, reduced CBF, and increased MTT, a phenomenon known as misery perfusion. The rate of oxygen metabolism in the brain remains stable regardless of perfusion pressure. Once the compensatory mechanism of increased OEF reaches a maximum, further decrease in perfusion pressure will result in ischemia.

Table 23.1 Computed Tomography Perfusion Findings Interpretation Guide

	Specific Pathologic Conditions				
CT Perfusion Parameters	**Normal**	**Arterial Stenosis/ Occlusion with Excellent Collateral Compensation**	**Oligemic Tissue that Likely Will Survive**	**Oligemic Tissue at Risk**	**Tissue that Likely Is Irreversibly Damaged**
MTT	Normal	Prolonged	Prolonged	Prolonged	Markedly prolonged
CBF	Normal	Normal	Mild to moderate reduction	Markedly reduced	Severely reduced
CBV	Normal	Normal	Normal to minimally reduced	Moderately reduced	Severely reduced
Intervention		Not needed	May require acetazolamide challenge to determine need for intervention	Most useful	Unlikely to be useful to salvage the tissue

Abbreviations: MTT, mean transit time; CBF, cerebral blood flow; CBV, cerebral blood volume; Mild to moderate, one to two color scale change; Severe, two or more color scale change.

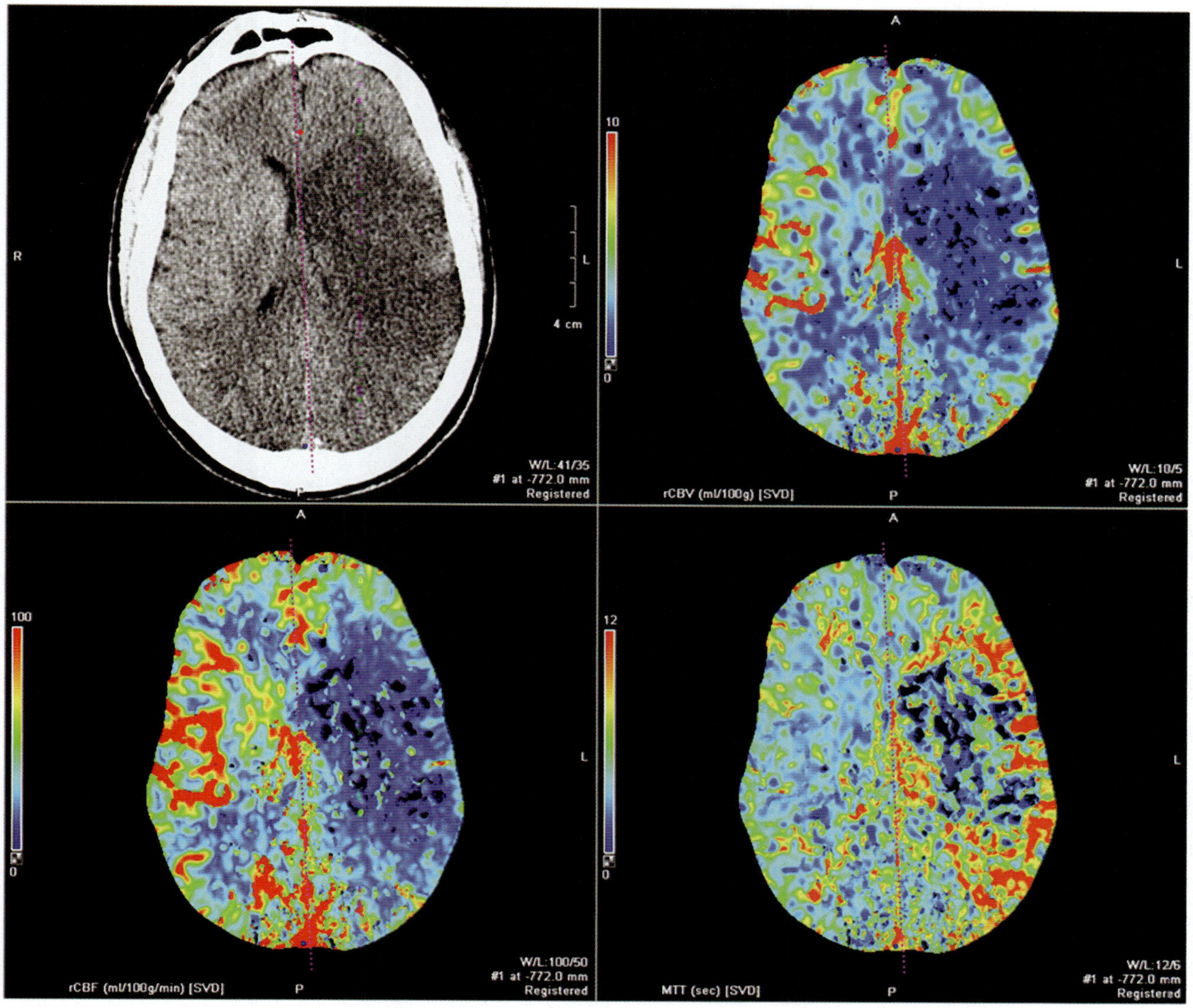

A

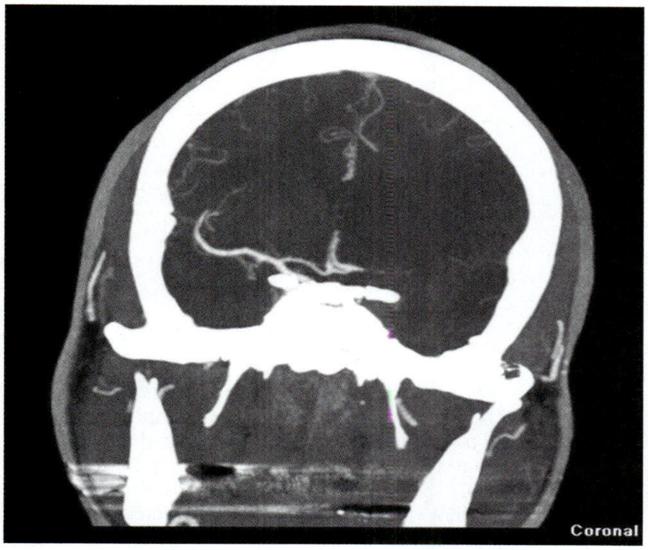

B

Fig. 23.2 **(A)** CT perfusion shows prolonged mean transit time, decreased cerebral flow and volume in the left middle cerebral artery (MCA) territory, consistent with an infarct. The core of this infarct, the left basal ganglia, shows no prolongation of mean transit time but rather decreased cerebral blood flow and cerebral blood volume. This spurious color is possibly due to complete occlusion of supplying arteries with no detectable flow. **(B)** Maximum intensity projection (MIP) coronal CT angiogram shows complete occlusion of left internal carotid artery and middle cerebral artery with poor to no collateral flow. Cytogenic edema in left middle cerebral artery territory can be seen.

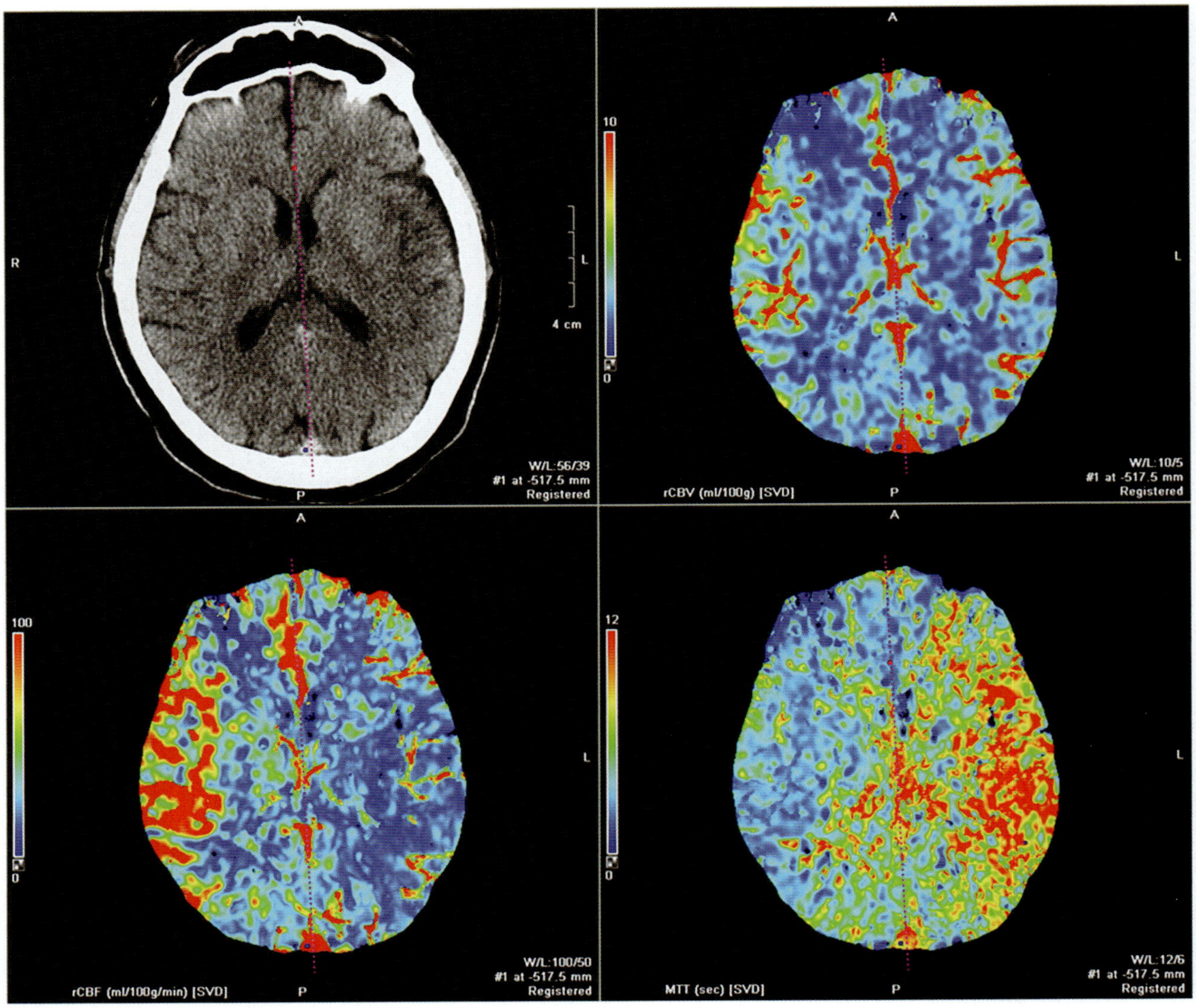

A

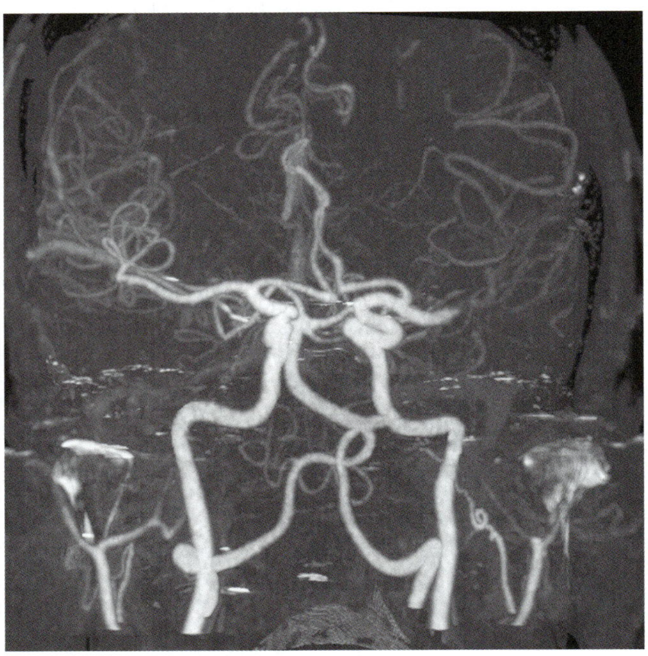

B

Fig. 23.3 **(A)** This patient presented with acute symptoms. CT perfusion maps show prolonged mean transit time in the left middle cerebral artery (MCA) territory as well as the left anterior cerebral artery–MCA and MCA–posterior cerebral artery watershed territories. The cerebral blood flow is moderately reduced and cerebral blood volume is mildly reduced. These findings are consistent with oligemia and tissue at risk. **(B)** Subtracted CT angiogram in three-dimensional volume display shows complete occlusion of the distal M1 segment of left middle cerebral artery with paucity of distal M3 and M4 vessels indicating less collateral flow. (Compare with **Fig. 23.4B**.)

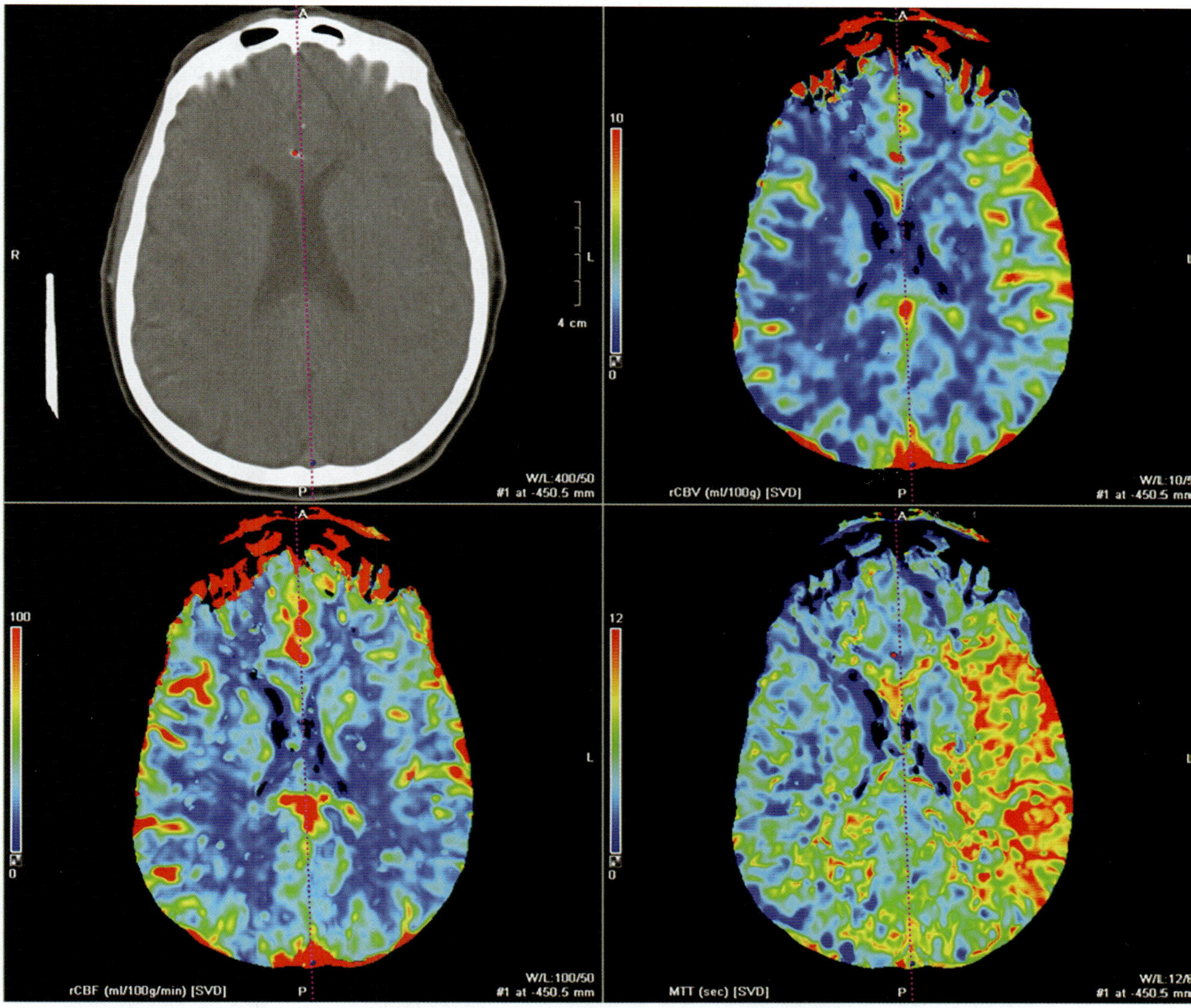

A

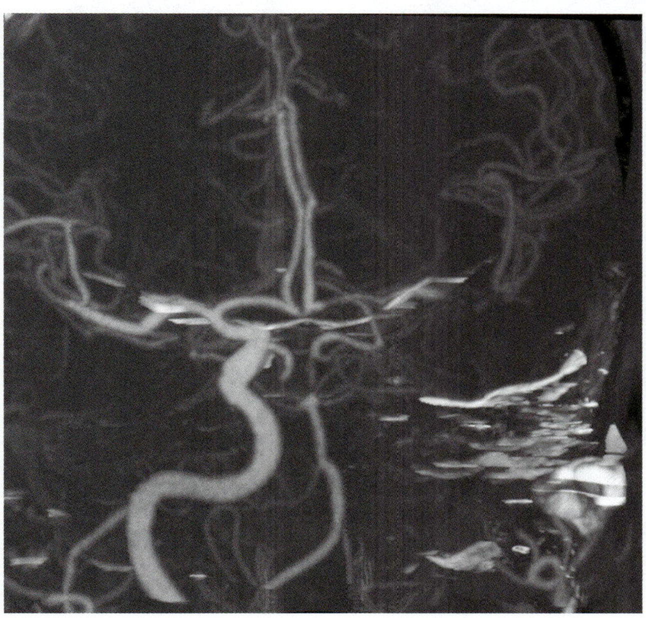

B

Fig. 23.4 **(A)** CT perfusion study shows prolonged mean transit time, with maintained cerebral blood flow and mildly increased cerebral blood volume (CBV) in left middle cerebral artery (MCA) territory. The increased CBV is a compensatory phenomenon due to mild degree of oligemia (luxury perfusion). **(B)** Subtracted CT angiogram in three-dimensional display shows complete occlusion of the left internal carotid artery and MCA but with good retrograde filling of distal MCA vessels. In fact, the M3 and M4 vessels on the left are marginally larger in caliber compared with the right, explaining the luxury perfusion on color maps.

OEF and cerebral metabolic rate of oxygen consumption can be measured directly with PET. However, the test is expensive, as the radioisotopes required have a very short half-life and need to be created at a nearby cyclotron. A major use of PET is therefore in validation studies of other modalities. Another complex test that has been used to quantitatively measure CBF is xenon CT, but this is not FDA-approved for clinical use.[11]

Three types of responses of cerebral perfusion during the ACZ study have been described.[12] Type I patients have normal CBF at baseline, and increased CBF after ACZ. These patients are not significantly compromised by their vessel stenosis. Type II patients have decreased CBF at baseline and increased CBF after ACZ. These patients have adequate cerebral vascular reserve. Type III patients have decreased CBF at baseline and a further decrease in CBF after ACZ. These patients do not have cerebrovascular reserve as they have already maximally vasodilated in the affected vascular territory at baseline. These patients are at increased risk for infarction and may be candidates for surgical revascularization (**Fig. 23.5**).

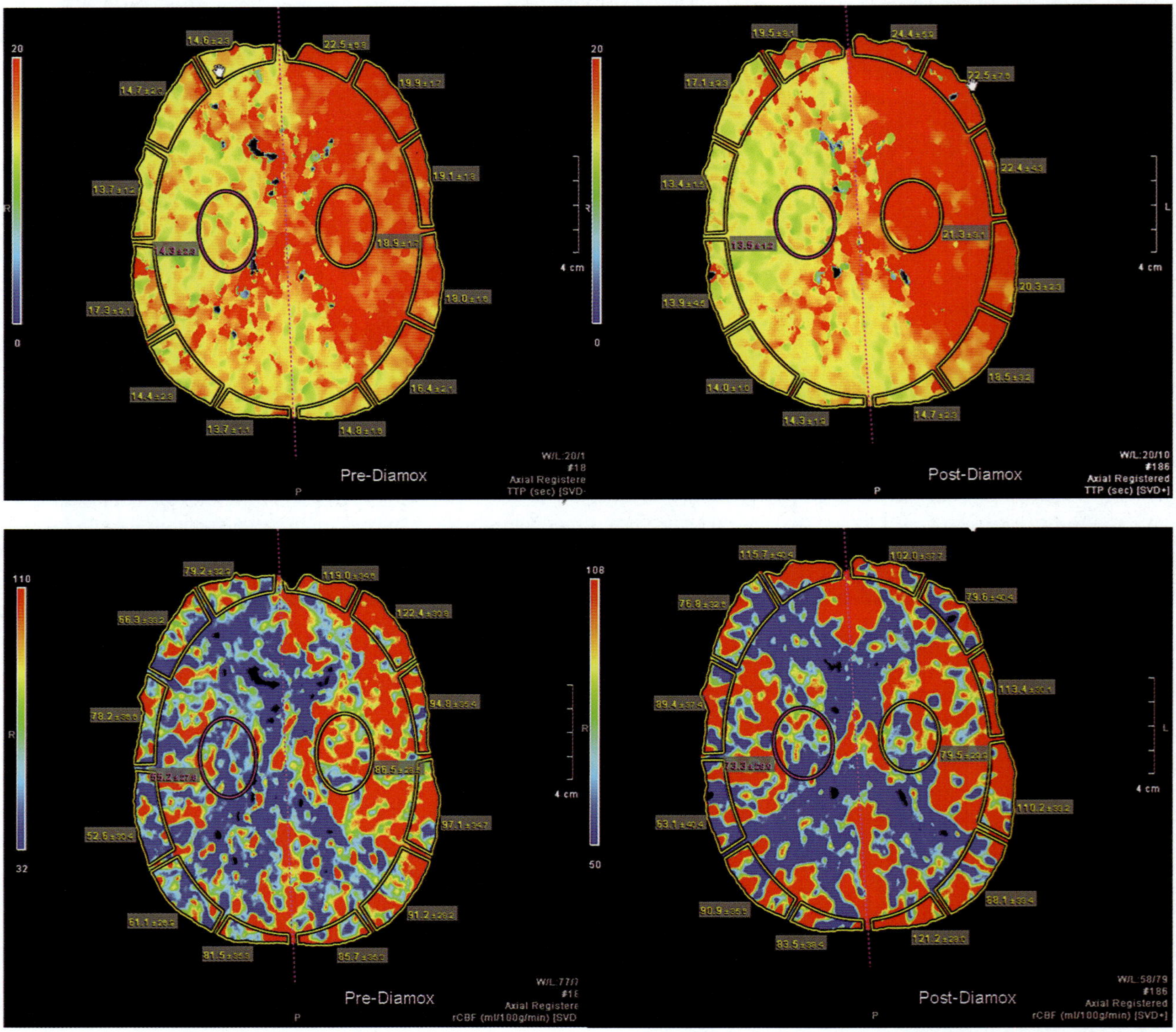

A

B

Fig. 23.5 CT perfusion maps of preacetazolamide and postacetazolamide study of time to peak (TTP), cerebral blood flow (CBF), and cerebral blood volume (CBV), respectively, in a patient with complete occlusion of left internal carotid artery (ICA). **(A)** Preacetazolamide *(left)* and postacetazolamide *(right)* TTP. The prolonged TTP in the left anterior cerebral artery (ACA) and middle cerebral artery (MCA) territories in the preacetazolamide study indicates filling by collaterals. The TTP is further prolonged on postacetazolamide study, especially in the left basal ganglia and the ACA-MCA and MCA–posterior cerebral artery (PCA) watershed territories. **(B)** Preacetazolamide *(left)* and postacetazolamide *(right)* CBF. There is good flow at rest, but flow decreases in the postacetazolamide study in the left basal ganglia and the ACA-MCA and MCA-PCA watershed territories. *(continued)*

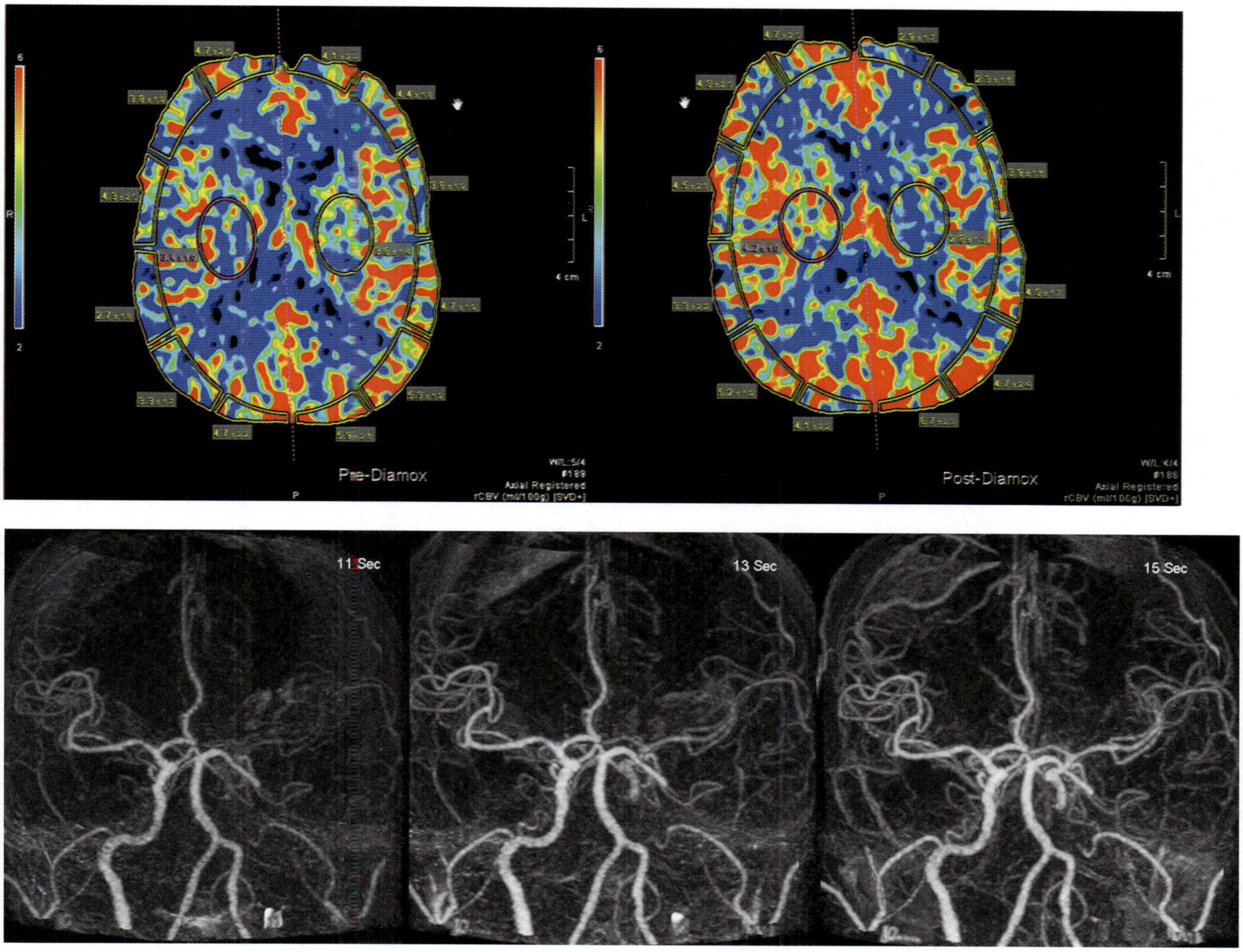

C

D

Fig. 23.5 *(continued)* **(C)** Preacetazolamide *(left)* and postacetazolamide *(right)* CBV. There is normal to mildly increased volume in the affected region at rest. On the postacetazolamide study, however, there is a corresponding decrease in the CBV in the left basal ganglia and the ECA-MCA and MCA-PCA watershed territories. These findings are consistent with the lack of central reserve in the above-described regions, suggesting a need for bypass surgery. **(D)** Digitally subtracted CT angiogram three-dimensional volume rendered views of the same patient at 11, 13, and 15 seconds. The left supraclinoid ICA and MCA show delayed contrast opacification and retrograde filling by anterior communicating and ophthalmic arteries. These findings correlate well with the perfusion abnormality.

◆ Future Directions

Technical advancements in physiologic imaging are progressing at a rapid rate. In the realm of CT perfusion, software packages are being developed to fully automate processing of CT perfusion maps. Current map creation requires selection of an arterial input function, which makes the assumption that all contrast in the brain arrives at the same time as it is measured at that data point. This obviously is not always the case, such as if there is severe carotid stenosis and poor collaterals. Newer map construction techniques correct for this delay by using a circulant deconvolution algorithm eliminating this potential source of error.[1,13] This is particularly important for maps generated with the acetazolamide challenge for determining cerebral blood flow reserve. In general, how the data are presented needs to become standardized. Set thresholds for abnormalities need to be determined with accurate quantitative data and validated with outcome studies so that more informed and accurate decisions can be made from the perfusion images.

Additional data may also be possible with CT and MR perfusion techniques. For example, CT perfusion image acquisition can be continued for an additional 2 minutes after the initial 75 to 90 seconds, with one image collected every 10 to 15 seconds to generate blood–brain barrier permeability maps. Increased permeability may identify patients at increased risk of hemorrhage following thrombolysis, and permeability may correlate with stroke outcome.

Further developments with MRI will also continue to generate new techniques for identification of vascular territories and watershed regions.[4] Some of these, such as selective arterial spin labeling, are completely noninvasive and are already entering clinical practice. Physiologic imaging is likely to become the standard of care in the treatment of many cerebrovascular disease conditions.

References

1. Konstas AA, Goldmakher GV, Lee T-Y, Lev MH. Theoretic basis and technical implementations of CT perfusion in acute ischemic stroke. Part 1: theoretic basis. AJNR Am J Neuroradiol 2009;30(4):662–668
2. Zaharchuk G. Theoretical basis of hemodynamic MR imaging techniques to measure cerebral blood volume, cerebral blood flow, and permeability. AJNR Am J Neuroradiol 2007;28(10):1850–1858
3. Vagal AS, Leach JL, Fernandez-Ulloa M, Zuccarello M. The acetazolamide challenge: techniques and applications in the evaluation of chronic cerebral ischemia. AJNR Am J Neuroradiol 2009;30(5):876–884
4. van Laar PJ, van der Grond J, Hendrikse J. Brain perfusion territory imaging: methods and clinical applications of selective arterial spin-labeling MR imaging. Radiology 2008;246(2):354–364
5. Momjian-Mayor I, Baron JC. The pathophysiology of watershed infarction in internal carotid artery disease: review of cerebral perfusion studies. Stroke 2005;36(3):567–577
6. Powers WJ, Zazulia AR. The use of positron emission tomography in cerebrovascular disease. Neuroimaging Clin N Am 2003;13(4):741–758
7. Tissue plasminogen activator for acute ischemic stroke. The National Institute of Neurological Disorders and Stroke rt-PA Stroke Study Group. N Engl J Med 1995;333(24):1581–1587
8. Schaefer PW, Barak ER, Kamalian S, et al. Quantitative assessment of core/penumbra mismatch in acute stroke: CT and MR perfusion imaging are strongly correlated when sufficient brain volume is imaged. Stroke 2008;39(11):2986–2992
9. Konstas AA, Goldmakher GV, Lee T-Y, Lev MH. Theoretic basis and technical implementations of CT perfusion in acute ischemic stroke. Part 2: technical implementations. AJNR Am J Neuroradiol 2009;30(5): 885–892
10. Murphy BD, Fox AJ, Lee DH, et al. White matter thresholds for ischemic penumbra and infarct core in patients with acute stroke: CT perfusion study. Radiology 2008;247(3):818–825
11. Wintermark M, Sesay M, Barbier E, et al. Comparative overview of brain perfusion imaging techniques. J Neuroradiol 2005;32(5):294–314
12. Rogg J, Rutigliano M, Yonas H, Johnson DW, Pentheny S, Latchaw RE. The acetazolamide challenge: imaging techniques designed to evaluate cerebral blood flow reserve. AJR Am J Roentgenol 1989;153(3):605–612
13. Sasaki M, Kudo K, Ogasawara K, Fujiwara S. Tracer delay-insensitive algorithm can improve reliability of CT perfusion imaging for cerebrovascular steno-occlusive disease: comparison with quantitative single-photon emission CT. AJNR Am J Neuroradiol 2009;30(1):188–193

Index

A

Index

I

Q

R

S

W